ANNALS OF THE NEW YORK ACADEMY OF SCIENCES

Volume 283

THE BEHAVIOR OF BLOOD AND ITS COMPONENTS AT INTERFACES

Edited by Leo Vroman and Edward F. Leonard

The New York Academy of Sciences
New York, New York
1977

Library of Congress Cataloging in Publication Data

Main entry under title:

The Behavior of blood and its components at interfaces.

(Annals of The New York Academy of Sciences; v. 283)

"The result of a conference . . . held by The New York Academy of Sciences, and co-sponsored by the Columbia University Seminar on Biomaterials, on March 24, 25, and 26, 1976."

1. Blood—Congresses. 2. Biomedical materials—Congresses. I. Vroman, Leo, 1915- . II. Leonard, Edward F. III. New York Academy of Sciences. IV. Columbia University Seminar on Biomaterials. V. Series: New York Academy of Sciences. Annals; v. 283. [DNLM: 1. Hematology—Congresses. 2. Surface properties —Congresses. 3. Biocompatible materials—Congresses. 4. Blood vessel prosthesis—Congresses. W1 AN626YL v. 283/WH100 B419 1976] Q11.N5 vol. 283 [QP91] 508'.1s [599'.01'13]

ISBN 0-89072-029-0 77-895

PCP

Printed in the United States of America

ISBN 0-89072-029-0

ANNALS OF THE NEW YORK ACADEMY OF SCIENCES

VOLUME 283

February 10, 1977

THE BEHAVIOR OF BLOOD AND ITS COMPONENTS AT INTERFACES *

Editors and Conference Organizers
LEO VROMAN AND EDWARD F. LEONARD

CONTENTS

* This series of papers is the result of a conference entitled The Behavior of Blood and its Components at Interfaces, held by The New York Academy of Sciences and cosponsored by the Columbia University Seminar on Biomaterials on March 24, 25, and 26, 1976.

Part VIII. The Comparison and Classification of Materials

Robert J. Wineman and Hirotsugu K. Yasuda, *Chairpersons*

Part IX. Evaluation of Artificial Interfaces

A. *In Vitro* Evaluation

Reginald G. Mason and Robert R. Stromberg, *Chairpersons*

B. *Ex Vivo* and *In Vivo* Evaluations

Robert E. Baier, John J. Brash, Leo Vroman, A. U. Daniels, and Robert S. Litwak, *Discussion Leaders*

Part X. Summary

Leo Vroman and Edward F. Leonard, *Chairpersons*

Financial assistance was received from:

- THE NATIONAL HEART, LUNG, AND BLOOD INSTITUTE (GRANT NO. 1 R13 HL 18872–01)

- EXTRACORPOREAL MEDICAL SPECIALTIES, INC.
- MERCK & CO., INC.
- RUDOLPH RESEARCH
- UNION CARBIDE CORPORATION

OPENING REMARKS

Leo Vroman

Interface Laboratory
Veterans Administration Hospital
Brooklyn, New York 11209

This Conference was sponsored by The New York Academy of Sciences, and cosponsored by the Columbia University Seminar on Biomaterials. The Seminar's Chairman of this year, Prof. E. F. Leonard, is cochairman of this Conference. A steering committee, selected from the seminar members, helped us shape this program. The Conference was partly supported by a grant from the National Heart and Lung Institute, National Institutes of Health. Thanks are also due to the several contributing organizations listed elsewhere in this volume.

Five years ago, at a Symposium on Problems in Evaluating the Blood Compatibility of Biomaterials sponsored by the New York Academy of Medicine, eleven of our present participants also spoke. One person sadly missed at the present Conference is Dr. Bert Kusserow. We will do less well without his gentle yet inspired approach to *in vivo* testing of blood compatibility, a style that distinguished him. The main question posed then was a practical one: on what basis can we make, and test, blood-compatible materials? Some guidelines suggested even earlier by certain convenient hypotheses have led to fabrication of materials that embody them and thus allowed us to test them. Without the diversity of those inspiring views—be they right or wrong—there would not have been the range of materials on which to observe the complexity of blood/surface interactions.

Now, we are looking for coherence among the successive reactions following the exposure of blood to this variety of surfaces: the adsorption of specific plasma proteins, the interaction of these adsorbates with the plasma that had deposited them, the effect of products resulting from these interactions upon platelets and white blood cells, and the effect of their adhesion on the formation of gross aggregates. This program is arranged to reflect the chronology of such a sequence, first as if in stagnant, then in flowing, blood, first *in vitro,* then *ex vivo* and *in vivo*. Finally, efforts are described to use this information for improving development and testing of biomaterials that are tolerated in the bloodstream.

Part I. Overview

BLOOD AND BIOMATERIALS: A GLIMPSE AT THE ELEPHANT *

Theodore H. Spaet

Hematology Division, Department of Medicine
Montefiore Hospital and Medical Center
The Bronx, New York 10467
Albert Einstein College of Medicine
The Bronx, New York 10461

In February of 1971, the keynote address to the predecessor of the present sessions was given by Dr. Vincent Gott.[1] In it he concluded that the time was ripe for application of the scientific method to the field of biomaterials. This was a conclusion to which we could heartily add "amen"! The specific implementation of this injunction was less clear. In the subsequent five years, a considerable increment of science has, in fact, been added. Some of this has derived from investigators specifically interested in prosthetic devices; perhaps even more has been contributed by those whose interests intersect only incidentally. I have no doubt that these sessions will produce some pleasant surprises. However, the exercise of putting together the program demonstrated to those responsible for it that the discipline of biomaterials was best subjected to subdivision, whereby the specific application under investigation determined the branches of science to be involved. The organization of the program reflects our attempt to recognize appropriate relationships.

When blood encounters a "foreign" surface, a sequence of events is initiated. Some of these begin virtually instantaneously; depending upon the use of the surface, the consequences may be relatively brief, or of extreme duration. In all cases, the relationship between blood and the normal vessel wall may serve as the basis for comparison.

The normal vessel wall is illustrated in Figure 1. In large veins and arteries it is covered completely with a sheet of endothelial cells that are in apposition, with junctions that act as an effective seal to particles and macromolecules. There is a relatively trivial passage of plasma and its components through pinocytotic vesicles; smaller proteins and low molecular weight compounds pass directly through the cells at a much greater rate.[2] As long as the vessel is so covered with normal endothelium, it is nonthrombogenic: neither platelets nor the products of blood coagulation deposit on it. The reason for this property is unknown, but an important possibility for its basis is that the living cell actively renews its membranes. Since normal erythrocytes and leukocytes are similarly nonreactive, nonthrombogenicity may well be a property of normal cells in general; hemostatic reactions may require the presence of appropriate extracellular materials. If these considerations prove to be the case, the search for a nonthrombogenic biomaterial based upon the properties of physiological surfaces may well be fated for inevitable failure. Of course, an artificial material may ultimately become "physiological" if it is overgrown with endothelium.

* Supported by USPHS grant no. HL 16387–01 from the National Heart and Lung Institute.

A second property of the normal vessel wall is its stability with respect to proliferative activity. Vascular cells under baseline conditions in adult animals have a very low level of labeling with tritiated thymidine, although they may undergo a dramatic proliferative response following injury.[3] The importance of these considerations will become evident later in this presentation.

The earliest reaction between blood and a foreign surface is evidently the adsorption of plasma proteins onto it. In the deendothelialized vessel, perhaps

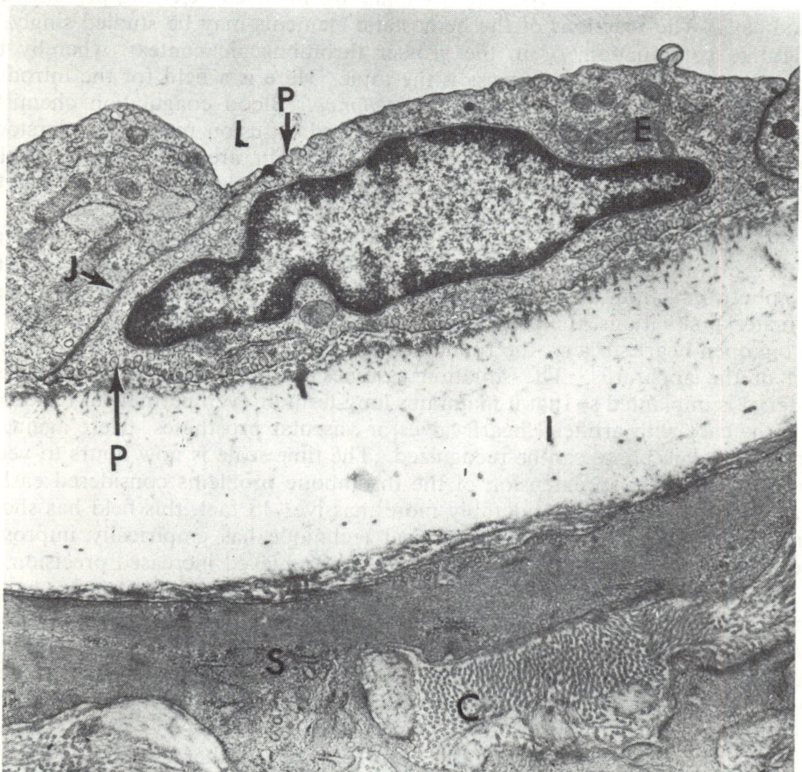

FIGURE 1. Electron micrograph of rabbit aortic intima. C=collagen fibrils; E=endothelial cell; I=internal elastic lamina; J=junction between endothelial cells; L=vessel lumen; P=pinocytotic vesicles; S=smooth-muscle cell. (×13,500).

a considerable portion of the exposed surface already has undergone these reactions in the course of normal plasma transport, as noted above; however, the injury responsible for the loss of endothelium may also lead to uncovering of virgin material, so that an unknown degree of fresh reaction may occur. Nevertheless, potential differences between vessel and biomaterials may be based upon these considerations, and any general conclusions drawn must allow for them.

In the sessions to follow, various methods that have been used to characterize these early reactions will be described, and the applicability of studies with simple reagents will be contrasted to those in which mixtures of proteins or plasma are used. In each case, there will be the stated or implicit question pervading the program, as to the applicability of the observations and conclusions to real life: How will the data favor the development of more efficacious devices?

Adsorption of hemostatic blood components follows quickly upon the previous step, which deals with the general principles of nonspecific protein-surface reactions. Two classes of reactants are involved: clotting proteins and blood cells. The reactions of the hemostatic elements may be studied singly, in ballet-like combination, or in the grosser thrombogenic context, whereby the formation of the thrombotic mass is the topic. Here is a field for the introduction of interdisciplinary activity *par excellance!* Blood coagulation chemistry needs assistance from surface physics; flow and diffusion must be understood; platelets, formerly the monopolists of the cell spotlight, are receiving competition from leukocytes and perhaps even erythrocytes; platelets are affected by the coagulation process, and in turn, they exert significant effects back upon it.

The reactions that have been considered so far are short-term, in that the surface events may be measured in terms of fractions of a second, and the thrombotic reactions take place for periods of minutes and hours. For many biomaterial situations, the problems go no farther. In the renal dialysis unit or during open heart surgery, the fundamental problems terminate with disconnection of the apparatus. The situation assumes a new dimension when a biomaterial is implanted so that it maintains long-term or even permanent residence, as is the case with artificial heart valves or vascular prostheses. Here again, an early and a late phase can be recognized. The time scale is now hours to years. The early phase is an extension of the thrombotic problems considered earlier, but now the deposit is considerably more massive. In fact, this field has shown considerable recent progress, as surgical technique has empirically improved, and rational use of antithrombotic therapy has achieved increased precision.

The hyperplastic response of the blood vessel constitutes the greatest long-term problem leading to failure of heart valves and vascular grafts. As noted earlier, the injured blood vessel responds promptly with a proliferative response. The classic studies of Ross and Glomset[4] have shown that vascular smooth-muscle cells are stimulated to proliferate, at least in part, by materials carried in blood platelets. This proliferative response results largely, if not entirely, in intimal hyperplasia, and thereby encroachment of the new tissue into the lumen. The new tissue is often particularly liable to the pathological changes that characterize atherosclerosis, and thereby result in the production of a highly thrombogenic surface. Thus, graft failure may be consequence of a tissue overgrowth reaction not predicted by the previous tests used to evaluate biomaterials, nor by the flow characteristics in the region of the implant, nor by the impact of the biomaterial upon hemostatic reactions.

In the past five years, the various elephant feelers have applied themselves scientifically to their parts, and their descriptions have achieved a degree of scope and precision that should be most gratifying to Dr. Gott. It is hoped that this conference will enable these investigators to compare notes so that he entire animal is given a degree of perspective not hitherto possible. We know already that the elephant is large, that he has a thick skin, and that he is difficult to manage. We know, further, that his tusks are valuable. If the

Conference goes according to plan, the next time we meet, it will be to congratulate each other that he has been tamed.

REFERENCES

1. GOTT, V. C. 1972. The second decade of biomaterials development and evaluation: A time to apply the scientific method. Bull. N.Y. Acad. Med. **48:** 216.
2. PALADE, G. E. Recent studies on the vascular endothelium. Ann. N.Y. Acad. Sci. In Press.
3. SPAET, T. H. & I. LEJNIEKS. 1967. Mitotic activity of rabbit blood vessels. Proc. Soc. Exper. Biol. Med. **125:** 1197–1201.
4. ROSS, R. & J. GLOMSET. 1974. Studies of primate arterial smooth muscle cells in relation to atherosclerosis. *In* Arterial Mesenchyme and Arteriosclerosis. W. D. Wagner and T. B. Clarkson, Eds. : 265. Plenum Press. New York, N.Y.

PROPERTIES OF MATERIALS AFFECTING THE BEHAVIOR OF BLOOOD AT THEIR SURFACES

Edward W. Merrill

Chemical Engineering Department
Massachusetts Institute of Technology
Cambridge, Massachusetts 02139

Blood/Surface Contact: Adsorption, Solution, Activation

Upon contact of blood with a surface other than the endothelial lining of a vessel, it is well recognized that the following events occur:

Molecular species adsorb on, or dissolve into, the surface. Plasma proteins interact with the surface in specific ways; this initial interaction can set off the series of activations of the intrinsic system that culminates in network formation of fibrin monomer. Plasma lipids probably play an important role.

At the cellular level, any of three major classes—erythrocytes, leukocytes, and platelets—can temporarily adsorb onto a surface. The platelets, especially, will adsorb to any surface (though they cannot dissolve into it, like the proteins), as shown by Leonard and his associates.[1] The platelets, having adsorbed on the surface, seem to interrogate it to ascertain if it is friend or foe. The surface more often appearing to be the latter, the platelets summon reinforcements of their kind, and a platelet thrombus develops.

It is natural to suppose that manifestation at the cellular level reflects a sequence of special molecular events, in which some of the participating molecules belong to the membranes of the cells. Although platelets are clearly the most active, leukocytes can play a synergistic role by strongly adsorbing so as to stabilize growth of a thrombus. It seems reasonable to suppose that if, via the intervention of Maxwell's demon at the molecular level, or by means of a "transpired boundary layer," contact of the surface by protein molecules or platelets were absolutely prevented, there would be no activation of the clotting systems. Finally, it must be recalled that the erythrocytes are coated with fibrinogen. Thus, their presence is probably important in the transport of fibrinogen to a surface undergoing thrombotic attack.

Smoothness—Relative to What

As will be brought out in other communications, the scale of roughness of the surface is important in at least two respects: entrainment of cells, and stabilization of molecular biochemical activation sequences against dilution to subcritical levels. Ordinarily the surface of interest forms part of a conduit for flow of blood, and this flow is usually laminar and nearly one-dimensional.

If the scales of surface roughness is of the order of tens of microns "peak to peak λ_1" and "peak to valley λ_2," as shown in FIGURE 1, erythrocytes and leukocytes are easily retained, insuring amplification of the processes of activation via platelets or the intrinsic clotting systems.

Because of the yield shear stress inherent in blood (resulting from red cell-fibrinogen-red cell interactions) the plane of shear is defined by the peaks and not the mean level from peak to valley.[2]

Thus a surface smooth with respect to blood cells should have characteristic λ_1 and λ_2 values of the order to 1 μ or less. Various evidence, including cinephotomicrography, indicates that at flow rates attainable in the arterial circulation, the shear stress at the surface of cylindrical tubes could be sufficient to thwart adhesion, unless the surface is rough in the sense described. Using the same ratio, about ten, of λ_1 or λ_2 to absorbed species diameter as an index of roughness, one would compute that a surface *rough* to globular protein molecules (diameter ca 100 Å) would have λ_1, λ_2 values around 1/10 micron. As shown in FIGURE 2, a spherical protein molecule on a smooth surface is exposed to a wall stress τ_w fixed by the pressure gradient $\Delta P/L$ and the radius of the tube (or vessel) r_w. If this "sphere" were a formed element (e.g. red cell), it

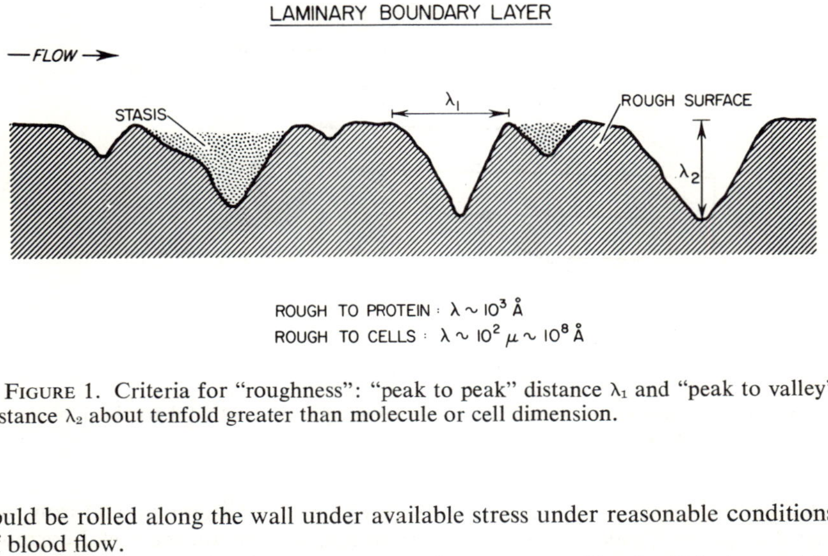

FIGURE 1. Criteria for "roughness": "peak to peak" distance λ_1 and "peak to valley" distance λ_2 about tenfold greater than molecule or cell dimension.

could be rolled along the wall under available stress under reasonable conditions of blood flow.

If one computes the shear stress operating, not on a blood cell but a protein molecule adsorbed at the wall of a cylinder, even the most miniscule forces will suffice to keep the molecule there against any shear stress conceivable. Thus the surface need not be rough in order that protein molecules can adsorb. However, the successive activation of clotting factors will be thwarted (held to subcritical levels) if the adsorption begins on a truly smooth surface exposed to rapid flow. Roughness at the molecular scale will favor advance of the clotting cascade, possibly to the ultimate fibrin layer.

These considerations thus suggest that, since coagulation is favored by stasis (if activation of platelet or intrinsic clotting systems has occurred), "smooth" surfaces free of gross pits and fissures must be sought.

A separate paper could be written on the subject of thrombosis at junctions between implanted conduit and living vessel, where the central problem is flow separation, stagnation, and recirculation downstream of the junction.

METALLICS, CERAMICS, "POLYMERICS"

It is useful to consider materials under three categories: *metallic, ceramic/ glass,* and *organic polymer,* allowing the last-named to include graphite and pyrolytic carbon.

The use of metals in prolonged direct contact with blood is of limited interest on the following accounts: their stiffness is inconsistent with the living vascular system, except under very special conditions such as a frame for valve; and only a few metals (platinum, titanium, tantalum) are unreactive toward 0.30 N NaCl solution at pH 7.04 (blood plasma). Aluminum, magnesium, copper, and iron as pure elements are all hopelessly reactive. To the extent that they can be protected by organized, dense, unreactive metal oxide surfaces, by alloying, anodizing, and so on, they should be considered as ceramic-glasses. We note that "stainless steel" owes its corrosion resistance to a stable, dense,

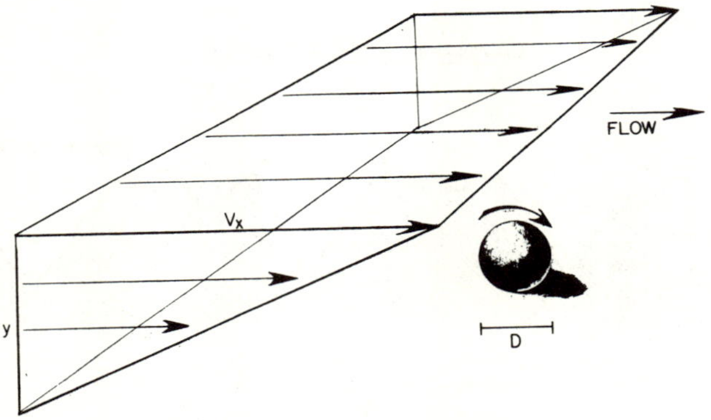

$$\text{TORQUE} \sim (\text{Viscosity}) \times \frac{\Delta V_x}{\Delta y} \times D^3$$

FIGURE 2. Fluid shear at surface produces torque proportional to third power of diameter of adsorbed sphere.

relatively impermeable oxide layer formed with nickel, chromium, and iron, and that this layer is rendered porous by nitrate ion, whereupon the metal corrodes away.

As is well known, compounds of metal oxides such as alumina and borosilicate glasses withstand indefinitely exposure to the "salt water" part of blood. The ceramics as a class, however, have such high moduli in bending that periodic deformation of any sort is inconceivable.* Like the metals, they are impermeable to any component of blood (unless intentially created with porosity, such as sintered powder metal compacts, etc.).

We then come to the third category—organic high polymers—of which one can at least say that by appropriate design they can be matched to whatever degree one wants with the gross mechanical properties of the living vessel wall, i.e., in density, viscoelastic response ("compliance," "softness," "loss factor," "elastic extensibility," and so on).

* Filamentary metals (wire) and ceramics would not be so limited.

Polymers: States of Aggregation

The most important states of aggregation of organic polymers are *"perfect" crystal, spherulitically crystalline,* and *randomly disordered,* with subdivisions in the latter according to mobility of polymer chains.

Apart from single crystals of polyethylene grown from solution, irrelevant to this discussion, pyrolytic carbon with its graphitic crystalline surface is an approximate example of a "perfect crystal."

The surface of pyrolytic carbon will be smooth as judged by the two criteria noted. The secondary force fields normal to the two-dimensional polycarbon network are low; the network atoms are rigidly placed relative to each other. Proteins and other blood components can adsorb to, but *not mix with,* the surface. The surface is impenetrable to any component of blood, water included.

The highly crystallizing polymers—nylon, polyethylene, polypropylene—are given to spherulitic crystallization. Spherulitically crystallized polymers can undergo extensive molecular rearrangement under tensile or other stresses (tension, flexing, exposure to solvent). For this reason they can readily develop pits and fissures. In addition, the polymeric segments at the surface that happen to be part of crystallites must constitute sites for stable adsorption of protein molecules; i.e., they provide a stable two-dimensional lattice of atoms analogous to but not identical with the hexagonal layered crystal of graphite. The noncrystalline area of the surface is permeable (in principle) to all the small molecule components of blood, and thus "equilibrium" with blood poses the question of solution in the polymer as well as adsorption on it.

It is especially this class of polymer which, upon solidifying, will force to its surface low-molecular species of itself by reason of the inability of the short mobile species to remain mixed with the long-chain molecules as they undergo crystallization.[3] Hence, in polyethylene, the surface usually consists of paraffin waxlike molecules, not necessarily highly active toward blood, but different from the bulk interior.

Amorphous Polymers

In contrast to crystalline polymers, wherein molecular chains are mutually organized over extensive distances in specific geometrical array, the disposition of molecular chains in amorphous polymers is governed solely by bond angles between connected chain atoms and energy barriers to rotation, internal to each chain.[4]

Paul Flory brilliantly proposed the concept that in bulk, nonsolvated polymer—in the absence of crystallization—each molecular chain has a configuration known as the "unperturbed random walk."[5] Figure 3 shows a computer calculation[6] of the projection on the XZ axis of 200 steps of a polyethylene chain in the bulk molten state, based on appropriate values of bond lengths and angles and energy barriers to rotation. The consequence of this configuration is that *each polymer chain approximates* an open coil of great size compared to its own volume, a coil so "open" that more than 95% of its volume is filled with segments of chains *other* than the one considered. This leads to enormous entanglement of chains and such properties as high viscosity, elastic elongation, and so on. Recent work by Benoit and others, who

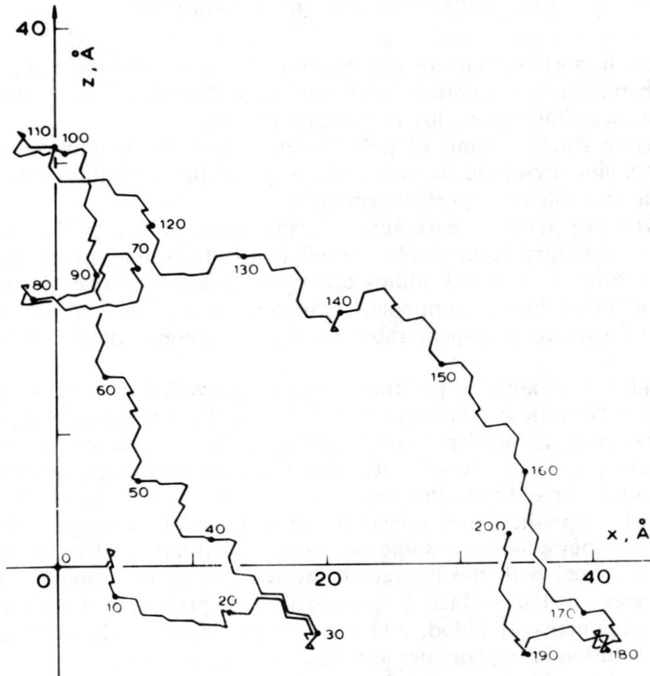

FIGURE 3. Compute calculation of first 200 steps in random walk of polyethylene chain, projected on X-Y axis.

used neutron scattering, has confirmed Flory's prediction beyond question. Furthermore, it has been shown conclusively that the chain configuration is essentially the same whether the substance is above or below its glass transition. The difference is that in the rubbery state the chains are randomly fluctuating; stated another way, segments of the chains diffuse through each other, limited only by the constraint that these segments are parts of strong chains; thus the larger the scale of the diffusion, the greater the number of segments that must cooperatively move. Even after cross-linking (as by sulfur vulcanization), chain segments diffuse locally among each other.

In our view this has an important bearing on the manner in which plasma proteins interact with the surface.

A Maxwell's demon, riding on a protein molecule, which approached the surface of a polymer in the rubbery state, might well conclude that the surface was that of a liquid, since it has two major attributes of a liquid: no systematic order among atoms, and fluctuations of positions of atoms—therefore fluctuations of density.

The protein molecule could attempt to mix with or dissolve into this surface by altering its native configuration composed of α-helical sequences so as to become itself a random-coiling polymer.

FIGURE 4 refers to the liquid lattice underlying the statistical thermodynamic theory of Flory[7] pertaining to mixtures of random-coiling polymers with solvents and with other polymers. Shown herein is a particular polymer chain randomly placed in a succession of sites in the lattice (black circles). Other lattice sites could be occupied by solvent molecules (in the case at hand: water, lipid) or by "denatured" protein molecules.

As Flory has shown on thermodynamic arguments,[8] complete mixing of two *polymers,* in contradistinction to *one* polymer and a *small* molecule solvent, is extremely unlikely because of the highly negative entropy of mixing, but this could be offset if the heat of mixing of segments were strongly exothermic. However, incomplete mixing at a protein-polymer interface to a depth of several tens of angstrom units is *not* foreclosed by any thermodynamic principle, regardless of the heat of mixing.

Let the temperature fall below the glass transition T_g of the substance and motion of the main chains ceases, or nearly ceases. The substance is now glassy.

However, the Maxwell's demon inspecting the surface of such a polymer could still be confused, to a certain degree. If the substance is at a temperature less than its α transition (T_g) but above its β transition, there could be vigorous wagging and rocking of groups of atoms attached to the sides of chains, like a field of flowers blown by the wind. The demon might well regard this as a quasiliquid surface.

If, on the other hand, atomic motion of all kinds has mainly ceased (as would be the case of polystyrene at 37° C), the observing demon would perceive a surface of atoms in random but relatively fixed positions. This is one condition favoring adsorption of a plasma protein. Indeed, one can now identify the protein interaction as being that of adsorption only, since solution is impossible. (One must qualify such an assertion with the postulate that lipids or other small-molecule blood components do not dissolve into the polymer, thereby creating a polymer-solvent solution which causes the β and α (T_g) transitions to drop below 37° C).

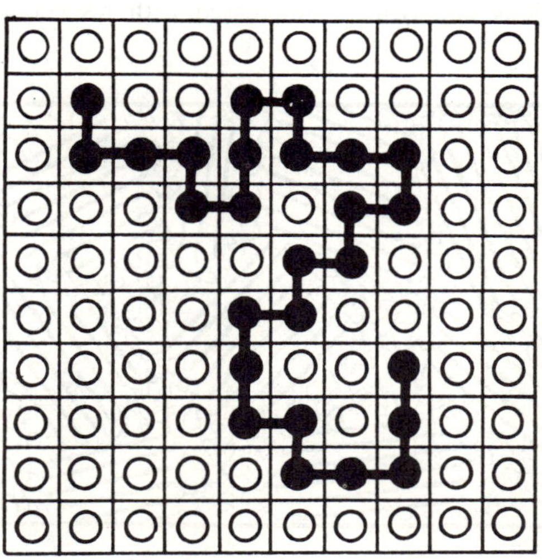

FIGURE 4. Liquid lattice underlying statistical thermodynamic analysis of polymer-solvent mixing. (By permission of Cornell Univ. Press, Ithaca, N.Y.[7])

Amorphous Polymers Containing a Separated, Dispersed Phase

This brings us to two related states, involving random-coiling polymer chains, in which the *continuous* phase presumably consists of the random-coiling chains. The separated and discontinuous phase is, in each instance, a cross-linking or network-forming phase, acting like chemical cross-linking to prevent viscous flow.

Some polymers undergo a very limited crystallization which results in the fringed micelle state. The "fringed" micelle crystallites are like soap micelles in the sense that sequences of carbons are packed in fully extended configuration and that the total length of the crystal *in the direction* of the chain axis is relatively small.

FIGURE 5, taken from Flory, is a schematic representation of the fringed micelle state of crystallization. The volume fraction of crystallization herein represented is probably far greater than occurs in the polymers noted below.

Unlike the soap micelle, the polymer crystal micelle has a continuation via its molecular chains into the surrounding "amorphous" polymer which forms a continuous phase. Abandoned a few years ago by many polymer physicists, the concept has been revived, since all evidence indicates that it is the correct model for such polymers as polyvinyl chloride (including its plasticized states), cellulose acetate, and sundry other polymers.

Unlike the spherulitic crystal polymer, the fringed micelle polymer is more likely to bury its crystal micelles under randomly organized chains. The random or amorphous polymer chains can be either in the glassy or in the rubbery state. Plasticized polyvinyl chloride is an example of the latter.

Crystallites as micelles are not uniquely necessary to create a network. The same result can be achieved with a separated phase that "holds together" because its molecular components are glassy. Triblock copolymers of styrene with butadiene or isoprene are examples of a network formed by phase separation. FIGURE 6 shows[9] schematically how, as the volumetric ratio of component A of a block copolymer is increased with respect to the other com-

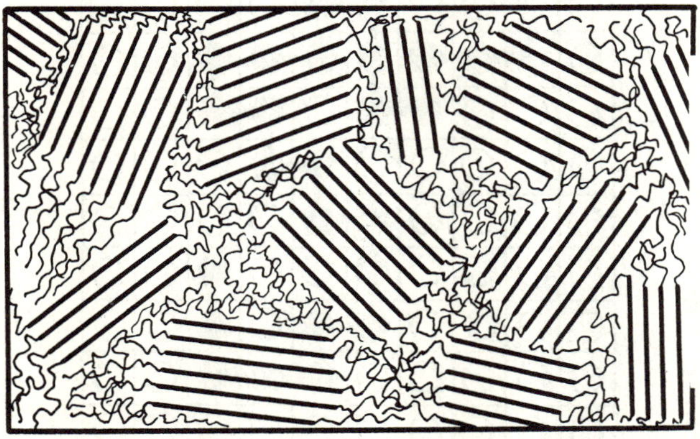

FIGURE 5. "Fringed" micelle model of crystallites in a polymer, emphasizing ordered chain sequences in micelles (crystals) as dispersed phase, connected by random coiling chain sequences constituting the continuous phase.

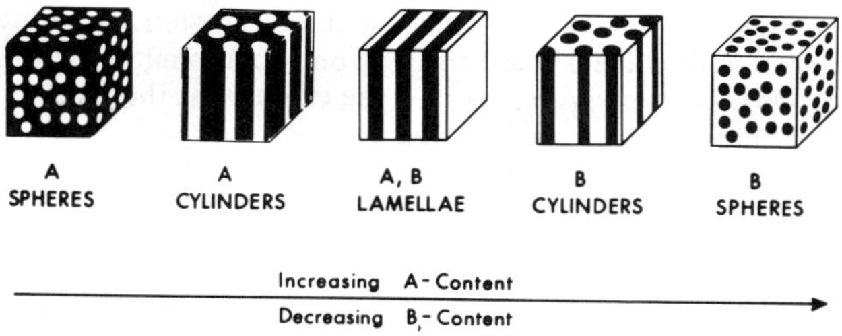

FIGURE 6. Models of phase-separated polymers emphasizing forms of aggregations of dispersed and continuous phases. (By permission of the Plenum Publishing Co., New York, N.Y.[9])

ponent B, the A phase, initially dispersed as spheres in a continuum of B, can ultimately become the continuous phase, with B dispersed in it as spheres. Between these two states lie the lamellar states shown. Of particular interest is the case of glassy polystyrene, as the "A" phase, dispersed in the rubbery, continuous butadiene phase "B," forming a network which holds the latter together. Application of statistical thermodynamics, with the liquid lattice previously mentioned (FIGURE 4), to components A and B of a block copolymer leads to the conclusion previously noted with respect to denatured protein molecules and amorphous sythetic polymer: although total mixing is unlikely from entropy considerations, limited mixing at the interface is not impossible.

"Polyurethanes" include a wide range of quite different polymeric substances. Some of these, of interest in blood contact, are usefully regarded as block copolymers, as the terminology "hard segment," "soft segment" implies.

The central question, then, regarding fringed micelle or block copolymers, is whether the dispersed phase is at an interface with blood, or buried under it by random-coiling, liquidlike chain segments.

The answer must involve both thermodynamics and kinetics. For example, if the bulk polymer is cooled against a solid surface that will nucleate crystallization or phase separation, it may be expected that in the finally cooled substance there could be *at this interface* fringed micelle crystallites, or "hard segment" entities, respectively, but at an air interface, a polymeric mass upon cooling past its phase transition may be expected to place the amorphous random-chain segments outside.

SPECIAL STATES

Before considering more specifically interactions of blood with polymers in the rubbery amorphous state, for the sake of completeness we note the tightly cross-linked, glassy state characteristic of phenolic and other "hard" resins. This corresponds to glassy polymer at a temperature below its β, as well as its glass transition (α), temperatures. We expect that adsorption of proteins is at least possible but that mixing at the interface is impossible. It is also reasonable to suppose that permeability to any small-molecular component of blood, including water, will be essentially zero. In other words, no blood components can "mix into" the polymer surface.

"Extended chain polymers," which include polytetrafluorethylene, have greatly extended coil dimensions arising from rotational energy barriers between successive carbon chain atoms. To the extent that these polymers crystallize, the crystallization is anomalous and cannot be classified as either spherulitic or micellar.[10] Another example of this kind is the aromatic polyamides with 1,4 linkage of benzene rings.

Reactivity of Molecular Groups at the Surface

From the foregoing discussion it appears that the activatable factors in blood (the plasma proteins) can be "activated" if they diffuse to a solid surface capable of adsorbing them so as to alter their native configuration, or if they diffuse to a "liquid-solid" surface, as exemplified by the rubbery, random polymer, in which they can, by partially mixing, alter their native configuration.

As will be apparent in subsequent discussion, the activatable protein molecules have a *wide variety* of *molecular groups* that they can bring to a synthetic polymer surface, far *more* groups than has the synthetic polymer. The protein groups consist of bound anions, cations, hydroxyls, alkyl chains, and sulfhydryls, not to mention "parasitic" lipid of various kinds.

How activation can be prevented we shall learn more of in this conference. A few generalizations seem possible (noting the necessity always to distinguish between platelet activation and intrinsic clotting activation.)

Ultrapure dimethyl silicone has been found to be relatively inert toward the intrinsic clotting system.[11] By exposing the uncross-linked polymer to ionizing radiation, while rigorously excluding oxygen—for example, by maintaining the specimen under nitrogen or argon—cross-linking *without* oxidation is accomplished by coupling of radical methylene groups. The activity toward the intrinsic clotting system is significantly increased by accidental placement of oxidized groups on the surface, as occurs in heat curing. Infrared shows these groups to include carbonyls. Thrombogenic activity is drastically increased further by the presence of colloidal silica used as reinforcing agent.

Aside from the filler, this observation teaches us that strongly hydrogen bonding groups *may* be activating. This is borne out by investigations of polymers containing nitrile groups ($-C{\equiv}N$). On the other hand, alkyl ester groups, weakly hydrogen-bonding, seem relatively passive.

Ionic groups on the polymer always present a problem, because they are likely to be violently thrombogenic unless first equilibrated against the ionic components of serum (Na^+, K^+, Ca^{++}, HCO_3^-, Cl^-, etc.). If not so equilibrated, upon first contact with blood they are capable of changing local pH to 1 or 13, or otherwise drastically altering the local ionic environment of protein molecules at the surface. We also recall that while all proteins and cells are electrophoretically negative, they are not, in general, repelled by negative surfaces. And why not? Because they in fact have a surface mosaic of positive and negative groups, with the latter exceeding the former in number.

It is difficult from the published evidence to draw conclusions about the merits of hydrogels, which generally may be considered to be hydroxyl-bearing, amorphous, hydrated polymers.

From the viewpoint of the Flory-Huggins liquid lattice theory of thermodynamics,[7] and aside from ion-ion interactions between a protein molecule and a polymer surface, the tendency of a moiety on the protein to dissolve into the polymer surface will be maximum when the interaction parameter (χ_1) goes to zero. That is when the cohesive energy density of the protein moiety matches that of the moieties on the polymer (say methyl acrylate).

Since, however, the protein contains a variety of moieties of widely differing CED, some are capable of mixing into a polymer surface regardless of what it is, provided the polymer is not glassy.

Since the sequence of moieties on the protein are rarely known, one is nearly completely ignorant of how to design the polymer surface to thwart activation of activatable proteins that arrive at the surface. The apparent success of ultrapure silicone may teach us that the lipidlike, low CED of the methyl groups is advantageous in preventing mixing, but it is also true that the chain segments of the silicones are among the most liquidlike (mobile) of any polymer, and this may affect the kinetics of adsorption of proteins as much as the equilibrium thermodynamic relation.

One does know that polymeric substances become coated with protein molecules after exposure to blood *in vivo* and that in some instances a stable layer of protein is finally achieved that renders the polymer passive.

This may reflect a need for a polymer to allow partial admixture into itself of plasma lipids and/or nonactivatable plasma proteins, in order that a stable passive layer be achieved.

Polymeric surfaces to which heparin is bound represent a totally different state of affairs, and such surfaces may become passive, or resist thrombogenesis, by specific interaction with circulating antithrombin. This important topic will be addressed by others in this conference. We conclude by noting that, in the end, it is the material in the first few hundred angstrom units below a blood interface that govern what the blood will do, and thus, on the one hand, one can bury reinforcing filamentary material of any kind without affecting the surface reactions, and on the other hand, adventitious contamination or oxidation or other transformation of a polymer surface may provoke activation however pure the interior material may be, just below the surface.

Acknowledgment

I am indebted to Dr. Edwin W. Salzman as a long-time friend, colleague, and collaborator who aroused my interest in thrombogenesis and got me started in trying to find out how polymers interact with blood. Without his encouragement and guidance over the years, I would not be in a position to present this paper.

References

1. Leonard, E. F., L. I. Friedman, H. Liem, E. F. Grabowski & C. W. McCord 1970. Trans. Am. Soc. Artif. Intern. Organs **16:** 63–73.
2. Cokelet, G. C., E. W. Merrill, E. R. Gilliland, H. Shin, A. Britten & R. E. Wells, Jr. 1973. Trans. Soc. Rheology, **7:** 303–317.
3. Flory, P. J. 1953. Principles of Polymer Chemistry : 563 ff. Cornell Univ. Press. Ithaca, N.Y.
4. Flory, P. J. 1968. Statistical Mechanics of Chain Molecules. McGraw Hill. New York, N.Y.

5. Flory, P. J. 1953. Principles of Polymer Chemistry : 602. Cornell Univ. Press. Ithaca, N.Y.
6. Mark, J. E. Private communication. Univ. of Michigan. Ann Arbor, Mich.
7. Flory, P. J. 1953. Principles of Polymer Chemistry : 497. Cornell Univ. Press. Ithaca, N.Y.
8. Flory, P. J. 1953. Principles of Polymer Chemistry : 554. Cornell Univ. Press. Ithaca, N.Y.
9. Molau, G. E. 1970. Colloidal and Morphological Behavior of Block and Graft Copolymers, in Block Copolymers. S. L. Aggarwal, Ed. Plenum Press. New York, N.Y.
10. Bunn, C. W. & E. R. Howells. 1954. Nature **174:** 549.
11. Weathersby, P. K., T. Kolobow & E. W. Stool. 1975. J. Biomed. Mat. Res. **9:** 561.

THE ORGANIZATION OF BLOOD COMPONENTS NEAR INTERFACES

Robert E. Baier

Calspan Corporation
Buffalo, New York 14221

The arrangement of blood elements near their border with intact vascular endothelial cells is poorly understood. However, the order and succession of blood components arriving at nonphysiologic boundaries has been experimentally determined. After essentially instantaneous transitions occur in the interfacially bound layer of water and ions, specific blood proteins, usually fibrinogen, adsorb immediately. The strange interface is coated by a 50-Å thick film within five seconds, "converting" to a more complex mixture of components with increasing contact time. Blood platelets arrive continuously, but little cell adhesion occurs until the "conditioning" film of protein achieves a critical—but nonequilibrium—state, about 200-Å deep. Within two minutes of first blood contact, most platelets adhere in a nearly random and discontinuous monolayer. White cells, mainly neutrophils, are chemotactically activated toward the adherent platelets (and aggregates) within five minutes, adding to the growing white thrombus mass, in most cases. Thrombi extend into the blood flow, accelerating fibrin formation and red cell entrapment to result in a typical red clot. At some interfaces, white cells assist in detaching platelets to leave a "passive" blood-compatible proteinaceous film.

Natural Blood Interfaces

Natural blood conduits, including the arteries and veins of mammalian vasculature, are known to be coated on their blood-contacting faces with a pavement of closely packed spindle-shaped cells. Called the endothelial cellular lining, this living monolayer has by evolution become specialized for its role of separating blood components from the structural matrix of the vessel itself. Until recently, this layer has been poorly depicted in its natural arrangement and morphological state because of the extreme lability of the cells. Endothelial cells exhibit ready damage and sloughing under the most modest stresses induced during dissection or chemical treatment. The intact endothelial lining has been even more poorly described in terms of those interfacial properties we would hope to mimic with synthetic materials for blood-contact applications.

Figure 1 provides a collection of scanning electron microscopic views of an intact human endothelial layer as fixed immediately upon delivery of an umbilical cord, without traumatizing the vessel by its dissection from the surrounding Wharton's jelly and umbilical arteries prior to chemical stabilization. Critical point drying was required for the excellent preservation of the three-dimensional morphology of this vascular lining, as depicted in Figure 1. Even with excellent chemical fixation, air-drying of blood vessel specimens leads to severe flattening, disruption, and peeling away of this endothelial cellular lining, in most instances. Close inspection of some of the views in Figure 1

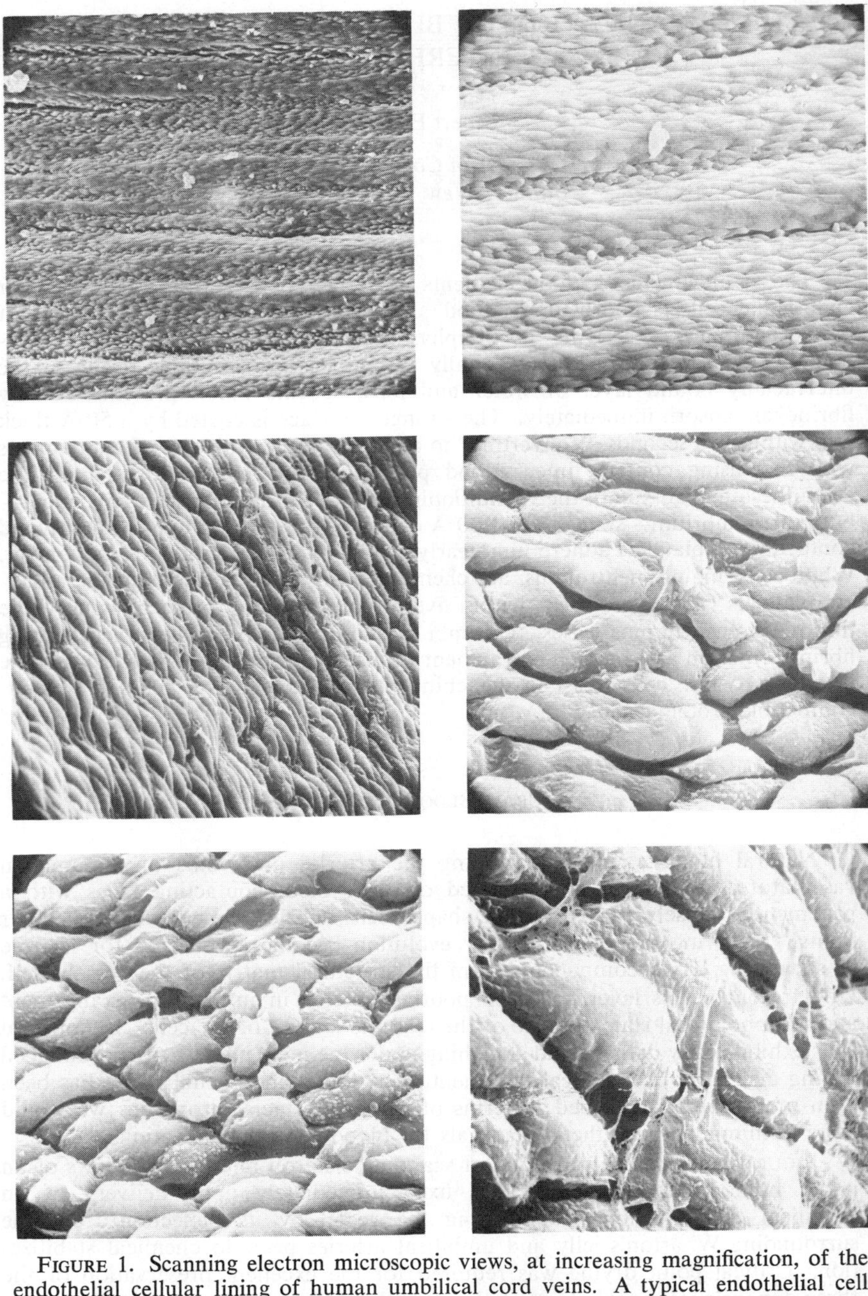

FIGURE 1. Scanning electron microscopic views, at increasing magnification, of the endothelial cellular lining of human umbilical cord veins. A typical endothelial cell dimension is 20 μm $\times$ 5 μm, and the cells are organized with their long dimensions parallel to the original blood flow. Note the adherent platelets in most views, with pseudopods reaching between endothelial cells to attach to the basement membrane. (Specimen kindly provided by Michael Wodka, Meadox Medicals, Inc., Oakland, N.J.)

will reveal that, where cell-to-cell separation did occur, and even in regions where no such separation is obvious, blood platelets have sequestered themselves (or their pseudopods) between the endothelial cell margins to guarantee the "environmental seal" and selective permeability of the cellular lining.

Thus, given healthy natural blood vessel linings, platelet adhesion is not necessarily to be correlated with adverse consequences in all cases. In fact, platelet adhesion to the subendothelial lining beneath the endothelial cells seems to be a perfectly tolerable circumstance with regard to establishing blood-compatible substitute conduits to replace diseased natural blood vessels. We have recently shown that neither the endothelial cells—damaged or undamaged—nor the subendothelial lining need remain viable to exhibit long-term physiologically tolerable responses in contact with fresh flowing human blood, with no adverse thrombogenic or immunogenic consequence.[1] The most highly magnified view of the endothelial cell layer provided in FIGURE 1 shows a thin polymeric veil, perhaps contiguous with, but more likely coated upon, the endothelial cellular membranes, which represents the natural blood-contact interface of apparently healthy blood vessels. If this material is synthesized as an exudate of the endothelial cells, it is then equally likely that an equivalent exudate occupies the zone beneath the cells, separating them from the internal elastic and medial components of the blood vessel wall, and is responsible for the chemical properties of the subendothelial lining.

In this sense, the endothelial cells can be implicated in the synthesis of their own basement membrane, or in the provision of the proteinaceous carpet upon which they rest. When detached, then, the remaining subendothelial lining may continue to exhibit physiologically tolerable—even if platelet-adhesive, temporarily—interactions with fresh flowing blood. Beyond these speculative remarks, we cannot yet provide further details of the sequence or arrangement of blood components adjacent to the interface that nature has provided, and must turn our attention to the synthetic structural and engineering materials that we are constrained to utilize for the next five years or more in biomedical devices having blood-contact applications.

Synthetic Solid/Blood Interfaces

For most nonphysiologic materials proposed for blood contact applications, there are three major descriptors of the surface properties which can and should be considered. These parameters relate to the texture, the surface charge, and the surface chemistry of each solid or semisolid (e.g. hydrogel) substrate brought into contact with blood. The interplay of these factors has already been described at a conference held in 1971 [2] on this same subject.

Surface Texture

We have since presented preliminary evidence [3] that surface textural irregularities at a scale less than a micron or so can be tolerated, given the caveat that all of the surface irregularities, including voids, must be thoroughly prewetted before contact with protein-containing solutions. Complete wetting (alternatively, outgassing) is required to prevent adverse thrombus-initiating events of protein adsorption and denaturation at remnant pockets of gas (at gas/liquid interfaces). The apparent mechanism by which this tolerance of a reasonably heterogenous surface geometry is manifested involves the adsorption and geometrical leveling provided by the earliest deposited biological macromolecules.

Surface Charge

With respect to surface charge as a parameter of blood compatibility, the prevailing theory for three decades has been that of Sawyer and co-workers [4, 5] that net negatively charged surfaces are antithrombogenic. It can be argued, however, that measurements of net negative surface charges or negative surface potentials have been only incidentally, rather than absolutely, correlatible with nonthrombogenic outcomes. Blood-component adhesion and aggregation at some net negatively charged substrates are probably overlooked because either erosion or corrosion takes place at the substrate interfaces to project thromboemboli and, probably, unwanted substrate components downstream. This interpretation implies that observation of net negativity for a substrate in contact with blood (or with physiologically balanced electrolyte solutions) successfully predicts apparent thromboresistance at the site of that implant only because such net negativity also correlates with a high corrosion potential for that material. Among metals, the reactive aluminum and magnesium specimens that have been reported as thromboresistant are examples. Among anionic polyelectrolytes, the apparently thromboresistant polyethylene/acrylic acid copolymers that slowly erode in contact with blood are examples.[6, 7] Otherwise, both nonmetallic and metallic surfaces which do not lose mass to the bloodstream, regardless of their initial surface charge or surface potential, are probably thrombus-inducing to a degree greater than that which would be obtained with a neutral surface for the same generic materials. In the special case of glass, which for centuries has been considered a strong clot-inducing contact surface, glow discharge treatment, and incubation in distilled water before blood contact can also predispose its surface to erosion into the flowing bloodstream. Thromboresistance at the implant site,[8] but not freedom from thromboembolism,[9] can be demonstrated.

In a conference on the topic of "Moving Blood at Interfaces" at the beginning of this decade, other surface charge- and surface potential-related features of synthetic materials, the vascular endothelium, and potentially adherent blood components were described.[10] One conclusion from considerations of computed interaction energies at various distances of separation between planar surfaces and blood platelets or erythrocytes was that the kinetic energy (or equivalent velocity of the cells toward the wall) required to establish contact in even the "secondary minimum" for stable cell-to-surface adhesion was in an unrealistically high range.[11]

Fluid Dynamics

Reviews of the fluid mechanical factors favoring and/or preventing cells from reaching interfaces of tubes through which blood flows also provide strong theoretical arguments that cells are preferentially excluded from the zone near the tube wall.[12, 13] Adhesive interactions with smooth walls require exceptional inputs of energy (or momentum transfer) to augment transverse velocities.

Unconventional mechanisms, such as the paddle motion provided by the rotating erythrocytes, are currently invoked to impart an additional velocity toward the wall (through the fluid mechanically forbidden zone) to the blood platelets known to be the first cellular elements involved in thrombus formation. Alternatively, many workers propose that probes of low radii of curvature are extended from the cell to overcome the electrostatically and fluid mechanically forbidden zones between the cell bodies and the solid substrates to which cells do, in fact, attach. This invocation has the unsettling consequence of requiring that the cell respond at a distance to the existence of a wall by undergoing a profound morphological change that allows it to reach closely enough to that wall to come into its adhesive "sphere of influence." Rather than adopting this teleological view of cells anticipating their coming adhesive interactions with solid substrates, it has been suggested that the equivalent of the required probes of low radii of curvature arise, instead, from the substrate side of the pending biological joint. This occurs by the spontaneous adsorption of biological macromolecules—predominately glycoproteins—to the prerequisite thickness to simply geometrically overcome the distance between the walls and the zone where cell arrival, without any anticipatory shape changes, is facile.[14] Here we find a convincing, if not compelling, explanation for the observation that *no* cell adhesion to solid substrates occurs without an intervening thin film of spontaneously or deliberately deposited macromolecular material.[15] This is especially true in all blood contact phenomena involving synthetic materials.

Surface Chemistry

Probably the most important parameters of surface properties for substrates brought into contact with blood are those related to their interfacial reactivities. The existing surface charge distribution does, in many ways, impart specific surface energetic states to each substrate, with the general finding being that either anionically or cationically charged materials are of higher surface free energy than their neutral counterparts. Nevertheless, surface free energy, or parameters thereof, is the most useful descriptor of the actual suface chemical identity of those many organic and polymeric materials dealt with in practical biomedical devices or prostheses. As introduced and described earlier,[16] one empirical parameter of surface free energy called the "critical surface tension" has correlated well with the true outermost atomic constitution of low-energy organic materials. It has been hypothesized that a particular zone of critical surface tension correlates best with biological compatibility in general and with blood compatibility in particular.[17, 18]

The general theme has been that specific chemical groupings at interfaces between solids and biological phases must dictate the pattern and binding strength of the first adsorbed proteins and thus secondarily determine the initial adhesive interactions of the first arriving cells. In the case of blood, these initial cells are platelets. The adhesional lifetime of the first adherent cells or cellular aggregates is also related to the original surface chemical array. In the case of blood, platelet aggregates or microthrombi (which also involve white cells) would be surface-bound with varying degrees of tenacity, depending upon the initial chemical groups available. The hypothesis has been that an appropriate critical surface tension, as a "flag" of the appropriate surface chemical distribution, results in minimal distortion and therefore adhesion of the spontaneously adsorbed proteins. Minimizing of protein distortion then favors shorter adhesional lifetime of the first deposited cells, and there is a smaller aggregate size of detached thrombus masses and a decreased likelihood of untoward embolic consequences downstream.

SEQUENCE AND ORGANIZATION OF BLOOD COMPONENTS AT FOREIGN INTERFACES

Simultaneous and sequential nondestructive analytical techniques are available to deduce the consequences of exposure of a variety of metallic and nonmetallic interfaces to biological systems or biological fluids such as blood. These techniques include the use of internal reflection spectroscopy to deduce molecular structure of interfacial films; of ellipsometry to deduce the thickness and refractive index of those same layers; of contact potential devices to measure the surface charge and surface potential features in noncontacting circuits; of contact angle measurements to infer critical surface tension as a parameter of surface free energy and surface chemical constitution; and of scanning electron microscopy to assess the microtextural features and patterns of cellular deposition or cell morphology. These techniques, and more, are reviewed with numerous examples from the many fields of biological adhesion research in a recent publication in the *Advances in Chemistry Series*.[19]

Regarding the organization of blood components at interfaces, these methods have already clearly demonstrated that within a few seconds of first blood contact, all nonphysiologic materials acquire a rapidly thickening film of essentially pure protein, most likely fibrinogen, which dramatically changes the surface texture, surface charge, and surface chemistry of these substrates. A critical stage is reached (usually when the protein thickness is between 100 and 200 Å) about one minute after first blood contact with a buffer-wetted solid, at which point the platelets arriving in the vicinity of that surface can make their first adhesive liaison with it.[20–23]

When the arriving platelets are thus enabled, through this mandatory conditioning film of protein, to respond to the presence of the solid surface, they do so specifically and individually. Their population density in the first incompletely packed layer of cells is not very different on different substrates, but their morphological changes (or lack of changes) then trigger a thrombogenic (or thromboresistant) outcome through a secondary sequence of events. The general observation, of course, has been that the first arriving platelets flatten, degranulate, and become very sticky toward their subsequently arriving siblings to form platelet aggregates. These aggregates grow in pyramidal shapes into the blood volume, and have blunted teardrop profiles in the plane of the surface aligned with the prevailing blood flow direction. Within about four minutes (in the usual case) of first blood contact with a foreign-material surface, white blood cells are then chemotactically stimulated (in abundance) toward the already debris-strewn solid/liquid boundary. The white cells adhere to and around the growing platelet aggregates and enter the growing cellular mass to form microthrombi now capable of seriously perturbing the near-surface-flow field. These flow perturbations, coupled with the chemical modifications of degranulating platelets and probably surface activation of sensitive proteins, accelerate the coagulation process, forming frank fibrin strands that entrap and enmesh the red blood cells still moving at some distance from the solid/liquid interface. The result is a typical red blood clot. This description of the organization of blood components at a thrombogenic interface clearly defines the event known popularly as blood clotting to have been initiated at least two structural levels beneath the red blood cell/fibrin mesh which casual observation provides as an indicator of blood incompatibility.

On an ultimately thromboresistant material the initial sequence of events and organization of blood components seem to be identical. Protein adsorption—most probably the same protein or small groups of proteins—precedes platelet adhesion. The clear difference in platelet morphology is the first obvious signal that a thromboresistant surface, or physiologically tolerable surface, has been encountered. On the most tolerable blood contact surfaces, the platelets remain rounded or discoid, exhibiting few pseudopods and no degranulation. With occasional exceptions, these undistorted cells are resistant to three-dimensional aggregation with subsequently arriving platelets or white cells. Yet it is clear that some chemical change has occurred, because within a few minutes the chemotactic stimulation of white cells—almost exclusively segmented neutrophils at this time—toward the surface is observed. These white cells tend to surround and in many cases overlap with the originally attached, only moderately distorted, platelets, and through some poorly understood process assist in their removal into the flowing stream. Since segmented neutrophils are known as phagocytic cells, there is perhaps some phagocytic activity associated with this process. The phagocytic process would be frustrated by the relatively large platelet particles and the infinitely large surface area of the substrate. In response to this biological frustration, exogenous enzymatic products are provided by the white cells which can disrupt, digest, or hydrolyze the tentative anchor provided to the adherent platelets by a fibrinogen-dominated conditioning film. Thence, the prevailing shear from blood continuously flowing over the surface can wash away platelets, microthrombi, and white cells on "rafts" of detached protein film. The more native the components of the conditioning film, the looser will be its structure and the greater its amenability to disruption by exudates from the arriving white cells. Simple shear detachment as platelet aggregates form and couple more efficiently with the near-surface flow field can then result. With heparinized surfaces, or heparinized blood volumes, the sequence of blood components arriving and organizing at the strange interface is held to be similar. The anticoagulant prevents the transformation of the fibrinogen in the initially adsorbed film to a modified, probably fibrin-like layer, which provides the more permanent interfacial cement for the initially adherent platelets, aggregates, and microthrombi. In heparinized blood flows, the initial platelet aggregates, protein deposits, and secondarily involved white cells can be peeled back into large rug-like and wedge-shaped conglomerates which readily detach and move downstream, where they can be demonstrated to exist in abundance by simple trapping with filters.[24, 25] The redeeming feature of anticoagulation, at least with heparin, seems to be that these conglomerates can dissipate in the recipient's vascular system to provide recirculating platelets, at least, to the blood volume. Nevertheless, the notion that heparinization of blood supresses the initial events of thrombus formation at foreign material interfaces is erroneous.

Examples of Thrombogenic and Thromboresistant Interfaces with Blood

A useful biomedical elastomer that is marginally acceptable in long-term blood contact applications is the polyether-type polyurethane known as Biomer, or, in its spandex fiber form, as Lycra. This elastomer has a critical surface tension at the boundary between the zone of 20–30 dynes/cm, which has been defined as biocompatible, and 30–40 dynes/cm, which has been defined as incompatible, by our measurements during the past decade.[26, 27] In long-term blood contact applications, such as in circulatory assist devices used to pump unmodified calf blood for many weeks, this polymer remains in dynamic equilibrium with the flowing blood through an intervening layer of protein, the composition of which remains to be defined. Given the dynamic nature of this surface (undergoing cyclic stretch—relaxation in contact with blood from a living animal) and the only marginally good surface chemistry of the material, one would expect there to be numerous events of platelet adhesion and microthrombi shedding from time to time and place to place on the blood contact surface of these pumping chambers. FIGURE 2 provides a scanning electron micrograph illustrating such cellular activity at a surface location that does not often go on to full thrombus formation. It will be noted, in FIGURE 2, that many platelets are adherent to the subjacent protein mat (which mat masks the elastomeric surface from view), but the platelets are quite rounded and undistorted. Numerous white cells are secondarily adherent to the platelet/protein composite. These white cells are apparently capable, in circumstances such as that illustrated, of coping with the process of platelet deposition at a rapid enough rate to assure a long-term "clean up" of the surface to provide only a cell-free passive film of protein in contact with the flowing blood.[28, 29]

FIGURE 3 provides a scanning electron microscopic view of a region of the

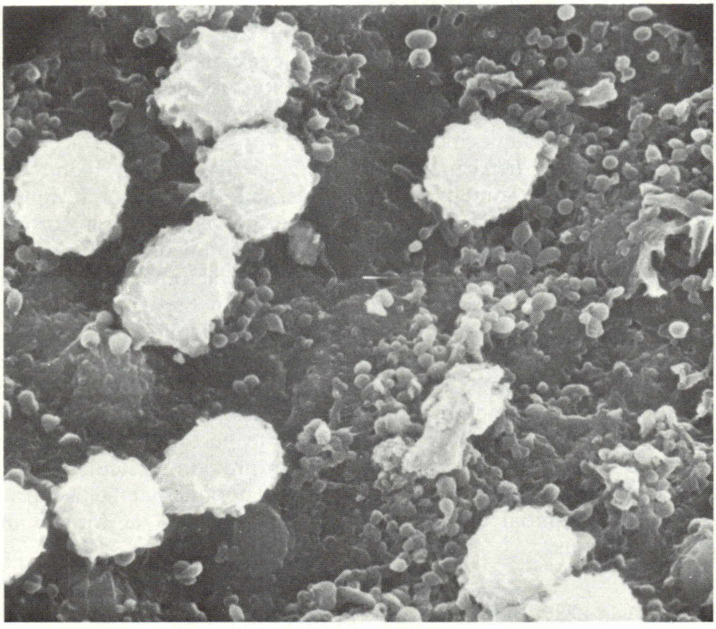

FIGURE 2. Polyether-type polyurethane sac from circulatory assist device in dynamic equilibrium with unmodified calf blood. Note white cells in process of detaching adherent layer of platelets. (Specimen kindly provided by Dr. William Pierce, University Medical Center, Hershey, Pa.) (×1500.)

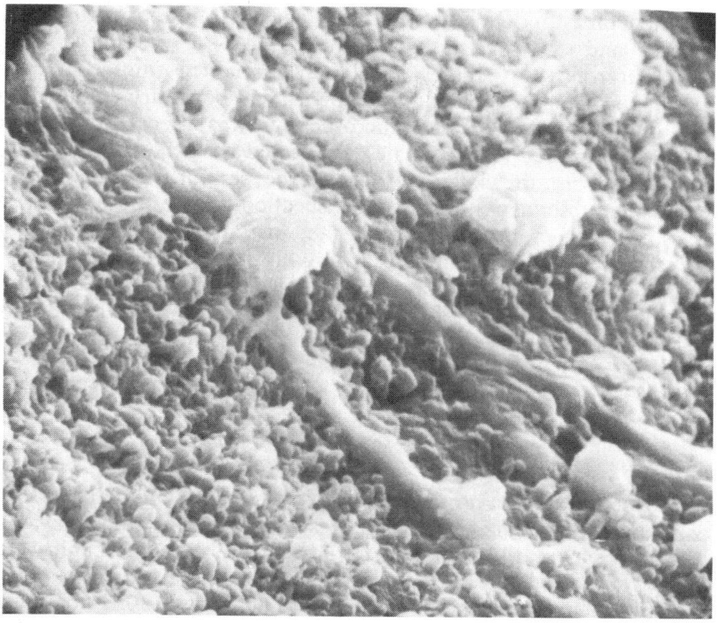

FIGURE 3. Organizing laminar thrombus on polyether-type polyurethane sac from circulatory assist device, in region near flex point. Note aggregated platelets and incorporation of white cells into growing thrombus mass. (Specimen kindly provided by Dr. William Pierce, Hershey Medical Center, Hershey, Pa.) (×1500.)

same elastomeric blood-pump surface contacting blood in a region that is predisposed, by geometrical and flow conditions, to full thrombus formation. Note the greater abundance of adherent platelets and their aggregation with one another to form a closely knit platelet thrombus which also incorporates fibers and white cells. White cells are always present on the upper face of these early thrombi, but their activity in phagocytosis or exudation of lytic enzymes seems insufficient to overcome the continuous buildup of cellular mass to form an accumulating and permanently attached thrombus. The contrast between FIGURE 2 and FIGURE 3 quite well represents the difference between thromboresistant and thrombogenic surfaces seen within minutes of first blood contact with various materials exposed to blood in stagnation-point flow experiments used to model this process for many years.[23, 30]

Another specific example of the organization of blood components near an interface which, because of local imperfections, can exhibit both thromboresistant and thrombogenic behavior is provided from recent studies of a variety of polymeric coatings.

Beginning in 1968, large numbers of potentially useful coatings for biomaterials applications were evaluated in contact with blood and blood components. One of the materials, available in commercial quantities, which showed the least detrimental effect on blood components and no shortening of blood-clotting time was a material based upon the reaction of polyvinyl alcohol and octadecylisocyanate. Thin coatings of this moderately low surface-energy polymer were superior to similar coatings of both lower and higher surface energies when measured by stypven time, partial thromboplastin time, hemoglobin release, and ATP release.[31]

During our follow-up studies on acutely implanted rings coated with this material, which included application of the critical point drying technique prior to viewing in the scanning electron microscope, it was discovered that one of the dehydrating agents used (amylacetate) interacted with the polymer and caused its detachment from the solid surface of the supporting ring. It was also observed during subsequent microscopic inspection that, in those few areas where thrombosis had, in fact, occurred on the face of the coating, the thrombus mass could be partially detached from the coating layer to allow examination of both the blood-contacting and substrate-contacting faces of the initial thrombotic deposits. This study, therefore, was among the most revealing of numerous similar observations with explanted vena cava rings in that microscopic detail could be assessed for the earliest phases of thrombosis.

Materials

The polymeric reaction product of polyvinyl alcohol and octadecylisocyanate which was used to provide the thromboresistant coatings studied was supplied under the experimental designation "L-3051" by the 3M Central Research Laboratories in St. Paul, Minn. It became apparent early in the investigation that the halogenated hydrocarbon solvent used with the L-3051 coating material would significantly attack the thrombogenic plastic implantable cylinders originally selected as the supporting structure for the coating. Thus, it became necessary to choose an alternative substrate that was also intrinsically thrombogenic. Glass cylinders, which typically thrombose completely within two hours

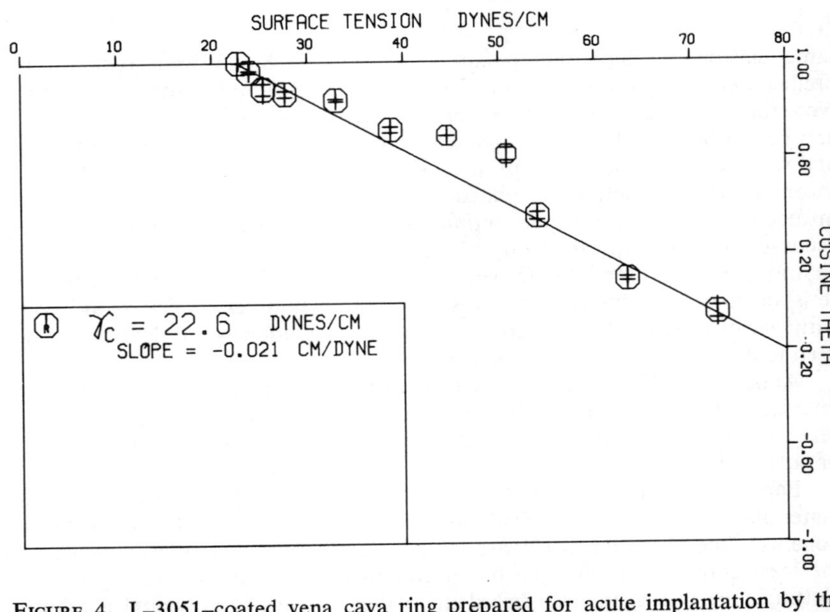

FIGURE 4. L–3051–coated vena cava ring prepared for acute implantation by the 3M Central Research Laboratories, St. Paul, Minn. Points with small symbols not included in straight-line fit.

TABLE 1

AVERAGE CONTACT ANGLES OBTAINED ON L-3051-COATED VENA CAVA RINGS

Liquid	Surface Tension @20° C	Average Contact Angle (Degrees)
Water	72.8	92.
Glycerol	63.4	85.
Thiodiglycol	54.0	69.
Methylene Iodide	50.8	52.
I-Bromonaphthalene	44.6	46.
α-Methyl naphthalene	38.7	44.
Dicyclohexyl	33.0	33.
Hexadecane	27.7	30.
Dodecane	25.4	27.
Decane	23.9	16.
Nonane	22.8	0.

of canine inferior vena cava implantation (if not previously glow discharge-treated) were used as the substrates and dip-coated with the L-3051 material. FIGURE 4, together with TABLE 1, characterizes by wettability criteria the coated lumen surface of the first batch of rings as prepared for acute implantation. The indicated critical surface-tension value of about 22 dynes/cm insures that the actual chemical structure exposed to the freshly flowing blood during implantation was that of closely packed methyl terminal groups from the octadecyl side chains of the coating agent.

ACUTE IMPLANTATION RESULTS

TABLE 2 presents the postimplantation ring diagrams illustrating the patent condition of three such coated glass specimens after two hours in canine inferior vena cavae. Tests performed on these postimplanted rings to assess the lability and surface activity of the lumenal coating acquired *in vivo* showed that a proteinaceous film was present. Labile components of the coating depressed the contact angle of pure distilled water on Teflon® from its normally high value of 110° C to an average value of 94° C. Thus, termination of the implantation experiment can be taken to represent only the "freezing" of a dynamic process occurring at the coating/blood interface.

FIGURE 5 presents scanning electron micrographs of one of the small thrombus masses that did form against the L-3051 substrate film. Since, during the critical point drying of this specimen, the substrate with its attached thrombotic deposits peeled from the glass ring itself, we were able to obtain views of all aspects of this initial deposit. It will be noted from inspection of the views in FIGURE 5 that the substrate was very smooth except where it had replicated the small pits that are regularly found on the internal surfaces of glass tubing. The lower electron micrographs in this figure show cross-sectional views of the early

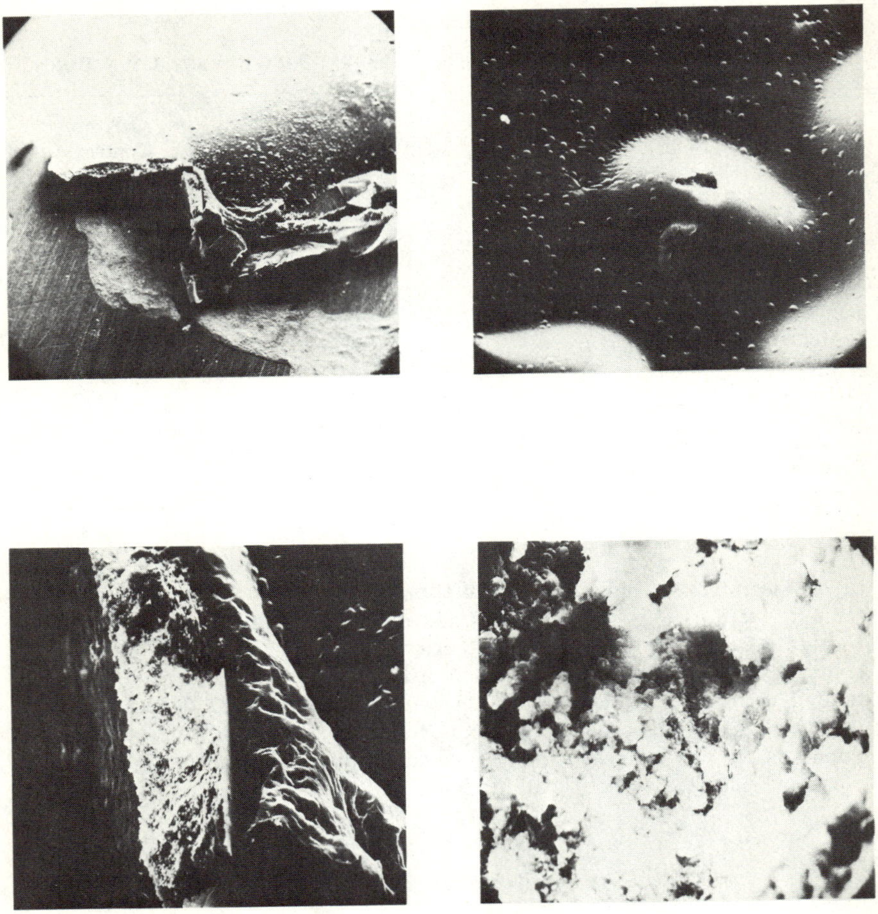

FIGURE 5. Scanning electron microscopic examination of thrombus mass still attached to 3M–3051 substrate film, as separated from glass ring during critical point drying. *Upper left:* substrate side up. (×11.4.) *Upper right:* 3M–3051 substrate as separated from glass ring. Note that bumps reflect pits in glass. (×2170.) *Lower left:* cross section of thrombus as it appears detached from plastic substrate. Note solvent-distorted substrate at right. (×93.) *Lower right:* cell distribution across mass of thrombus. (×1138.)

thrombus and the differential cell distribution across the mass of the thrombus from an initiating interface out toward the blood. FIGURE 6 shows other scanning electron microscopic views of this initial thrombotic deposit in which it can be clearly seen that the blood-contacting face of the fully developed thrombus mass was dominantly populated by platelets, whereas the substrate-contacting face of that same thrombus mass—where the adhesive events had been initiated—was essentially free of cells. These views serve to emphasize the presence of a "conditioning" layer of protein that forms on even nominally thromboresistant coatings prior to platelet adhesion and platelet aggregation.

With the exception of the small thrombotic deposits noted in these figures and in the ring diagrams, the entire remainder of the ring interior surfaces was free of cells at the two-hour termination of the acute implantations. It did, of course, retain an amorphous-appearing proteinaceous mat.

After leaching of all labile components (analytically, reasonably pure proteins) with physiologic saline for two minutes, a remnant film of cell-free protein remained. Contact angle characterizations of that remaining coating indicated it to be just at the upper boundary of the 20 to 30 dynes/cm critical surface-tension zone which was earlier suggested to correlate with significant thromboresistance.[17, 18] On thrombogenic surfaces, similar measurements always

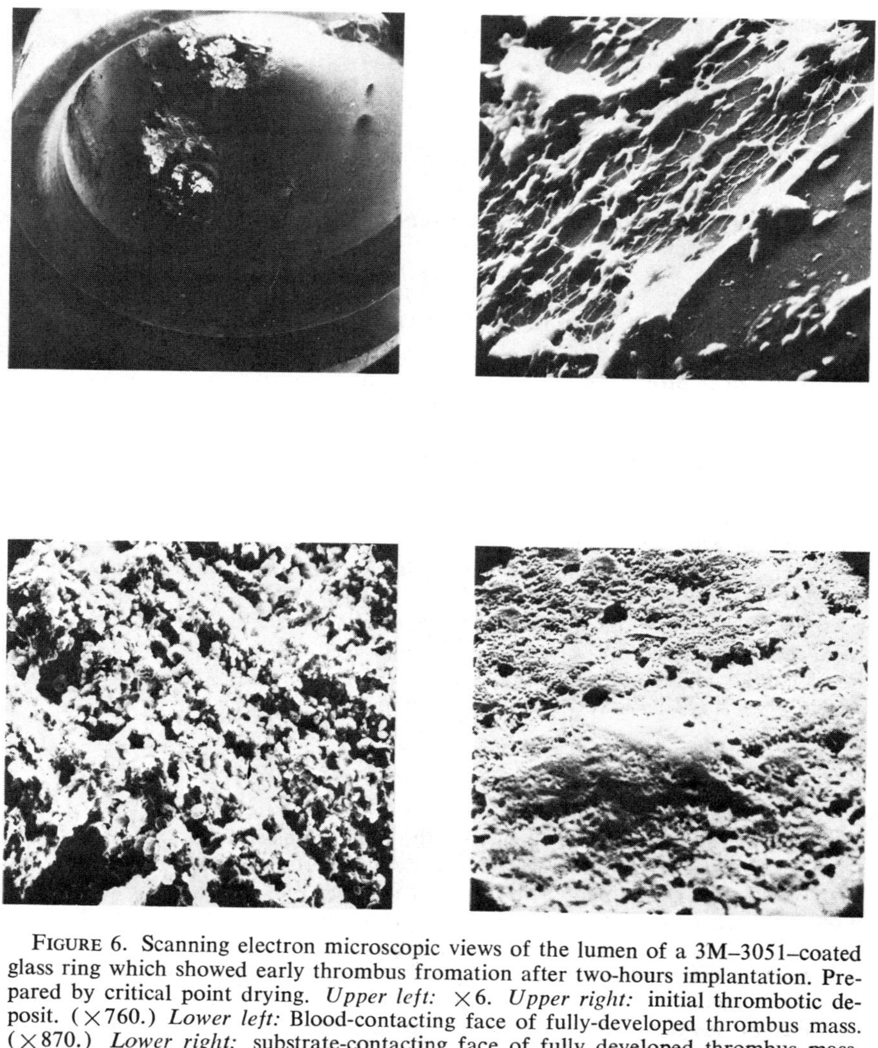

FIGURE 6. Scanning electron microscopic views of the lumen of a 3M–3051–coated glass ring which showed early thrombus fromation after two-hours implantation. Prepared by critical point drying. *Upper left:* ×6. *Upper right:* initial thrombotic deposit. (×760.) *Lower left:* Blood-contacting face of fully-developed thrombus mass. (×870.) *Lower right:* substrate-contacting face of fully developed thrombus mass. Note freedom from cells. (×4350.)

TABLE 2

GLASS RINGS COATED c̄ 3M-3051 POLYMER
IMPLANTATION RESULTS

Acute (Time 2 Hr)				
Material	Date of Implant	Sterilization	Ring Appearance	
	10–29–73	ethylene oxide		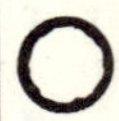
3M–3051	10–29–73	ethylene oxide	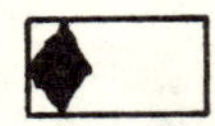	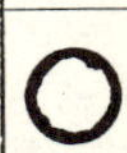
	10–29–73	ethylene oxide	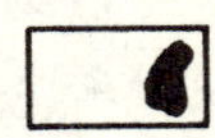	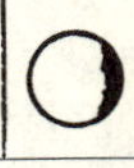

show critical surface tensions for the acquired protein mats to be in the mid to high 30s dynes/cm.

CHRONIC IMPLANTATION RESULTS

Given these promising acute test results, a second batch of L-3051 coated glass rings was prepared at the 3M Company for chronic implantation. These rings were not as favorably dominated by closely packed methyl groups in the blood-contacting layer of the coating as had been the batch prepared for acute implantation. Thus, a potential problem of reproducibly preparing nominally thromboresistant coatings was suggested. When, however, as with the rings prepared for acute implantation, ethylene oxide sterilization showed no apparent degradation of the coating in place on the glass rings, the decision was made to proceed with chronic implantation of the rings supplied. TABLE 3 presents the postimplantation findings for these chronic implants, demonstrating results that have been considered in the past to indicate at least moderate thromboresistance for a candidate biomaterial. Only one of the chronically implanted L-3051-coated glass rings, however, was completely patent in this two-week test.

DISCUSSION

FIGURE 7 shows infrared spectra of the material easily extracted into saline from the lumens of completely patent acute and chronic implants of glass rings coated with this experimental material. It is noted that the extracts are mainly proteinaceous, containing no significant quantities of lipoidal or carbohydrate material. Since electron microscopic inspection showed the surfaces to be essentially cell-free in all these cases, it is reasoned that the passive behavior of such coated rings in fresh flowing blood was predicated upon continued equilibrium of blood proteins with the labile protein components in residence at the coating/blood interface. Given the good performance of this coating in the acute tests and the moderately good performance of poorer versions of the coating in the severe chronic test, the tentative conclusion from this study is that the initiation of thrombus very likely reflects coating defects or damaged areas rather than a general propensity to thrombosis of properly applied films of this material. Independently of the merits of this coating, its novel features, when handled by the critical point drying technique, allowed multiple aspects of early thrombotic deposits to be viewed by scanning electron microscopy.

Gas/Liquid Interfaces

One does not fairly describe the organization of blood components at interfaces without at least brief mention of the gas/liquid interface. Such interfaces exist in blood reservoirs or storage vessels, or at the surfaces of most exposed organs during surgery or during wound healing. The work of Fred Leonard on surgical adhesives has made it strikingly clear that the gas/liquid interface of blood with air is not dominated by high-surface-free-energy or by hydrophilic components. Rather, it is hydrophobic in the sense that fluid phases contacting it from the air side will strongly interact only if they are dominated more by hydrophobic components than hydrophilic moieties.[32, 33]

The blood/gas interface which is prolifically generated in bubble-type blood oxygenators has been so often described and discussed in terms of the resulting untoward effects on blood components that no further description need be given here.

Liquid/Liquid Interfaces

Finally, it should be mentioned that a number of fluorocarbon and organic fluids have been proposed as "artificial blood," and liquid/liquid interfacial studies with these materials are required. Such studies are now in progress to eludicate the sequence and organization of blood components at liquid/liquid boundaries.[34]

TABLE 3

GLASS RINGS COATED c̄ 3M-3051 POLYMER
IMPLANTATION RESULTS

Chronic (Time 2 Weeks)				
Material	Date of Implant	Sterilization	Ring Appearance	
L–3051	6–4–74	ethylene oxide		
Sterilized	to	ethylene oxide	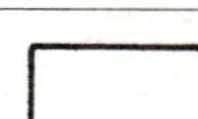	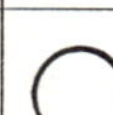
Et_2O	6–18–74	ethylene oxide		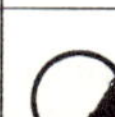

Summary, Conclusions, Remaining Questions

We can define a biomaterial to be any material designed to replace, supplement, store, or otherwise come into intimate contact with living biological cells

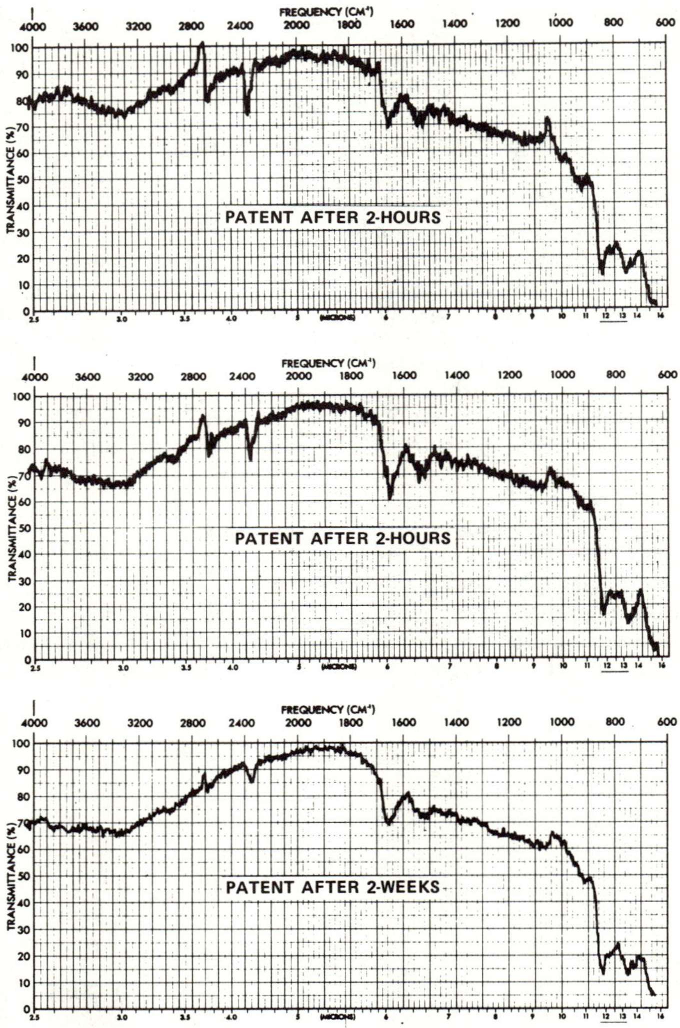

FIGURE 7. Infrared spectra of extracts into saline from the lumens of patent L-3051-coated glass rings after acute and chronic implantation.

or biological fluids. Here the concern is with materials' research problems related to diagnostic, prosthetic, or therapeutic applications where the material must exhibit long-term compatibility with blood.

Blood/material contact phenomena fall into the following three time domains:

1. Immediate, defined as that time period of blood contact prior to the adhesion of the first-formed elements of blood (usually platelets). Although dependent on specific flow circumstances, this time period does not usually exceed two minutes from first blood contact.

2. Short-Term, defined as that time period of blood contact during which cellular accumulation at surfaces (as in thrombogenesis) or protein modification (as in coagulation) are dominant factors in determining the continued function of the system. This time period does not usually exceed two weeks.

3. Long-Term, defined as that time period of blood contact during which continued cell accumulation and shedding (as in thromboembolism), cell proliferation (as in endothelialization or oncogenesis), or cell stimulation (as in inflammation or immune reactions) determines the continued function of the system. This time period extends to years. Known events during blood contact with strange interfaces, and the key research needs, may be listed (in part) as follows:

1. Immediate. On all materials, spontaneous adsorption of proteinaceous matter from blood precedes platelet adhesion, platelet aggregation, and fibrin formation. Protein adsorption does not proceed to equilibrium, but only to a thickness (usually about 200 Å) sufficient for the attachment of a first layer of platelets. The morphology, reactivity, and aggregation potential of the first adherent platelets differs on different materials. Secondary adhesion of white cells around individual adherent platelets or aggregated platelet clusters is always noted. We need answers to the following questions: What is the composition of the adsorbed film? What is its degree of organization? Molecular configuration? Is complete surface coverage achieved? How do these factors depend on surface chemistry of the original material? Surface Charge? Texture? Prevailing flow conditions? What is critical about the thickness or composition achieved which makes platelet adhesion possible? Why do platelets respond differently to films on different substrates? How is the influence of the substrate felt through the protein-dominated mat? Or does the platelet "see" the substrate through pores? Of what size? How, specifically, does platelet morphology depend upon substrate and film conditions? How does platelet aggregability depend on surface conditions? What attracts white cells, and why? How do white cells assist in detachment of single platelets or small aggregates? What goes on in the regions between originally attached platelets? Surface-induced coagulation?

2. Short Term. Once the first attached layer of platelets and secondary surrounding white cells (usually segmented neutrophils) are in place, two divergent routes are followed, depending upon the properties of the biomaterial surface. Most often, the first random layer of adherent platelets is flattened, pseudopodial, and degranulated, and adheres quantitatively with subsequently arriving platelets. Numerous pyramidal mounds of platelets grow by accretion, with many white cells participating, out into the flowing bloodstream. Along the surface, the early thrombi assume a teardrop shape with the blunt edge broadening and thickening on the upstream side. Sufficient flow perturbations, especially including near-surface eddy formation, are caused by the aggregated platelet + white cell mounds that fibrin strands collect—with numerous entrapped erythrocytes—in the regions between and above the original platelet thrombi. Given venous flow rates or vessel sizes less than 4 millimeters in diameter, this process continues until flow has ceased. Given larger vessel diameters and arterial flow conditions, the surface layer of thrombi, fibrin, and enmeshed red cells undergoes slow remodeling to form a pseudointimal layer in apparent long-term equilibrium with flowing blood.

In a minority of cases, the originally adherent platelets are not morphologically distorted and do not form large aggregates with subsequently arriving cells. The secondarily attached white cells assist in the detachment of the initially adherent platelets, and the adsorbed proteinaceous film converts to a thromboresistant passivating layer that remains cell-free and in apparent equilibrium with blood over the long term. Gently deendothelialized blood vessels subjected to arterial flows provide a natural model for this process, which otherwise occurs on only a few available biomaterials.

3. Long-Term. Autogenous blood vessels, the graft material of choice, are usually spontaneously deendothelialized by the time they are reinserted in the vascular tree. This has been clearly demonstrated with human veins, which exhibit a 70%–90% patency when used in arterial reconstructive surgery. Therefore, the best available model for synthetic blood-compatible grafts is the deendothelialized blood vessel surface, and not the native, endothelialized vessels.

On ultimately thromboresistant, smooth and nonporous, surfaces, the initially attached platelets and white cells are shed spontaneously during continuing contact with flowing native blood. On these same surfaces, a residual protein-dominated layer builds to equilibrium thickness and apparently "passivates" the surface against further thromboembolic episodes. What is the nature of this "passivating" layer, formed in native and anticoagulated blood?

Acknowledgments

The scanning electron micrographs included in this manuscript were kindly provided by Dr. C. K. Akers and Dr. V. A. DePalma of Calspan Corporation, Dr. V. L. Gott, cardiac surgeon-in-charge at Johns Hopkins Hospital, Baltimore, Md., directed the vena cava ring implantations. The L-3051 coating material discussed was provided by C. Dahlquist of 3M Corporation. B. J. Spahr prepared the final manuscript.

References

1. Baier, R. E., C. K. Akers, S. Perlmutter, H. Dardik, I. Dardik & M. Wodka. 1976. Processed human umbilical cord veins for vascular reconstructive surgery. Trans. Amer. Soc. Artif. Int. Organs **22:** 514–524.
2. Baier, R. E. 1972. The role of surface energy in thrombogenesis. Bull. N.Y. Acad. Med. **48:** 257–272.
3. De Palma, V. A., R. E. Baier, J. W. Ford, V. L. Gott & A. Furuse. 1972. Investigation of three surface properties of several metals and their relation to blood compatibility. *In* Biomaterials for Skeletal and Cardiovascular Applications. C. Homsy & C. D. Armeniades, Eds. : 37–75. Interscience Publications, New York, N.Y.
4. Sawyer, P. N. 1964. Bioelectric phenomena and intravascular thrombosis: The first 12 years. Surgery **56:** 1020–1026.
5. Sawyer, P. N., K. T. Wu, S. A. Wesolowski, W. H. Brattain & P. J. Boddy. 1965. Long-term patency of solid-wall vascular prostheses. Arch. Surg. **91:** 735–742.

6. Costello, M., B. Stanczewski, P. Vriesman, T. Lucas, S. Srinivasan & P. N. Sawyer. 1970. Correlations between electrochemical and antithrombogenic characteristics of polyelectrolyte materials. Trans. Amer. Soc. Artif. Int. Organs **16:** 1–6.
7. Baier, R. E. 1976. Adverse behavior of synthetic polyelectrolytes towards blood. J. Bioeng. In press.
8. Baier, R. E., V. A. De Palma, A. Furuse, V. L. Gott, G. W. Kammlott, T. Lucas, P. N. Sawyer, S. Srinivasan & B. Stanczewski. 1975. Thromboresistance of glass after glow discharge treatment in argon. J. Biomed. Mater. Res. **9:** 547–560.
9. Baier, R. E., C. Akers, S. Perlmutter, V. L. Gott & J. O'Riordan. 1976. Interfacial Biophysics of Materials in Contact with Blood. Report No. NO1-HB-2953–2. National Technical Information Service, 5285 Port Royal Road, Springfield, Va. 22151. 101 pp.
10. Varco, R. L., Ed. 1971. Mechanical Surface and Gas Layer Effects on Moving Blood. Federation of Amer. Societies for Experimental Biology. Bethesda, Md. 227 pp.
11. Weiss, L. 1971. Biophysical aspects of initial cell interactions with solid surfaces. Fed. Proc. **30:** 1649–1662.
12. Brenner, H. & P. M. Bungay. 1971. Rigid-particle and liquid-droplet models of red cell motion in capillary tubes. Fed. Proc. **30:** 1565–1576.
13. Keller, K. H. 1971. Effect of fluid shear on mass transport in flowing blood. Fed. Proc. **30:** 1591–1599.
14. Baier, R. E. 1975. Blood compatibility of synthetic polymers: Perspective and problems. *In* Polymers in Medicine and Surgery. R. L. Kronenthal, Z. Oser and E. Martin, Eds. : 139–159. Plenum Press. New York, N.Y.
15. Baier, R. E. 1975. Applied chemistry at protein interfaces. *In* Applied Chemistry at Protein Interfaces. R. E. Baier, Ed. : 1–25. Advances in Chemistry Series 145. American Chemical Society. Washington, D.C.
16. Zisman, W. A. 1964. Relation of the equilibrium contact angle to liquid and solid constitution. *In* Contact Angle, Wettability and Adhesion, F. M. Fowkes and R. F. Gould, Eds. : 1–51. Advances in Chemistry Series 43. American Chemical Society. Washington, D.C.
17. Baier, R. E. 1970. Surface properties influencing biological adhesion. *In* Adhesion in Biological Systems. R. S. Manly, Ed. : 15–48. Academic Press. New York, N.Y.
18. Baier, R. E. & V. A. De Palma. 1971. The relation of the internal surface of grafts to thrombosis. *In* Management of Arterial Occlusive Disease. W. A. Dale, Ed. : 147–163. Year Book Medical Publishers, Inc. Chicago, Ill.
19. Baier, R. E., Ed. 1975. Applied Chemistry at Protein Interfaces. Advances in Chemistry Series 145. American Chemical Society. Washington, D.C.
20. Baier, R. E. & R. C. Dutton. 1969. Initial events in interactions of blood with a foreign surface. J. Biomed. Mater. Res. **3:** 191–206.
21. Dutton, R. C., A. J. Webber, S. A. Johnson & R. E. Baier. 1969. Microstructure of initial thrombus formation on foreign materials. J. Biomed. Mater. Res. **3:** 13–23.
22. Baier, R. E., G. I. Loeb & G. T. Wallace. 1971. Role of an artificial boundary in modifying blood proteins. Fed. Proc. **30:** 1523–1538.
23. Dutton, R. C., R. E. Baier, R. L. Dedrick & R. L. Bowman. 1968. Initial thrombus formation on foreign surfaces. Trans. Amer. Soc. Artif. Int. Organs. **14:** 57–68.
24. Dutton, R. C. & L. H. Edmunds, Jr. 1974. Formation of platelet aggregate emboli in a prototype hollow fiber membrane oxygenator. J. Biomed. Mater. Res. **8:** 163–183.
25. Dutton, R. C., L. H. Edmunds, Jr., J. C. Hutchinson & B. B. Roe. 1974. Platelet aggregate emboli produced in patients during cardiopulmonary bypass

with membrane and bubble oxygenators and blood filters. J. Thorac. Cardiovasc. Surg. **67:** 258–265.

26. Baier, R. E., V. L. Gott & A. Furuse. 1970. Surface chemical evaluation of thromboresistant materials before and after venous implantation. Trans. Amer. Soc. Artif. Int. Organs. **16:** 50–57.
27. Baier, R. E., R. C. Dutton & V. L. Gott. 1970. Surface chemical features of blood vessel walls and of synthetic materials exhibiting thromboresistance. Adv. Ex. Med. Biol. **7:** 235–260.
28. Boretos, J. W., W. S. Pierce, R. E. Baier, A. F. Leroy & H. J. Donachy. 1975. Surface and bulk characteristics of a polyether urethane for artificial hearts. J. Biomed. Mater. Res. **9:** 327–340.
29. Baier, R. E., V. A. De Palma, W. S. Pierce & J. W. Boretos. 1976. Surface chemical evaluation of a segmented polyether-type polyurethane after long-term contact with blood. J. Bioeng. In press.
30. Madras, P. N., W. A. Morton & H. E. Petschek. 1971. Dynamics of thrombus formation. Fed. Proc. **30:** 1665–1676.
31. Mason, R. G., D. E. Scarborough, S. R. Saba, L. D. Ikenberry, J. J. Kearney & H. G. Clark. 1969. Thrombogenecity of some biomedical materials: Platelet-interface reactions. J. Biomed. Mater. Res. **3:** 615–644.
32. Leonard, F., J. A. Collins & H. J. Porter. 1966. Interfacial polymerization of n-alkyl alpha-cyanoacrylate homologs. J. Appl. Poly. Sci. **10:** 1617–1623.
33. Leonard, F., J. W. Hodge, Jr., S. Houston & D. K. Ousterhout. 1968. Alpha-cyanoacrylate adhesive bond strengths with proteinaceous and nonproteinaceous substrates. J. Biomed. Mater. Res. **2:** 173–178.
34. Wallace, H., W. Asher & R. E. Baier. Unpublished observations.

Part II. Adsorption and Reaction of Blood Protein at Interfaces

BLOOD ELEMENTS AT FOREIGN SURFACES: A BIOCHEMICAL APPROACH TO THE STUDY OF THE ADSORPTION OF PLASMA PROTEINS *

Shaul Kochwa, Robert S. Litwak,
and Richard E. Rosenfield

Mount Sinai School of Medicine
The City University of New York
New York, New York 10029

Edward F. Leonard

Artificial Organs Research Laboratory
Columbia University School of Engineering
New York, New York 10027

When a foreign surface, solid, liquid, or gas, is brought into contact with a protein solution, a certain amount of the dissolved protein will be adsorbed to the surface. This process is consistent with the Gibbs theory of surface energy and may be described by the adsorption isotherms of Freudlich or Langmuir.[1] The amount of protein adsorbed and the characteristics of the protein monolayer depend mainly on the nature of the foreign surface and the structure and concentration of the proteins in solution. It is impossible in the frame of this presentation to cover the vast amount of data on protein adsorption that has accumulated over the past two decades, but reference will be made to two of several excellent reviews that have been published on this subject.[2, 3] Despite development of sophisticated experimental methods, it is not yet possible to infer, from the behavior of a surface (metal, glass, or polymer) in one system, its response in another. This unpredictability is unfortunate in the context of this conference, because an extrapolation from the behavior of surfaces *in vitro* to their thrombogenic behavior *in vivo* would allow prediction of the clinical usefulness of candidate biomaterials.

Before a protein molecule can be adsorbed to a surface it must become located at a distance from the surface that will allow interaction between the molecular forces associated with the surface and the protein molecule. This approach is governed by diffusion, but the characteristics of the adsorbing surface also determine the nature of the bond and what changes may take place in the configuration of the bound protein molecule.

Protein molecules in aqueous solution are compact structures, globular or fibrillar, depending on characteristics of their polypeptides. The effect of dissolution on the hydrophobic and hydrophilic amino acid residues of a polypeptide chain is reduction of the number of hydrophobic amino acids on its surface and exposure of hydrophilic amino acids. Hydrogen bonds, hydrophobic interactions, ionic and polar forces facilitate such conformational changes, so that the final result is a hydrated, compact protein molecule with an increased number of surface hydrophilic groups, many hydrophobic groups

* Supported by Contract NO1–HB–3–2910 from the National Heart, Lung, and Blood Institutes, NIH.

having been internalized. When a molecule, so adapted to an aqueous environment approaches a foreign surface it must undergo some conformational changes to allow its adsorption.[4] During this process the adsorbed and ordered water molecules that surround both the foreign surface and the protein molecules are displaced to allow direct contact between the surface and the protein molecules, and appropriate side-chain groups are selected from the protein molecule, especially inner hydrophobic amino acid residues that become part of the adsorptive bond.

Measurement of protein conformational changes such as these is complicated. In the past, we have utilized potentiometric titration as a measurement of increasing numbers of titrable groups occurring during adsorption of γ-globulin by polystyrene Lytron particles.[5] We found that the number of titrable groups increases as the density of protein molecules on the particle surface decreases, indicating a direct relationship between unfolding of molecules and the results of potentiometric titration. We were also able to show that the nature and composition of the foreign surface influences the number of groups titrated. On a hydrophobic surface, Lytron 617, the unfolding, as measured by the number of titrable groups, is much higher than when carboxyl groups are present, such as on Lytron 615 and 612.

Proof that a protein molecule tends to maximize the area it shares with a Lytron particle was obtained when a pentamer of γG [6] was studied. This pentamer was a molecule of γG myeloma protein of about 880,000 molecular weight, but it dissociated at pH 3.0 into 7S IgG monomers. When Lytron particles carrying adsorbed pentamer on their surface were similarly exposed to pH 3.0, all monomers that were not in direct contact with, and bound tightly to, the Lytron surface were removed (FIGURE 1). At low surface densities of pentamer, practically no protein molecules were dissociated at pH 3.0, but as the density of bound pentamer was increased, either one or two monomers were released, indicating that only part of the pentamer was in contact with Lytron surface, and that a concentration-dependent change in the orientation of the bound pentamer had occurred. The final surface density of the bound protein molecule was similar to that of the monolayer formed by γG.[5]

Brash and Lyman [7] suggested that such titration data might be interpreted as complexing of ionic groups instead of unfolding. But critical evidence for unfolding dependent on surface concentration was provided by immunochemical studies of the Lytron-adsorbed protein.[5] Immune responses of rabbits injected intravenously with Lytron particles carrying different surface saturations of IgG revealed that antibodies incited in rabbits by Lytron covered with IgG at low density resulted in the same type of antibodies as were incited both by Lytron covered with heat-aggregated IgG at high density and IgG in complete Freund adjuvant. Heat-aggregation and emulsification in Freund adjuvant are known to cause conformational changes in protein molecules.[8]

Conformational changes in protein molecules that occur during adsorption do not necessarily destroy the biological properties of the adsorbed protein. We have found [9] that Lytron-bound actomyosin retains its Ca^{++} and Mg^{++} ATPase activity and that components of actomyosin, actin and myosin, may be sequentially bound to Lytron, indicating preservation not only of the enzymatically active site, but also of the attachment site of myosin for actin.

All of these data were obtained by measurement of the decrease of protein concentration in the surrounding solution. Thus, the experiments required a very high area of foreign surface per unit volume, such as is available when particles of 0.2 μM diameter are used. When materials are available only in film form, a different approach is necessary. The proteins to be studied either can be labeled before adsorption with isotopes like ^{125}I, or can be detected and measured after adsorption by use of labeled antibodies specific for the adsorbed proteins. We shall present data using both approaches. Stanford Research Institute polyurethane was chosen as a representative material, and both static and kinetic uptake of proteins from solution was studied.

Three proteins, albumin, γ-globulin, and fibrinogen were applied both sequentially and simultaneously from a mixture to determine preferential binding

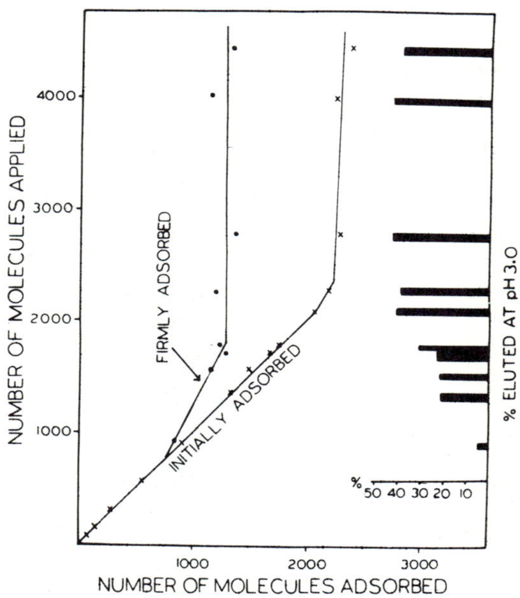

FIGURE 1. Lytron 615 particles were coated with varying concentrations of IgG pentamer,[6] as described in Ref. 5. The initial adsorption is plotted on the abscissa as a function of the number of molecules applied (ordinate). After adsorption, Lytron particles were washed, exposed to glycine buffer pH 3.0, the quantity of protein removed detremined spectrophotometrically, and firmly adsorbed protein calculated as the difference and also plotted on the abscissa. On the right, % removed protein is presented as bars.

(TABLE 1). The results are expressed as the percentage of decrease in the amount of radioactively labeled protein that was taken up, either sequentially by a disc previously exposed to unlabeled protein, or simultaneously from a mixture of two unlabeled and one labeled protein.

When SRI polyurethane was first exposed to unlabeled protein and then to labeled protein, the prior exposure was always found to decrease the uptake of the labeled protein over that observed for the labeled protein on a virgin surface. The greatest blocking effect was obtained with fibrinogen where over 80% of the polymer surface became inaccessible to the labeled fibrinogen. Similarly,

IgG blocked the sequential application of labeled IgG by over 50%. Smaller degrees of blocking were observed when nonidentical proteins were applied.

In application of protein mixtures to discs of polyurethane, where only one of the components was radioactive, whenever fibrinogen was used in unlabeled form the uptake of albumin and IgG was decreased by 50%. However, albumin and IgG blocked only 20% of the uptake of fibrinogen. It seems clear from this set of data, although the study was limited to one polymer, that there is a blocking effect of one protein on the uptake of another, and when the proteins are taken up from a mixture, uptake of fibrinogen is preferential to uptake of IgG and albumin.

TABLE 1

INHIBITION OF THE UPTAKE OF ^{125}I-LABELED PROTEIN BY OTHER PROTEINS *

	Unlabeled	Labeled	% Decrease in Uptake
Sequential Adsorption	albumin	albumin	20
		γG	46
		fibrinogen	38
	γG	γG	51
		albumin	27
		fibrinogen	38
	fibrinogen	fibrinogen	81.5
		albumin	30
		γG	36
Simultaneous Adsorption	fibrinogen + γG	albumin	49
	γG + albumin	fibrinogen	19
	albumin + fibrinogen	γG	48

* Discs, one centimeter diameter, were cut from polyurethane sheets (segmented polyether urethanes, Stanford Research Institute, Palo Alto, Calif., $3-\left(\frac{1000}{425}\right)-\frac{70}{30}-1-x$) and exposed for 1 hr either sequentially to unlabeled followed by ^{125}I-labeled serum protein, or simultaneously to a mixture of three proteins, one of which was ^{125}I-labeled. Protein concentration = 1 mg/ml. Inhibition is expressed as percent decrease in the uptake of labeled protein when compared with direct uptake of a single ^{125}I-labeled protein.

Similar results were obtained in time-varying studies using a spinning disc apparatus [10] developed to mimic the effect of blood flow. Adler [11] used this apparatus for a detailed study of the interaction between fibrinogen and polyurethane. A typical curve of kinetic uptake of fibrinogen by polyurethane discs is depicted in FIGURE 2 (upper broken line). This uptake is partially blocked by previous exposure of the disc to unlabeled albumin (lower solid line). Although the kinetics are not changed, the final concentration of fibrinogen taken up is lower and compares favorably with the results of static experiments (TABLE 1).

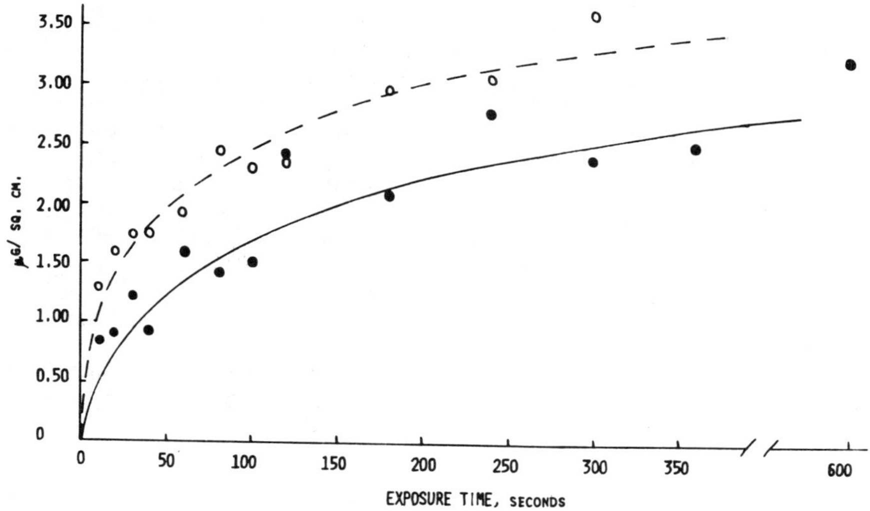

FIGURE 2. Time-varying studies of blocking of the uptake of human fibrinogen by human serum albumin. Polyurethane discs (size and type as in TABLE 1) were exposed in spinning-disc apparatus at 400 rpm to 1.1 mg/ml ^{125}I-fibrinogen for varying periods of time. Discs were washed and counted (upper curve - - -). The lower curve (——) depicts the effect of preexposure of discs for 30 sec at 400 rpm and 90 sec stationary to 1.1 mg/ml albumin followed by ^{125}I-labeled fibrinogen.

As a closer approach to what happens when a biomaterial is exposed to blood, the kinetic uptake of fibrinogen from plasma trace-labeled with ^{125}I-tagged fibrinogen was determined. As FIGURE 3 shows, after an initial short rise in bound fibrinogen, a decline with very low residual radioactivity was observed. To ascertain that this unexpected result was not due to elution or exchange of plasma fibrinogen, discs of polyurethane were exposed for five minutes to a

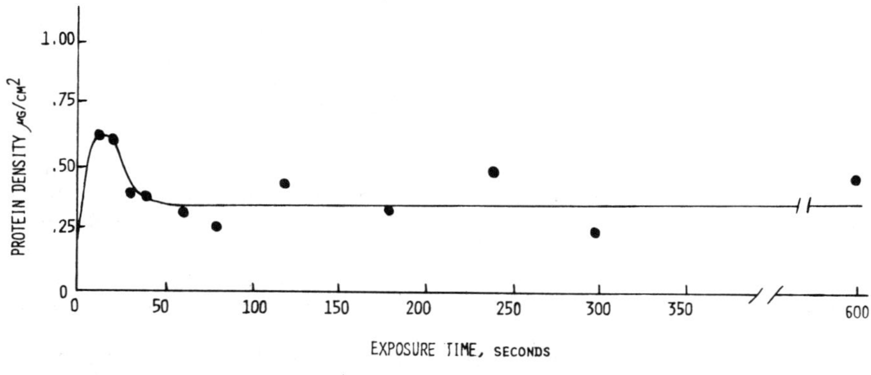

FIGURE 3. Uptake of ^{125}I-fibrinogen from human plasma. Human plasma was trace-labeled with ^{125}I-fibrinogen and used for adsorption to polyurethane discs in spinning apparatus.

solution of ^{125}I-labeled fibrinogen. After establishing a uniform plateau of radioactivity, discs were exposed (FIGURE 4) for various periods of time to fibrinogen solution or saline, but no change in the radioactivity on the different discs was found. However, when polyurethane discs precoated with ^{125}I-labeled fibrinogen were kinetically tested in human plasma, in a period of a few minutes the amount of radioactivity decreased to about 50%. These results suggest enzymatic action; it is likely that plasma enzymes attack fibrinogen molecules that have undergone an appropriate conformational change after their adsorption by polyurethane. Since the same plasma did not affect ^{125}I-labeled fibrinogen added in solution, digestion occurred only after adsorption. In an observation that may be related, Vroman,[12] using elipsometric methods, reported a decrease in the thickness of a surface-bound fibrinogen layer after exposure to plasma.

When artificial surfaces are exposed to a mixture of proteins, such as human plasma, it is not feasible to determine the nature of adsorbed proteins by addi-

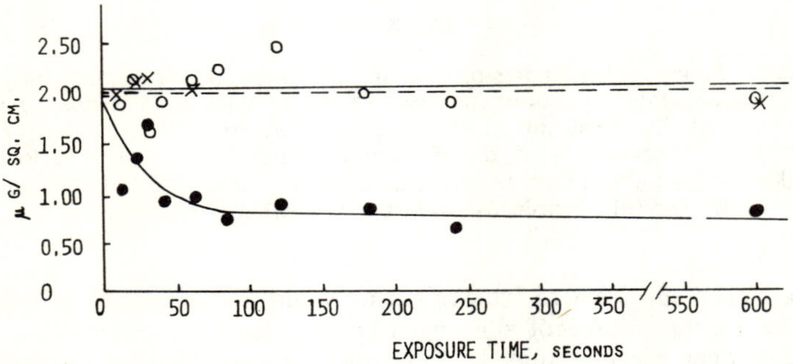

FIGURE 4. Effect of plasma on fibrinogen adsorbed to poylurethane. Polyurethane discs were coated with ^{125}I-labeled fibrinogen and subsequently exposed in spinning disc apparatus to human plasma (●), saline (○), and 1.1 mg/ml unlabeled fibrinogen (×).

tion of a single radioactive protein to the mixture. Antibodies to single proteins were used for such studies. The antisera were chromatographed on DEAE cellulose[13] to isolate their 7S IgG, and this material was appropriately labeled with ^{125}I. Cold normal IgG of the same species was added to reduce background radioactivity.

Discs of polyurethane (705A) and hydrogel (707A) were exposed to human ACD and heparin plasma, and to fibrinogen solution. After being washed, these discs were incubated with a solution of ^{125}I-labeled antibodies. The results (TABLE 2) show clearly that less radioactivity was picked up by hydrogel disc, which is known to adsorb less protein from solution.[14] This was true for fibrinogen, IgG, and albumin. Additionally, uptake of fibrinogen from plasma was lower than uptake from a pure fibrinogen solution. This corresponds to the results of kinetic studies of the uptake of ^{125}I-labeled fibrinogen from plasma and the effect of plasma on fibrinogen adsorbed on discs. We were also able to show that the uptake of antifibrinogen antibodies by discs exposed to heparin plasma was higher than on those exposed to ACD plasma. It is

TABLE 2

UPTAKE OF ^{125}I-LABELED ANTIBODIES BY DISCS OF SEGMENTED POLYETHER URETHANES *

	Antifibrinogen		Anti-γG		Antialbumin	
	705A	707A	705A	707A	705A	707A
Heparin plasma	4897	2581	2945	775	1233	302
ACD plasma	2862	2159	2159	821	861	977
Fibrinogen	13302	5406	1764	349	198	311

* Stanford Research Institute, Palo Alto, Calif. $3-\frac{1000}{425}-\left(\frac{70}{30}\right)-1-\times$(705A) and Polyscience Inc. hydrogel. 40% (w/v) acrylamide on polyurethane 705 (707A) exposed for 1 hr to heparin plasma, ACD plasma, and fibrinogen 1.1 mg/ml.

known that heparin inhibits several enzymes present in plasma (e.g. thrombin and complement components),[15, 16] and a possibility exists that one of these enzymes is responsible for some of the plasma effects reported.

An attempt was made to quantify the amount of protein adsorbed to the surfaces of polyurethane discs (TABLE 3). Artificial mixtures were made of fibrinogen and IgG. Discs were exposed, washed, and then incubated with either antifibrinogen or anti-IgG. The uncorrected counts shown indicate, first, that a considerable background exists. This nonspecific uptake probably repre-

TABLE 3

UPTAKE OF ^{125}I-LABELED ANTIBODIES BY DISCS OF SEGMENTED POLYETHER URETHANES *

Mixture %		Φ/γG Antifibrinogen		Φ/γG Anti-γG		Φ/albumin Antifibrinogen		Φ/albumin Antialbumin	
		705A	707A	705A	707A	705A	707A	705A	707A
100	—	26,596	17,992	1,026	1,083	29,377	12,818	5,253	4,493
95	5	30,927	14,864	5,463	1,797	22,589	8,626	6,869	4,990
90	10	30,024	18,092	6,811	1,839	32,737	9,935	6,962	2,312
80	20	43,608	9,888	7,051	1,568	31,315	8,609	7,557	3,879
70	30	26,394	14,588	10,290	2,568	26,651	10,486	6,012	6,092
50	50	14,132	25,782	9,760	2,902	21,081	9,245	8,569	2,319
30	70	17,928	29,400	10,635	2,546	26,247	7,253	14,519	2,741
20	80	19,816	24,954	16,255	4,073	29,427	6,451	10,000	3,065
10	90	15,695	7,062	18,689	4,096	14,341	7,722	11,699	2,835
5	95	17,190	11,864	16,841	8,304	18,108	7,945	18,189	5,216
—	100	6,241	6,502	22,961	13,654	9,738	5,427	19,951	2,820

* SRI $3-\frac{425}{1000}-\left(\frac{70}{30}\right)-1-\times$(705A) and Polysciences Inc. hydrogel 40% (w/v) acrylamide on 705 (707A) exposed to mixtures of fibrinogen and γG and fibrinogen and albumin. Protein concentration = 1.1 mg/ml. Counts are not corrected for nonspecific adsorption of antibodies. Φ = fibrinogen.

sents nonantibody IgG, consequent to the fact that the labeled IgG fractions contain less than 1% of specific antibodies. Secondly, there is a poor correlation between the number of adsorbed antibody counts and the amount of applied fibrinogen or IgG. When fibrinogen or IgG was applied at high concentrations, more counts were picked up than at lower concentrations, but it was not possible to establish a clear relationship between the counts obtained and the ratio of fibrinogen to IgG. Of special interest is the fact that the maximum uptake of antifibrinogen did not occur when only fibrinogen was applied, but when 90 or 80% mixtures were present. A possible explanation of this phenomenon is that the adsorption of fibrinogen from pure solution is accompanied by binding of antifibrinogen antibodies to two adjacent bound molecules in a bridging pattern so as to utilize both antibody-combining sites, whereas when γ-globulin is present the fibrinogen molecules may be interspersed in some areas with IgG molecules so that each molecule of fibrinogen binds separate molecules of antifibrinogen. This type of adsorption would result in the higher counts seen with 90/80 and 80/20 mixtures.

TABLE 4

UPTAKE OF ^{125}I-LABELED γG FROM MIXTURES WITH 7S γG AND HEAT-AGGREGATED γG *

	^{125}I-Labeled 7S γG (cpm)			
	1	2	3	4
7S γG, control	18909	15251	20019	22229
Aggregated γG	12285	11473	14253	15782
% decrease	35	25	29	29

* Protein concentration = 1.1 mg/ml. Adsorbing surface segmented polyether urethanes SRI $3-\frac{1000}{425}-\left(\frac{70}{30}\right)-1-\times$. Time = 1 hr.

Such an observation is not limited to fibrinogen-IgG mixtures, but is found with fibrinogen-albumin mixtures as well. Until now, we have not been able to prepare antibodies pure enough to provide a background low enough to allow us to convert this qualitative method into a quantitative one.

In all these experiments we encountered a certain variability in the amount of radioactivity that was detected on the surface of exposed polyurethane, irrespective of specific activities, amounts applied, and the source and time of preparation of the proteins used. As shown in FIGURE 5, the standard deviation of results from ten typical tests, amounts to about 15%. To explain such variability, two hypotheses were tested: that the protein undergoes aggregation during the iodination procedure, and that large aggregates are randomly deposited on test discs, or that the surface of the polyurethane is uneven in its ability to adsorb proteins so that a random blotchy adsorption pattern results. To investigate the possibility that the labeling procedure induces aggregation, we have investigated the effect of heat-aggregated, nonradioactive γ-globulin on the uptake of radioactively labeled 7S IgG. It is well known that more IgG adsorbs to a surface when aggregated than when in the native state. Four separate tests, the results of which are summarized in TABLE 4, all have shown

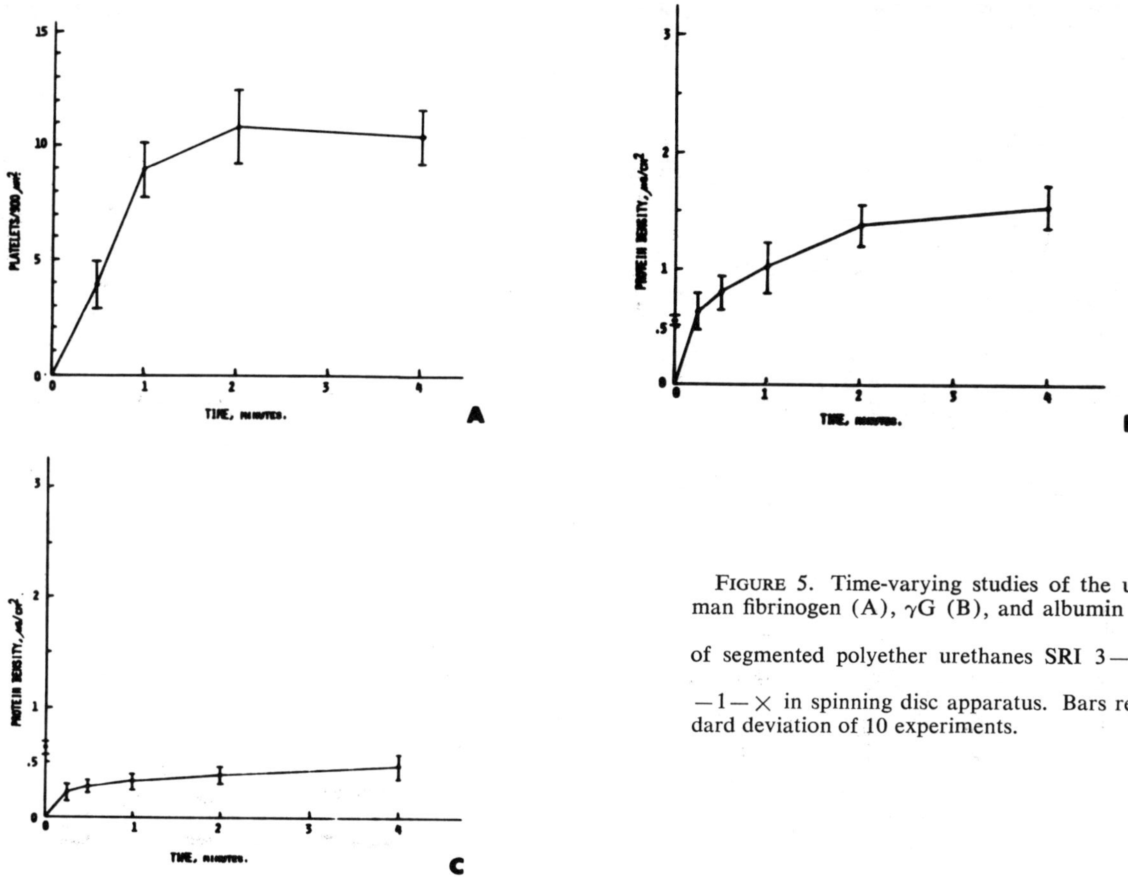

FIGURE 5. Time-varying studies of the uptake of human fibrinogen (A), γG (B), and albumin (C) by discs of segmented polyether urethanes SRI $3-\frac{1000}{425}-\left(\frac{70}{30}\right)-1-\times$ in spinning disc apparatus. Bars represent standard deviation of 10 experiments.

that radioactivity on the surface is decreased by about 30% when the surface is exposed to heat-aggregated IgG. If the labeled IgG were agggregated, no such decrease would be expected.

Such aggregates should show, on autoradiography, distinct black spots of intense radioactivity. To test this possibility, five discs were exposed to the same batch of radioactive fibrinogen. Upon counting, these discs showed an expected variation of 15% and the autoradiography revealed two types of artifacts. One was an occasional excessive accumulation of radioactivity on the edges of the disc caused probably by imperfections in the cutting process, whereas the second was lightly shaded areas of large size relative to molecular and cellular scales that appeared to be relatively free from radioactive protein (FIGURE 6). Although the discs came from the same sheet of polyurethane, different patterns of irregularities can be seen on them. If it is true that protein adsorption precedes all other events that lead to thrombus formation, these results suggest that the approach to synthesizing artificial foreign surfaces should be reassessed with an effort to identify and synthesize homogeneous materials that will have the properties of those parts of polyurethane films that remain bare.

Until now, this paper has been concerned solely with the interaction of proteins and solid surfaces, the latter as the sole significant recipient of proteins from solutions. In certain clinical conditions, however, especially during open-heart surgery, interfaces of gas and protein-containing solution exist. Liquid-gas interfaces are characterized by the constant changing of one of the constituents, air, because bubbles of gas are constantly formed and constantly disappear. Therefore, we must look for changes in proteins in the bulk of the solution itself.

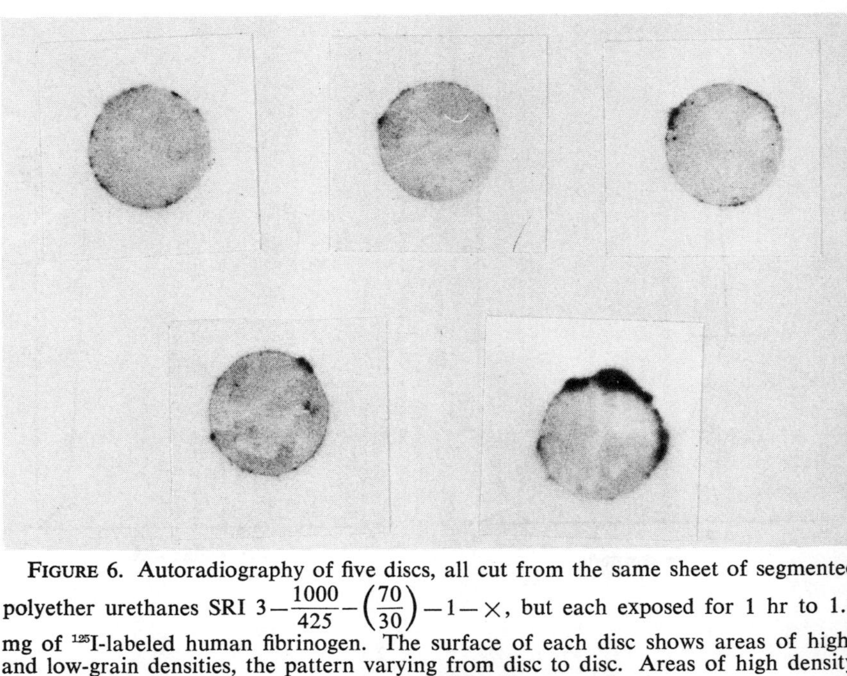

FIGURE 6. Autoradiography of five discs, all cut from the same sheet of segmented polyether urethanes SRI $3-\frac{1000}{425}-\left(\frac{70}{30}\right)-1-\times$, but each exposed for 1 hr to 1.1 mg of ^{125}I-labeled human fibrinogen. The surface of each disc shows areas of high- and low-grain densities, the pattern varying from disc to disc. Areas of high density on the edges of each disc represent irregularities disc to cutting.

TABLE 5

EFFECT OF THE BLOOD-GAS INTERFACE ON AGGREGATION OF PLASMA ALBUMIN *

		1 Unit		10 Units	
Direct	15′	−4.6±2.44	1.89	−3.0±1.08	2.78
	1 hr	−3.0±5.20	1.29	−15.5±8.39	3.70
	2 hr	−3.0±5.92	1.13	−12.8±2.56	4.98
	4 hr	−2.6±4.34	1.34	−9.8±5.12	2.56
	6 hr	−1.2±1.64	1.63	−11.3±6.21	1.81
Indirect	15′	1.0±1.00	1.0	−1.7±0.88	1.89
	1 hr	0		−2.7±1.76	1.51
	2 hr	0		−3.7±1.86	1.98
	4 hr	0		−2.0±2.00	1.00
	6 hr	1.3±1.25	1.0	−4.3±1.10	3.61

* For details, see text.

To explore this problem we have tested two devices used in extracorporeal circulations: the Bentley oxygenator and the Modulung. The first device is based on direct gas-liquid interfaces that are constantly forming and disappearing; the second provides an exchange of oxygen through a fixed membrane so that the gas-liquid interfaces are stable and indirect. Whole heparinized blood was pumped through these devices at 37° C for a period of up to six hours, with gas pressures and flow rates identical to those in clinical use. Samples were taken at starting time, ¼, 1, 2, 4, and 6 hours later. To mimic conditions of extracorporeal circulation, where sometimes up to ten units of blood are used for perfusion, an artificial mixture of blood from ten donors of the same ABO type was constructed and treated in the same way as the blood of one donor. The volume used in both instances was 600 ml. Following exposure to these extracorporeal devices, the blood plasma was separated and studied by acrylamide gel electrophoresis and gradient ultracentrifugation. Both procedures showed that aggregation of some plasma proteins had occurred. A full report of studies of eight plasma proteins is in preparation, and a detailed statistical analysis of immunodiffusion data showing the effects of both direct and indirect gas-liquid interfaces on plasma albumin is given in TABLE 5. The numbers indicate the mean and standard deviation of samples obtained at different times, with t values for comparisons of later results with those obtained at zero time.

The data presented show clearly that the changes occurring in plasma albumin during exposure to direct gas interfaces are more extensive than those occurring with indirect interfaces. In fact, such changes are minimal when oxygenation occurs indirectly. There are also significant differences between the changes seen in the plasma of a single unit of blood and the plasma from a mixture of ten bloods, the latter being much more susceptible to changes by direct oxygenation.

It is clear that the interaction of foreign surfaces with mixed proteins in solution is a very complex phenomenon, especially when one is concerned not only with the extent of adsorption, but with subsequent consequences of that adsorption.

To understand the interactions of plasma proteins with biomaterial surfaces in regard to initiation of thrombogenesis, one must understand first how the chemical homogenity of the surface will affect the individual proteins adsorbed from pure solutions. This problem contains unanswered questions about conformation and reversibility. Second, one should understand competitive adsorption of independent proteins. Here, too, questions of reversibility and conformation exist. Third, one must consider both the enzymatic activity of adsorbed proteins, and the acquired susceptibility of adsorbed proteins to enzyme action. Finally, the macroscopic nonhomogeneity of the protein adsorption by many artificial surfaces must be considered and will necessarily complicate analysis of all of the three steps just enumerated. In this report, we have shown that all of these phenomena occur, but much more needs to be done before an orderly understanding of the biochemistry of surface-initiated thrombogenesis will be clarified.

Summary

Protein molecules at a solid-liquid interface exist on the solid surface in amounts and a molecular configurations different from those of protein molecules in the bulk solution, and cannot be considered to be in equilibrium with the dissolved proteins. Competition between proteins in a mixture, or variation of the sequence in which different protein solutions are introduced to a solid surface, affect the end result. The kinetics of adsorption from unstirred systems differ from those with controlled stirring (i.e., a spinning disc developed to mimic blood flow), both in rate of uptake and composition of the steady-state adsorbed layer. Surface concentration of adsorbed proteins does not reflect their relative concentration in the supernatant solution. Concentration of adsorbed proteins can be assessed by either radiotracers or specific antibodies; nonuniformity of the protein layer can be analyzed by autoradiography; and configuration of bound protein molecules can be determined by potentiometric titration, retention of enzymatic activity, and variations in antigenicity. Gas-liquid interfaces affect the integrity of protein molecules and result in aggregation or fragmentation that can be detected in the liquid phase.

Acknowledgment

The authors gratefully acknowledge the excellent technical assistance of Estelle Makuku in performing the protein adsorption and autoradiographic procedures.

References

1. Kipling, J. J. 1965. Adsorption from solutions of non-electrolytes. Academic Press. New York, N.Y.
2. The Chemistry of Biosurfaces. 1971. Michael L. Hair, Ed. Vol. 1, 2. Marcel Decker. New York, N.Y.
3. Medical Applications of Plastics. 1971. H. P. Gregor, Ed. Symp. 1. J. Biomed. Mater. Res.
4. Hoffman, A. S. 1974. Principles governing biomolecule interactions at foreign interfaces. J. Biomed. Mater. Res., Symp. **5**(Part 1): 77.

5. KOCHWA, S., M. BROWNELL, R. E. ROSENFIELD & L. R. WASSERMAN. 1967. Adsorption of proteins by polystyrene particles. I. Molecular unfolding and acquired immunogenicity of IgG. J. Immunol. **99:** 981.
6. KOCHWA, S., E. SMITH, M. BROWNELL & L. R. WASSERMAN. 1966. Aggregation of IgG globulin in vivo. II. Physicochemical properties of the isolated protein. Biochemistry **5:** 2777.
7. BRASH, J. L. & D. J. LYMAN. 1971. Adsorption of proteins and lipids to non biological surfaces. *In* The Chemistry of Biosurfaces. Michael L. Hair, Ed. : 177–229. Marcel Decker. New York, N.Y.
8. SCIBIENSKI, R. J. 1973. Denaturation of lysozyme by Freund's complete adjuvant. J. Immunol. **111:** 117.
9. PUSZKIN, S., S. KOCHWA, E. G. PUSZKIN & R. E. ROSENFIELD. 1975. A solid liquid biphasic model for characterization of properties of muscle and platelet contractile proteins. J. Biol. Chem. **250:** 2085.
10. TURITTO, V. & E. F. LEONARD. 1972. Platelet adhesion to a spinning surface. Trans. Am. Soc. Artif. Intern. Organs **18:** 34.
11. ADLER, M. A. 1969. Protein adsorption to artificial biomaterial surfaces: An investigation involving the spinning disc apparatus. M.S. thesis. 1975. Columbia Univ. New York, N.Y.
12. VROMAN, L. & A. L. ADAMS. 1969. Identification of rapid changes at plasma solid interfaces. J. Biomed. Mater. Res. **3:** 43.
13. KOCHWA, S., R. E. ROSENFIELD, L. TALLAL & L. R. WASSERMAN. 1961. Isoagglutinin associated with ABO erythroblastosis. J. Clin. Invest. **40:** 874.
14. KOCHWA, S., R. S. LITWAK, R. E. ROSENFIELD & E. F. LEONARD. This volume.
15. BRADSHAW, R. A. & S. WESSLER. 1975. Heparin, structure, function and chemical implications. Plenum Press. New York, N.Y.
16. COLTEN, R. & R. STRUNK. 1976. Inhibition of the enzymatic activity of the first component of complement by heparin. Clin. Immunol. **6:** 248.

THE ADSORPTION AND CONFORMATION OF PLASMA PROTEINS: A PHYSICAL APPROACH *

Bruce W. Morrissey

Institute for Materials Research
National Bureau of Standards
Washington, D. C. 20234

The rapid adsorption of plasma proteins is the initial event in a complex series of reactions that occurs upon introduction of a synthetic material into the cardiovascular system. This protein surface layer has been shown to modify the interaction of various blood components at interfaces. The activity of soluble enzymatic factors involved in coagulation can be established, as in the case of factor XII,[1] or greatly enhanced as occurs following prothrombin adsorption to lipid vesicles.[2] Thrombosis may be induced through the rapid adsorption and desorption of denatured thrombin,[3] by alteration of the adhesion of platelets [4–6] and red blood cells,[7] or the hemolysis of red blood cells.[8] Although the relative importance of coagulation and thrombosis remains at issue, protein adsorption has a central role in each case. The parallel mechanisms are illustrated schematically in FIGURE 1.

In view of the ever-increasing use of artificial materials in the body, better techniques and information are required to characterize the major events occurring at the blood-implant interface. If the properties of proteins adsorbed at the solid/solution interface were known, the compatibility of synthetic materials *in vivo* might be predictable and subject to greater control. The ability to minimize thrombosis by an informed selection or design of materials might prevent such clinical problems as the formation of deposits impairing the mechanical function of heart valves, the shedding of emboli, or, in the case of large surface area dialyzers and oxygenators, the removal of blood factors from the circulation.

This article summarizes recent quantitative studies concerning the surface chemical properties of plasma proteins. The review is not exhaustive, but it is hoped that most of the current concepts and approaches are indicated. Although the adsorption of plasma proteins and its role in surface-induced thrombosis are emphasized, many of the techniques described would be equally applicable to investigations of matrix insolubilized enzymes, clinical analysis by antibody flocculation, and cellular adhesion and aggregation.

PROTEIN ADSORPTION MEASUREMENTS

The characterization of adsorbed serum albumin has been a long-term continuing interest of Bull and his coworkers. An early study [10] of adsorption on crushed Pyrex® glass using solution-depletion techniques established that the isotherm was apparently of the Langmuir type, with a plateau adsorbance of

* This work was supported in part by the Biomaterials Program of the National Heart and Lung Institute.

4 $mg \cdot m^{-2}$ occurring at an equilibrium concentration of 2 $mg \cdot ml^{-1}$. The adsorbance for a given serum albumin concentration varied with pH and showed a broad maximum at pH 4–5, near the isoelectric point of the protein. Despite the fact that extensive rinsing experiments indicated that serum albumin adsorption was only partially reversible, Bull derived equations for the Gibbs energy changes in order to calculate the force area curve for the protein "spread" at the solid/solution interface. Although Bull clearly stated the limitations of this procedure, its subsequent application by many investigators is indicative of the desire to abstract structural information from strictly adsorbance measurements. Whether one assumes that the plateau adsorbance corresponds to a close-packed monolayer, thereby calculating the area per adsorbed molecule, or whether one uses the above procedure to calculate limiting areas, it is the conformation of the adsorbed protein that is desired. By assuming a density of 1.37 for adsorbed serum albumin films, Bull calculated thicknesses of 11–35 Å.

An early study of protein adsorption on a hydrophobic substrate was carried

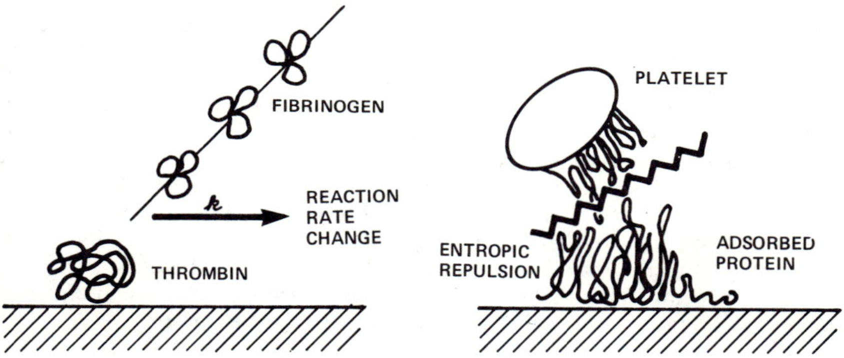

FIGURE 1. Protein adsorption can result in activation or loss of enzymatic activity and in passivation of a surface toward platelet adhesion. Analogies with colloidal stabilization by polymer adsorption [9] suggest the importance of entropy changes arising from protein segment interpenetration.

out by Oreskes and Singer [11] for the human γ-globulin-polystyrene latex system. The adsorbance was determined as a function of latex particle size and pH, and was analyzed with use of a modified Langmuir equation. The results indicated that adsorption apparently occurred in two steps characterized by different binding constants. The authors speculated that either multilayer adsorption of γ-globulin occurred, or that adsorption of protein just prior to full surface coverage produced a change in the orientation of the adsorbing molecule to occupy the remaining available space. Inexplicably, the use of different-sized particles altered the binding characteristics of the protein. Maximum adsorption of γ-globulin occurred at the pH closest to the isoelectric point where the protein net charge, and hence the electrostatic repulsion between adsorbed γ-globulin molecules was the least. The effect of a constant negative surface charge on the latex particles played a negligible role and emphasized the importance of protein-protein interactions on the surface.

The solution-depletion techniques described above are limited by the necessity of working with finely divided substrates. The uncertainty of determining the available area/gram of material for the adsorption of large protein molecules can make it difficult to normalize the adsorbance to unit area, although the geometry of the substrate can affect protein adsorption characteristics, as noted above by Oreskes and Singer.[11] Since the characterization of materials for use in synthetic implants is an important goal of protein-adsorption studies, techniques for dealing with low surface area planar substrates are required.

An important study of the adsorption of fibrinogen, γ-globulin, and serum albumin on a variety of hydrophobic polymers was carried out by Brash and Lyman.[12] By applying the technique of internal reflection spectroscopy, the surface concentration of the adsorbed protein was related to the intensity of the amide I band. The intensity of an infrared band of the substrate polymer was used to normalize the protein spectrum and remove artifacts due to variable contact area between the germanium internal reflection element and the protein film.

The adsorption isotherms for each protein at pH 7.4 were quite similar for adsorption on polystyrene, polyethylene, silicone rubber, and fluorinated ethylene-propylene copolymer (FEP). Plateau surface concentrations were approximately 0.8, 1.2, and 1.5 $mg \cdot m^{-2}$ for serum albumin, γ-globulin, and fibrinogen, respectively, with saturation achieved at solution concentrations of only 0.1–0.15 $mg \cdot ml^{-1}$, indicating high affinity of the proteins for polymer surfaces. Despite the dubious validity of the correspondence between the plateau adsorbance with a close-packed monolayer,[13] the authors calculated average areas/adsorbed molecule and minimum film thicknesses in order to determine if denaturation occurred upon adsorption. The general conclusion from this analysis was that the plasma proteins investigated were not drastically changed in conformation upon adsorption. Recent advances in internal reflection techniques, including spectrum-averaging and smoothing with Fourier transform spectrophotometers, may provide a more sensitive infrared analysis of adsorbed protein.[14]

Using infrared internal reflection techniques similar to those applied by Brash and Lyman, Lee and Kim [15] have studied the effect of time and flow rate on the adsorption of serum albumin, γ-globulin, and prothrombin to silicone rubber, FEP, and a segmented polyether urethane. Adsorption was, in general, found to be rapid, with adsorbance values dependent on the substrate, not the adsorbing protein. In the case of albumin adsorption on silicone rubber, the plateau adsorbance increased, with flow rate showing a sixfold increase between the static and 12 $ml \cdot sec^{-1}$ conditions. For albumin adsorption on a polyether urethane, flow rate had no effect on the ultimate adsorbance, although adsorption was slower at higher flow. No general feature of the systems studied could account for the different behaviors noted.

Since fibrinogen [5] or γ-globulin [6] adsorption is believed to be required for platelet adhesion, and thereby presumably for surface-induced thrombosis, the study of the adsorption of these proteins from protein mixtures or plasma might provide a prediction of biocompatibility. Spectroscopic methods are of little use in this case, since the techniques cannot discriminate between the various possible adsorbed proteins. Radiotracer techniques using labeled proteins have therefore evolved to measure rates of adsorption and surface concentrations to characterize adsorption from complex mixtures. Such techniques are simple conceptually, although one must carefully test [16] for artifacts arising from improper rinsing, labeling effects including protein denaturation and preferential adsorption, and variations in surface roughness.

An extensive investigation of competitive effects of plasma proteins adsorbed on hydrophobic polymers has been carried out by Lee and coworkers.[17] Using [^{125}I]-labeled albumin, γ-globulin, and fibrinogen, the rates of adsorption of each protein were measured separately and from mixed solutions, and the composition of the protein film at the plateau of the isotherm determined. As expected, the adsorbance of each protein in adsorption from mixed solutions decreased, compared to that of single-component solutions. Fibrinogen was generally the most rapidly adsorbed, and in addition, was preferentially adsorbed for mixtures on all substrates considered. The time required to achieve plateau adsorbance was very similar for single-component and mixed solutions, except for adsorption on FEP where fibrinogen and γ-globulin plateau adsorption times decreased by an order of magnitude, whereas albumin adsorption required twice the time.

Using different techniques, Lyman and coworkers [18] have studied the relation of the adsorbed protein composition to the extent of surface-induced thrombosis. Recirculation tubes fabricated from various materials were implanted in dogs for varying periods up to an hour. Following explantation of the tubes and rinsing with water to remove nonadsorbed material, the tubes were soaked in detergent solution to remove the remaining protein. With use of acrylamide gel electrophoresis, the amount of albumin, γ-globulin, and other globulins adsorbed on a series of polyether urethanes, silicone rubber, and FEP was determined. The *in vivo* results for the materials which they considered indicated that surfaces with low evidence of thrombogenicity adsorbed predominately serum albumin, whereas thrombogenic materials adsorbed large amounts of globulins. Since *in vitro* studies of platelet interactions with proteinated surfaces [6, 18] have implicated adsorbed γ-globulin as causing increased adhesion, the *in vivo* studies of Lyman and coworkers would then imply that low adsorption of globulins relative to serum albumin might be useful as a design criterion for cardiovascular implant materials.

Protein Desorption and Exchange

Desorption studies are necessary to establish the reversibility of protein adsorption in order to justify the use of thermodynamic equations of state to describe the adsorbed phase, as well as to establish the mechanisms by which changes occur in the composition of protein films adsorbed from mixtures. Rates of desorption can also provide information on the adsorbed conformation of proteins, since removal of a molecule is a function of the number of attached segments.

Early studies by Bull [10, 19] showed that extensive washing could remove adsorbed albumin from pyrex glass. The fraction remaining varied greatly with the pH of the wash medium; protein removal was most difficult at pH values near the albumin isoelectric point.[20]

More recently, Brash and colleagues [21] have investigated the desorption and exchange of serum albumin adsorbed on various polymers. The substrates were tubes through which radiolabeled albumin solutions were pumped. The amount adsorbed was followed by direct counting of the surface following a 24-hour rinsing procedure. Adsorption on polyethylene was quite rapid, although a plateau adsorbance was not defined for the isotherm. Desorption and exchange experiments were carried out for polyethylene tubes having albumin films adsorbed from solutions of 0.1 mg·ml.$^{-1}$ No detectable albumin was removed by desorption into water or exchange with nonlabeled albumin at 0.1 $mg \cdot ml^{-1}$ solution concentration. At a solution concentration of 3.7 $mg \cdot ml^{-1}$, an exchange of adsorbed protein for albumin in solution occurred with a turnover of approximately 10% in the first hour and 85% in 220 hours. These studies indicate that exchanges mediated by protein-protein interaction can occur, thereby providing a basis for postulating adsorption, activation, and release of clotting factors at surfaces.

Using isotopically labeled albumin in conjunction with rapid rinsing techniques, Grant et al.[16] and Stromberg et al.[22] have studied the adsorption, desorption, and exchange of protein, using both hydrophobic and hydrophilic substrates. Desorption of albumin initially adsorbed at 2.5 $mg \cdot ml^{-1}$ solution concentration into buffer is quite different for the two types of materials. As observed by Brash et al.,[21] adsorption on polyethylene is irreversible, with no change in surface concentration over a three-hour period. Adsorption on

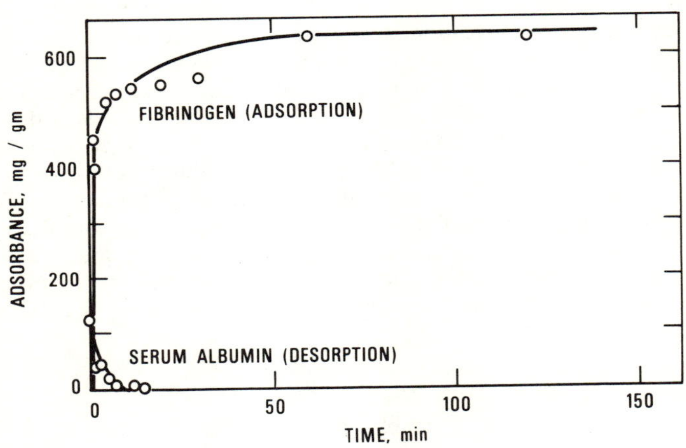

FIGURE 2. Displacement of bovine serum albumin initially adsorbed at 126 mg/gm by bovine fibrinogen at 6.5 mg/ml solution concentration.

chromium, a representative high-energy surface, is quite labile, with up to 25% of the adsorbed protein removed in the first minute. The desorption of albumin was also extremely rapid from silica, with 40% removed in the first minute and 50% at ten minutes. Most importantly, the rate of exchange for the albumin-silica system at a solution concentration of 2.5 $mg \cdot ml^{-1}$ was identical to the desorption rate.

Competitive effects modifying protein desorption behavior have been studied by Fenstermaker et al.[23] With solution-depletion techniques and the advantage of the biological properties of fibrinogen to analyze mixed solutions, the adsorption of native, nonlabeled fibrinogen and albumin on finely divided silica was measured. Fibrinogen completely dominated the adsorbed film when adsorption occurred from initially equimolar mixtures. Albumin adsorption became significant only at high concentration ratios (10:1). FIGURE 2 shows that previously adsorbed albumin is rapidly and completely displaced by fibrinogen from solution, despite the finding that serum albumin adsorbed at the same surface concentration shows only a desorption of 70% under identical conditions. These results indicate that fibrinogen has a much greater affinity than albumin for the silica surface.

The possibility that surface activation and desorption of clotting factors might occur has been studied by Waugh and coworkers,[3] who used thrombin adsorption on glass as a model system. The clotting time of standardized fibrinogen solutions was used as a measure of the native thrombin concentration. The activity of thrombin in glass vessels measured relative to a large poly(methylmethacrylate) reservoir of thrombin indicated that an initial rapid adsorption occurred on the glass followed by a slow, continuous inactivation of 2.5% of the adsorbed molecules/minute. This data is consistent with a model of adsorption, denaturation, and desorption of inactive thrombin and establishes the possibility of similar mechanisms for other clotting factors interacting with surfaces.

Conformation of Adsorbed Protein

The adsorption, desorption, and exchange properties of plasma proteins at the solid/solution interface are important considerations for describing blood-material interactions. The amount adsorbed and the composition of adsorbed protein films do not, however, account for the variation in biocompatibility observed for some materials.[24] The adsorbed conformation and conformational changes of plasma proteins have therefore received attention as a possible means of predicting the effect of interactions with the surface.

Polymers are adsorbed to surfaces by the attachment of various segments along the chain. Attached segments can occur singly or in runs with loops extending out from the surface into the solution. The size and distribution of the extension of the loops depend upon the molecular weight of the polymer and the segment-surface interaction energy. Statistical mechanics has been successfully applied to the problem of independent polymer molecules adsorbed on planar surfaces [25] resulting in predictions of the distribution of segments normal to the adsorbing surface, the fraction of bound segments, and the average number of loops. In the case of adsorbed proteins, numerous internal constraints due to disulfide cross-links and hydrophobic and electrostatic interactions limit the accessible set of conformations and make a prediction of the adsorbed conformation very difficult. In this context, only experimental measures can determine the dependence of the adsorbed protein conformation upon various parameters.

Nyilas and colleagues [26] have developed sensitive microcalorimeters to determine the thermodynamic functions for the adsorption of γ-globulin on glass particles. From the experimental measurement of ΔH, and the calculation of ΔG from the adsorption isotherm,[10] one can calculate ΔS and obtain an estimate of the protein conformational changes associated with adsorption. It was felt that the heat of adsorption could trigger conformational changes. The net heat of adsorption for γ-globulin adsorbed on glass powder (corrected for the substrate heat of immersion but not the buffer ionization) showed a sharp maxima at the surface concentration corresponding to the plateau value. The net heat decreased rapidly as additional protein was adsorbed, supposedly in multilayers. These data, in conjunction with relatively large apparent areas per adsorbed molecule, indicated that γ-globulin molecules in the first adsorbed layer undergo substantial conformational changes.

Lyklema and Norde [27] have used enthalpy of adsorption data in a somewhat different manner. They recognized that the experimentally measured enthalpy is a sum of contributions that includes effects from the displacement of water from the substrate or adsorbing protein, changes in the state of aggregation, buffer ionization, the binding of ions to the substrate due to pH changes upon adsorption, and changes in protein conformation, as well as the actual surface-segment interaction energy. Since the adsorbed protein conformation is unknown, it is impossible to predict *a priori* the magnitude of the various contributions to the measured enthalpy of adsorption. One must therefore work from the opposite view of determining what factors could lead to the observed results and thereby obtain indirect information on the adsorbed protein conformation.

With these considerations in mind, Lyklema and Norde have determined the enthalpy of adsorption for serum albumin adsorbed on polystyrene latices as a function of pH and substrate surface charge. At physiological conditions, the enthalpy of adsorption is exothermic and the adsorbance large, despite the fact that both the protein and surfaces are negatively charged. Interestingly, at pH 5 near the isoelectric point where the adsorbance is a maximum, the net enthalpy is highly endothermic. This finding indicates that entropic factors are of dominant importance in the adsorption of serum albumin to polystyrene and suggests that changes in conformation occur as a function of the pH of the adsorbing solution.

Circular dichroism (CD) has been utilized by McMillin and Walton [28] to study the conformation of fibrinogen and factor XII adsorbed on quartz. By adsorbing the proteins on a stack of thin quartz plates, standard transmission techniques could be applied to measure spectra of both wet and dried adsorbed films, which were compared to solution spectra. The assumption was made that the product of the concentration and path-length for a protein solution producing the same measured ellipticity as the adsorbed system could be used to normalize the data for the adsorbed protein and calculate molar ellipticities to characterize the adsorbed conformation. Dried, adsorbed films of fibrinogen produced a spectrum very similar to that of fibrinogen in solution, leading to the conclusion that fibrinogen does not change conformation upon adsorption. Spectra for solution and adsorbed factor XII, both wet and dried, showed major differences. The authors concluded that the binding of water is conformationally important and may be involved in the activation of factor XII. Further analysis would be required, however, to determine the extent of the actual conformation changes upon adsorption.

The molecular unfolding and acquired immunogenicity of γ-globulin molecules concomitant with adsorption to a polystyrene latex has been studied by Kochwa et al.,[29] using potentiometric titrations. Conformational changes accompanied by the rupture of intramolecular bonds and exposure of additional titrable groups should result in an increased acid uptake per adsorbed molecule. Determinations of the number of acidic groups per adsorbed IgG molecule as a function of pH and concentration during adsorption established an inverse linear relationship between the logarithm of the surface population and the number of titrable groups per adsorbed molecule. The effect was maximal at a pH of 6.8, indicating that additional histidine and free amino groups are exposed upon adsorption. The inverse nature of the relationship shows that adsorption under conditions of low surface coverage apparently leads to a molecular unfolding. These conformational changes of IgG were reinforced by the finding that IgG adsorbed at low concentration behaves immunogenically like heat-denatured material, but that adsorbed at high concentrations behaves normally.

An interesting study of the adsorption of haemoproteins to polystyrene latex particles was carried out by Benko and colleagues,[30] using broad-line NMR. Since the resonances of bound protein nuclei are greatly broadened, high-resolution techniques are, in general, unsuccessful. The authors noted, however, that the environment of the iron atom in the heme pocket determined the relaxation time of the solvent protons. Upon adsorption of the protein, the relaxation rate of the water protons changed significantly, indicating a change in conformation that affected the heme portion of the molecule.

Two studies in which novel techniques were used have recently been carried out to determine the conformation of adsorbed serum albumin. Harrick and Loeb [31] have developed internal reflectance fluorescence techniques to measure the surface concentration of dansyl chloride-labeled protein at the quartz/ solution interface *in situ*, using visible light. Their results were consistent with the presence of an adsorbed monolayer of unmodified albumin. Izmailova and coworkers [32] measured the modulus of elastic deformation for albumin adsorbed on the disk of a Couette-type viscometer. Changes in modulus as a function of shear were interpreted as conformational changes of the protein. Neither of these techniques are, at the present moment, very sensitive for the measurement of adsorbed protein conformation.

Fenstermaker et al.[23] and Smith et al.[33] have used *in situ* ellipsometry to determine the adsorbance and extension of fibrinogen, prothrombin, and serum albumin adsorbed on a variety of surfaces. Using physiological conditions, they typically observed a rapid adsorption on materials varying in surface free energy from platinum to polyethylene with little or no change in extension with time. The adsorbance was sometimes found to increase about 20% over the three-to-four-hour adsorption period. Apparently there is little or no rearrangement of adsorbed molecules, and late arrivals at the interface merely fill in the unoccupied areas without adopting a different conformation from the majority of previously adsorbed molecules.

The steady state properties of the above three proteins adsorbed on different materials exhibited two interesting features. Characteristically the extension of the adsorbed protein molecule increased with decreasing surface free energy (estimated by the critical surface tension for wetting). Typically, as observed for fibrinogen, the film thickness increased from 32 to 59 nm over the range encompassed by platinum, chromium, quartz, carbon, and polyethylene. The adsorbance was variable, but not in a discernible pattern for the various materials. For fibrinogen, the average adsorbance value of 4.5 ± 0.6 $mg \cdot m^{-2}$ was obtained, and similar patterns were found for prothrombin and serum albumin. The lack of variation in the adsorbance values for different materials is similar to the observations of Horbett and Hoffman.[24] The increase in extension with decreasing surface energy would be consistent with flat, tightly held conformations on the high-energy surfaces and open, extended conformations on the low-energy substrates.

Upon interaction with a surface, the amide I infrared absorbance band of the carbonyl chromophore of proteins shifts approximately 20 cm^{-1}. From the intensities of the shifted and unshifted bands measured by difference techniques, the bound fraction, i.e., the fraction of carbonyl groups of an absorbed molecule directly interacting with the surface, can be measured and used to calculate the number of surface attachments. The bound fraction can therefore provide essential information characterizing the conformation and changes in conformation of adsorbed proteins.

Using this technique, Morrissey and Stromberg [13] and Fenstermaker et al.[23]

have studied the conformation of prothrombin, serum albumin, and fibrinogen as a function of surface concentration, time of adsorption, pD, and ionic strength. As shown in FIGURE 3, there is no change or trend apparent in the bound fraction of either prothrombin or serum albumin measured along their respective isotherms. The average value of 0.11 for both proteins indicates that approximately 80 carbonyl attachments to the surface exist. A bound fraction of approximately 0.1 for both serum albumin and prothrombin indicates that most segments of the bound molecules remain in solution away from the interface. These results, in conjunction with the finding that the bound fraction does not change with time of adsorption (for $t > 45s$), suggest that conformational changes or rearrangements upon adsorption are minimal. The internal bonding of prothrombin and serum albumin is apparently sufficient to preserve the basic tertiary structure of the molecules. These results do not, however, rule out changes in conformation concomitant with adsorption. The conceptual importance of these changes for understanding the nature of the interaction of blood with foreign surfaces led to further studies with modified serum albumin.

By reacting the protein with diethyl malonimidate dihydrochloride (DEM), using the method of Dutton et al.,[34] approximately 21 additional internal cross-links were introduced. The resulting material has been shown to be unchanged in conformation as judged by measurements of antigenicity. Rearrangements

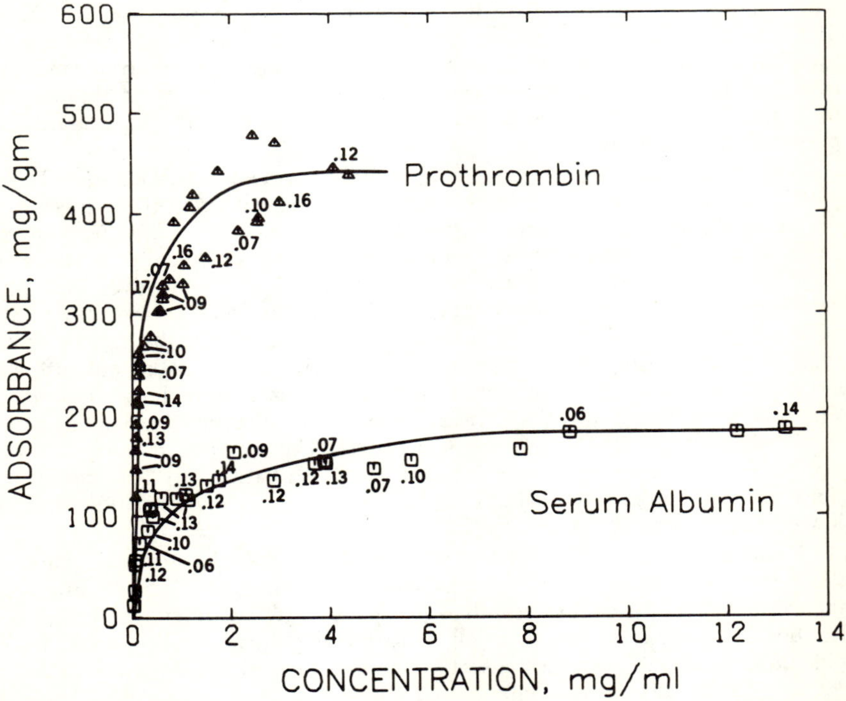

FIGURE 3. Adsorption isotherms for bovine serum albumin and prothrombin at pD 7.4 on silica. Values of bound fraction given for isotherm points.

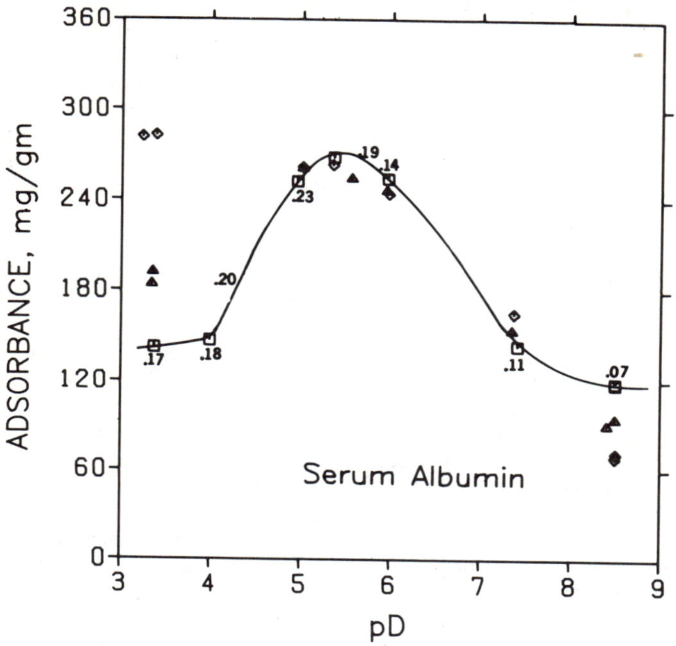

FIGURE 4. Adsorbance vs. pD for bovine serum albumin at 0.1 (□), 0.2 (△), and 0.5 (◇) ionic strength. The curve is for ionic strength 0.1 and the values along the curve are the average bound fractions at the given pD. (Courtesy of the publishers of J. Colloid Interface Sci.[13])

of the molecular conformation upon adsorption are therefore unlikely, since the protein molecule is more rigid. The cross-linked serum albumin gave a bound fraction that was experimentally indistinguishable from that of the native material. Since no increment in the bound fraction due to rearrangement upon adsorption could be detected, it was concluded that no change in conformation of serum albumin occurred.

The bound fraction technique can also be used to determine the effect of surface charge on the adsorbed conformation of plasma proteins.[13] As shown in FIGURE 4, there is a maximum observed in the adsorbance as a function of pD at moderate ionic strength. The experimentally measured bound fraction, and hence the conformation, was found to depend only on the pD and exhibited a broad maximum from approximately pD 4–5.5. The coincidence in the profiles of adsorbance and bound fraction with maxima near pD 5.2, the isoelectric point of bovine serum albumin in D_2O, indicates the importance of protein-protein electrostatic interactions on the adsorbing surface. At the isoelectric point where these repulsions are a minimum, more protein can adsorb with a somewhat flatter conformation.

The effect of surface charge on protein adsorption has more recently been investigated by Stromberg et al.,[22] and Morrissey et al.,[35] who ascertained the effect of applied potential on the conformation of adsorbed plasma proteins. Ellipsometric measurements carried out *in situ* showed the existence of an anodic potential at which enhanced adsorption occurred, and a cathodic potential at which a conformational change occurred as evidenced by a large increase in the extension. For example, the case of fibrinogen adsorbed on platinum at pH 7.4, the application of a sequence of potentials beginning at —0.2 V/SCE (voltages relative to the saturated calomel electrode) resulted in no change in the steady state, rest potential value of adsorbance until +0.4 V/SCE was reached. At this potential and above, a rapid increase in adsorbance occurrred, the rate of which was roughly proportional to the applied potential. The extension, measured concomitantly with the adsorbance, showed a large increase at —0.2 V/SCE and subsequently decreased back to the initial rest potential value as the potential was incremented in the anodic direction. Additional studies indicated that the conformational changes were reversible, although no desorption of protein was observed.

Data obtained for serum albumin and γ-globulin indicated a similar behavior with potentials for enhanced adsorption of +0.6 V and +0.8 V/SCE, respectively. At physiological pH, all proteins studied exist with a net negative charge. The observed behavior is therefore consistent with electrostatic repulsion at cathodic potentials causing the increase in extension, and electrostatic attraction at anodic potentials causing he enhanced adsorption. The details of the protein conformation are, however, important, since the potentials of enhanced adsorption do not correlate with the protein isolectric points.

In contrast to earlier studies of serum albumin and prothrombin, γ-globulin has been found to undergo changes in conformation as a function of surface concentration.[36] As shown in FIGURE 5, the bound fraction of γ-globulin adsorbed on pyrogenic silica varied from 0.2 at low concentration of 0.02 on the plateau of the isotherm. This change in bound fraction corresponds to a decrease from 270 to 30 carbonyl surface attachments and indicates the molecule is held in a flattened conformation at low-surface coverage. These conformational changes were further investigated with ellipsometry to measure

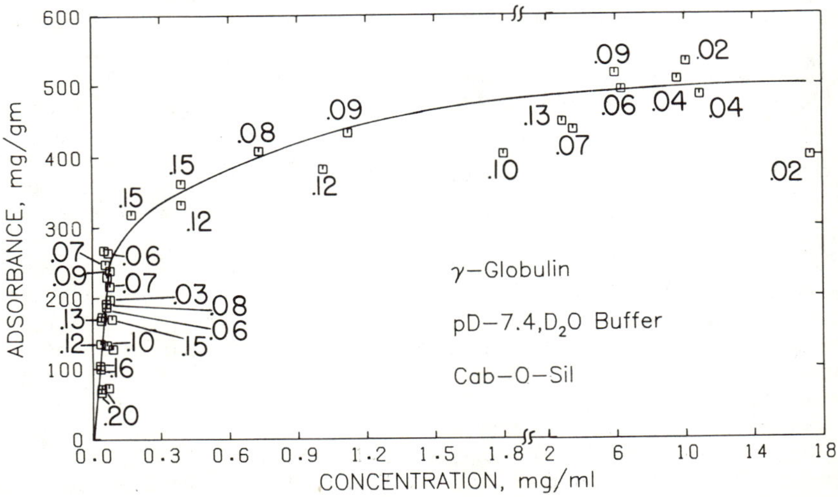

FIGURE 5. Adsorption isotherm for bovine γ-globulin adsorbed at pD 7.4 on silica. Values of bound fraction given for isotherm points.

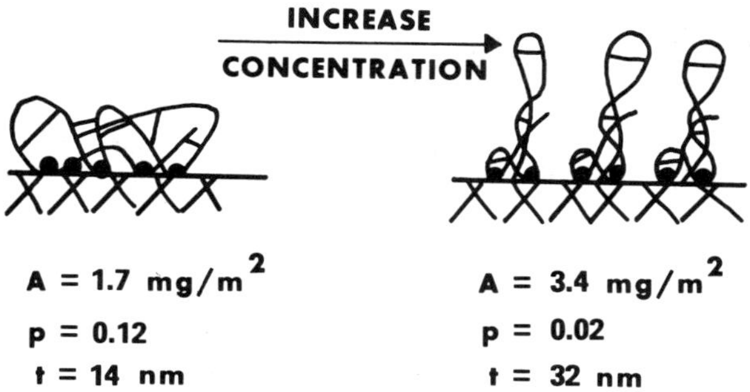

FIGURE 6. Schematic representation of effect of surface concentration on adsorbed γ-globulin conformation. Parameters reported are the adsorbance (A), bound fraction (p), and extension (t).

the extension of γ-globulin adsorbed on planar fused silica. For this study, the protein solution concentrations were selected to correspond to two regions of the adsorption isotherm which exhibited a large difference in bound fraction. As indicated in FIGURE 6, the extension of adsorbed γ-globulin is higher for adsorption from the higher concentration solution. At 0.3 and 10.0 $mg \cdot ml^{-1}$ bound fractions (p) of 0.12 and 0.02 were measured, while extensions (t) of 14 ± 3 and 32 ± 11 nm were observed, respectively. The molecule assumes a more extended conformation at high-surface concentration where competition for adsorption sites is great. These results are consistent with studies mentioned earlier using calorimetry [26] and potentiometric titrations.[29]

None of these results (bound fraction, ellipsometry, calorimetry, or potentiometric titrations) for native γ-globulin actually establish at what point along the adsorption isotherm the adsorbed protein is most nearly native. Studies by Fontana [37] of synthetic polyelectrolytes adsorbed at the solid/solution interface establish that adsorbate-adsorbate interactions generally determine both the adsorbance and conformation. Since lateral surface interactions are clearly present for adsorbed γ-globulin, distortions in conformation can occur at both low and high surface coverage. To determine the adsorbed conformation that corresponds most closely to the native conformation in solution, both ellipsometric and bound fraction studies were carried out using DEM cross-linked γ-globulin. Since the conformation of the cross-linked protein is unchanged from the native material,[34] adsorption studies where the molecule cannot freely rearrange on the surface will indicate the most native adsorbed conformation. The results indicated that adsorbed γ-globulin is most like the solution protein conformation at intermediate surface concentrations. Distortions of the native conformation therefore occur at both low and high adsorbance. At low surface coverage, lack of competition for surface adsorption sites results in a flatter adsorbed conformation, while at high surface coverage, repulsions cause a more extended conformation with fewer surface attachments.

In summary, our experimental studies of adsorbed plasma proteins have shown that they are rapidly adsorbed to a variety of surfaces with a significant number of surface attachments. Changes in conformation of γ-globulin, but not serum albumin or prothrombin, can occur as a function of surface concentration. The extension of all adsorbed plasma proteins increased with decreasing surface energy of the substrate. Studies of the effect of applied potential show that an enhanced adsorption and reversible conformational changes occur at voltages determined by the protein and substrate. Finally, rates of adsorption and desorption have established that the surface composition is different from that of the adsorbing solution, and that displacement and desorption of proteins can occur from silica and chromium, but not polyethylene.

Overview

Although a significant effort has been mounted to characterize the interaction of plasma proteins with materials to provide a basis for predicting the nature of the interaction of blood with artificial devices, there remains much to be learned and understood. Confirmation of the properties of adsorbed proteins using new techniques such as circular dichorism and quasielastic light scattering will increase confidence in the reported dimensions and behavior. The conceptual importance of short time (less than 10 seconds) measurements of plasma protein adsorbance and conformation for the development of models of the initiation mechanism for coagulation or thrombosis cannot be minimized. Efforts are currently under way to carry out such measurements with the automatic recording ellipsometer. Finally, the development of correlations between the physicochemical and biological properties of adsorbed proteins will determine the ultimate utility of such data. Since the orientation of an adsorbed enzyme can be used only to explain decreases in enzymatic activity, recent investigations showing large increases in the activity of adsorbed enzymes [2, 38–42] establish the biological importance of conformational changes upon adsorption. The relation of adsorbed plasma protein conformation and biocompatibility may provide guidelines for the development of nonthrombogenic materials and an understanding of the events that trigger surface-induced coagulation.

Acknowledgment

The author thanks Dr. L. E. Smith and Dr. R. E. Dehl for helpful suggestions.

References

1. Salzman, E. W. 1972. Surface effects in hemostasis and thrombosis. *In* The Chemistry of Biosurfaces. M. L. Hair, Ed. Vol. **2:** 489–522. Marcel Dekker, Inc. New York, N.Y.
2. Gitel, S. N., W. G. Owen, C. T. Esmon & C. M. Jackson. 1973. A polypeptide region of bovine prothrombin specific for binding to phospholipids. Proc. Nat. Acad. Sci. USA. **70:** 1344–1348.
3. Waugh, D. F., L. J. Anthony & H. Ng. 1975. The Interaction of thrombin with borosilicate glass surfaces. J. Biomed. Mater. Res. **9:** 511–536.
4. Salzman, E. W., E. W. Merrill, A. Binder, C. F. W. Wolf, T. P. Ashford & W. G. Austen. 1969. Protein-platelet interaction on heparinized surfaces. J. Biomed. Mater. Res. **3:** 69–81.

5. ZUCKER, M. B. & L. VROMAN. 1969. Platelet adhesion induced by fibrinogen adsorbed onto glass. Proc. Soc. Exp. Biol. Med. **131:** 318–320.
6. KIM, S. W., R. G. LEE, H. OSTER, D. COLEMAN, J. D. ANDRADE, D. J. LENTZ & D. OLSEN. 1974. Platelet adhesion to polymer surfaces. Trans. Amer. Soc. Artif. Int. Organs **2:** 449–455.
7. MOHANDAS, N., R. M. HOCHMUTH & E. E. SPAETH. 1974. Adhesion of red cells to foreign surfaces in the presence of flow. J. Biomed. Mater. Res. **8:** 119–136.
8. NICHOLS, A. R. & M. C. WILLIAMS. 1976. Suppression of shear-induced hemolysis by three plasma proteins. Biomat., Med. Dev., Artif. Organs **4:** 21–48.
9. VINCENT, B. 1974. The effect of adsorbed polymers on dispersion stability. Adv. Colloid Interface Sci. **4:** 192–277.
10. BULL, H. B. 1956. Adsorption of bovine serum albumin on glass. Biochim. Biophys. Acta **19:** 464–471.
11. ORESKES, I. & J. M. SINGER. 1961. The mechanism of particulate carrier reactions. Adsorption of human γ-globulin to polystyrene latex particles. J. Immunol. **86:** 338–344.
12. BRASH, J. L. & D. L. LYMAN. 1969. Adsorption of plasma proteins in solution to uncharged, hydrophobic polymer surfaces. J. Biomed. Mater. Res. **3:** 175–189.
13. MORRISSEY, B. W. & R. R. STROMBERG. 1974. The conformation of adsorbed blood proteins by infrared bound fraction measurements. J. Colloid Interface Sci. **46:** 152–164.
14. MATTSON, J. S., C. A. SMITH & K. E. PAULSEN. 1975. Infrared internal reflection spectroscopy of aqueous protein films at the germanium-water interfaces. Anal. Chem. **47:** 736–738.
15. LEE, R. G. & S. W. KIM. 1974. Adsorption of proteins on hydrophobic polymer surfaces. Adsorption isotherms and kinetics. J. Biomed. Mater. Res. **8:** 251–259.
16. GRANT, W. H., L. E. SMITH & R. R. STROMBERG. 1976. Radiotracer technique for protein adsorption measurements. J. Biomed. Mater. Res. In press.
17. LEE, R. G., C. ADAMSON & S. W. KIM. 1974. Competitive adsorption of plasma proteins onto polymer surfaces. Thrombosis Res. **4:** 485–490.
18. LYMAN, D. J., L. C. METCALF, D. ALBO, JR., K. F. RICHARDS & J. LAMB. 1974. The effect of chemical structure and surface properties of synthetic polymers on the coagulation of blood. III. In vivo adsorption of proteins on polymer surfaces. Trans. Amer. Soc. Artif. Intern. Organs **20:** 474–478.
19. BULL, H. B. 1957. Adsorbed monolayers of egg albumin. Arch. Biochem. Biophys. **68:** 102–111.
20. MACRITCHIE, F., also. 1972. The adsorption of proteins at the solid/liquid interface. J. Colloid Interface Sci. **38:** 484–488.
21. BRASH, J. L., S. UNIYAL & Q. SAMAK. 1974. Exchange of albumin adsorbed on polymer surfaces. Trans. Amer. Soc. Artif. Intern. Organs **20:** 69–76.
22. STROMBERG, R. R., B. W. MORRISSEY, L. E. SMITH, W. H. GRANT & C. A. FENSTERMAKER. 1975. Interaction of Blood Proteins with Solid Surfaces. PB 241–267 (Available from NTIS). Annual report prepared for the Biomaterials Program, National Heart and Lung Institute, NIH, Bethesda, Md.
23. FENSTERMAKER, C. A., W. H. GRANT, B. W. MORRISSEY, L. E. SMITH & R. R. STROMBERG. 1974. Interaction of Plasma Proteins with Surfaces. PB 232–629 (Available from NTIS). Annual report prepared for the Biomaterials Program, National Heart and Lung Institute, NIH, Bethesda, Md.
24. HORBETT, T. A. & A. S. HOFFMANN. 1975. Bovine plasma protein adsorption to radiation grafted hydrogels based on hydroxyethylmethacrylate and N-vinylpyrolidone. *In* Applied Chemistry at Protein Interfaces. R. E. Baier, Ed. Advances in Chemistry Series No. 145. ACS. Washington, D.C.
25. DIMARZIO, E. A. & R. J. RUBIN, for example. 1971. Adsorption of a polymer chain between two plates. J. Chem. Phys. **55:** 4318–4336.

26. NYILAS, E., T-H. CHIU & G. A. HERZLINGER. 1974. Thermodynamics of native protein/foreign surface interactions. I. Calorimetry of the human γ-globulin/glass system. Trans. Amer. Soc. Artif. Intern. Organs **20:** 480–490.
27. LYKLEMA, J. & W. NORDE. 1973. Biopolymer adsorption with special reference to the serum albumin-polystyrene latex system. Croatica Chem. Acta **45:** 67–84.
28. MCMILLIN, C. R. & A. G. WALTON. 1974. A circular dichroism technique for the study of adsorbed protein structure. J. Colloid Interface Sci. **48:** 345–349.
29. KOCHWA, S., M. BROWNELL, R. E. ROSENFIELD & L. R. WASSERMAN. 1967. Adsorption of proteins by polystyrene particles. I. Molecular Unfolding and Acquired Immunogenicity of IgG. J. Immunol. **99:** 981–986.
30. BENKO, B., S. VUK-PAVLOVIC, G. DEZELIC & S. MARICIC. 1975. A proton magnetic relaxation study of methaemoproteins bound to monodisperse polystyrene latex particles. J. Colloid Interface Sci .**52:** 444–451.
31. HARRICK, N. J. & G. I. LOEB. 1973. Multiple internal reflection fluorescence spectrometry. Anal. Chem. **45:** 687–691.
32. IZMAILOVA, V. I., I. G. ALEKSEEVA, E. D. SHCHUKIN & P. A. REBINDER. 1972. Rheological investigation of interfacial adsorption layers of proteins and surface-active polymers. Dokl. Akad. Nauk. SSSR **206:** 1150–1153.
33. SMITH, L. E., C. A. FENSTERMAKER & R. R. STROMBERG. 1970. Adsorption of blood proteins from solution. ACS Polymer Preprints **11:** 1376–1377.
34. DUTTON, A., M. ADAMS & S. J. SINGER. 1966. Bifunctional imidoesters as crosslinking reagents. Biochem. Biophys. Res. Commun. **23:** 730–739.
35. MORRISSEY, B. W., L. E. SMITH, R. R. STROMBERG & C. A. FENSTERMAKER. 1976. Ellipsometric investigation of the effect of potential on blood protein conformation and adsorbance. J. Colloid Interface Sci. **56:** 557–563.
36. MORRISSEY, B. W. & C. A. FENSTERMAKER. 1976. Conformation of adsorbed γ-globulin and β-lactoglobulin. Effect of surface concentration. Trans. Amer. Soc. Artif. Intern. Organs **22:** 278–283.
37. FONTANA, B. J. 1971. Adsorption of biological analog molecules on nonbiological surfaces. Polymers. *In* The Chemistry of Biosurfaces. M. L. Hair, Ed. Vol. **1:** 83–142. Marcel Dekker, Inc. New York, N.Y.
38. GABEL, D., I. Z. STEINBERG & E. KATCHALSKI. 1971. Changes in conformation of insolubilized trypism and chymotrypsin followed by fluorescence. Biochemistry **10:** 4661–4669.
39. MANECKE, G., G. GUNZEL & H. J. FORESTER. 1970. Enzymes covalently bound to various polymers and the effects on the properties of these enzymes. J. Poly. Sci. **30C:** 607–613.
40. SIEGEL, B. Z. & S. M. SIEGEL. 1960. Enhancement of peroxidase action by polysaccharides. Nature **186:** 391.
41. BERNATH, F. R. 1973. The effect of micelles on enzymatic reactions. *In* Biomedical Applications of Polymers. H. P. Gregor, Ed. Vol. **7:** 17–31. Plenum Press. New York, N.Y.
42. DIMARZIO, E. A. & M. BISHOP. 1974. The nature of the helix-coil transition of biological macromolecules attached to a surface. Biopolymers **13:** 2331–2348.

REACTIONS OF FORMED ELEMENTS OF BLOOD WITH PLASMA PROTEINS AT INTERFACES *

Leo Vroman, Ann L. Adams, Madeleine Klings, Gena C. Fischer, Priscilla C. Munoz, and Regina P. Solensky

Interface Laboratory
Veterans Administration Hospital
Brooklyn, New York 11209

We have seen from the preceding how complex the behavior of single proteins and their simple combinations can be. There is no way of studying the behavior of the same proteins in unmodified whole blood: all man-made surfaces, unlike the blood vessel wall, cause activation of clotting or adhesion of platelets and white blood cells. It is true that certain changes imposed upon a sample of blood by the walls of its artificial container can be prevented by additives, but then we are adding one artifact to another. In the carefully planned *in vitro* test systems where no anticoagulant is used, such as in brief exposure of a biomaterial-lined space to native blood,[1, 2] or where blood is allowed to flow directly from blood vessel to material surface,[3, 4] whatever is being measured must be some early effect of the triggered clotting process. In systems where anticoagulants are used, the effect of these additives is often unpredicted. Only quite recently the discovery was made that removal of calcium ions (e.g. by addition of citrate) promoted secondary aggregation of platelets,[5] whereas the more reasonable explanation had been that it was inhibited by addition of heparin. The diversity in action of these two anticoagulants should not be surprising, since they inhibit clotting in quite different ways. For this reason, in experiments where they differ in action less from each other than from a third added variable, we can claim to be observing the effects of that third variable and not of anticoagulant. For example, we found that both in heparinized and in citrated plasma, activation by contact with glass or diatomaceous earth reduced the ability of plasma to modify its own deposit on a glass-like surface.[6–8] In this case we may presume that the anticoagulants did not affect this property of intact plasma. We may even presume that plasma, being intact in the body, also has this property in *vivo.* Similarly, under certain conditions platelet retention is affected more by the retaining material surface than by the anticoagulant used; [9] again, this would give us hope that the same material will do *in vivo* without anticoagulant what it did *in vitro* with anticoagulants.

Casting aside the effects of anticoagulants in the belief that we control them, and building on our knowledge of protein adsorption, we face the task of finding the few among thousands of plasma and platelet or white cell membrane proteins involved in the various surface/blood interactions. Fortunately,

* This work was supported in part by Interagency Agreements YO1–AM–7–X012 with the Artificial Kidney-Chronic Uremia Program, National Institute of Arthritis, Metabolism and Digestive Diseases, and Y01–HB50001–01 with the Biomaterials Program, Division of Heart and Vascular Diseases, National Heart and Lung Institute, National Institutes of Health.

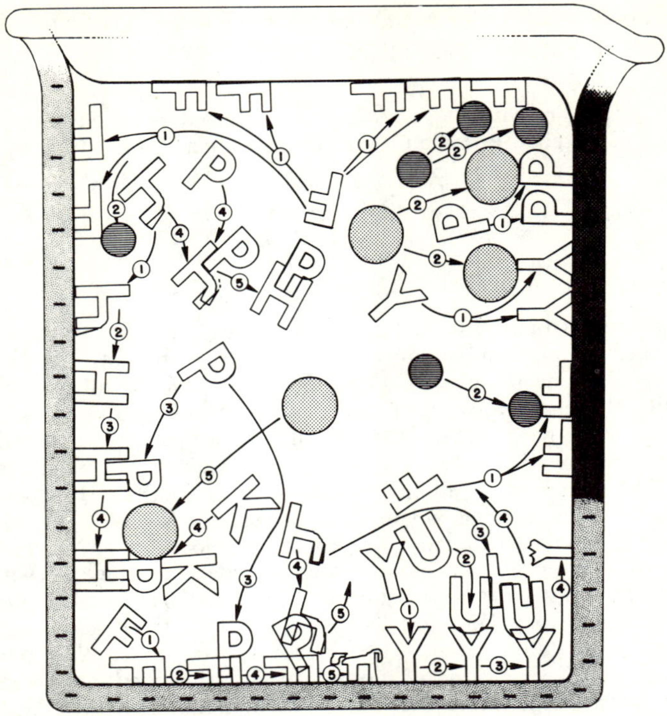

FIGURE 1. A beaker with negative surface charges (—) but also with a hydrophobic area (0) (under spout) containing intact blood. Proteins discussed in text are shown as: F=fibrinogen; h=intact factor XII (Hageman factor); H=activated Hageman factor; K=kininogen (of high mol wt.); P=(pre)kallikrein; U=unknown protein; Y=γ-globulins (the stem of the Y representing the Fc fragment, and the arms the Fab area). Platelets are indicated as (unproportionally) small shaded discs, granulocytes as larger ones. Numbered arrows indicate the following events.

1. Primary adsorption of: a) fibrinogen at air/blood interface (top), at negatively charged surface (bottom and left top), and hyrophobic surface (right) in various orientations; b) intact Hageman factor (fr. XII) at negatively charged surface; c) γ-globulins at negatively charged surface (bottom, right), possibly (for explanation, see text) with Fc fragment attaching to surface; and at hydrophobic surface possibly with Fab adhering to surface; d) (pre)kallikrein perhaps adhering most actively to hydrophobic surface.

2. Interactions of blood with primary films: a) platelets adhere to unconverted fibrinogen film wherever they find it (at interfaces with air and with hydrophobic surfaces, and, if arriving early, at the negatively charged surfaces); b) Hageman factor is activated if adsorbed onto a negatively charged surface; c) (2 and 3) prekallikrein (or some other intact surface factor but not Hageman factor) is adsorbed onto fibrinogen at negatively charged substrate.

3. a) Activated Hageman factor adsorbs prekallikrein; b) Prekallikrein (or other intact non-Hageman factor) adsorbed onto fibrinogen, converts it; c) intact Hageman factor is adsorbed onto the unknown matter that covers the gamma globulins on negatively charged substrate.

4. a) Activated kallikrein, gone into solution, combines with intact Hageman factor in solution; b) activated kallikrein, while still adsorbed on activated Hageman factor, in turn adsorbs high molecular weight kininogen; c) intact Hageman factor is ad-

nature provides us with patients who congenitally lack a single protein. We found that the platelets in blood of patients who have no fibrinogen adhere to glass only where fibrinogen had been preadsorbed; normal platelets suspended in plasma rendered fibrinogen-free by heating [7] or in serum [10] behave similarly. The adhesion of platelets, however, rendered predictable by the removal of the fibrinogen from their normal environment, will then serve no better use than as an indicator—a "biological stain"—of fibrinogen deposits. The behavior of platelets in media that are even more lacking deviates even more from normal.[11] Our findings in such experiments are briefly described below and will be published in more detail elsewhere.[12] As in most studies of live systems, it seems that the more artificial and controlled they are, the more statistically significant and the less biologically significant are the results they produce.

A similar problem of interpretation arises when we try to derive the behavior of plasma at a certain interface from the behavior of three or four purified proteins studied singly or even in combination at that interface.[13, 14]

Certainly, thrombus formation on an implanted device *in vivo* cannot be predicted from the behavior of a few proteins on its surface *in vitro.* Some authors do equate protein adsorption [15] or gross clotting [16] with thrombogenicity. Yet, glow discharge-treated glass tubes implanted in the venous flow of dogs often perform well,[17] though the clotting time of blood on glass is shorter than on most biomaterials. The role of blood-clotting enzymes in the behavior of blood at interfaces is still not known, but some bonds between certain of these factors and the behavior of platelets and white cells must exist. For example, onto cuprophane under certain conditions human (but perhaps not canine) blood deposits leukocytes.[18] Possibly, the conversion of prekallikrein by surface-activated factor XII (to be described later by Dr. Ratnoff and Dr. Kaplan; also see Ref. 19) causes chemotactic activity that will attract neutrophils.[20] Interactions between platelets and white cells may well be initiated by interfaces: platelet aggregation appears to cause as well as to be caused by complement activation and chemotaxis.[21] Platelets are phagocytized by neutrophiles.[22] This area of the "tangled web" [23] of interactions represents only part of the system that faces us.

Our own work is based on the hope that this involved performance by the blood can be analyzed by allowing it to perform only brief, traceable acts at one time. Coagulationists do this too: they have pinpointed the location of single factors in the scheme of clotting by observing where the process stopped in deficient plasmas and how it resumed upon reconstitution. On the basis of work we have done so far, several overlapping phases of interaction between blood and solid surfaces can be presumed to exist. For example, one surface will exert its influence in several ways (FIGURE 1). It may affect one area of one protein so that this molecule is adsorbed and interacts with another protein molecule, and so on. The diagram shows how various interactions among proteins on or near the interface will help or hinder platelet and granulocyte adhesion and their subsequent spreading.

If this is indeed the kind of interplay that takes place, and if protein species

---

sorbed onto converted fibrinogen film; d) intact Hageman factor removes matter (including some globulin) of unknown nature that had been deposited onto the globulin film.

5. a) Activated kallikrein activates Hageman factor in solution; b) intact Hageman factor removes converted fibrinogen; c) granulocytes adhere to the kallikrein that had been adsorbed by film of activated Hageman factor.

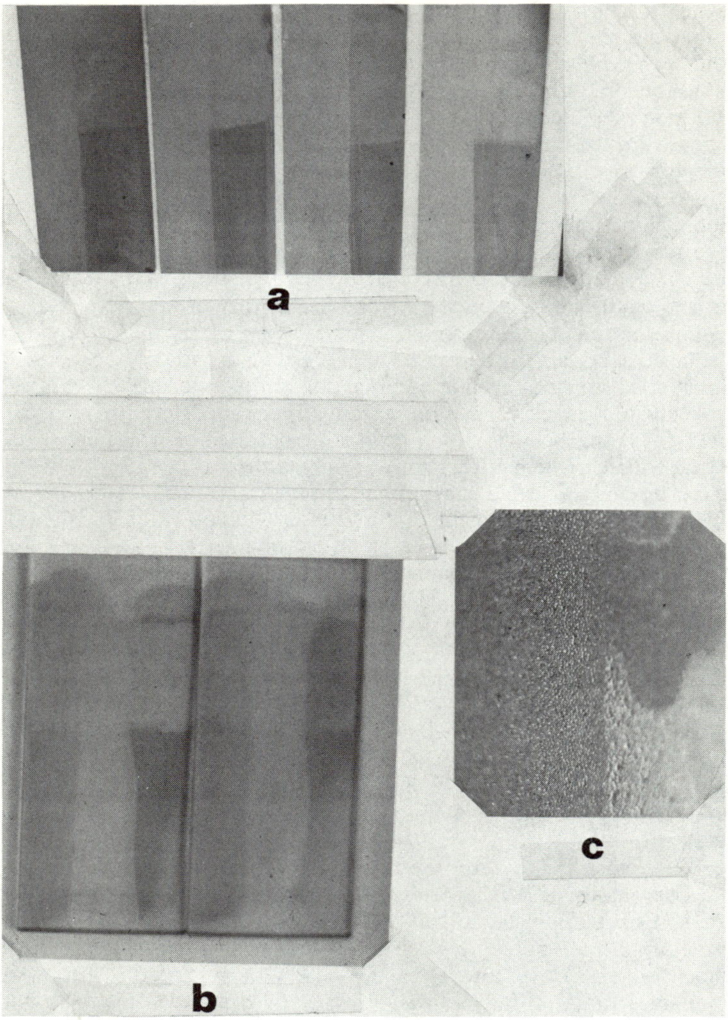

FIGURE 2. Evidence that normal intact plasma deposits fibrinogen and then converts it on glass-like surfaces. Substrates used: anodized tantalum (FIGURE 2a) and glass (b and c). Intact plasmas had resided on slides for 10 min (upper areas of all figures) or for a few sec only (lower areas). After rinse with buffer and water, all dried surfaces were covered over entire right-hand sides with rabbit antiserum to fibrinogen; left sides of slides in FIGURE 2b also were covered with antiserum to γ-globulins. All were rinsed a few min later with buffer and then with water. The human intact plasmas used were, from left to right: FIGURE 2a, normal, Fletcher-deficient, XI-deficient, and factor XII-deficient. FIGURE 2b, normal and Fletcher-deficient; FIGURE 2c, normal only. Deposition of antibody was detected and photographed as follows: FIGURE 2a, by interference color on anodized tantalum, where right lower areas shown darkest were deep purple; note rather dark right upper area on Fletcher-deficient plasma deposit indicating incomplete conversion of fibrinogen by this plasma; FIGURE 2b, by staining with Coomassie Brilliant Blue R, showing deepest blue in right lower

participate that are rarely if ever missing in human blood, then the following kind of experiment is required to discover this interplay. The test surface is exposed to normal intact plasma for various periods and is then rinsed with buffer, and the nature and significance of the remaining adsorbate are studied in essentially two ways. a. The proteins remaining adsorbed are identified either by their enzymatic activity (their ability to correct the clotting of certain clotting factor-deficient plasmas) or by their antigenicity (their ability to adsorb matching antibody out of antisera). Conclusions from these experiments are based on our presumption that the adsorption of a protein is of significance only if its enzymatic activity or its antigenicity is maintained or generated. We do not believe that retention of a protein, usually demonstrable only by passage over powder to expose a large enough surface area, need be related to the function of that protein at the material/plasma or solution interface.

b. Instead of proceding as under a, we expose the surface that had been preexposed to plasma, now to whole blood that was anticoagulated with citrate in one series and with heparin in another; after various periods of exposure the coated slide is rinsed and fixed to observe adhesion of formed elements and fibrin. Thus far, methanol appears the fixative to be preferred, since we found it affects antigenicity of adsorbed proteins less than do formalin and glutaraldehyde, so that it may allow us to study the identity of proteins, as well as of formed elements adhering to a surface.

Usually, we expose areas of one surface (such as a 2 $\times$ 3-inch microscope slide) to various conditions, e.g., by adsorbing one protein in one area and another one elsewhere; this treatment may be followed by exposure of the entire half of the slide (including half of each area) to plasma and then of the entire buffer-rinsed and wet slide to whole blood. This allows us to compare the effects of the various adsorbed proteins, with and without their being exposed to plasma, upon the adhesion of formed elements in whole blood, while their adhesion to the untreated areas of the slide serves as a control. At all times, air/liquid/solid interfaces are avoided: a protein solution will form a film at the liquid/air interface, and where the solution advances over a hydrophobic substrate, it will "print out" this film onto the substrate. On blood, this film may be fibrinogen, and platelets may adhere to it either before or after the film is transferred to the solid.[24] This would explain the high loss of platelets by blood advancing over a hydrophobic solid in air.[25] Often, we avoid air interfaces as follows. A drop of buffer is placed on one area of a slide. Plasma is placed in it. After the desired period of contact, a drop of buffer is placed elsewhere, is then allowed to flow into the plasma + buffer drop, and the entire slide is rinsed rapidly with more buffer, then with water if tests described under 1 are to follow, or it is left wet with buffer for those described under 2.

We developed three simple ways of detecting antibody deposition on preadsorbed protein films,[26] based on interference color, stainability, and wettability of the antigen/antibody complex (FIGURE 2). Under suitable conditions, these methods allow qualitative identification, but thus far do not yield quantitative data. These are provided by ellipsometry,[27] especially in conjunction with

areas where antiserum to human fibrinogen had resided on area of brief contact with plasma; again, Fletcher-deficient plasma did not appear to convert fibrinogen deposit (upper right area being darker than same area of normal plasma-treated glass); also note some conversion of deposited globulins (lower left areas being darker than upper left areas); FIGURE 2c, water-vapor condensation, showing larger drops in lower right area where antiserum to fibrinogen had left wettable deposit.

antibody adsorption (FIGURE 3).[6, 7, 14, 28] However, substrates that adsorb water, that are themselves stainable, and that are too thick or uneven to show interference colors or to allow ellipsometry on a reflecting substrate, will not allow any of these methods to be applied. Perhaps to some, internal reflection spectroscopy [29] can be applied, but efforts to identify adsorbed proteins with this technique in conjunction with immune detection have not yet been published.

A large amount of our data was obtained with our various methods on two small families of surfaces: 1) glass, anodized tantalum, and oxidized silicon crystal slices, all being wettable and more or less "negatively charged"; and 2) polyvinyl chloride slides, and glass and anodized tantalum slides that had been rubbed with a solution of ferric stearate in petroleum ether, all being nonwettable. Unoxidized silicon crystal slices also behave as if belonging to this group. In our present efforts to combine and interpret all of these data, we

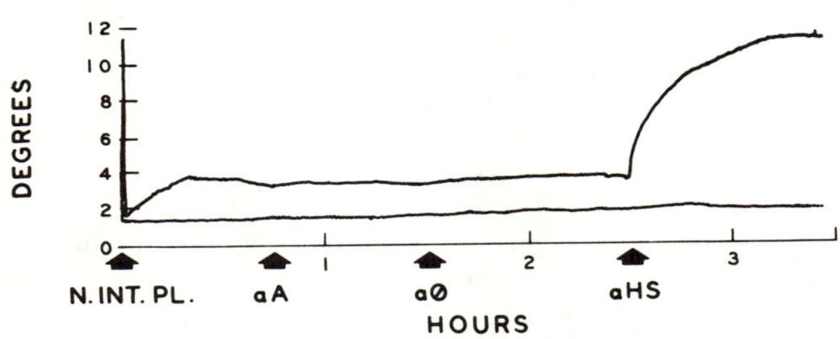

FIGURE 3. Automated ellipsometer recording of azimuth (upper curve) and ellipticity (lower curve); changes are shown in degrees (with arbitrary 0). Substrate: oxidized polished silicon crystal slice. Rectangular cuvette contained 15 ml veronal-buffered saline at 37° C, in light incident at 70°. At "n.int.pl.," 0.1 ml normal intact plasma was added. Note rapid rise of azimuth (returns to 2 to remain on scale). Forty-five min later, at "aA," cuvette contents were replaced 3 × with fresh buffer, and 0.1 ml antiserum was added to human albumin. At aϕ, replacements were followed by antiserum to fibrinogen, and at aHS, by antiserum to whole human serum. Note that only out of the latter, matter was adsorbed, indicating the film contained no albumin and no more fibrinogen, but other proteins.

presume that, e.g., reactions detectable only with the ellipsometer and therefore only on a reflecting surface, will also occur on other surfaces within the family. Also, we will presume that the rapid yet subtle reactions we discovered using ellipsometry and very dilute plasma samples, occur even more rapidly at the interface of the same material with undiluted plasma and blood. We do have some evidence [28] that this presumption is correct.

BEHAVIOR OF NORMAL PLASMA ON NONWETTABLE SURFACES

The following sequence of events takes place.

1. Fibrinogen is deposited by the plasma in less than 2 sec, whether or not the plasma is intact. Some γ-globulins are also adsorbed, possibly adhering to the hydrophobic substrate with their Fab parts. There is evidence

for [30] and some against [31] the belief that the Fab part is more hydrophobic, the Fc part more hydrophilic. Our own finding that the antibody/antigen complex is more wettable than the film of antigen by itself [26] supports this view: on antigen, the antibody would attach itself with its most hydrophobic area (Fab), exposing its more hydrophilic (Fc) "tail" to the liquid. Neither albumin nor activatable factors XII and XI are adsorbed out of plasma. (However, Teflon does adsorb albumin.)

2. Very slowly, the fibrinogen deposited on the hydrophobic surface is modified ("converted") by the plasma, if the plasma is intact. Fibrinogen film that had been formed at the plasma/air interface and "printed out" onto the hydrophobic substrate by the advancing plasma cannot be converted. Under conversion of an adsorbed protein film, we classify any loss of activity or antigenicity of the film without significant change in its thickness. It may be caused by distortion or by displacement of the entire protein by another. Very little adsorbed γ-globulin is converted on the hydrophobic substrate by plasma. Activated plasma converts neither fibrinogen nor globulin films.

Behavior of Normal Plasma on Glass-like Surfaces

The following sequence of events takes place.

1. Fibrinogen, some γ-globulin, and factor XII are all adsorbed in less than 2 seconds. (The consequences of factor XII adsorption will be described by others.) There seems to be no mutual interference or evidence of competition between fibrinogen and factor XII in plasma for the available surface.[8] No albumin is deposited.
2. The intact plasma that had deposited the fibrinogen within 2 sec converts it completely at room temperature or at 37° C within about 20 sec on glass and on oxidized silicon crystal slices, and within a few minutes on anodized tantalum. Conversion by activated plasma is slower. A factor other than factor XII or XI—perhaps kallikreinogen—may be required. Conversion of the fibrinogen film is followed by some removal of matter if intact factor XII is present; this process is relatively slow.
   On oxidized silicon crystal slices preexposed to γ-globulins, the ellipsometer shows that plasma deposits matter; then, if intact factor XII was present either in this added deposit or in the plasma, removal of the deposit and/or some of the underlying globulin follows.[6, 14]
   Where fibrinogen, rather than globulin, is preadsorbed onto oxidized silicon crystal slices, or onto glass, and is then exposed to plasma, it undergoes the same changes as does the fibrinogen deposited by plasma itself; on anodized tantalum, conversion of preadsorbed fibrinogen occurs more slowly even than of the fibrinogen deposited by plasma.

Behavior of Platelets in Normal Plasma or Blood at Nonwettable versus Wettable Surfaces

The possibility that platelets are transferred from the air/blood to the blood/hydrophobic solid interfaces along with fibrinogen film was described above. Out of suspension, platelets adhere on the fibrinogen that is already deposited by the plasma around them well before the platelets can "see" the solid surfaces. Platelets arriving minutes later will still find unconverted fibrinogen to adhere to, since on the hydrophobic surfaces, conversion is delayed. On a glass-like, wettable surface this period of fibrinogen availability is much shorter. If platelets do adhere even after fibrinogen film has been converted, maybe they do so by some other mechanism, such as the release of matter by the adhering platelets, that causes other platelets to stick to them. This mechanism will be described by others. Paradoxically, platelets in intact whole blood or plasma will adhere more to "bare" glass—where the surrounding plasma has just deposited fibrinogen—than where we had preadsorbed fibrinogen: the latter can be converted by the plasma before platelets land on it.

Under our experimental conditions, such as exposure of surfaces to blood for no more than about one hour, and with a minimum of flow, platelets do not adhere to a wettable or nonwettable surface that had been preexposed to albumin.[32] Others, using controlled flow, found that they adhere after some delay.[33]

Behavior of Granulocytes in Normal Plasma or Blood

Under the conditions of our experiments, very few lymphocytes ever adhere either to wettable or to nonwettable surfaces, but granulocytes do. Quite recently,[12] we found very large numbers of neutrophils adhering and spreading where gamma globulin had been adsorbed from solution (fraction II) onto hydrophobic surfaces. Adsorbed onto hydrophilic ones, the globulins had no such effect.

Quite preliminary data indicate that normal intact plasma, resting briefly on glass or polyvinyl chloride, leaves a deposit that will cause granulocytes in heparinized blood to adhere; but where the plasma has remained for 60 minutes on glass (rather than on the nonwettable plastic), fewer granulocytes adhere than on the "bare" glass.

This relationship of granulocytes toward preadsorbed globulins and perhaps toward the globulin deposited by the surrounding plasma itself seems to parallel that of platelets toward fibrinogen. Possibly even the ability of intact plasma to convert its own deposit of globulin on glass-like surfaces parallels the fate of its fibrinogen and serves to render the adsorbed globulin only briefly available to the granulocytes for their adhesion, with the difference that the availability of deposited fibrinogen to platelets does not last as long. Also, like platelets, white cells suspended in buffer instead of plasma behave differently. When we list these qualitative results (FIGURE 4), the variability of effects on platelet and granulocyte adhesion is most striking: wettability of the substrate, nature of the preadsorbed protein, and of the suspending medium, all have profound influences. Clearly, too, platelet and granulocyte adhesion appear not to be caused by identical events. A parallel experiment to suspending platelets in a fibrinogen-free medium such as serum would be the suspension of granulocytes in a globulin-free plasma. At present, other studies are being carried out to discover how adsorbed γ-globulins are oriented. We can combine the fact that the granulocyte membrane carries Fc receptors[34] that cause adhesion to the Fc part of globulin, and our finding that granulocytes adhere to γ-globulin adsorbed onto hydrophobic rather than hydrophilic surfaces, as well as at least some of our findings indicating that antibody adhering upon an adsorbed film of antigen renders it more wettable. This set of notes suggests that granulocytes adhere to γ-globulin on nonwettable surfaces because the molecule attaches itself to the solid with its Fab portion and exposes its Fc portion to the liquid containing the white cells. Under these conditions, with the orientation of the globulin mimicking its orientation in immune reactions, complement and kallikreinogen may also become involved. (See also FIGURE 1.)

The predominance of granulocytes as the formed elements adhering during

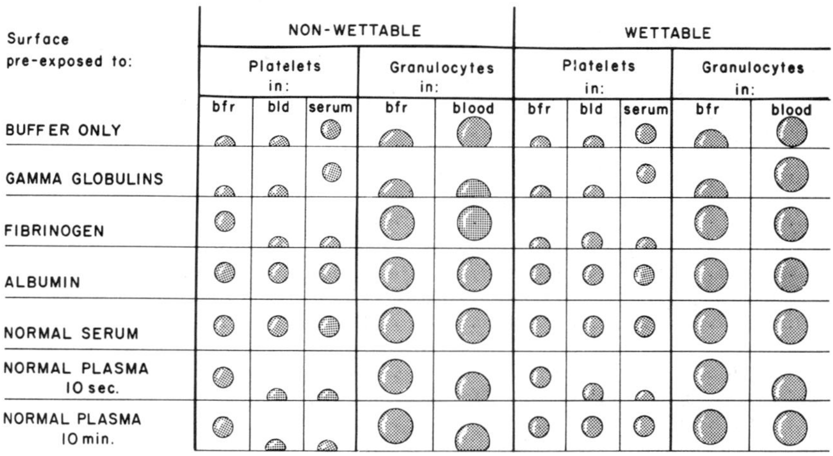

FIGURE 4. Effect of substrate wettability and of its protein covering, and effect of suspending medium, upon adhesion of platelets and granulocytes. Wettable surfaces: glass, and anodized tantalum-sputtered glass. Nonwettable surfaces: the same, but rubbed with ferric stearate in petroleum ether; and clean polyvinylchloride slides. Substrates were exposed to solutions of 8 mg γ-globulin (fraction II), 3 mg fibrinogen or 20 mg albumin/ml Veronal buffered saline (VS), or to serum or citrated plasma (left-hand column). All were rinsed with VS afterwards and covered with one of the following: columns marked "bfr": supernatant (containing platelets and white cells) collected from settled blood taken into EDTA; formed elements washed 3 times with VS and resuspended in VS; columns marked "serum": as above, but formed elements resuspended in serum; columns marked "bld" and "blood": blood collected in heparin (Becton-Dickinson, Rutherford, N.J., 4783 lot 815B 216) and, without further manipulation, used about 30 min to two hr after collection. After 30 min in moist chamber at room temperature, all slides were rinsed with VS and fixed with glutaraldehyde. Numbers of formed elements adhering are indicated by degree of contact (ranging from none, up to squatting).

hemodialysis to the device's membranes is now well known.[35, 36] The activation of kallikrein in situ [37] may be responsible, but there is a rich variety of shape and configuration to be found on the various parts of dialyzers, drip chambers, filters and tubing after use, with groups of leukocytes looking like webs of granulated starbursts in one area, like dense hairy bodies, or schools of spread discs elsewhere.[38] More than a few factors must govern this diversity of granulocyte/interface reactions.

Relationship of these Findings to *In Vivo* Events

We have so far investigated small numbers of samples of a large number of biomaterials. There seems to be a broad spectrum of material/plasma/blood interactions displayed when carefully observed *in vitro* that must be correlated with the necessarily rather gross observations obtained after prolonged implantation. We must presume no two materials fail or succeed in identical ways. We are distant giants to our own blood cells; to say that all thrombi look alike is like saying all foreigners do. It has been stated [39] that a well-designed artificial heart may perform well *in vivo* no matter what material it is made of. If sufficient evidence can ever be collected for statistical proof, our blood must have the ability to modify the surface of each material in the highly varied ways of behavior we are discovering, and render each compatible with blood in its own way. Such extremely "forgiving" behavior of blood would in itself be worth studying.

References

1. Mason, R. G., D. E. Scarborough, S. R. Saba, K. M. Brinkhous, L. D. Ikenberry, J. J. Kearney & H. G. Clark. 1969. Thrombogenicity of some biomedical materials: platelet-interface reactions. J. Biomed. Mater. Res. **3:** 615.
2. Mason, R. G. 1972. Some methods for *in vitro* estimation of the blood compatibility of biomaterials. Bull. New York Acad. Med. **48:** 407.
3. Petchek, H. E., A. R. Kantrowitz & D. Adamis. 1967. Effect of flow on thrombus formation. Proc. Ann. Conf. Engin. Med. Biol. **9:** 19.6.
4. Dutton, R. C., R. E. Baier, R. L. Dedrick & R. L. Bowman. 1968. Initial thrombus formation on foreign surfaces. Trans. Amer. Soc. Artif. Intern. Organs **14:** 57.
5. Mustard, J. F., D. W. Perry, R. L. Kinlough-Rathbone & M. A. Packham. 1975. Factors responsible for ADP-induced release reaction of human platelets. Amer. J. Physiol. **228:** 1757.
6. Vroman, L. & A. L. Adams. 1969. Identification of rapid changes at plasma-solid interfaces. J. Biomed. Mater. Res. **3:** 43.
7. Klings, M., A. L. Adams & L. Vroman. 1972. Effects of protamine sulfate, polybrene and heparin on the behavior of plasma, plasma proteins, platelets and factor XII activity at interfaces. Thromb. Res. **1:** 507.
8. Vroman, L. & A. L. Adams. 1971. Peculiar behavior of blood at solid interfaces. J. Polymer Sci. **34:** 159.
9. Mohammad, S. F., M. D. Hardison, C. H. Glenn, B. D. Morton, J. C. Bolan & R. G. Mason. 1975. Adhesion of human blood platelets to glass and polymer surfaces. I. Studies with platelets in plasma. Haemostasis **3:** 257.
10. Zucker, M. B. & L. Vroman. 1969. Platelet adhesion induced by fibrinogen adsorbed onto glass. Proc. Soc. Exp. Biol. Med. **131:** 320.
11. Packham, M. A., G. Evans, M. F. Glynn & J. F. Mustard. 1969. The effect of plasma proteins on the interaction of platelets with glass surfaces. J. Lab. Clin. Med. **73:** 686.
12. Vroman, L., A. L. Adams & G. C. Fischer. To be published.
13. Brash, J. L. & D. J. Lyman. 1969. Adsorption of plasma proteins in solution to uncharged hydrophobic polymer surfaces. J. Biomed. Mater. Res. **3:** 175.
14. Vroman, L., A. Adams, M. Klings & G. Fischer. 1975. Fibrinogen, globulins, albumin and plasma at interfaces. Adv. Chem. Series **145:** 255.
15. Leininger, R. I., C. W. Cooper, R. D. Falb & G. A. Grode. 1966. Nonthrombogenic plastic surfaces. Science **152:** 1625.

16. WEATHERSBY, P. K., T. KOLOBOW & E. W. STOOL. 1975. Relative thrombogenicity of polydimethylsiloxane and silicone rubber constituents. J. Biomed. Mater. Res. **9:** 561.
17. BAIER, R. E., V. A. DEPALMA, A. FURUSE, V. L. GOTT, G. W. KAMMLOTT, T. LUCAS, P. N. SAWYER, S. SRINIVASAN & B. STANCZEWSKI. 1975. Thromboresistance of glass after glow discharge treatment in argon. J. Biomed. Mater. Res. **9:** 457.
18. SCHWARTZ, A., K. H. STENZEL, I. KOHNO, D. AST, T. MIYATA & A. L. RUBIN. 1975. Deposition of blood cells on collagen and cuprophane membranes. J. Biomed. Mater. Res. **9:** 453.
19. KAPLAN, A. P., A. B. KAY & F. AUSTEN. 1972. A Prealbumin activator of prekallikrein. III. Appearance of chemotactic activity for human neutrophils by the conversion of human prekallikrein to kallikrein. J. Exp. Med. **135:** 81.
20. WEISS, A. S., J. I. GALLIN & A. P. KAPLAN. 1974. A diminished rate of Hageman factor activation caused by absence of prekallikrein with abnormalities of coagulation, fibrinolysis, chemotactic activity, and kinin generation. J. Clin. Invest. **53:** 622.
21. WEKSLER, B. B. 1974. The platelet in inflammation: Interaction with complement to promote chemotaxis. *In* Platelets: Production, Function, Transfusion, and Storage. M. G. Baldini & S. Ebbe, Eds. : 277. Grune & Stratton. New York, N.Y.
22. SHIRASAWA, K. & A. B. CHANDLER. 1971. Phagocytosis of platelets by leukocytes in artificial thrombi and in platelet aggregates induced by adenosine diphosphate. Amer. J. Pathol. **63:** 215.
23. RATNOFF, O. D. 1971. A tangled web. The interdependence of mechanisms of blood clotting, fibrinolysis, immunity and inflammation. Thromb. Diathes. Haemorrh. Suppl. **45:** 109.
24. VROMAN, L., A. ADAMS, M. KLINGS & G. FISCHER. 1975. Blood and air. *In* Blood Bubble Interaction in Decompression Sickness. DCIEM Conf. Proc. 73–CP–960. Defence and Civil Inst. of Environmental Med. K. N. Ackles, Ed.
25. LYMAN, D. J., D. G. KLEIN, J. L. BRASH & B. K. FRITZINGER. 1970. The interaction of platelets with polymer surfaces I. Uncharged hydrophobic polymer surfaces. Thromb. Diath. Haemorrh. **23:** 120.
26. ADAMS, A. L., M. KLINGS, G. C. FISCHER & L. VROMAN. 1973. Three simple ways to detect antibody—antigen complex on flat surfaces. J. Immunol. Meth. **3:** 227.
27. VROMAN, L. 1964. Effects of hydrophobic surfaces upon blood coagulation. Thromb. Diath. Haemorrh. **10:** 455.
28. VROMAN, L. & A. L. ADAMS. 1969. Findings with the recording ellipsometer suggesting rapid exchange of specific plasma proteins at liquid/solid interfaces. Surface Sci. **16:** 438–446.
29. BAIER, R. E. 1975. Applied chemistry at protein interfaces. *In* Applied Chemistry at Protein Interfaces, Advances in Chemistry Series. R. E. Baier, Ed. **145:** 1. Amer. Chem. Soc. Washington, D.C.
30. KABAT, E. A. 1968. Structural Concepts in Immunology and Immunochemistry. Holt, Rinehart and Winston, Inc. New York, N.Y.
31. VAN OSS, C. J., C. F. GILLMAN & A. W. NEUMANN. 1975. Phagocytic engulfment and cell adhesiveness as cellular surface phenomena. Marcel Dekker, Inc. New York, N.Y.
32. VROMAN, L., A. L. ADAMS & M. KLINGS. 1971. Interactions among human blood proteins at interfaces. Fed. Proc. **30:** 1494.
33. FRIEDMAN, L. I., H. LIEM, E. F. GRABOWSKI, E. F. LEONARD & C. W. MCCORD. 1970. Inconsequentiality of surface properties for initial platelet adhesion. Amer. Soc. Artif. Intern. Org. **16:** 63.
34. ISHIZAKA, K., H. TOMIOKA & T. ISHIZAKA. 1970. Mechanisms of passive sensitization. I. Presence of IgE and IgG molecules on human leukocytes. J. Immunol. **105:** 1459.

35. Brubaker, L. H. & K. D. Nolph. 1971. Mechanisms of recovery from neutropenia induced by hemodialysis. Blood **38:** 623.
36. Marschall, J. W., D. J. Ahearn, R. J. Nothum, J. Esterly, K. D. Nolph & J. F. Maher. 1974. Adherence of blood components to dialyzer membranes; morphological studies. Nephron **12** :157.
37. Wardle, E. N. & D. A. Piercy. 1972. Studies of contact activation of blood in haemodialysis. J. Clin. Pathol. **25:** 1045.
38. Klings, M. Morphology of formed element distribution on various hemodialyzers and associated blood/interface areas after normal use. To be published.
39. Kolff, W. J. 1976. Personal communication.

ELLIPSOMETRIC STUDY OF PROTEIN FILM ON CHROMIUM

P. A. Cuypers, W. T. Hermens, and H. C. Hemker

Department of Biophysics
Biomedical Centre
State University Limburg
Maastricht, The Netherlands

Introduction

The ellipsometer is an optical instrument that measures thickness and refractive index of thin transparent layers deposited on a reflecting surface. When a polarized light beam is reflected on such a surface the polarization state of the light (i.e., azimuth and ellipticity) change. These changes are measured by the changes of the analyzer and polarizer position. It is possible to calculate the thickness and refractive index of the transparant layer from these measurements. We developed an automatized ellipsometer suitable for the monitoring of the adsorption and interaction of proteins and lipids at interphases.

Instrument

We modified a Rudolph ellipsometer, type 43303–200 E. The instrument is automatized by computer-steered stepping motors on the analyzer and polarizer. The program steers these motors in such a way as to find the analyzer and polarizer positions at which light transmission is minimal. The minimalization procedure is based on the fact that the light intensity not too far from the minimum is a parabolic function of both the polarizer and analyzer angular displacement. The procedure consists of finding the analyzer position giving minimal tight transmission at fixed polarizer position; then the analyzer is fixed and the polarizer changed, and so on. This procedure continuously follows changes of the minimum up to a velocity of about 1.5 degree per second. The changes observed in actual experiments do not exceed 0.2 degree per second. By this method of automatization we can measure one position every two or three seconds. The accuracy and reproducibility is within 0.01 of a degree. The complete description of the apparatus and the method we use is given in References 1 and 2.

Calculation Technique

To interprete analyzer and polarizer positions in terms of thickness (d) and refractive index (n), we made computer simulation graphs of the theoretical dependence of analyzer and polarizer of n and d of a growing layer at the prevailing wavelength (632.8 nm), angle of incidence (68), refractive index of the medium (1.3335), and optical parameters of the reflecting surface (calculated from initial analyzer and polarizer positions). By plotting the experimental behavior of analyzer and polarizer (Δ, ψ) in the same graph, we could read the thickness and refractive index of the growing layer in the experiment. The technique was checked by using it in measuring a series of barium stearate layers of known n and d. From 1 to 50 layers (i.e., d 28–1400 Å at n = 1.48) the experimental and theoretical behavior coincided to within about 3%.

Materials

As a reflecting surface we used chromium-sputtered glass slides manufactured by Stabilix, The Hague, Holland.

Human fibrinogen (lyophilized, grade L) was obtained from Kabi A.B., Stockholm, Sweden. Antifibrinogen (precipitating antiserum Batch KH18–05–PO_2) was obtained from Centraal Labratorium Bloedtransfusiedienst van het Nederlandse Rode Kruis, Amsterdam, Holland. Serum was obtained from normal human blood by clotting for two hours and centrifugation during 30 min at 12,000 × *g*.

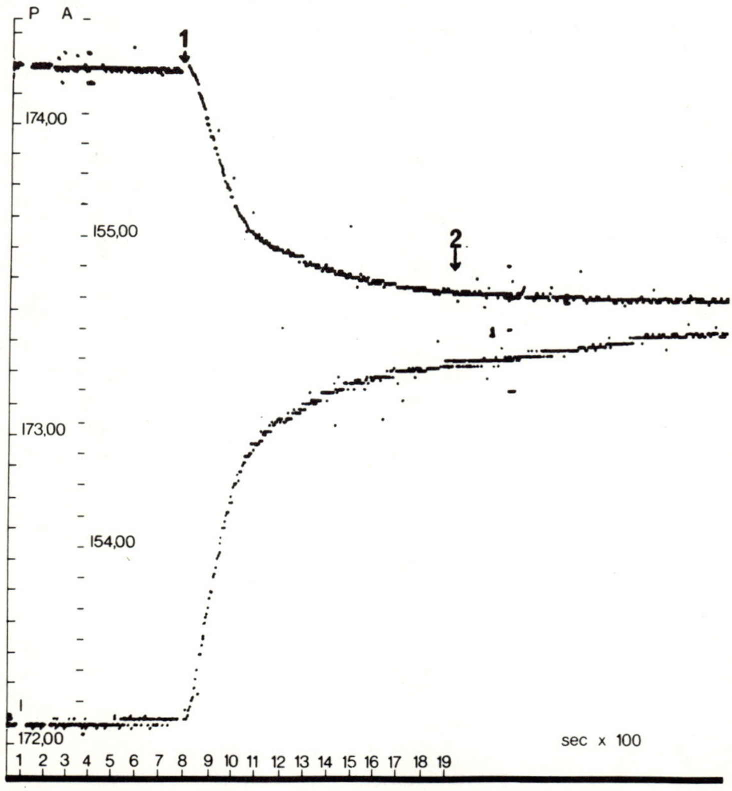

FIGURE 1. Fibrinogen adsorption. Hard copy of the memory scope recording of the change in analyzer and polarizer after two additions[1,2] of 100 μl of fibrinogen 1 mg/ml. Surface: chromium oxide n = 2,7525–2,6544 i.

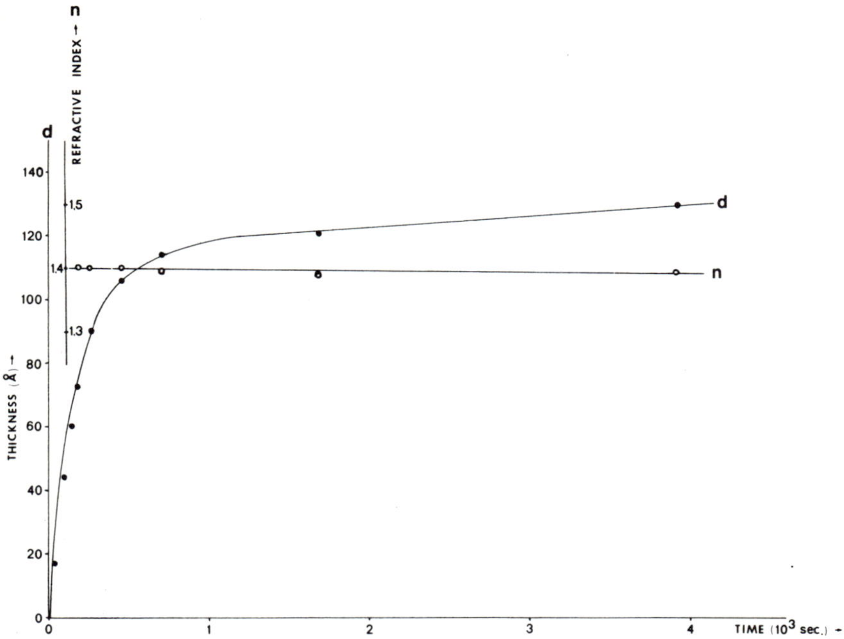

FIGURE 2. Behavior of thickness and refractive index as a function of time during the adsorption of fibrinogen (10 μg/ml) in 0.01 M Tris-HCl buffer pH 7.0 onto a chromium oxide (hydrophilic) surface.

RESULTS

Adsorption of Fibrinogen on a Hydrophilic Chromium Surface

The chromium-sputtered glass slides which are hydrophobic can be made hydrophilic by treatment with hot chromic acid. In this way a polar chromic oxide layer is formed that binds water. The cuvet was filled with buffer (Tris-HCl 0.01 M pH 7.4) and the slides were measured in two different zones to determine their initial optical properties. After about 800 seconds, 0.1 mg of fibrinogen was added (100 μl of a mg/ml solution). After this addition the polarizer (Δ) and analyzer (ψ) changes are recorded in time (FIGURE 1). After the moment of addition the polarizer and analyzer change rather rapidly, and an end level is reached after about 600 seconds for both analyzer and polarizer. Further addition of fibrinogen does not cause any further changes.

The calculated behavior of n and d as a function of time is given in FIGURE 2. This figure shows that the refractive index does not change much during the adsorption. The thickness follows the saturation behavior of a monolayer adsorption (type 1 of Winterbottom [3]). After about 4000 seconds the thickness stabilizes about 130 Å. The refractive index then is 1.38.

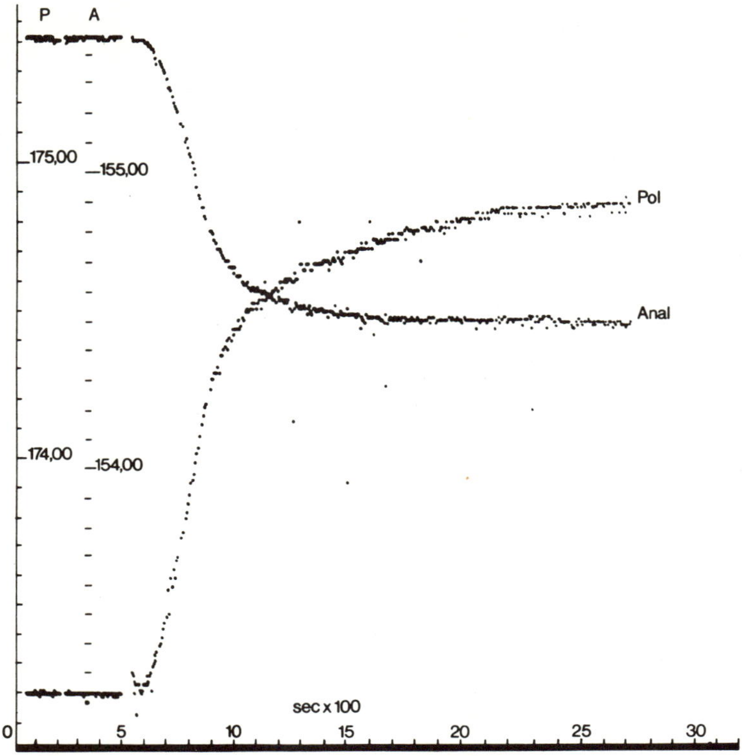

FIGURE 3. Fibrinogen adsorption of hydrophobic chromium.

Hydrophobic Chromium Surface

The adsorption of fibrinogen on chromium which is hydrophobic is done under the same experimental conditions as the foregoing experiment. The adsorption behavior of analyzer and polarizer are shown in FIGURE 3. In this graph one immediately observes that at 1600 seconds the analyzer does not change any more, whereas the polarizer is not yet stable. This indicates that processes other than adsorption of a layer of constant refractive index must be going on.

During the first 150 seconds, the thickness grows at constant refractive index n = 1.8. Then the refractive index lowers and the thickness still increases. The thickness grows up to about 68 Å, while the refractive index lowers to about 1.5. From this point on, the layer gets thinner and optically denser. The layer stabilizes at d = 35 Å and n = 1.8 (FIGURE 4).

CONCLUSIONS

The difference in character of adsorption on hydrophobic and hydrophilic surfaces depends upon the interaction of the protein and the surface. The interaction with hydrophobic surfaces is much stronger than with hydrophilic ones. This is to be expected, since a hydrophilic surface resembles to a certain extent the natural surroundings of a protein in solution. Our explanation of the adsorption behavior is as follows: The first fibrinogen molecules adsorb onto the surface with the whole length of the molecules fixed to the surface. This gives a thin layer that is optically very thick, so we have a high refractive index. After some time the surface is partly covered, and it is no longer possible for the molecule to attach to the surface directly over its whole length. Thus, we get a layer of random-orientated fibrinogen molecules partly attached to the surface. This results in a thick layer which is loosely packed, i.e., a layer with a high water content and a low refractive index. These random-oriented molecules reorientate, giving a layer that is closely packed with a high refractive index and a thickness of about 40 Å. This thickness may indicate a layer of one denaturated molecule if we accept the dimensions of the molecule being 375–450 Å in length and with a mean traverse diameter of 60–90.

Fibrinogen-Antifibrinogen Interaction

In the study of these interactions we used the same experimental conditions and surfaces as described in the foregoing experiment. We first adsorbed the fibrinogen. When the analyzer and polarizer did not change any further, the content of the cuvet was washed twice with new buffer. Because the polarizer

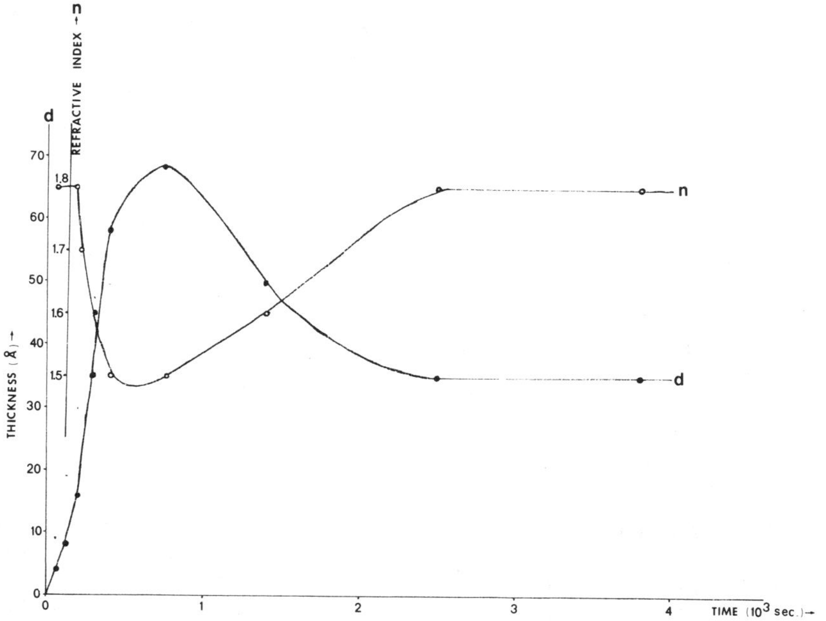

FIGURE 4. Behavior of thickness and refractive index as a function of time during the adsorption of fibrinogen (10 μg/ml) in 0.01 M Tris HCl buffer pH 7.0 onto a chromium oxide (hydrophobic) surface.

and analyzer did not change during this washing, the fibrinogen layer remained unchanged on the chromium. After this washing the antifibrinogen was added and the polarizer and analyzer started to change (FIGURE 5). The thickness and refractive index, calculated as shown before, are given in FIGURE 6. In this figure we see a thickness of the fibrinogen of 100 Å at a refractive index of 1.40. The addition of antifibrinogen gives a change in thickness of about 400 Å, with a refractive index of 1.366.

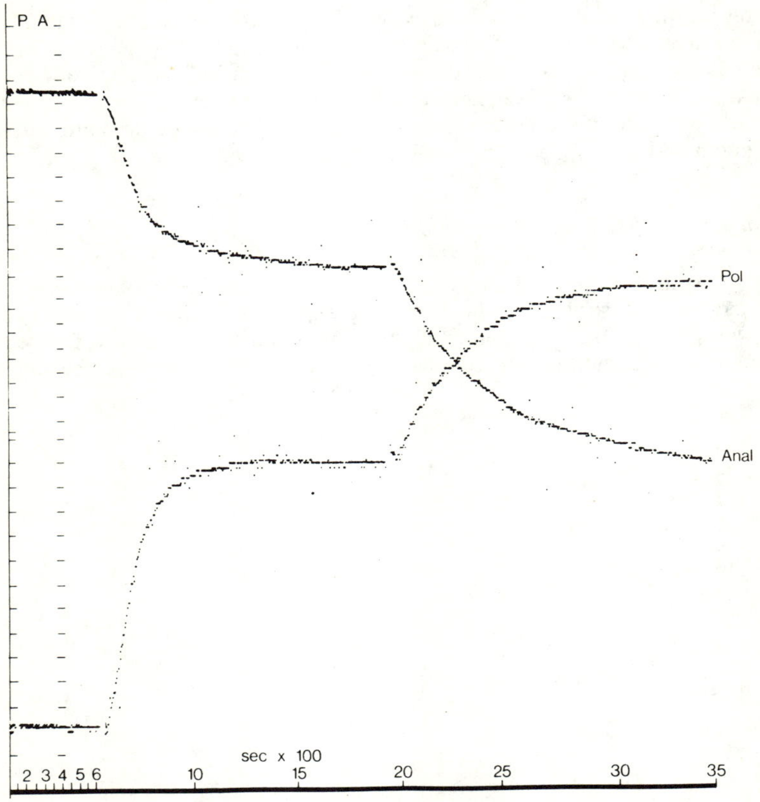

FIGURE 5. Fibrinogen-antifibrinogen interaction.

Displacement of Serum Proteins by Fibrinogen on a Chromium Surface

The serum protein was added to a final concentration in the cuvet of 10 μg/ml. After the adsorption of serum, the fibrinogen was added. In FIGURE 7 we see the changes in polarizer and analyzer. FIGURE 8 shows the thickness and refractive index as a function of time. Addition of serum gives an adsorption of about d = 180 Å and n = 1.36. After refreshing the contents of the cuvet, the optical constants remain the same. Addition of fibrinogen causes a change in polarizer and analyzer (FIGURE 7) that must be interpreted (FIGURE 8) as a

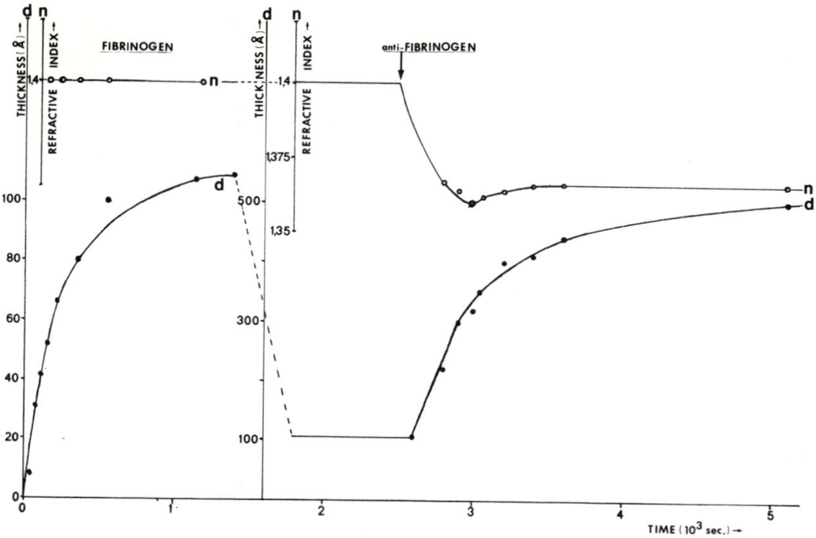

FIGURE 6. Fibrinogen-antifibrinogen interaction.

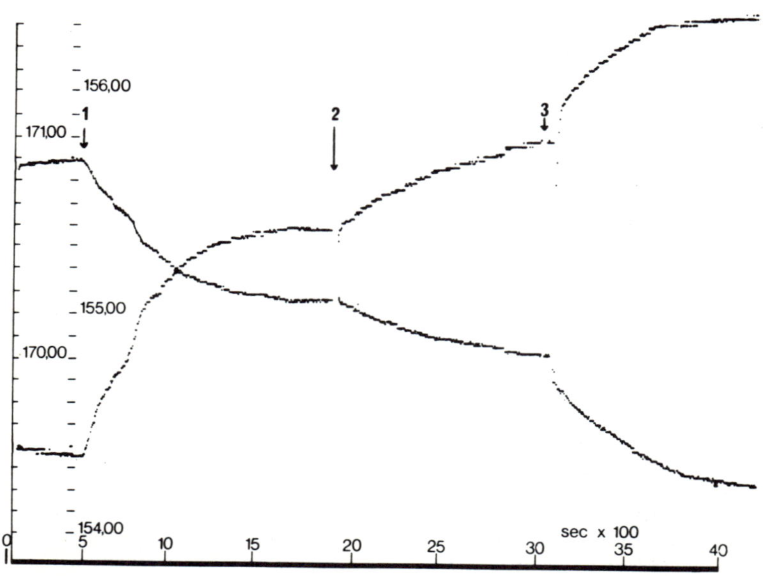

FIGURE 7. Displacement of serum proteins by fibrinogen. 1) Addition of serum proteins, final concentration=10 μg/ml; 2) addition of fibrinogen, final concentration=10 μg/ml; 3) addition of antifibrinogen.

change in the refractive index only. After washing, addition of antifibrinogen causes a large change in thickness. This indicates that fibrinogen replaced the adsorbed serum proteins. This is further supported by the observation that antifibrinogen does not interact with the adsorbed serum proteins (first layer) and anti-whole serum does not interact with the layer generated after addition of fibrinogen (second layer).

The same type of experiments have been done with an ellipsometer in which the transmitted light is recorded.[4-7] In principle, the same conclusion applied. Our observations extend these results in that (1) interpretation is no longer dependent upon the assumption of a constant refractive index of the adsorbed layer (which indeed, as we and others show, is not correct,[8-9] and (2) we give a determination of the thickness of the layers involved.

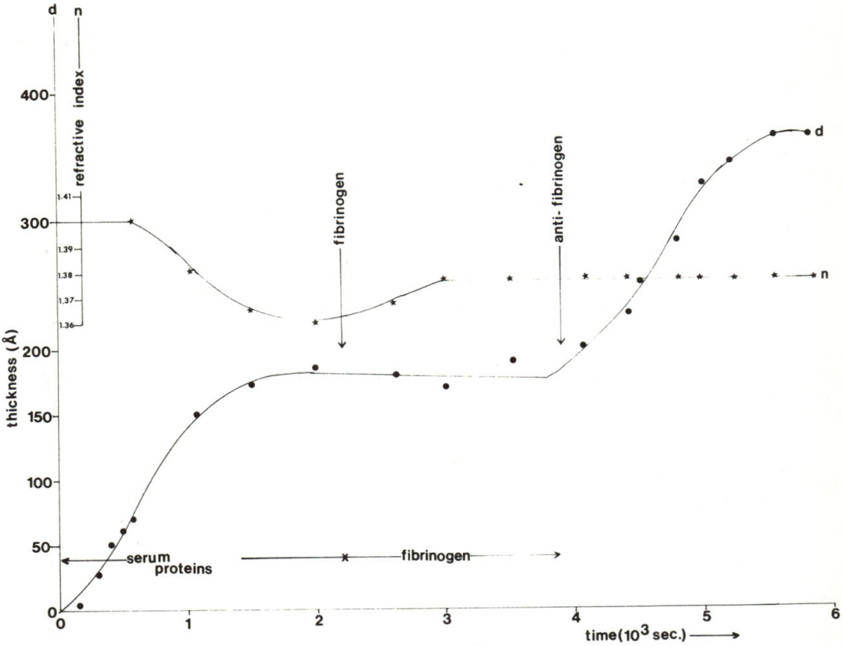

FIGURE 8. Displacement of serum proteins by fibrinogen.

REFERENCES

1. CUYPERS, P. A. 1976. Dynamic ellipsometry, biochemical and biomedical applications. Ph.D. thesis. State University Limburg. Maastricht, The Netherlands. (Available upon request.)
2. CUYPERS, P. A., W. T. HERMENS & H. C. HEMKER. Dynamic ellipsometry, biochemical and biomedical applications. Anal. Biochem. Submitted for publication.
3. WINTERBOTTOM, A. B. 1946. Trans. Faraday Soc. **41:** 487–501.
4. VROMAN, L. 1964. Thromb. Diathes. Haemorrh. **10:** 455–493.
5. VROMAN, L. 1962. Nature **196:** 476–477.

6. VROMAN, L. & A. L. ADAMS. 1967. Thromb. Diathes. Haemorrh. **18:** 510–524.
7. ZUCKER, M. B. & L. VROMAN. 1969. Proc. Soc. Exp. Biol. Med. **131:** 318–320.
8. POSTE, L. & C. MOSS. 1972. The study of surface reactions in biological systems by ellipsometry. Progress in Surface Science. Vol. II, part 3. Pergamon Press. New York, N.Y.
9. FENSTERMAKER, C. A., W. H. GRANT, B. W. MORRISSEY, L. E. SMITH & R. R. STROMBERG. 1974. Interaction of plasma proteins with surfaces. Natl. Bureau of Standards, Washington, D.C. N.B.S.I.R. : 74–470.

DISCUSSION

DR. NYILAS: Adsorbed proteins will never see the original surface, because each of those proteins has a hydration shell of bound water; through that cloud of water, a protein molecule will interact with the metal surface.

DR. HOFFMAN: We have seen some unusual reversals of adsorption of fibrinogen from isotonic buffered saline solutions versus that from plasma. Do any of the speakers know if there is something special about fibrinogen? Also, what plasma factors might get to the surface before fibrinogen and might mediate its adsorption on surfaces?

DR. MORRISSEY: Fibrinogen is indeed somewhat different from other plasma proteins. It is a very effective flocculating agent. It destabilizes colloidal suspensions, maybe because it is a long rodlike molecule; it does behave differently from globular proteins when they adsorb. Many other molecules adsorb more quickly. From our early data, prothrombin adsorbed at the same equimolar concentration as fibrinogen onto silica to its plateau seven or eight times more rapidly. Fibrinogen does, however, have a large molecular weight and a high affinity for the surface, and, as the data shown by Dr. Cuypers indicate, fibrinogen can displace albumin from the surface. We have similar data, and I know Dr. Vroman does also.

DR. VROMAN: I think reversibility of fibrinogen adsorption is very complex, being slower, for example, on hydrophobic than on wettable surfaces, and one intact clotting factor may be involved in its conversion, while another is involved in removal of the product.

DR. SILBERBERG: Dr. Cuypers' data do suggest that the physical state of the surface would be of very much importance to the behavior of the fibrinogen adsorbed.

DR. CUYPERS: When adsorption of fibrinogen onto a hydrophobic surface has stabilized, on a dense layer there will be a less dense one, some of which will be removed.

DR. M. FROJMOVIC (*McGill University, Montreal, Canada*): I was wondering whether there are any differences between exposing blood or plasma in air to surfaces and going to great pains not to have air exposure.

DR. VROMAN: We have studied this problem in connection with a meeting on decompression sickness where gas bubbles form in the blood. Fibrinogen may be adsorbed at this gas interface; platelets may adhere and even migrate to this film. At a hydrophobic surface Langmuir—Blodgett transfer occurs; the fatty skin of the drop is rolled out on the fatty surface and sticks there, causing a great loss of platelets, especially at air/hydrophobic surfaces. Very wettable surfaces, I think, are always wet; it has been shown that they always have some water on them, and I don't think this transfer happens so easily on them, but even there, air interfaces may do harm.

DR. MORRISSEY: In some recent work, Grant, Stromberg, and Smith of the Bureau of Standards used radio tracer techniques to study competitive adsorption; they tested the effect of overflow techniques versus direct withdrawal of the substrate from the adsorbing solution. If the substrate is wetted by the medium, then there is indeed no difference, and the gas/liquid interface presents no problem. When it's hydrophobic and not wetted, you have to worry. But when you expose a hydrophobic polymer to a protein, the adsorbed protein makes the surface hydrophilic, so one can generally avoid the problem.

DR. P. N. SAWYER: Would any of the speakers care to speculate on the relationship of their presentations this morning to the real world of thrombogenesis?

DR. VROMAN: At the end of this conference I think we will all decide whether or not any of it is meaningful.

DR. MORRISSEY: I think blood is certainly a complex tissue; unless you attempt to unravel some of the interactions into some of its components and study the interaction of those components, you will never carry out a synthesis to describe the behavior of the whole system. Over the last three years or so, some important relations between the physical chemical surface properties of these proteins, lipoproteins or lipids, which are being studied, and their interaction with formed cellular elements, which we feel is closer to thrombogenicity of the surface, will be explored. At present we know that there are a number of enzymes whose enzymatic activity can increase by a factor of fifty upon interaction with a surface.

DR. STEWART: Fibrinogen is the only protein in the plasma that, when minimally modified by enzyme action or modified by the charged groups, will undergo polymerization. Simply adding protamine sulfate causes a limited polymerization. Altering only one molecule, such as by adsorption, may cause it to complex with various other fibrinogen molecules; this may be very important in the real world.

PART III. INTERFACE-INTRODUCED COAGULATION REACTIONS

COAGULATION FACTORS AND THE ROLE OF SURFACE IN THEIR ACTIVATION *

Oscar D. Ratnoff † and Hidehiko Saito

Department of Medicine
Case Western Reserve University School of Medicine
University Hospitals of Cleveland
Cleveland, Ohio 44106

A critical moment in the development of knowledge concerning mammalian blood coagulation was the observation of Bordet and Gengou [1] that the clot-promoting property of glass was exerted, at least in part, by an action upon cell-poor plasma. Over the years, many attempts were made to localize the effect of glass to one or another component of plasma. Borrowing methods that had been developed by Margolis [2] and by Shafrir and deVries,[3] we were able to demonstrate that the clot-promoting effect of glass was related to an action upon Hageman factor (factor XII), an agent deficient in the plasma of an asymptomatic individual, Mr. John Hageman.[4, 5]

Since then, a large number of insoluble agents have been discovered that appear to initiate the clotting process through an action upon Hageman factor, including, for example, kaolin, diatomaceous earth, and talc.[6] All of these substances have the property of adsorbing Hageman factor from plasma. After suitable washing, these solids with their adsorbed Hageman factor can then correct the defective clotting of individuals deficient in Hageman factor, as if the adsorbed Hageman factor had been converted from an inert to an activated form.

How the activation of Hageman factor comes about is only partially understood. Hubbard and Lucas [7] demonstrated that a wide variety of substances that initiated coagulation bore, on their surfaces, a negative ionic charge. A reasonable assumption, then, is that such substances activate Hageman factor by reacting in some unknown way with amino acid residues of the Hageman factor molecule that are positively charged. Analysis of purified preparations of human Hageman factor demonstrate that each molecule contains approximately 27 arginine, 23 lysine, and 23 histidine residues,[8] any of which might be affected by negative charges. Takahashi [9] reported that under appropriately mild conditions, phenylglyoxal hydrate would react specifically with arginine residues. Using his conditions, we found that this compound would so alter Hageman factor that it could no longer be activated by kaolin. If the Hageman factor had first been adsorbed to kaolin, however, this inhibitory property of phenylglyoxal hydrate was no longer manifest.[10] These experiments do not tell us the way in which clot-promoting surfaces activate Hageman factor, nor even if these residues are the only sites upon which charged surfaces act, but they do suggest a rational basis for further studies.

* Supported by grant HL 01661 from the National Heart and Lung Institute, the National Institutes of Health, USPHS, and in part by grants from the American Heart Association, and the Northeast Ohio Affiliate of the American Heart Association.

† Career investigator of the American Heart Association.

We are more in the dark concerning the nature of the alteration in the Hageman factor molecule brought about by negatively charged surfaces that allows this agent to exert its biological effects. Vroman [11] and Margolis [12] suggested that activation of Hageman factor reflected a conformational change in its molecule that might make it more hydrophobic than in its native state. An early experiment of Donaldson [13] seemed to be in agreement with this view. Her preparations of Hageman factor had a sedimentation constant of 5.0 and an apparent molecular weight of about 80,000, as determined by Sephadex gel filtration. In contrast, Hageman factor, activated in a variety of ways, sedimented to the bottom of sucrose gradient tubes and was excluded from columns of Sephadex G–200. One possible explanation for this change in Hageman factor, which we have been able to confirm once again, is that the molecules of Hageman factor are so altered by activation that they have become more hydrophobic, as had been predicted. Alternatively, activated Hageman factor cannot be separated from its activator, and the complex is insoluble.

More recently, a clearer understanding has come from studies performed with Dr. Carl McMillin et al.[8] that utilized the technique of circular dichroism to examine the secondary structure of Hageman factor. In brief, we activated Hageman factor by adsorption to quartz or by adding solutions of ellagic acid, a derivative of tannic acid that appears to activate Hageman factor while in the liquid phase. Interpretation of the conformational changes detected by circular dichroism is somewhat controversial. But both quartz and ellagic acid seemed to alter the structure of the molecule in such a way that the conformation of aromatic residues, particularly tyrosine, was particularly perturbed. The changes brought in the Hageman factor molecule by quartz were more extensive than those induced by solutions of ellagic acid. This suggests that several different portions of the Hageman factor molecule may stick to insoluble substances, and that not all of these sites are involved in converting Hageman factor to its clot-promoting form. Support for this comes from the observation that Hageman factor that has been inactivated by phenylglyoxal hydrate will, nonetheless, stick to kaolin.[10]

Once Hageman factor has been activated, it promotes coagulation via both the intrinsic and extrinsic pathways. Its role in the intrinsic pathway, probably first described by Soulier,[14] is to convert plasma thromboplastin antecedent (PTA, factor XI) to its activated form. In our early experiments, this activation process appeared to be enzymatic.[15, 16] Our reagents were not as well purified as those now available, and we did not realize that the situation was, in fact, more complicated.

Newer insights derive from the discovery that two asymptomatic disorders of clotting—Fletcher trait [17] and Fitzgerald trait [18]—are localized functionally to the earliest steps of the clotting process. In each case, the activated partial thromboplastin time is strikingly prolonged, and other surface-mediated reactions dependent upon activated Hageman factor—kinin generation, fibrinolysis, augmentation of the activity of factor VII, and elaboration of the property of diluted plasma enhancing vascular permeability (that is, PF/Dil)—are all impaired.[19–23] In each case, these defective reactions have been ascribed to the deficiency of hitherto unrecognized clotting factors, Fletcher factor and Fitzgerald factor, respectively. A major step in our understanding of the various surface-mediated reactions came when Wuepper [19] demonstrated that Fletcher factor, recognized for its coagulant properties, was identical to a plasma prekallikrein. Prekallikrein is a substrate of activated Hageman factor that, once converted to plasma kallikrein, liberates biologically active kinins from their plasma precursors, the kininogens. Two groups of kininogens have been described, separated into those of relatively high and low molecular weights.[25] It was therefore especially exciting when several groups of investigators demonstrated that a high molecular weight kininogen was apparently identical to the factor missing in Mr. Fitzgerald's plasma.[18, 23, 26–28]

The manner in which Fletcher factor (that is, a prekallikrein) and Fitzgerald factor (that is, a high molecular weight kininogen) promote clotting has not yet been clarified. We do know that the addition of activated Hageman factor corrects the defect in Fletcher-trait plasma, but not that of Fitzgerald-trait plasma. The addition of activated PTA corrects both defects. Thus, Fitzgerald factor appears to act after the activation of Hageman factor and before the step in which activated PTA participates, but the action of Fletcher factor is obscure. But beyond this, present data do not provide a clear picture. Let us summarize some of this disjointed information.

The most challenging observation, originally made by Hathaway et al.,[17] is that the abnormally long partial thromboplastin time of patients with Fletcher trait shortens to normal if the plasma is exposed for a prolonged period to a clot-promoting surface such as kaolin before the addition of calcium ions. Thus, in Fletcher-trait plasma, either the activation of Hageman factor or the action of this agent upon PTA is defective. We have already noted, however, that the addition of activated Hageman factor corrects the clotting defect in Fletcher-trait plasma. Activated Hageman factor was prepared for these experiments by addition of ellagic acid, and then repurified to remove excess ellagic acid; the activated material, as we mentioned earlier, has the characteristics of a macromolecule, as though Hageman factor were complexed to its activator. In this form, it appears to circumvent the defect in Fletcher-trait plasma.

In agreement with this view, no time-dependent reaction can be demonstrated in a mixture of Hageman factor, prekallikrein, PTA, and kaolin. These observations, contradicting our early conclusions with crude materials, were reported by Schiffman and Lee,[29] and our own data are entirely in agreement. Cochrane and his associates [30] and Weiss and his colleagues [20] believe that plasma kallikrein activates Hageman factor. Their data, in fact, are not in disagreement with those we have reviewed. It is entirely possible that in whole plasma, Fletcher factor is needed for the activation of Hageman factor. When Hageman factor is purified, perhaps because the separation process modifies the molecule, a role for Fletcher factor can no longer be demonstrated.

In further support of this conception, Schiffman and Lee [31] reported that when they added plasma containing Fitzgerald factor to the mixture of Hageman factor, prekallikrein, kaolin, and PTA, activated PTA was generated. Fitzgerald factor supplied the ingredient missing in her earlier experiments. But our more recent experiments are still more intriguing. We find that partially purified Hageman factor, activated by ellagic acid, will convert PTA to its activated form if, and only if, Fitzgerald factor is present.[32] It must be emphasized that in these experiments we did not knowingly provide a source of Fletcher factor.

Still other clues may lead to a unifying explanation. Kaplan [33] and others separated a fragment of the Hageman factor molecule that readily converts prekallikrein to kallikrein, but is relatively weak in procoagulant activity. When we tested such Hageman factor fragments for their capacity to convert PTA to its activated form, we found, to our surprise, that Fitzgerald factor no longer influenced the reaction. In short, Fitzgerald factor was needed for the activation of PTA by activated Hageman factor (presumably complexed to its activator), but not by the fragment of the molecule containing its functionally active groups. This leads to the speculation that the preparations of Hageman factor with which we were able to activate PTA without the addition of Fletcher factor or Fitzgerald factor may have contained Hageman factor fragments. In support of this view, we reported that our early preparations of Hageman factor increased vascular permeability in guinea pig skin; only about two or three percent of the Hageman factor in these preparations was in the activated form, as determined by coagulant assays.[34] Further activation of the preparations did not increase their capacity to enhance vascular permeability.[35] Thus, the agent increasing vascular permeability was not identical with that enhancing clotting, and may well have been a fragment of Hageman factor.

And, finally, we have an incomplete clue. Solutions of prekallikrein can digest the synthetic chromogenic amide α-*N*-benzoyl-L-proline-L-phenylalanine-L-arginine-*p*-nitroanilide.[36] This function of plasma kallikrein can be inhibited by kaolin.[37] In turn, the inhibitory properties of kaolin can be blocked by the addition of Fitzgerald factor. Thus, in this highly artefactual system, the role of Fitzgerald factor is to protect plasma kallikrein—that is, activated Fletcher factor. Nonetheless, we have not been able to demonstrate that Fitzgerald factor can influence the action of Fletcher factor in kaolin-treated plasma.[32]

It is on this note that we wish to stop. Deficiencies of Hageman factor, prekallikrein, or high molecular weight kininogen are associated neither with evidence of a bleeding tendency nor of abnormal inflammatory responses. Every experiment demonstrating the function of these agents is necessarily based upon artefactual situations. We deal with substances altered by the very act of withdrawing them from the body, and their role in nature still eludes us. If what we have described seems unimportant in the normal physiologic processes of hemostasis, perhaps its interest lies in the reactions between plasma and synthetic prosthetic materials that may in some way activate the clotting process. Fortunately, the experiments we have reviewed tell us a great deal about what remains to be done.

References

1. Bordet, J. & O. Gengou. 1901. Ann. Inst. Pasteur **15:** 129.
2. Margolis, J. 1956. Nature **178:** 805.
3. Shafrir, E. & A. deVries. 1956. J. Clin. Invest. **35:** 1183.
4. Ratnoff, O. D. & J. E. Colopy. 1955. J. Clin. Invest. **34:** 602.
5. Ratnoff, O. D. & J. M. Rosenblum. 1958. Am. J. Med. **25:** 160.
6. Ratnoff, O. D. 1966. Progr. Hematol. **5:** 204.
7. Hubbard, D. & G. L. Lucas. 1960. J. Appl. Physiol. **15:** 265.
8. McMillin, C., H. Saito, O. D. Ratnoff & A. G. Walton. 1974. J. Clin. Invest. **54:** 1312.
9. Takahashi, K. 1968. J. Biol. Chem. **243:** 6171.
10. Ratnoff, O. D. & H. Saito. 1975. Proc. Soc. Exp. Biol. Med. **148:** 177.
11. Vroman, L. 1965. Nature **205:** 496.
12. Margolis, J. 1963. Ann. N.Y. Acad. Sci. **104:** 133.
13. Donaldson, V. H. & O. D. Ratnoff. 1965. Science **150:** 754.
14. Soulier, J. P., O. Wartelle & D. Ménaché. 1958. Rev. franç. Ét Clin. Biol. **3:** 263.

15. Ratnoff, O. D., E. W. Davie & D. L. Mallett. 1961. J. Clin. Invest. **40:** 803.
16. Ratnoff, O. D. & E. W. Davie. 1962. Biochemistry **1:** 967.
17. Hathaway, W. E., L. P. Belhasen & H. S. Hathaway. 1965. Blood **26:** 521.
18. Waldmann, R., J. P. Abraham, J. W. Rebuck, J. Caldwell, H. Saito & O. D. Ratnoff. 1975. Lancet **1:** 949.
19. Wuepper, K. D. 1972. *In* Inflammation: Mechanisms and Control. I. H. Lepow & P. A. Ward, Eds. : 93. Academic Press. New York, N.Y.
20. Weiss, A. S., J. I. Gallin & A. P. Kaplan. 1974. J. Clin. Invest. **53:** 622.
21. Saito, H., O. D. Ratnoff & V. H. Donaldson. 1974. Circulation Res. **34:** 641.
22. Donaldson, V. H., H. Saito & O. D. Ratnoff. 1974. Circulation Res. **34:** 652.
23. Saito, H., O. D. Ratnoff, R. Waldmann & J. P. Abraham. 1975. J. Clin. Invest. **55:** 1082.
24. Saito, H. & O. D. Ratnoff. 1975. J. Lab. Clin. Med. **85:** 405.
25. Jacobsen, S. 1967. Brit. J. Pharm. Chem. **29:** 25.
26. Donaldson, V. H., H. I. Glueck, M. A. Miller, H. Z. Movat & F. Habal. 1976. J. Lab. Clin. Med. **87:** 327.
27. Wuepper, K. D., D. R. Miller & M. J. Lacombe. 1975. J. Clin. Invest. **56:** 1663.
28. Colman, R. W., A. Bagdasarian, R. C. Talamo, C. F. Scott, M. Seavey, J. A. Guimaraes, J. V. Pierce & A. P. Kaplan. 1975. J. Clin. Invest. **56:** 1650.
29. Schiffman, S. & P. Lee. 1974. Br. J. Haematol. **27:** 101.
30. Cochrane, C. G., J. D. Revak & K. D. Wuepper. 1973. J. Exp. Med. **138:** 1564.
31. Schiffman, S. & P. Lee. 1975. J. Clin. Invest. **56:** 1082.
32. Saito, H. 1976. Unpublished observations.
33. Kaplan, A. P. & K. F. Austen. 1971. J. Exp. Med. **133:** 696.
34. Ratnoff, O. D. & A. A. Miles. 1964. Brit. J. Exp. Pathol. **45:** 328.
35. Ratnoff, O. D. 1962. Unpublished observations.
36. Amundsen, E., L. Svendsen, A. M. Vennerød & K. Laake. *In* Proc. Internat. Conf. Chemistry & Biology of Kallikrein-Kinin System in Health & Disease. In press.
37. Ratnoff, O. D. & H. Saito. 1976. Blood **47:** 243.

REQUIREMENTS FOR CONTACT ACTIVATION OF HUMAN HAGEMAN FACTOR

Henry L. Meier,*† Cheryl F. Scott,§ Robert Mandle, Jr.,*
Marion E. Webster,‡ Jack V. Pierce,‡ Robert W. Colman,§
and Allen P. Kaplan *¶

**Allergic Diseases Section, Laboratory of Clinical Investigation*
National Institute of Allergy and Infectious Diseases
Bethesda, Maryland 20014
‡ Section on Physiologic Chemistry Hypotension-Endocrine Branch
National Heart and Lung Institute, National Institutes of Health
Bethesda, Maryland 20014
§ Coagulation Unit of the Hematology-Oncology Section
Department of Medicine, University of Pennsylvania
Philadelphia, Pennsylvania 19104

Introduction

Activation of the intrinsic coagulation pathway is initiated by negatively charged surfaces. The plasma protein that is bound and activated upon these surfaces was discovered in 1955 and is called Hageman factor (factor XII).[1] Hageman factor-deficient plasma, however, not only has a very prolonged partial thromboplastin time (PTT) but it also fails to support surface initiated fibrinolysis [2, 3] as well as the generation of bradykinin.[4] These pathways have been shown to be mediated by the various Hageman factor substrates. Activation of factor XI (Precursor Plasma Thromboplastin Antecedent or Pre-PTA) is required for the coagulation pathway to proceed,[5] conversion of a plasminogen proactivator to plasminogen activator is followed by cleavage of plasminogen to yield the fibrinolytic enzyme plasmin,[6] and Hageman factor activation of human prekallikrein [7] generates the enzyme kallikrein, which digests kininogen to liberate the vasoactive peptide bradykinin.

Recent studies have demonstrated that the proteins of the kinin-forming sequence, namely, prekallikrein and a high molecular weight form of human kininogen, are required for Hageman factor-dependent coagulation and fibrinolysis. In this paper we summarize the functional abnormalities associated with prekallikrein and high molecular weight (HMW) kininogen deficiency and, using purified components, present evidence that HMW kininogen is a cofactor required for surface-dependent activation of Hageman factor. HMW kininogen was found to enhance the function of activated Hageman factor in the fluid phase and to potentiate the function of the proteolytic site of surface-bound Hageman factor, and it is a cofactor required for the activation of Hageman factor by kallikrein.

† Predoctoral student, Department of Biochemistry, Georgetown University, Washington, D.C. 20037.

¶ Reprint requests to Dr. Allen P. Kaplan, National Institutes of Health, NIAID, LCI, Building 10, Room 11N–246, Bethesda, Md. 20014.

Results

HMW Kininogen Deficiency

In the past year, a protein that is required for the surface activation of Hageman factor in whole plasma was independently identified by two groups to be a high molecular form of human kininogen (HMW kininogen). This was determined utilizing plasmas of patients named Williams [8] and Flaujeac,[9] which possessed unique abnormalities of the Hageman factor-dependent pathways. Two other patients, Fitzgerald [10] and Washington,[11] have also been shown to possess the same functional abnormalities present in Williams-trait plasma and have also been shown to lack HMW kininogen.[11] Williams-trait plasma corrected the coagulation defect present in Hageman factor-deficient plasma, demonstrating that it did contain functionally viable Hageman factor. Kaolin activation of Williams-trait plasma, however, generated no bradykinin; therefore, the plasma level of the other proteins required for kinin formation were determined. No functional or antigenic kininogen was found (FIGURE 1), which provided a ready explanation for the inability to generate kinin. However, when the ability of kaolin to initiate kallikrein formation was determined by an arginine esterase assay,[8] essentially no conversion of prekallikrein to kallikrein was evident. Yet Williams-trait plasma possessed 43–45% of normal antigenic prekallikrein, and this prekallikrein could be isolated chromatographically and activated in the fluid phase by the Hageman factor fragments. In addition, kaolin activation of a mixture of equal volumes of plasma containing no prekallikrein with Williams-trait plasma yielded approximately 40% of the normal

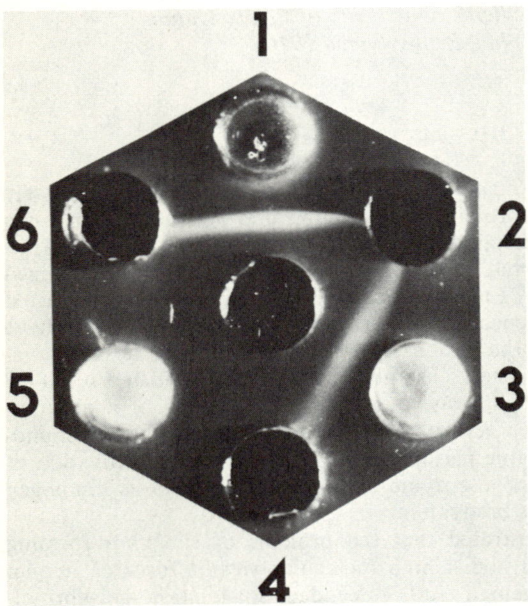

FIGURE 1. Oucterlony analysis of Williams-trait plasma with antibody to low molecular weight kininogen. Sheep antikininogen is in the center well. Well 1 contains normal plasma, well 3 contains a 1:4 dilution of normal plasma, and well 5 contains Williams-trait plasma. Wells 2, 4, and 6 are empty.

one-minute arginine esterase activity, which is consistent with its prekallikrein content of 45%. Thus two abnormalities of kinin generation were defined including a functional defect in the conversion of prekallikrein to kallikrein and the absence of any functional or antigenic kininogen. Since Williams-trait plasma contained both Hageman factor and prekallikrein, it appeared that the inability of kaolin to lead to conversion of prekallikrein to kallikrein might be secondary to a defect in the formation of active Hageman factor.

Although Williams-trait plasma contained a normal level of coagulation factors I through XIII, it possessed a prolonged partial thromboplastin time as well as a markedly diminished generation of Hageman factor-dependent fibrinolysis. These pathways are dependent upon Hageman factor substrates other than prekallikrein, lending further support to the thesis that the major defect in Williams-trait plasma was an abnormality in the activation and/or function of the patient's Hageman factor.

When normal plasma was fractionated by QAE-Sephadex, SP-Sephadex, and Sephadex G–150 gel filtration, an α-globulin with an estimated molecular weight of 200,000 was identified which corrected the coagulation, fibrinolytic, and kinin-generating defects present in Williams trait plasma. The chromatographic properties of this factor coincided with a peak of antigenic kininogen that corresponded to a form of human kininogen designated "high molecular weight kininogen." [12, 13] When highly purified kininogen was prepared by DEAE-cellulose batch adsorption, passage over an antikininogen immunoadsorbent, chromatography on DEAE cellulose, and gel filtration on Bio-Gel A–0.5m, kininogens could be further resolved by charge and size.[14] The corrective factor was primarily associated with the fractions of molecular weight 160,000–225,000, although a minor component of molecular weight 80,000 was also capable of correcting the functional abnormalities.[8] Together, these fractions comprised only 15–20% of the total plasma kininogen and correspond to those molecular forms that are the preferred substrate for plasma kallikrein.[12–15] The predominant plasma kininogen, low molecular weight kininogen (80,000 by gel filtration), did not possess this corrective activity.

Prior to the discovery of these deficient plasmas, two reports suggested that a plasma cofactor for surface activation of Hageman factor was necessary. The first presented evidence that surface-bound Hageman factor did not activate prekallikrein,[16] and the second, that surface-bound Hageman factor did not activate factor XI.[17] Subsequent studies by each group have shown that normal plasma possesses the missing factor, whereas plasmas deficient in kininogen do not.[18, 19] Furthermore, purified HMW kininogen was shown to correct this abnormality in the activation of prekallikrein [19] and a "contact activation cofactor" required for factor XI activation has been partially purified that possesses the physiochemical properties of HMW kininogen.[20]

Potentiation of the Function of Surface-Bound Hageman Factor

We have recently reported that surface-bound Hageman factor activity is markedly enhanced by the addition of HMW kininogen as assessed by the subsequent activation of the Hageman factor substrates mediating coagulation, fibrinolysis, and kinin generation.[21] An example of this effect with prekallikrein as the substrate is shown in FIGURE 2. For a given amount of Hageman factor, an increasing dose of high molecular weight kininogen was shown to yield an incremental increase in the quantity of prekallikrein that is converted to kallikrein.[19, 21] A similar phenomenon has been reported for factor XI activation[20] suggesting that the quantity of Hageman factor activated is a linear function of the quantity of kininogen added.

Potentiation of the Function of Hageman Factor Fragments by HMW Kininogen

If a fluid-phase form of activated Hageman factor (Hageman factor fragments) is assayed for its ability to activate prekallikrein (i.e. with no surface present) as assessed by either kinin formation or ability to cleave synthetic substrates, a two- to threefold enhancement is observed upon addition of HMW kininogen.[22] FIGURE 3 shows that HMW kininogen also enhances the activity of the Hageman factor fragments upon the synthetic substrate acetyl-glycyl-lysyl-methyl-ester by approximately 25%, suggesting that this effect of HMW kininogen is upon the Hageman factor rather than upon its natural substrates.

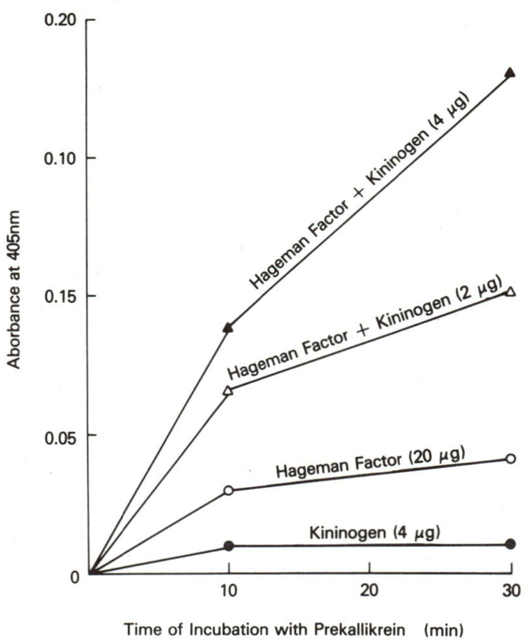

FIGURE 2. Effect of high molecular weight kininogen upon surface-mediated activation of Hageman factor. Twenty μg of Hageman factor in the presence or absence of HMW kininogen were bound to 5 mg of supercell, the suspension was washed, and a time course of prekallikrein activation by the bound Hageman factor was determined as assessed by the ability of generated kallikrein to liberate *p*-nitrophenol from *N*-Benzoyl-L-phenylalanyl-L-valyl-L-arginine-*p*-nitroanilide HCl. Four μg of HMW kininogen alone yielded no significant prekallikrein activation; however, the addition of 2 μg or 4 μg of HMW kininogen to the surface-bound Hageman factor yielded proportionate increases in the generation of prekallikrein-activating activity.

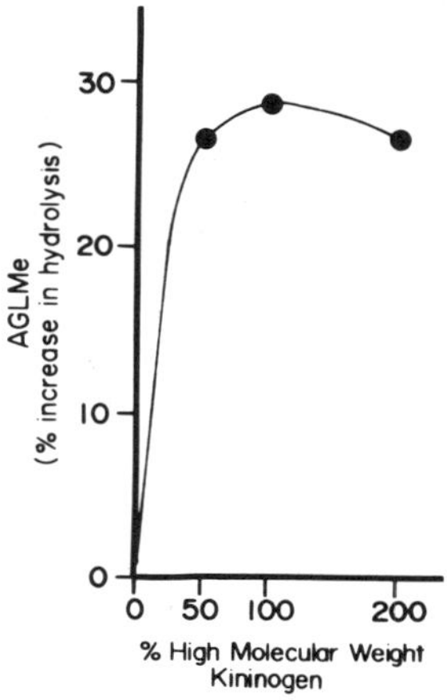

FIGURE 3. Twenty-five μg of Hageman factor fragments were incubated at 23° for 5 minutes with varying concentrations of high molecular weight kininogen (100% equals the amount of 1 ml of normal plasma by coagulant assay). The enzyme mixture was then added to acetyl-glycine-methyl-ester (ABLMe) (final concentration 5 mM) in 0.1 M sodium phosphate buffer pH7.0. The hydrolysis of AGLMe was measured by the amount of methanol released at 37° during 90 minutes as determined by the chromotropic acid method. The percentage of increase in the hydrolysis due to kininogen over that due to Hageman factor fragments alone is plotted on the ordinate.

Prekallikrein Deficiency

Another protein required for a normal rate of activation of Hageman factor is prekallikrein, the proenzyme from which the kininogen-cleaving enzyme kallikrein is derived. In 1965, Fletcher trait deficiency was described as an autosomal recessive disorder characterized by a diminished rate of surface-mediated coagulation.[23] This plasma possessed an unusual abnormality in that the partial thromboplastin time returned to normal as the time of incubation with kaolin was increased. The factor in normal plasm that corrected the deficiency was partially purified and eluted near factor XI on CM-cellulose.[24] In 1972, the corrective protein was identified as prekallikrein.[25] The Fletcher trait plasma also possessed an abnormality in the rate of surface-mediated fibrinolysis [26] and generated no bradykinin upon incubation with kaolin. The last abnormality is expected if the plasma contained no prekallikrein, but one would not have readily predicted an effect upon the coagulation and fibrinolytic pathways. The presence of both these abnormalities again suggested an effect upon Hageman factor, the one protein common to each pathway. Correction of both the coagulation and fibrinolytic defects of Fletcher-trait plasma by activated Hageman factor in the absence of a surface demonstrated that the abnormality was a diminished rate of formation of activated Hageman factor.[26] Another study of Fletcher-trait deficiency found that reconstitution with activated Hageman factor yielded only a partial correction, suggesting that kallikrein alters the function of activated Hageman factor rather than the formation of activated Hageman factor.[27] In a subsequent paper describing Fitzgerald trait, however, activated Hageman factor did fully correct Fletcher-trait plasma but not the Fitzgerald-trait plasma.[10] The inability to correct fully the HMW kininogen deficiency with a fluid phase-activated Hageman factor may be related to the aforementioned ability of HMW kininogen to enhance the function of activated Hageman factor, an effect not observed with kallikrein.

Since kallikrein has been shown to convert unactivated Hageman factor to activated Hageman factor in the fluid phase,[28] a direct feedback activation of Hageman factor by kallikrein may account for the rapid rate of activation of the Hageman factor-dependent pathways in normal plasma compared to prekallikrein-deficient plasma. Yet the ability of kallikrein to activate Hageman factor in human plasma in the absence of a surface is negligible, suggesting that kallikrein acts only upon Hageman factor that is bound.[29] Prekallikrein and kallikrein correct Fletcher-trait deficiency equally well in the presence of a surface. However, as shown in FIGURE 4, DFP inhibits the ability of kallikrein to correct Fletcher-trait deficiency[30] but does not inhibit correction by prekallikrein, since the active site is not available.[31] DFP also has no effect upon the ability of HMW kininogen to correct William-trait deficiency (FIGURE 4). Thus it appears that conversion of prekallikrein to kallikrein by activated Hageman factor is required prior to this feedback activation of Hageman factor.

The rate of generation of kaolin-activatable fibrinolytic activity by these various deficient plasmas also reflects the relative rates of activation of Hageman factor. Essentially no activation is seen in Hageman factor-deficient plasma.

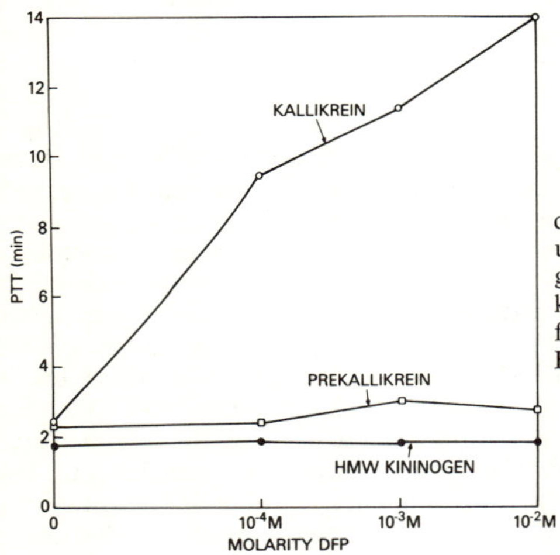

FIGURE 4. Comparison of the effect of varying concentrations of DFP upon the ability of 5 μg HMW kininogen, 1 μg prekallikrein, or 1 μg kallikrein to correct the coagulation defects of Williams-trait plasma and Fletcher-trait plasma, respectively.

Little activation is seen in Williams-trait plasma, indicating that in the absence of HMW kininogen, insufficient Hageman factor is activated to act upon any of the substrates.[8] The Fletcher-trait plasma has a diminished rate of generation of plasmin, which gradually approaches normal.[26] This slow generation of fibrinolytic activity is probably primarily the effect of HMW kininogen as well as enzymes such as plasmin or activated XI,[28, 32] which can also activate Hageman factor. Thus kallikrein generates most of the activated Hageman factor within the first few minutes, yet without HMW kininogen, this feedback is not observed.

The Effect of HMW Kininogen upon the Ability of Kallikrein to Activate Hageman Factor

We attempted to reproduce the abnormality present in Fletcher-trait plasma, utilizing purified components by tested mixtures of surface-bound Hageman factor, HMW kininogen, and kallikrein for their ability to activate Hageman factor. Interaction of surface-bound Hageman factor with kallikrein yielded a 30% increase in Hageman factor activity compared to that of the Hageman factor alone. Addition of HMW kininogen to the Hageman factor yielded a fourfold increase in Hageman factor activity. However, incubation of the Hageman factor—HMW kininogen mixture with the same dose of kallikrein yielded a tenfold increase in the quantity of activated Hageman factor. DFP-treated kallikrein had no effect upon the HMW kininogen-Hageman factor mixture, whereas prekallikrein or DFP-treated prekallikrein yielded the same enhancing ability as kallikrein.

Discussion and Summary

The number of kininogens circulating in plasma has been a controversial question. In 1965, two highly purified kininogens (I and II) were isolated that had a molecular weight of about 50,000, as estimated by gel filtration and sucrose density gradient ultracentrifugation.[33] Kininogen I appeared to have the bradykinin moiety at the C-terminus because it was inactivated by carboxypeptidase B, but kininogen II was not so inactivated and thus appeared to have the bradykinin within the molecule. Soon thereafter, Jacobsen demonstrated the presence of two different kininogens in various mammalian plasmas.[34] These consisted of a high molecular weight form of about 200,000 that was rapidly cleaved by plasma kallikrein, and a low molecular weight kininogen of 60,000, which was only slowly cleaved by plasma kallikrein but was rapidly cleaved by kallikreins of tissue origin.[10] Since then, several investigators have reported finding only the low molecular weight form in plasma,[35, 36] while others have found both high and low molecular weight forms in human[12, 13, 37] or bovine plasmas.[38, 39]

The discovery of plasmas that are deficient in kininogen (particularly HMW kininogen) have demonstrated that the two molecular weight forms do indeed exist in human plasma, and confirmed earlier observations that HMW kininogen represents approximately 15–20% of the total kininogen.[34] Both high and low molecular weight forms possess considerable microheterogeneity with charge differences as well as the presence or absence of bradykinin at the C-terminus.[40] It is of interest that recent studies of human LMW kininogen suggested that none of the bradykinin is at the C-terminus[41] in agreement with the finding reported for bovine LMW kininogen.[42] It has been suggested that bovine HMW kininogen containing C-terminal bradykinin may also be a cleavage product[40] contributing to the observed heterogeneity. Purification of human kininogens has revealed heterogeneity based upon size, charge,[12] and ability to correct Williams-trait deficiency.[8, 19] About one percent of the total kininogen isolated is a low molecular weight form that corrects Williams trait; however, it is not clear whether this and other described molecular species are native kininogens or have been formed during purification.

It is not known whether a single gene or two genes code for the high and low molecular weight forms of kininogen. Antibody to LMW kininogen gives a line of complete identity with HMW kininogen,[14, 15] suggesting that if one gene codes for both proteins, it is the LMW form that is derived from the HMW form. It is also possible that two separate genes can code for HMW kininogen (one of which codes for LMW kininogen) in a fashion analagous to an immunoglobulin light chain in which two polypeptide chains are linked during transcription or translation.

Human kininogen deficiency appears to be an autosomal recessive trait leading to a complete deficiency of HMW kininogen and partial deficiencies of LMW kininogen. Although LMW kininogen is not detectable in Williams' or Washington's plasma,[8, 11] the LMW kininogen level in Flaujeac- and Fitzgerald-trait plasmas are nine and fifty percent of normal, respectively.[9, 10] Apparently the genes coding for other factors in this pathway are closely linked to those coding for kininogen. Thus Fitzgerald-trait plasma has only 15% of normal prekallikrein and Williams-trait plasma has 45% of normal prekallikrein, but Flaujaec-trait and Washington-trait plasmas have normal levels of prekallikrein.

A diagram of the plasma-protein interactions required for the activation of Hageman factor is shown in FIGURE 5 indicating that prekallikrein and HMW kininogen are coagulation factors required for Hageman factor activation and function. HMW kininogen has no known enzymatic activity, but it facilitates the generation of a proteolytic site upon surface-bound Hageman factor. The Hageman factor activity measured is proportional to the HMW kininogen input. Studies of the interaction of HMW kininogen with Hageman factor fragments suggest that it can alter the active site of Hageman factor to yield a more

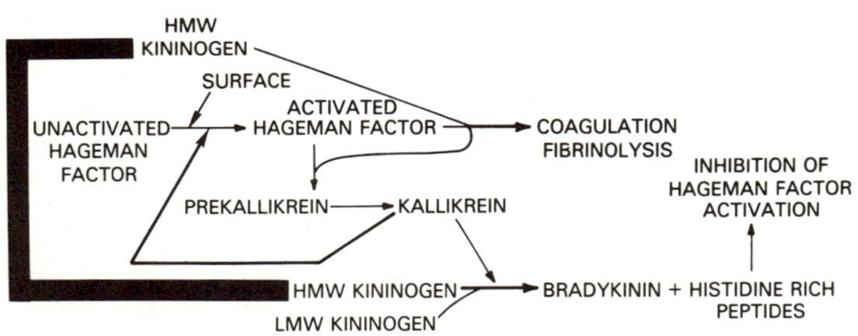

FIGURE 5. Diagram of the relationship of proteins of the kinin-generating pathway to the mechanism of activation of Hageman factor.

effective enzyme. Upon the surface, HMW kininogen also enhances the function of Hageman factor upon its substrates. The effect of kallikrein upon Hageman factor is presumed to be a direct one; however, HMW kininogen augments this interaction. It is also possible that a kallikrein-altered form of HMW kininogen might account for the ability of kallikrein to enhance the rate of Hageman factor activation. However, kallikrein-treated HMW kininogen is no more effective as a cofactor than the intact molecule.[8, 19] It therefore appears that upon a surface, kininogen is required to augment the function of activated Hageman factor which converts prekallikrein to kallikrein. The kallikrein then digests kininogen to yield bradykinin and enzymatically activates the Hageman factor; however, HMW kininogen facilitates the Hageman factor-kallikrein interaction. A byproduct of the cleavage of bovine kininogen by kallikrein is the release of a histidine-rich peptide, which has been shown to inhibit Hageman factor activation and may serve as an intrinsic regulatory mechanism.[43]

[NOTE ADDED IN PROOF: HMW kininogen and prekallikrein have been shown to circulate as a complex in human plasma (Mandle, R. J., R. W. Colman & A. P. Kaplan. PNAS, Nov., 1976) and are presumably bound to negatively charged surfaces together. They then interact with surface-bound Hageman factor. Griffin and

Cochrane have also recently reported that HMW kininogen is a cofactor in the reciprocal activation of Hageman factor and prekallikrein (PNAS **73:** 2554–2558).]

References

1. Ratnoff, O. D. & J. E. Colopy. 1955. A familial hemorrhagic trait associated with a deficiency of clot-promoting fraction of plasma. J. Clin. Invest. **34:** 602–613.
2. Niewiarowski, S. & O. Prou-Wartelle. 1959. Role du facteur contact (Facteur Hageman) dans la fibrinolyse. Thromb. Diath. Haem. **3:** 593–603.
3. Iatridis, S. G. & J. H. Ferguson. 1962. Active Hageman factor: A plasma lysokinase of the human fibrinolytic system. J. Clin. Invest. **41:** 1277–1287.
4. Margolis, J. 1958. Activation of plasma by contact with glass. Evidence for a common reaction which releases plasma kinin and initiates coagulation. J. Physiol. (Lond.) **144:** 1–22.
5. Ratnoff, O. D., E. W. Davie & D. L. Mallet. 1961. Studies on the action of Hageman factor: Evidence that activated Hageman factor in turn activates plasma thromboplastin antecedent. J. Clin. Invest. **40:** 803–819.
6. Kaplan, A. P. & K. F. Austen. 1972. The fibrinolytic pathway of human plasma. Isolation and characterization of the plasminogen proactivator. J. Exp. Med. **136:** 1378–1393.
7. Kaplan, A. P. & K. F. Austen. 1970. A prealbumin activator of prekallikrein. J. Immunol. **105:** 802–811.
8. Colman, R. W., A. Bagdasarian, R. C. Talamo, C. F. Scott, M. Seavey, J. A. Guimaraes, J. V. Pierce & A. P. Kaplan. 1975. Williams trait: Human kininogen deficiency with diminished levels of plasminogen proactivator and prekallikrein associated with abnormalities of the Hageman factor-dependent pathways. J. Clin. Invest. **56:** 1650–1662.
9. Wuepper, K. D., K. R. Miller & M. J. Lacombe. 1975. Flaujeac trait: deficiency of human plasma kininogen. J. Clin. Invest. **56:** 1663–1672.
10. Saito, H., O. D. Ratnoff, R. Waldmann & J. P. Abraham. 1975. Fitzgerald trait. Deficiency of a hitherto unrecognized agent, Fitzgerald factor, participating in surface-mediated reactions of clotting, fibrinolysis, generation of kinins, and the property of diluted plasma enhancing vascular permeability (PF/dil). J. Clin. Invest. **55:** 1082–1089.
11. Donaldson, V. H., H. I. Glueck, M. A. Miller, H. Z. Movat & F. Hamal. 1976. Kininogen deficiency in Fitzgerald trait; role of high molecular weight kininogen in clotting and fibrinolysis. J. Lab. Clin. Med. **87:** 327–337.
12. Jacobsen, S. & M. Kriz. 1967. Some data on two purified kininogens from human plasma. Br. J. Pharmacol. **29:** 25–36.
13. Pierce, J. V. 1968. Structural features of plasma kinins and kininogens. Fed. Proc. **27:** 52–57.
14. Pierce, J. V. & J. A. Guimaraes. Further characterization of highly purified human plasma kininogens. *In* The Chemistry and Biology of the Kallikrein Kinin System in Health and Disease. Fogarty Int. Center Proc. No. 27. J. J. Pisano and K. F. Austen, Eds. U.S. Government Printing Office. Washington, D.C. In press.
15. Habal, F. M., H. Z. Movat & C. E. Burrowes. 1974. Isolation of two functionally different kininogens from human plasma. Separation from proteinase inhibitors and interaction with plasma kallikrein. Biochem. Pharmacol. **23:** 2291–2302.
16. Webster, M. E. & J. V. Pierce. 1973. Activation of Hageman factor (factor XII): Identification and relationship to kallikrein-kinin system. Fed. Proc. (abstr.) **32:** 845.
17. Schiffman, S. & P. Lee. 1974. Preparation, characterization, and activation of

highly purified factor XI. Evidence that a hitherto unrecognized plasma activity participates in the interaction of factors XI and XII. Br. J. Haematol. **27:** 101–114.

18. SCHIFFMAN, S., P. LEE & R. WALDMANN. 1975. Identity of contact activation cofactor and Fitzgerald factor. Thromb. Res. **6:** 451–454.
19. WEBSTER, M. E., J. A. GUIMARAES, A. P. KAPLAN, R. W. COLMAN & J. V. PIERCE 1976. Activation of surface-bound Hageman factor: The critical role of high molecular weight kininogen and evidence for an additional factor. Adv. Exp. Med. Biol. **70:** In press.
20. SCHIFFMAN, S. & P. LEE. 1975. Partial purification and characterization of contact activation cofactor. J. Clin. Invest. **56:** 1082–1092.
21. MEIER, H. L., M. WEBSTER, C. Y. LIU, R. W. COLMAN & A. P. KAPLAN. 1976. Enhancement of surface dependent Hageman factor activation by high molecular weight kininogen. Fed. Proc. (abstr.) **35:** 692.
22. LIU, C. Y., A. BAGDASARIAN, H. L. MEIER, C. F. SCOTT, J. V. PIERCE, A. P. KAPLAN & R. W. COLMAN. 1976. Potentiation of the action of Hageman factor fragments (HF_f) by high molecular weight kininogen (HWM Kgn). Fed. Proc. (abstr.) **35:** 692.
23. HATHWAY, W. E., L. P. BELHAUSEN & H. S. HATHWAY. 1965. Evidence of a new plasma coagulation factor. I. Case report, coagulation studies and physicochemical properties. Br. J. Haematol. **26:** 521–532.
24. HATHWAY, W. E. & J. ALSEVER. 1970. The relation of "Fletcher factor" to factors XI and XII. Br. J. Haematol. **18:** 161–169.
25. WUEPPER, K. D. 1973. Prekallikrein deficiency in man. J. Exp. Med. **138:** 1345–1355.
26. WEISS, A. S., J. I. GALLIN & A. P. KAPLAN. 1974. Fletcher factor deficiency: Abnormalities of coagulation, fibrinolysis, chemotactic activity, and kinin generation attributable to absence of prekallikrein. J. Clin. Invest. **53:** 622–633.
27. SAITO, H., O. D. RATNOFF & V. H. DONALDSON. 1974. Defective activation of clotting, fibrinolytic, and permeability enhancing systems in human Fletcher trait plasma. Circ. Res. **34:** 641–651.
28. COCHRANE, C. G., S. D. REVAK & K. D. WUEPPER. 1973. Activation of Hageman factor in solid and fluid phases. A critical role of kallikrein. J. Exp. Med. **138:** 1564–1583.
29. KAPLAN, A. P., H. L. MEIER, L. D. YECIES & L. W. HECK. 1976. Hageman factor and its substrates: The role of Factor XI (PTA), prekallikrein, and plasminogen proactivator in coagulation, fibrinolysis, and kiningeneration. *In* The Kallikrein System in Health and Disease. Fogarty Int. Center Proc. No. 27. J. Pisano and K. F. Austen, Eds. U.S. Government Printing Office. Washington, D.C. In press.
30. KAPLAN, A. P., H. L. MEIER & MANDLE, R., JR. 1976. The Hageman factor dependent pathways of coagulation, fibrinolysis, and kiningeneration. Semin. Thromb. Haemostasis. In press.
31. KAPLAN, A. P., A. B. KAY & K. F. AUSTEN. 1972. A prealbumin activator of prekallikrein. III. Appearance of chemotactic activity for human neutrophlis by the conversion of human prekallikrein to kallikrein. J. Exp. Med. **135:** 81–97.
32. KAPLAN, A. P. & K. F. AUSTEN. 1971. A prealbumin activator of prekallikrein. II. Derivation of activators of prekallikrein from active Hageman factor by digestion with plasmin. J. Exp. Med. **133:** 696–712.
33. PIERCE, J. V. & M. E. WEBSTER. 1966. The purification and some properties of different kallidinogens. *In* Hypotensive Peptides. E. G. Erdös, N. Back, F. Sicuteri, and A. F. Wilde, Eds. : 130–136. Springer-Verlag. New York, N.Y.
34. JACOBSEN, S. 1966. Substrates for plasma kinin-forming enzymes in human, dog, and rabbit plasmas. Br. J. Pharmacol. **26:** 403–411.
35. SPRAGG, J. & K. F. AUSTEN. 1971. The preparation of human kininogen. II.

Further characterization of purified human kininogen. J. Immunol. **107:** 1512–1519.

36. WUEPPER, K. D. & C. G. COCHRANE. 1971. The biochemistry of the acute allergic reactions. Second Inter. Symp. K. F. Austen & E. L. Becker, Eds. Blackwell Scientific Publications, Ltd. Oxford, England.
37. HABAL, F. M. & H. Z. MOVAT. 1972. Kininogens of human plasma. Res. Commun. Chem. Pathol. Pharmacol. **4:** 477–486.
38. SUZUKI, T., Y. MIZUSHIMA, T. SATO & S. IWANAGA. 1965. Purification of bovine bradykininogen. J. Biochem. **57:** 14–21.
39. YANO, M., S. NAGASAWA, K. HARIUCHI & T. SUZUKI. 1967. Separation of a new substrate, kininogen I, for plasma kallikrein in bovine plasma. J. Biochem. **62:** 504–506.
40. KOMIYA, M., H. KATO & T. SUZUKI. 1974. Bovine plasma kininogens. II. Microheterogeneities of high molecular weight kininogens and their structural relationships. J. Biochm. **76:** 823–832.
41. SPRAGG, J. & K. F. AUSTEN. 1974. Preparation of human kininogen. III Enzymatic digestion and modification. Biochem. Pharmacol. **23:** 781–791.
42. KATO, H. & T. SUZUKI. 1968. The location and nature of the linkage of kinin moiety in bovine kininogen. II. Biochem. Biophys. Res. Commun. **32:** 800–805.
43. HAN, Y. N., M. KOMIYA, H. KATO, S. IWANAGA & T. SUZUKI. 1975. Primary structure of bovine high molecular weight kininogen. Chemical compositions of kinin-free kininogen and peptide fragments released by plasma kallikrein. FEBS Lett. **57:** 254–258.

BLOOD COAGULATION FACTORS AT PHOSPHOLIPID SURFACES

H. C. Hemker, M. J. Lindhout, and C. Vermeer

Department of Biochemistry
Biomedical Centre
State University Limburg
Maastricht, The Netherlands

The contact phase of blood coagulation results in activated factor XI.[1, 2] After that the reaction sequence leading to thrombin formation is as follows:

$$IX \xrightarrow{XI_a} IX_a$$

$$IX_a + VIII + \text{ph.lip.} + Ca^{++} \rightleftharpoons \text{"tenase"}$$

$$X \xrightarrow{\text{tenase}} X_a$$

$$X_a + V + \text{ph.lip.} + Ca^{++} \rightleftharpoons \text{"prothrombinase"}$$

$$II \xrightarrow{\text{"prothrombinase"}} II_a \quad (= \text{thrombin}).$$

Two features characterize this scheme:

1. *The cascade sequence:* the product of one reaction is (part of) the enzyme in the next.[3, 4]

2. *The complex enzymes.* Both the factor X-activating enzyme ("tenase") and the thrombin-forming enzyme ("prothrombinase") consist of two proteins (clotting factors) adsorbed to a phospholipid.

The activated forms of factor IX and factor X are serine proteases.[5–8] As such, they have hardly any tenase or prothrombinase activity.[9–13] To obtain this activity two other components are necessary: another protein (factor VIII or factor V, respectively) and a phospholipid, or rather, a micelle composed of a mixture of phospholipids.

The prevailing model of prothrombinase is the following: at the surface of a phospholipid micelle, factor X_a and factor V adsorb next to each other. At the same interphase the substrate, prothrombin, adsorbs. The active site in factor X_a attacks the vulnerable sites in prothrombin and so generates thrombin.

The evidence leading to this model is the following: 1) The proteins can be shown to adsorb onto the micelles. Activity generates when both adsorb onto the same micelle. Ca^{++} is necessary for the adsorption of factor X_a but counteracts the adsorption of factor V. Optimal activity is found when about equimolar quantities of both factor adsorb.[10, 11, 14–20] The dependence of the activity on the concentrations of the constituent moieties is in accordance with the following reaction scheme: [21, 22]

$$X_a + Ca^{++} + \text{ph.lip} \rightleftharpoons X_a - Ca - \text{ph.lip.}$$
$$V + \text{ph.lip.} \rightleftharpoons V - \text{ph.lip.}$$
$$V + X_a - Ca - \text{ph.lip.} \rightleftharpoons \text{prothrombinase}$$
$$X_a + Ca^{++} + V - \text{ph.lip.} \rightleftharpoons \text{prothrombinase}$$

For tenase, an analogous set of experiments has been carried out. Adsorption and Ca^{++} dependence [20, 23–25] adsorption on the same micelle [26] and the kinetics of the generation of activity [27] indicate a comparable reaction scheme:

$$IX_a + Ca^{++} + \text{ph.lip.} \rightleftharpoons IX_a - Ca - \text{ph.lip.}$$
$$VIII + \text{ph.lip.} \rightleftharpoons VIII - \text{ph.lip.}$$
$$VIII + IX_a - Ca - \text{ph.lip.} \rightleftharpoons \text{tenase}$$
$$IX_a + Ca^{++} + VIII - \text{ph.lip.} \rightleftharpoons \text{tenase}$$

We can elaborate upon this model on the basis of the existing evidence obtained on its various components.

The Active Site-Bearing Proteins (Factor X_a and Factor IX_a)

Both active site-bearing proteins are two-chain serine proteases.[5–8] The heavy chain shows extensive homologies to other members of the chymotrypsin family and contains the active serine.

The light chain is particularly interesting in that it contains several pairs of γ—COOH glutamyl residues. The dicarboxyl side chains generated bind Ca^{++} [28, 29] and via Ca^{++} bind to the phospholipid surface.[30] The study of the function of these groups in coagulation is facilitated by the fact that both factor IX and factor X (and factor II as well) have been demonstrated to exist in a form without carboxylated glutamic acids.[31, 32] The carboxylation of the glutamic acids is brought about by a vitamin K-dependent enzyme system. Consequently, in vitamin K deficiency or during administration of vitamin K antagonists, no carboxylation takes place. In that case, the uncarboxylated form of the protein comes into the circulation. These proteins induced by vitamin K absence (c.q. Antagonists) (PIVKAs) have no normal procoagulant function. Indeed, we discovered them [33] because they inhibit coagulation under certain circumstances. Recently, we isolated PIVKA-X, i.e. the uncarboxylated factor X from anticoagulated cows.[34] Like factor X, it can be activated by a protease from Russell's viper venom. Toward small synthetic substrates it shows esterolytic and peptidolytic activity similar to that of factor X_a. Like factor X_a it splits prothrombin in free solution. Unlike factor X, this activity cannot be enhanced by the addition of Ca^{++}, factor V, and phospholipid.[34] It thus seems that its active site, as well as its vulnerable site, is intact, but that due to an inability to bind to phospholipid it cannot partake in the normally active prothrombinase. Indeed, the only difference between the PIVKAs and the normal factors lies in the γ-carboxylation as has been demonstrated by Stenflo.[28, 29] He found γ-COOH groups as the only chemical difference between PIVKA-II and prothrombin. It is further emphasized by our recent finding that PIVKA-II can be converted into prothrombin in a vitamin K-dependent oxidative carboxylation by an enzyme system isolated from liver microsomes (Table 1).

The Paraenzymes (Factors V and VIII)

The function of the factors V and VIII is much less clear than those of the active site-bearing factors. Both factor V and factor VIII lack any known enzymatic property of their own.[35–38] Both occur in plasma as polymers; both are rendered more active by thrombin. Thrombin has been shown to favor the conversion of native factor V in more active moieties of ¼ of the original molecular weight, although small molecular weight factor V does occur without the action of thrombin, and then is also active. Thrombin-activated factor V readily inactivates in a reaction that is a dimerization or a higher order polymerization.[40] This suggests the following reactions:

$$V_t \leftrightharpoons 4V_{m.e} \xrightarrow{\text{thrombin}} 4V_{m.e} \rightleftarrows V_i.$$

t = tetramer; m = monomer; e = enhanced activity; i = inactive species.

The relative activities before and after thrombin action are unknown. Some

TABLE 1

CONVERSION OF PIVKA-II INTO PROTHROMBIN IN A CELL-FREE SYSTEM *

Component	Synthesis when Omitted	Replacement	Synthesis when Replaced
Microsomal protein	4	thromboplastin	5
Supernatant	33	—	
PIVKA–II	0	prothrombin	0
Vitamin K_1 (0.3 mM)	33	Warfarin (0.1 mM)	0
Mg (4 mM)	0	Ca (4 mM)	0
ATP (1.5 mM)	22	ADP (1.5 mM)	80
Creatine Phosphate (5 mM) +phosphokinase	89	—	
HCO_3^- (13 mM)	89	CO_3^{--} (13 mM)	11
O_2	—	N_2	38

* The activities are expressed as percentages of the synthesis rate in the complete mixture, i.e., 2 nM/hr. The complete system consists of: microsomal proteins, 0.2 OD_{280} units; microsomal supernatant, OD_{280} units; PIVKA–II, 0.16 units/ml; Tris-HCl, pH 8.5, 50 mM; Sucrose, 60 mM; and KCl, 30 mM. Thromboplastin (if present) 20% v/v Factor II (if present), 0.008 Units/ml, which causes a comparable clotting time as 0.16 U/ml of PIVKA–II. Mixtures of 0.1 ml were incubated for 1 hr at 37° C, diluted fourfold and assayed for factor II activity. The increase between the factor II activity at t=0 and t=60 min was a measure for the factor II synthesis. Microsomal proteins were partly purified on DEAE cellulose. PIVKA–II was partly purified on QAE Sephadex and adsorbed three times with an excess of $BaSO_4$ to remove the last traces of factor II.

reversibility of the inactivation has been demonstrated. It has also been demonstrated that the adsorption of factor V onto phospholipid enhances the adsorption of factor X_a. An interaction between factor V and factor X_a on the phospholipid surface is thus probable. This may also be deduced from the observation that prothrombinase and tenase develop slowly when a large phospholipid surface is offered.[22, 27] This may be interpreted as being due to a small chance for the two factors to interact, but persistent activity after interaction has taken place; i.e., the equilibrium in the formation of the complex must be at the side of the complex.

The biochemistry of factor VIII is even more complicated than that of factor V. As yet, no coherent picture of its mode of conversion and action can be given. The reader is referred to a recent review for further information.[41]

Both factor V and factor VIII do adsorb on hydrophobic powders. Factor V has been shown to retain a good deal of its activity when adsorbed, but will not elute from the powder.[42] This, together with the data on the influence of Ca^{++}-ions suggests that the binding of factor V to phospholipid may also be hydrophobic.

It has been demonstrated that factor V has a special affinity for a fragment of the prothrombin molecule.[43] Since factors V and VIII have no enzymatic activity of their own but specifically modify the enzyme with which they come in contact, we baptized them *paraenzymes.*

The Substrate

The substrate of prothrombinase is prothrombin. Prothrombinase brings about two cleavages of the primary structure, one at the Arg 373-Ile 374 bond. The active site-bearing β-chain of thrombin thus comes into being. The other is the Arg 274-Thr 275 bond that splits off thrombin α- and β-chain from the prothrombin molecule. The remainder of the molecule (the "pro"-part) contains the Ca^{++} and phospholipid-binding site; it can be again split by thrombin.[44-48]

PIVKA-II, which does not bind to phospholipid, is not a suitable substrate for prothrombinase, although it does contain normal thrombin[49] and will react like normal prothrombin when activated in free solution, either by proteolysis (Ecarin[50]) or by stoichiometric complexation with staphylocoagulase and subsequent change of tertiary structure.[51]

Factor X has been reported not to bind to phospholipid, but when it is activated, it does. It is not yet known if PIVKA-X is activated by "tenase."

The Phospholipid

Two types of protein-lipid interaction seem to be necessary: interaction of charged groups via Ca^{++} and hydrophobic interaction. The charge of the micelles will influence the possibilities for both Ca^{++} ions and charged proteins to approach the micelle and to attach to its surface by electrostatic forces. Since it has been shown that hydrophobic interactions do play a role too, the micelle also has to offer the possibility of hydrophobic interactions. Any micelle will do this, but to what extent depends on fatty acid chain length in the phospholipid as well as on the nature of the head groups. Therefore, apart from charge, *hydrophobicity* of the micelle will play a role in determining its coagulation activity.

The experiments on the formation of prothrombinase and tenase suggest that the lateral mobility of the adsorbed proteins will influence the activity of the enzymes.[27] This mobility will change with the "phase" of the micelle phospholipids; i.e., liquid, liquid crystalline, or solid. The phase at the ambient temperature is a function of the composition of the micelle.

Thus there are at least three properties of the micelle that will determine its effectiveness in these enzyme complexes: *phase, hydrophobicity,* and *charge.* All three vary with the composition of the micelle. This may explain why, in binary mixtures of pure phospholipids, there is a definite composition with optimal activity.[52-55]

The Role of the Phospholipid Surface

One can imagine at least three possible roles for the phospholipid surface in the generation of prothrombinase and tenase: 1) an increase in local concentration; 2) a reduction of the degrees of freedom of the movements of the proteins; and 3) induction of favorable changes in tertiary structure.

Increase in Local Concentration. The concentration of any protein at an interphase will be determined by the concentration of that protein in the surrounding solution and its affinity for the interphase. Proteins with a high affinity for a certain type of interphase will concentrate at that interphase. In fact, it has been shown that the concentration of clotting factors at the thrombocyte surface is high. One in every thousand or ten thousand protein molecules that a clotting factor meets is the partner for its function in coagulation. A local enrichment in concentration therefore seems essential. Yet there is reason to doubt that local concentration is the only factor involved, because 1) factor V enhances the adsorption of factor X_a, so there exists a cooperative interaction of these proteins; and 2) phillipin will interact with lipids in such a way as to enhance the adsorption of clotting factors but diminish its procoagulant activity.[56-57]

Local concentration at an interphase is a concept that should be used with some caution, because the amount of reacting species per unit volume is hardly a useful figure in this context. The possibility of interaction of the molecules is determined by the amount per surface and the mobility when adsorbed (c.q. via the fluid phase). Moreover, orientation effects will modify the percentage of meetings that lead to a reaction. This automatically leads to the following:

A Reduction of the Degrees of Freedom of the Movements of the Proteins. The active site of an enzyme and the vulnerable site of its protein substrate form only a small fraction of its total surface. A small portion of the collisions in free solution will therefore be effective. When enzyme and substrate are adsorbed at an interphase by a specific portion of their molecule they are orientated, and only a fraction of their surfaces can meet. Favorable orientation can enhance the possibility that the meeting surface contains the active and vulnerable sites. This orientation effect can be even more pronounced when a third molecule, the paraenzyme, brings about an orientation of substrate and enzyme in the plane of the interphase. There has recently been a discussion about the possibility that entropy changes favoring the "best fit" position could account for the final adjustment of positions just before the collision between enzyme and substrate. This entropy change would correspond to free energy changes in vibrational degrees of freedom. It was concluded that in bulk the translational degrees of freedom represent too much energy to allow this kind of regulation. These translational energies, however, are considerably lower for molecules adsorbed to an interface. We are at present investigating the possibilities that in that case this "entropy mechanism" might function. (W. T. Hermens, unpublished results.)

Induction of Favorable Changes in Tertiary Structure. Changes in tertiary structure will accompany any adsorption of a protein. That they are favorable in our case and if so, to what extent, is difficult to assess at this moment. One does not conclude from kinetic measurements that changes occur that are not readily reversible. This mechanism is of prime interest in the generation of contact product, but its role in the generation of tenase and prothrombinase waits for further elucidation.

REFERENCES

1. RATNOFF, O. D. 1976. This volume.
2. KAPLAN, A. P. 1976. This volume.
3. MACFARLANE, R. G. 1964. Nature **202:** 489–499.
4. DAVIE, E. & O. D. RATNOFF. 1964. 1310–1312.
5. FUJIKAWA, K., M. E. LEGAZ, H. KATO & E. W. DAVIE. 1974. Biochemistry **13:** 5208–5216.
6. RADCLIFFE, R. D. & P. G. BARTON. 1972. J. Biol. Chem. **247:** 7735–7741.
7. FUJIKAWA, K., M. E. LEGAZ & E. W. DAVIE. 1972. Biochemistry **11:** 4892–4898.
8. JACKSON, C. M. 1972. Biochemistry **11:** 4873–4881.
9. JACKSON, C. M., W. G. OWEN, S. N. GITEL & C. T. ESMON. 1974. Thrombos. Diathes. Haemorrh. (Suppl.) **57:** 273–293.
10. ESNOUF, M. P. & F. JOBIN. 1965. Thrombos. Diathes. Haemorrh. (Suppl.) **17:** 103–110.
11. JOBIN, F. & M. P. ESNOUF. 1967. Biochem. J. **102:** 666–674.
12. BANGHAM, A. D. 1961. Nature **4808:** 1197–1198.
13. CHUANG, T. F., R. B. SARGEANT & C. HOUGIE. 1972. Biochim. Biophys. Acta **273:** 287–291.
14. COLE, E. R., J. L. KOPPEL & J. H. OLWIN. 1965. Thrombos. Diathes. Haemorrh. **14:** 431–435.
15. COLE, E. R., J. L. KOPPEL & J. H. OLWIN. 1964. Can. J. Biochem. **42:** 1595–1603.
16. HANAHAN, D. J. & D. PAPAHADJOPOULOS. 1965. Thrombos. Diathes. Haemorrh. (Suppl.) **17:** 71–76.
17. PAPAHADJOPOULOS, D. & D. J. HANAHAN. 1964. Biochim. Biophys. Acta **90:** 436–439.
18. BARTON, P. G. & D. J. HANAHAN. 1969. Biochim. Biophys. Acta **187:** 319–327.
19. BULL, R. K., S. JEVONS & P. G. BARTON. 1972. J. Biol. Chem. **247:** 2747–2754.
20. HEMKER, H. C. & M. J. P. KAHN. 1967. Nature **215:** 1201–1202.
21. DEGGELLER, K. & J. VREEKEN. 1969. Thrombos. Diathes. Haemorrh. **22:** 45–67.
22. HEMKER, H. C., M. P. ESNOUF, P. W. HEMKER, A.C.W. SWART & R. G. MACFARLANE. 1967. Nature **215:** 246–251.
23. BARTON, P. G. 1967. Nature **215:** 1508–1509.
24. HEMKER, H. C., M. J. P. KAHN & P. P. DEVILEE. 1970. Thrombos. Diathes. Haemorrh. **24:** 214–223.
25. HOUGIE, C., K. W. E. DENSON & R. BIGGS. 1967. Thrombos. Diathes. Haemorrh. **18:** 211–222.
26. OSTERUD, B. & S. I. RAPAPORT. 1970. Biochemistry **9:** 1854–1861.
27. VARADI, K. & H. C. HEMKER. 1976. Thrombosis Res. **8:** 303–317.
28. STENFLO, J. 1975. *In* Prothrombin and Related Coagulation Factors. H. C. Hemker and J. J. Veltkamp, Eds. : 152–158. Leiden University Press. Leiden, The Netherlands.
29. STENFLO, J., P. FERNLUND, W. EGAN & P. ROEPSTORFF. 1974. Proc. Nat. Acad. Sci. USA **71:** 2730–2733.
30. ESMON, C. T., J. W. SUTTIE & C. M. JACKSON. 1975. J. Biol. Chem. **250:** 4095–4099.
31. REEKERS, P. P. M., M. J. LINDHOUT, B. H. M. KOP-KLAASSEN & H. C. HEMKER. 1973. Bioch. Biophys. Acta **317:** 559–562.
32. HEMKER, H. C., M. J. LINDHOUT & P. P. M. REEKERS. 1974. *In* Thrombosis, Pathogenesis and Clinical Trials. Trans. Plenary Sessions IVth Int. Congress Thrombosis and Haemostasis: 45–52. Vienna, Austria.
33. HEMKER, H. C., J. J. VELTKAMP, A. HENSEN & E. A. LOELIGER. 1963. Nature **200:** 589–590.
34. LINDHOUT, M. J. & B. H. M. KOP-KLAASSEN. 1975. Thrombos. Diathes. Haemorrh. **34:** 592.

35. BIGGS, R. & R. G. MACFARLANE. 1965. Brit. J. Haematol. **11:** 276–295.
36. NEWCOMB, T. F. & M. HASHIDA. 1965. Scand. J. Clin. Lab. Invest. (Suppl. 17) **84:** 61–69.
37. PRENTICE, C. R. & O. D. RATNOFF. 1969. Brit. J. Haematol. **16:** 291–302.
38. STENFLO, J. 1973. J. Biol. Chem. **248:** 6325–6332.
39. KAHN, M. J. P. & H. C. HEMKER. 1972. Thrombos. Diathes. Haemorrh. **27:** 25–32.
40. HEMKER, H. C. & M. J. P. KAHN. 1972. Thrombos. Diathes. Haemorrh. **27:** 33–42.
41. VAN MOURIK, J. A., B. N. BOUMA & I. A. MOCHTAR. 1975. *In* Handbook of Hemophilia. K. M. Brinkhous & H. C. Hemker, Eds. : 77–102. Excerpta Med. Amsterdam, The Netherlands.
42. KAHN, M. J. P. & H. C. HEMKER. 1969. Thrombos. Diathes. Haemorrh .**22:** 417–430.
43. ESMON, C. T. & C. M. JACKSON. 1974. J. Biol. Chem. **249:** 7791–7799.
44. HELDEBRANT, C. M. & K. G. MANN. 1973. J. Biol. Chem. **248:** 3642–3652.
45. OWEN, W. G., C .T. ESMON & C. M. JACKSON. 1974. J. Biol. Chem. **249:** 594–605.
46. MANN, K. G., C. M. HELDEBRANT & D. N. FASS. 1971. J. Biol. Chem. **246:** 6106–6114.
47. JESTY, J. & M. P. ESNOUF. 1973. Biochem. J. **131:** 791–799.
48. MAGNUSSON, S., L. SOTTRUP-JENSEN, T. ELLEBAEK-PETERSEN & H. CLAEYS. 1975. *In* Prothrombin and Related Coagulation Factors. H. C. Hemker & J. J. Veltkamp, Eds. : 25–47. Leiden Univ. Press. Leiden, The Netherlands.
49. HEMKER, H. C., A. D. MULLER & E. A. LOELIGER. 1970. Thrombos. Diathes. Haemorrh. **23:** 633–637.
50. KORNALIK, F. & B. BLOMBÄCK. 1975. Thrombos. Res. **6:** 53–63.
51. HEMKER, H. C., B. M. BAS & A. D. MULLER. 1975. Biochim. Biophys. Acta **379:** 180–188.
52. PAPAHADJOPOULOS, D., C. HOUGIE & D. J. HANAHAN. 1962. Proc. Soc. Exp. Biol. Med. **111:** 412–416.
53. MARCUS, A. J. 1966. Adv. Lipid Res. **4:** 1–37.
54. DAEMEN, F. J. M., C. VAN ARKEL, H. C. HART, C. VAN DRIFT & L. L. M. VAN DEENEN. 1965. Thrombos. Diathes. Haemorrh. **13:** 194–203.
55. BARTON, P. G. 1969. *In* Structural and Functional Aspects of Lipoproteins in Living Systems. E. Tria and A. M. Scanu, Eds. : 463–515. Academic Press. New York, N.Y.
56. VAN DER PLAS, P. M., L. KRAAN, G. VAN ES, J. STIBBE & H. C. HEMKER. 1974. J. Mol. Med. **3:** 1–8.
57. VAN DER PLAS, P. M., G. VAN ES, L. KRAAN & H. C. HEMKER. 1973. J. Mol. Med. **1:** 191–204.

DISCUSSION

Dr. Rosenberg: I think Dr. Hemker has pointed out the importance of cofactors in the coagulation mechanism. I might start out the discussion by asking both Dr. Ratnoff and Dr. Kaplan the following question: It seems to me that the high molecular weight kininogen-low molecular weight kininogen transition is a very critical one in allowing factor XII to activate its various substrates. We know that most of the kininogen circulates in the low molecular weight or inactive form. What do you think is responsible for running this process, and what effect does it have on the contact with blood?

Dr. Ratnoff: That's a charmingly easy question to answer. I don't know, but I would like to talk a little about high molecular weight kininogen. In my paper, I cut out description of an experiment that was close to but not identical with the one that Dr. Kaplan described; and I might say that his data and ours are in agreement about most things. The experiment that I didn't show runs something like this. Plasma kallikrein, as was first shown by others, digests a synthetic amide, and the result is a beautiful yellow color. This, I assume, is the same substrate used by Dr. Kaplan. Kallikrein will do this in a pure system in which you just have kallikrein and the substrate. The presence or absence of high molecular weight kininogen doesn't particularly matter. Now, kallikrein adsorbs onto insoluble substances, and it does this better than Hageman factor does. In its adsorbed state, kallikrein is a very poor digestor of this synthetic substrate. It's as if—perhaps as Dr. Hemker suggests—some of those active groups are turned upside down and can't get out. If one first treats the kaolin, the activator of Hageman factor (but there is no Hageman factor in this system now), and treats it with Fitzgerald factor, this kaolin-treated Fitzgerald factor will no longer inactivate plasma kallikrein. Prevention of inactivation thus looks like activation. I think, to get back to the last sentence of my talk, everything that Dr. Kaplan and I have been talking about is artifactual. In real life we haven't any idea how these agents interreact, and we know that we're missing the point because patients lacking Hageman factor, the Fitzgerald factor, and Fletcher factor are asymptomatic. Whales live out their whole long life times without any Hageman factor or any Fletcher factor.

Dr. Kaplan: There is so far no evidence that one can convert the high molecular weight kininogen to the low in a simple enzymatic way. The high is a substrate of plasma kallikrein. Nobody has succeeded yet in converting high molecular weight kininogen into low by digesting it with kallikrein; so one of the questions is: Are these two proteins synthesized by the same gene? Antibody to low molecular weight kininogen gives a complete line of identity with the high, so the structure of the low is essentially contained within the high, which would make you think that it's not synthesized by two genes. Tagged high molecular weight kininogen added to plasma shows no conversion to the low molecular weight kininogen, so there is no obvious proteolytic process, at least in plasma, by which the high is converted to the low. Finally, I would like to put forth the following notion: we know that to make an IgG molecule you have to have a minimum of four genes—two for the light chain and two for the heavy chain. The light chain is about 22,500 molecular weight. There is a gene for the antibody-binding region and a gene for the constant region, and somehow these are put together at the transcription level or the translation level. I would wonder whether, in fact, there is not one gene for low molecular weight kininogen and another gene for the part of the high that differs, and that the two are put together to form the high molecular weight kininogen; but there would be an excess on the part of the one that makes low, and that's what we see in the plasma. It is interesting to note that some of the patients with high molecular weight kininogen deficiency, like our patients, have no kininogen at all, zero high and zero low. But in the Fitzgerald patient, I believe total kininogen is almost 50%, yet all of it is the low form. So maybe he has that part of it but is completely missing the other half.

DR. VROMAN: How can we explain that the phospholipid micelles even when suspended in a lot of plasma protein to begin with, still seem to adsorb selectively only a couple of protein species during clotting? Do you presume that there is displacement of other proteins when you start adding calcium, for example, in your system? How can trace proteins such as factors VIII and IX compete with abundant proteins such as albumin and globulins?

DR. HEMKER: I think they would compete because of their equilibrium constants between their concentration in a free solution and the concentration adsorbed. I think there is a clear indication that at least the factors II, VII, IX, and X are provided with a specific binding group to bind to these phospholipids.

DR. B. ALEXANDER (*New York Blood Center, New York, N.Y.*): Dr. Hemker, there has been no allusion to the action of naturally occurring detergent agents such as bile salts. Would you care to speculate as to their possible role regarding the lipid micelles and their possible role in activation of some of the clotting factors.

DR. HEMKER: I have actually avoided discussing all types of physical and physicochemical circumstances that do alter the phospholipid surface, because things really get complicated.

DR. NOSSEL: There has been some suggestion that platelets may activate the Hageman factor system, and I wonder if Dr. Kaplan or Dr. Ratnoff has any sentiments about that phenomenon.

DR. RATNOFF: I suppose I have sentiments about everything. But as far as I know, the experiments by Dr. Walsh to which you refer have not been confirmed anywhere. And, as far as I know, there is no firm evidence that platelets will activate Hageman factor or PTA, in the presence or absence of ADP.

DR. NOSSEL: Does anybody want to contradict that?

DR. RATNOFF: Just remember I said "as far as I know." I didn't say it wasn't true.

DR. WEISS: We have tried to either confirm or not confirm Peter Walsh's studies, and we've had both some success on one hand and no success on the other. The contact system is activated by kaolin more readily in the presence of platelets than in the absence of platelets. However, we could not do the same with collagen.

DR. RATNOFF: Could we talk a little bit about terminology? High molecular weight kininogen, to the extent that we know at this point, is identical with the term "Fitzgerald factor," defined as being an agent missing in Fitzgerald trait. There are four other families that have been described in which high molecular weight kininogen is deficient. Three of these four families at least have a defect qualitatively different from Fitzgerald trait. The patients with William's trait lack not only high molecular weight kininogen—that is, Fitzgerald factor—but additionally, low molecular weight kininogen, as Dr. Kaplan said. The same is true of a family of a patient named Flaujeac, lacking both high and low molecular weight kininogen, and this has been referred to as "Flaujeac trait." The same is also true of the patients named Washington in Cincinnati described as having Fitzgerald trait, but in fact deficient both in the high molecular weight kininogen—that is, the Fitzgerald factor—and in low molecular weight kininogen. Hopefully, my colleagues and I will drop this rather charming nomenclature and stick to high and low molecular weight and combined kininogen deficiencies.

SURFACE-INDUCED PLATELET ADHESION, AGGREGATION, AND RELEASE * †

E. W. Salzman, J. Lindon, and D. Brier

Department of Surgery
Harvard Medical School
Boston, Massachusetts 02115
Department of Surgery
Beth Israel Hospital
Boston, Massachusetts 02215

E. W. Merrill

Department of Chemical Engineering
Massachusetts Institute of Technology
Cambridge, Massachusetts 02139

The secretion of intracellular constituents ("release reaction") and aggregation are common responses to stimulation of platelets by a variety of agonists and together constitute the major aspects of what Holmsen has termed "the basic platelet reaction."[1] These processes comprise the ultimate expression of a complicated series of biochemical reactions that have been extensively studied *in vitro* and about which much is known. There is evidence that an early event is activation of an endogenous phospholipase leading to hydrolysis of phospholipids in the platelet membrane, thought principally to involve phosphatidyl choline, with liberation of arachidonic acid.[2–4] Enzymatic conversion of this essential fatty acid to labile endoperoxide precursors of the stable prostaglandins, PGE_2 and $PGF_{2\alpha}$, can be blocked by aspirin and other nonsteroidal anti-inflammatory agents, which are powerful inhibitors of the release reaction and platelet clumping.[5–7] Samuelsson and associates have reported that prostaglandins are only a minor fraction of endoperoxide breakdown, quantitatively speaking, several orders of magnitude more of the endoperoxide molecules being converted to an unstable biologically active substance termed thromboxane A_2.[8, 9] This compound is postulated to be the principal effector in induction of the platelet release reaction, aggregation then resulting from the products of release. Prostaglandin E_2, which does not itself initiate platelet activity, apparently has an important amplifying effect on processes induced by other stimuli.[10, 11]

The release reaction of platelets in response to most stimuli is accompanied by a fall in the platelet content of cyclic AMP (cAMP).[12, 13] Like prostaglandin synthesis, this effect is blocked by aspirin. There is much evidence to suggest that cAMP is important in the regulation of platelet activity, although the details of its role are disputed. For example, marked inhibition of platelet function results from an increase in platelet cAMP, which may be produced in platelet-rich plasma by incubation with dibutyryl cAMP,[14] by inhibition of platelet

* This project was supported by National Institutes of Health grants HL 14322 and HL 11414.

† Abbreviations: PC=pyrolytic carbon; PVAc or PVA=polyvinyl acetate; PMA=polymethyl acrylate; PEA=polyethyl acrylate; AN=acrylonitrile; PS=polystyrene; PMMA=polymethyl methacrylate.

phosphodiesterase (e.g., by papaverine, dipyridamole, or caffeine),[14, 15, 16] or by stimulation of adenylate cyclase (e.g., by adenosine or PGE_1).[14, 17-20] The last-named is not a normal constituent of platelets, despite the fact that they possess the enzymatic machinery required for its synthesis. Its absence from the blood probably results from lack of its fatty acid precursor, dihomo-γ-linolenic acid. Recent evidence suggests that it may be produced in other tissues whose traffic with the blood could be significant for regulation of platelet function.[21]

In some instances, a reduction of platelet cAMP is paralleled by a rise in platelet cyclic GMP (cGMP). For example, increased cGMP has been demonstrated with collagen, ADP, epinephrine, thrombin, and arachidonic acid.[13, 22, 23]

The interrelations of the metabolism of platelet prostaglandins and their precursors and cyclic nucleotides are not entirely understood, but, as in other tissues, there is evidence to suggest an association.[24, 25] Low concentrations of PGE_2, in the range produced during platelet activation, enhance platelet clumping[11, 26] and lower cAMP.[12] Recently it has been reported that addition of prostaglandin endoperoxides to platelet-rich plasma lowers the platelet content of cAMP[24] and (in a suspension of washed platelets) raises cGMP.[22] Whether these alterations in cyclic nucleotide levels mediate the effects of prostaglandins and their precursors on platelets remains to be determined. Platelets contain cAMP-dependent protein kinases, the natural substrates of which have not been established with certainty.[27, 28] cGMP-dependent enzymes have not yet been identified in platelets.

Experiments with ionophores for divalent cations have indicated the importance of cytoplasmic calcium levels in the regulation of platelet function,[29, 30] and it is possible that cyclic nucleotides produce their effects by influencing calcium homeostasis. Unlike most other aggregating agents, calcium ionophores do not reduce platelet cAMP, but their actions are blocked by elevation of the platelet cAMP level.[24] Alternatively, Samuelsson has suggested that cAMP regulates the activity of platelet cyclo-oxygenase, the enzyme that converts arachidonic acid to endoperoxides.[31] A hypothetical scheme of the interrelations of these various processes has been proposed (FIGURE 1).[24]

Most of the evidence for the foregoing is from *in vitro* experiments, in which platelet activation was produced by soluble substances such as ADP, epinephrine, or thrombin. It is, however, clear that platelet activation can also occur in response to mechanical or other physical stimuli. The subsequent events apparently proceed through the same pathways.[32] For example, Lüscher and others[33-35] have initiated the platelet-release reaction by centrifugation of platelet-rich plasma, and similar effects have been seen with filtration of platelets through a column of Sepharose gel or by stirring with particles of kaolin or other substances.[32] Such stimuli have been shown to lead to the production of prostaglandins[32] and therefore presumably of endoperoxide prostaglandin precursors. Reduction of platelet cAMP in response to physical stimulation has also been reported.[32, 36] The magnitude of the response is a function of the intensity of the stimulus. For example, with centrifugation the production of prostaglandin E_2 and the decrease of cAMP are functions of the g force applied.[32] Elevation of platelet cGMP in response to centrifugation also occurs (FIGURE 2).

The responses of platelets to physical stimuli and to soluble substances have other similarities. When ADP, or epinephrine, or, in low concentration, thrombin are added to platelet-rich plasma the effects do not proceed immediately to release of platelet constituents and irreversible aggregation. Rather, there is

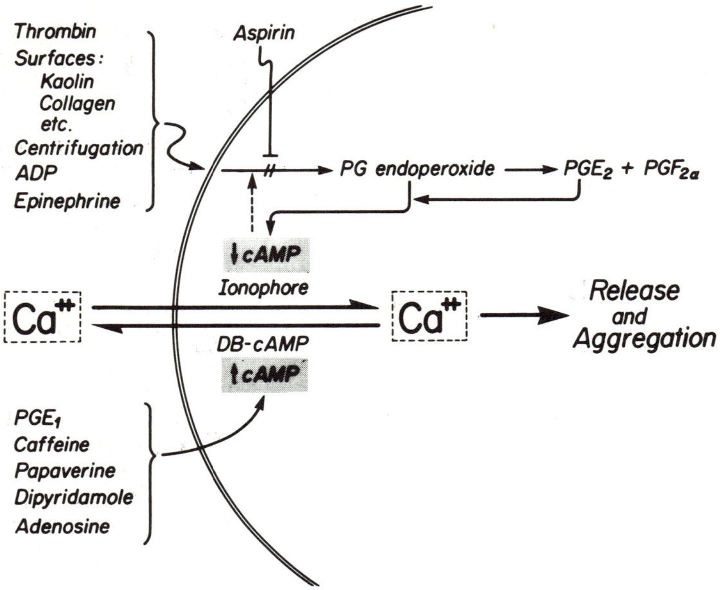

FIGURE 1. Hypothetical scheme of platelet reactions to a variety of stimuli. For description, see text.

first a reversible phase of platelet clumping that has been termed primary aggregation. During this interval, which in the case of ADP may last a minute or two, platelet release of serotonin or adenine nucleotides is said not to occur.[37] This point has been disputed recently.[37a] The release reaction appears to occur after the peak of primary aggregation, immediately preceding the second more

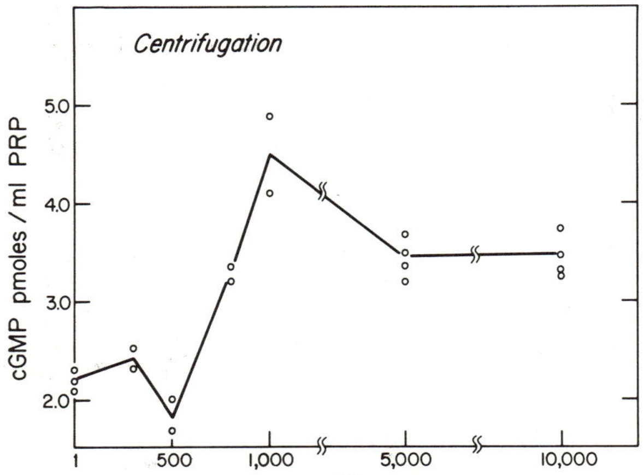

FIGURE 2. Cyclic GMP in citrated platelet-rich plasma (PRP) after centrifugation for 10 min at 20° (assayed by method of Steiner et al.)[48]

intense and generally irreversible phase of platelet aggregation. Inhibition of the release reaction by nonsteroidal anti-inflammatory agents eliminates the second but not the first phase of platelet clumping.[38] Thus, release and irreversible or second-phase aggregation might be attributed to reactions associated with activation of prostaglandin synthetic pathways, but the initial phase of platelet clumping would not seem to be dependent on these processes.

It seems possible that the platelet-platelet contact or propinquity of primary aggregation is in a sense a form of stimulation of the platelet by physical means, analogous to centrifugation or adsorption on an artificial surface. According to this hypothesis, deformation or other physical perturbations of the platelet membrane might be common pathways by which diverse agonists lead to phospholipase activation and inauguration of prostaglandin synthetic mechanisms and thus to the release reaction and irreversible aggregation.

The properties of a surface that determine its tendency to produce platelet adhesion and thus to set off the subsequent events, release and aggregation, are reviewed elsewhere in this symposium by Merrill.[39] We have studied these relationships *in vitro* with a method based on column chromatography. Beads of the material to be examined (diam 0.2–0.5 mm) are packed into a column through which anticoagulated blood is pumped from below at a fixed rate. Effluent blood is collected and examined for evidence of retention of platelets on the column, release of platelet constituents, hemolysis, and other effects. Air-blood contact is avoided. Materials tested have been especially synthesized under clean conditions and are substances of known composition free of plasticizers, mold release agents, surface polishes, and other contaminating artifacts. The surface-to-volume relationships are such that 3 ml of whole blood may be exposed to up to 1,600 square cm of bead surface, a severe test of blood-surface compatibility. The details of the method and its validation are presented elsewhere.[40]

Adhesion of a monolayer of platelets invariably occurs on materials we have studied and is often followed by the appearance of gradually enlarging masses of attached platelets that apparently develop by accretion (FIGURES 3A & 3B). In addition, platelet aggregation may occur in the bulk fluid phase; platelet clumps are sometimes found in the blood after passage through the bead column. The release of serotonin and adenine nucleotides can be demonstrated in this system. The extent of release varies with the material to be tested (FIGURE 4). With materials that are active in induction of the plaelet-release reaction, platelet aggregates in the effluent blood are more numerous. Some materials appear to retain many platelets despite minimal release of platelet constituents (e.g., pyrolytic carbon (FIGURE 4)). This point may be confused by reuptake of released serotonin by platelets retained on the column. Whether serotonin released by platelets retained in the column is taken up again by the same platelets or by other retained platelets that have not undergone release is not certain. To minimize the reuptake of serotonin by platelets on the column, imipramine 2.5 μM is added to the blood before it passes through the column of beads. At this concentration, imipramine does not inhibit the platelet-release reaction induced by ADP or thrombin but strongly inhibits platelet serotonin uptake.[41]

As has previously been suggested, materials in contact with the blood develop an adsorbed film of plasma constituents that seems to be important in the subsequent events.[42–44] Precoating the beads with fibrinogen solutions markedly augments their reactivity with platelets, whereas human serum albumin reduces the activity of most materials (FIGURES 5A & 5B). Preincubation with albumin solution decreases the extent of the release reaction and platelet aggregation that occur when blood is later passed through the column and also appears to reduce the adhesion of single platelets to the surface.

Some surfaces can be passivated by preliminary exposure to platelet-free

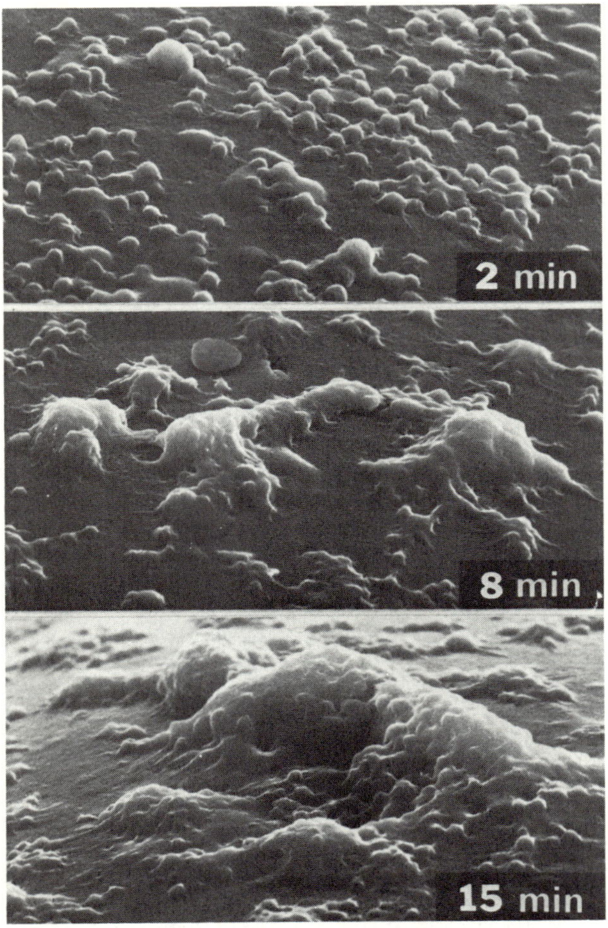

FIGURE 3A. Course of events during passage of citrated whole blood through a column of LTL pyrolytic carbon beads. Panels show scanning electron micrographs of the beads at intervals.

plasma. In the experiment illustrated in FIGURES 6A and 6B, 20 column volumes of citrated platelet-poor plasma were passed through the column, followed by whole blood. Reduction in platelet retention and release resulted, and electron microscopy demonstrated the absence of adherent platelets. This result was unexpected, since at first consideration, one might not expect exposure

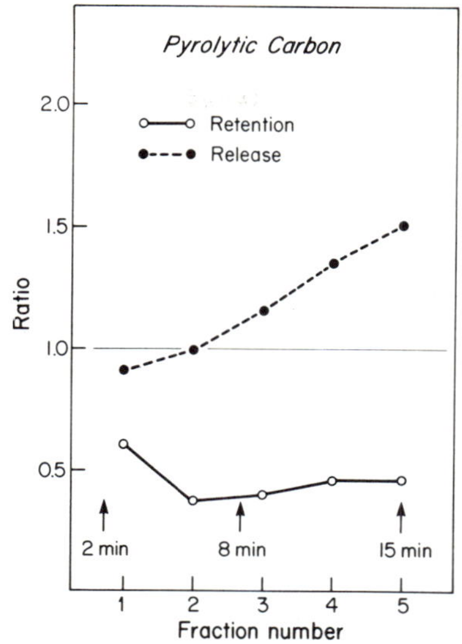

FIGURE 3B. See legend for FIGURE 3A. Upper tracing here and in subsequent figures illustrates release of [^{14}C]-serotonin in successive aliquots of blood passed through the column (expressed as a ratio of [^{14}C]-CPM in control plasma). Lower tracing here and in subsequent figures represents retention of platelets by the column (ratio of platelet count in effluent blood/platelet count in control blood). For details of methods, see Ref. 40.

of a surface to plasma followed by blood to differ in its effects from exposure to blood without preliminary plasma contact. It might reasonably be presumed that, when blood first entered the column of beads, the beads would acquire a coating film of plasma proteins before encountering any formed elements, all of which are less numerous and larger and therefore diffuse less rapidly than plasma-protein molecules. That a surface such as polymethyl acrylate can be passivated by relatively brief exposure to plasma before whole blood suggests rapid alterations in composition or configuration of the adsorbed protein film, with initial reactivity and subsequent development of an interface that is unattractive to platelets.

Other materials appear to achieve such a passive layer after a period of contact with whole blood, without preliminary exposure to plasma. Thus, polymethyl acrylate/acrylonitrile copolymer is one of the more reactive materials we have tested when it is initially exposed to blood, retaining most of the

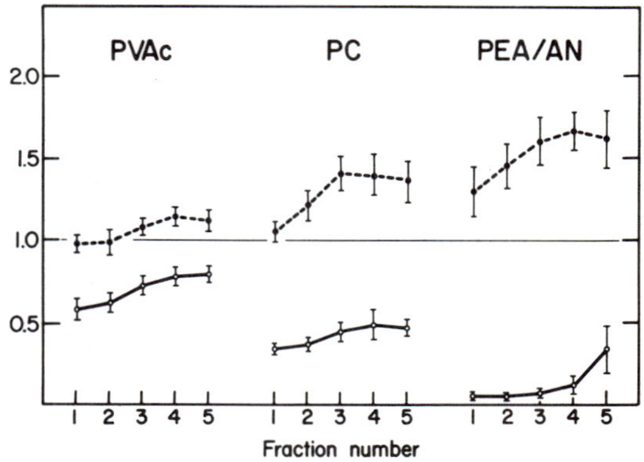

FIGURE 4. Comparison of three different materials. Values less than 1.0 in serotonin-release ratio presumably result from reuptake of released serotonin by platelets retained in the column despite the addition of 2.5 μM imipramine to the blood before the test.

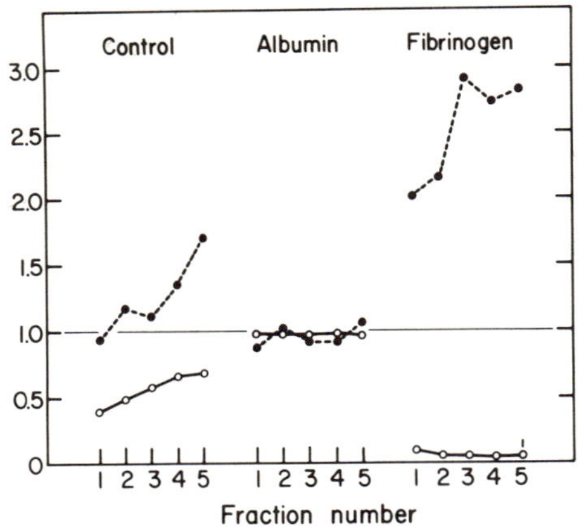

FIGURE 5A. Effect of preincubation of bead column (polystyrene) with human albumin (Hyland) 50 mg/ml or human fibrinogen (Kabi) 5 mg/ml in saline before passage of citrated whole blood through the column.

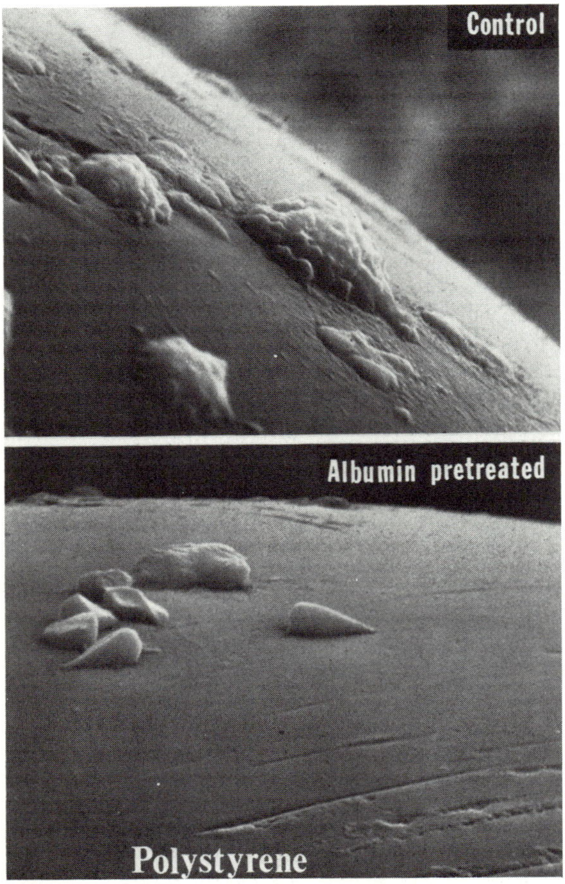

FIGURE 5B. See legend for FIGURE 5A. Scanning electron micrograph shows beads from control and albumin-coated samples after blood contact.

FIGURE 6A. Effects of passage of citrated platelet-poor plasma (PPP) 20 column volumes through a polymethyl acrylate bead column before whole blood. Period of pretreatment with plasma occupies 30 min and is followed by 20 column volumes of 0.145 M NaCl solution before the blood.

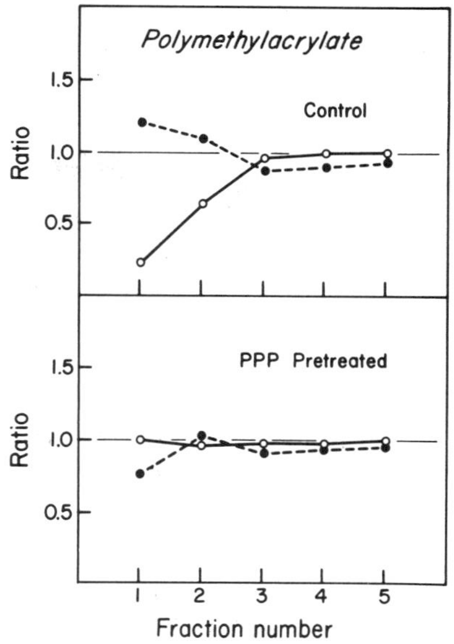

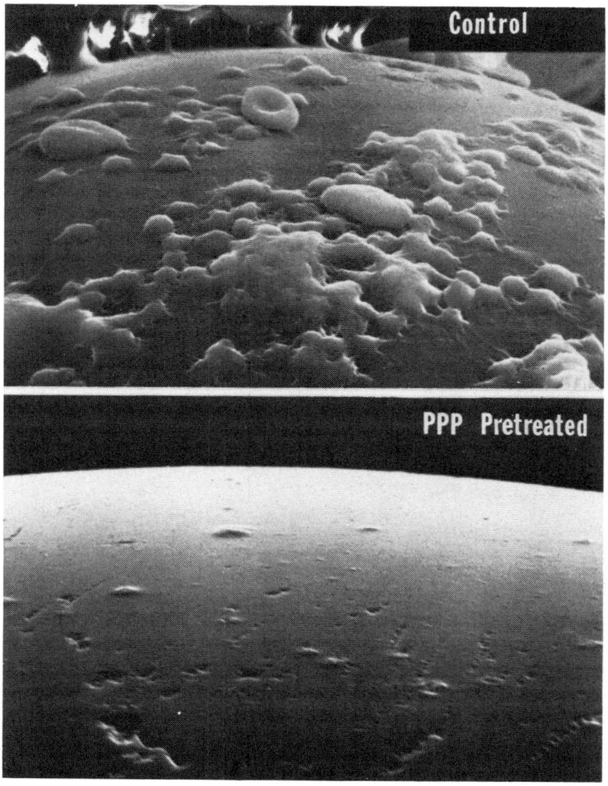

FIGURE 6B. See legend for FIGURE 6A.

TABLE 1

PLATELET RETENTION, CHANGE WITH TIME *

	Fraction 1 and 2 (mean)	Fraction 5
Surface		
PVA	.73±.22	.73±.37
PS	.75±.27	.62±.39
PC	.50±.20	.57±.27
PMA	.47±.29	.50±.43
PMA/AN Copolymer	.18±.17	.71±.26

* Each fraction=2 void volumes. Values=(1−fraction retained)±S.D.

platelets presented to it and producing a large release of serotonin (TABLE 1). By the time ten void volumes of blood have passed over the beads, however, the behavior of the polymer is quite different. Now, few platelets are removed from blood passing through the column, and serotonin release is not evident. By contrast, other polymers may not change appreciably in activity during the course of the experiment or may even become more reactive.

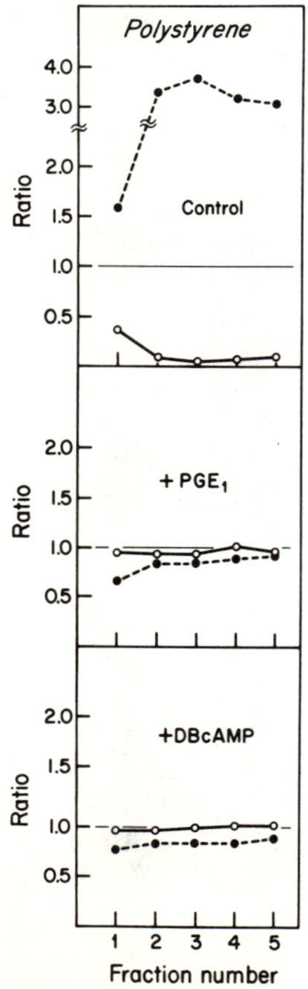

FIGURE 7A. Effect of prostaglandin E_1 1.0 μgm/ml or dibutyryl cyclic AMP 10^{-3} M added to whole blood immediately prior to passage through a column of polystyrene beads.

Addition to the blood of substances that increase platelet cAMP can totally eliminate adherence of platelets to surfaces. Effective agents include stimulants to adenylate cyclase such as prostaglandins E_1 or D_2 or adenosine, inhibitors of phosphodiesterase such as caffeine or dipyridamole, or more directly acting

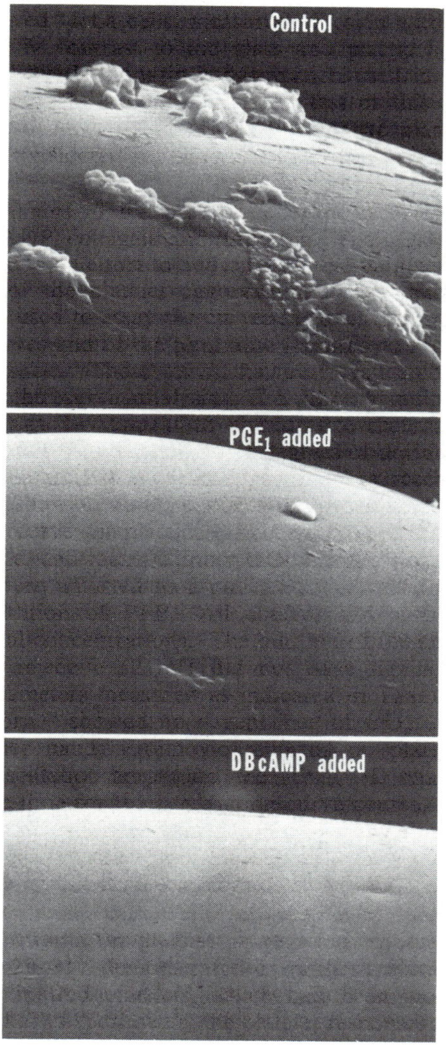

FIGURE 7B. See legend for FIGURE 7A.

agents such as dibutyryl cAMP (FIGURES 7A & 7B). In the case of these drugs, the platelet response is directly related to the concentration of the inhibitor. Release reaction and development of platelet thrombi are inhibited at lower concentrations, but adhesion of single platelets to the beads persists. To eliminate adhesion of platelets to surfaces requires higher concentrations of the drugs.

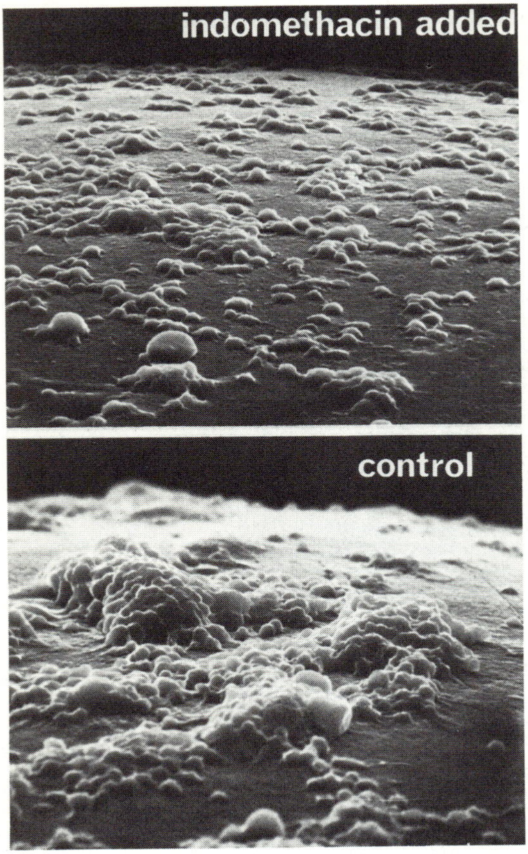

FIGURE 8A. Effect of indomethacin 10^{-4} M added to blood before passage through a column of beads. Scanning electron micrographs.

These results parallel the response of a platelet suspension or platelet-rich plasma to soluble aggregating agents in the presence of these inhibitors. The initial effect is reduction of release and of irreversible "second phase" aggregation. With increasing concentrations of the inhibitors and increasing cyclic AMP levels, primary aggregation is also blocked. These results provide an additional example of the similarity of platelet adhesion to surfaces and primary aggregation.

Release of platelet serotonin and therefore presumably of adenine nucleotides in response to surface contact can be blocked by nonsteroidal anti-inflammatory agents such as aspirin or indomethacin (FIGURES 8A & 8B). However, even at millimolar concentrations, these drugs do not prevent adhesion of platelets to artificial surfaces. Thus, the release reaction does not appear to be a necessary precursor for platelet adhesion to polymer surfaces.

Further, the platelet-release reaction does not seem to be essential for the development of platelet aggregates in response to platelet-surface interactions. In systems in which platelet release of serotonin and adenine nucleotides is strongly inhibited by indomethacin, extensive platelet aggregation may still occur, and clumps of platelets may be found on the surface of the beads

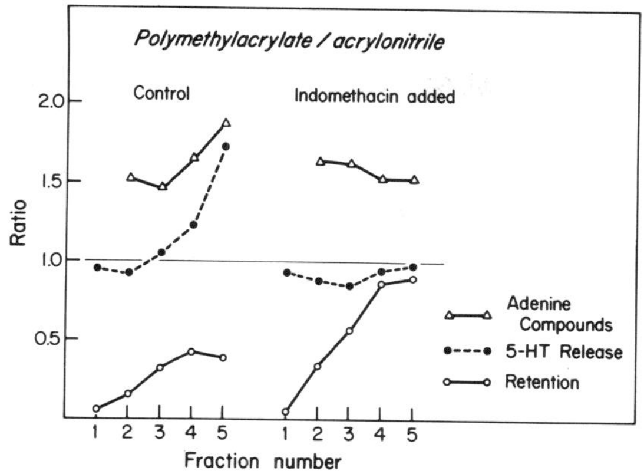

FIGURE 8B. See legend for FIGURE 8A. Tracing of release of [^{14}C]-5-hydroxytryptamine, adenine compounds in plasma, and platelet retention in the column.

(FIGURE 8A & 8B). Assay of plasma adenine nucleotides in the effluent blood demonstrates their presence in large quantities, despite the inhibition of serotonin release. These results suggest a source of plasma ADP other than the platelet, most likely from red cells as a consequence of their interaction with the artificial surfaces. Born, Bergqvist, and Arfors [45] have suggested a possible antithrombotic action for drugs that act by stabilization of the erythrocyte membrane. Allen and Rasmussen have reported that PGE_2 in low concentrations decreases the deformability of the red cell membrane and increases the red cell's sensitivity to hemolysis.[46] The effective PGE_2 concentrations in these experiments are in the same range as those produced by endogenous platelet prostaglandin synthesis after stimulation of platelets with aggregating agents and are similar to levels of PGE_2 that augment platelet activity, increase platelet thromboxane levels,[47] and reduce platelet cAMP.[12] It is possible that red cell-surface interactions have physiological importance as an additional control mechanism for modulation of platelet-surface reactivity.

Selection of polymer surfaces or of pharmacologic inhibitors permits one to eliminate the platelet release reaction and aggregation without impairment of the initial adhesion of platelets to artificial surfaces, but experiments in which adhesion is blocked invariably result in loss of release and aggregation. Adhesion of platelets appears to be a prerequisite for subsequent release and aggregation in response to surface contact. Surfaces to which platelets do not adhere because of albumin or plasma precoating, for example, do not induce platelet release, and platelet clumps are not observed on such beads within the column or in the effluent blood. Whether red cell-surface interactions are influenced by such pretreatment has not yet been clarified.

REFERENCES

1. HOLMSEN, H. 1974. Are platelet shape change, aggregation, and release reaction tangible manifestations of one basic platelet function? *In* Platelets: Production, Function, Transfusion, and Storage. M. Baldini & S. Ebbe, Eds.: 207–220. Grune & Stratton, New York, N.Y.

2. SMITH, J. B. & D. E. MACFARLANE. 1974. Platelets. *In* The Prostaglandins. P. Ramwell, Ed. Vol. **2:** 293–343. Plenum Press. New York, N.Y.
3. BILLS, T. K. & M. J. SILVER. 1975. Fed. Proc. **34:** 790.
4. SCHOENE, N. W. & J. M. IACNO. 1975. Fed. Proc. **34:** 257.
5. HAMBERG, M. & B. SAMUELSSON. 1973. Prco. Nat. Acad. Sci. USA **70:** 899.
6. WILLIS, A. L. & D. C. KUHN. 1973. Prostaglandins **4:** 127.
7. WEISS, H. J., L. M. ALEDORT & S. KOCHWA. 1968. J. Clin. Invest. **47:** 2169.
8. SAMUELSSON, B., M. HAMBERG, C. MALMSTEN & J. SVENSSON. 1976. The role of prostaglandin endoperoxides and thromboxanes in platelet aggregation. *In* Advances in Prostaglandin and Thromboxane Research. B. Samuelsson & R. Paoletti, Eds. Vol. **2:** 737–746. Raven Press. New York, N.Y.
9. HAMBERG, M., J. SVENSSON & B. SAMUELSSON. 1975. Proc. Nat. Acad. Sci. USA **72:** 2994–2998.
10. KLOEZE, J. 1967. Influence of prostaglandins on platelet adhesiveness and platelet aggregation. *In* Prostaglandins (Proceedings 2nd Nobel Symposium). S. Bergstrom & B. Samuelsson, Eds. : 241. Interscience. London, England.
11. SHIO H. & P. RAMWELL. 1972. Nature [New Biol.] **236:** 45–46.
12. SALZMAN, E. W. 1972. N. Eng. J. Med. **286:** 358.
13. CHIANG, T. M., E. H. BEACHEY & A. H. KANG. 1975. J. Biol. Chem. **250:** 6916.
14. SALZMAN, E. W. & L. LEVINE. 1971. J. Clin. Invest. **50:** 131.
15. MILLS, D. C. B. & J. B. SMITH. 1971. Biochem. J. **121:** 185.
16. VIGDAHL, R. L., J. MONGIN & N. R. MARQUIS. 1971. Biochem. Biophys. Res. Commun. **42:** 1088–1094.
17. ROBISON, G. A., A. ARNOLD & R. C. HARTMANN. 1969. Pharmacol. Res. Commun. **1:** 325.
18. WOLFE, S. M. & N. R. SHULMAN. 1969. Biochem. Biophys. Res. Combun. **35:** 265.
19. BALL, G., G. G. BRERETON, M. FULWOOD, D. M. IRELAND & P. YATES. 1970. Biochem. J. **120:** 709–718.
20. MOSKOWITZ, J., J. P. HARWOOD, W. D. REID & G. KRISHNA. 1971. Biochim. Biophys. Acta **230:** 279.
21. OSWALD, O., H. W. SEYBERTH, H. R. KNAPP & J. A. OATES. 1976. Effects of oral administration of dihomo-γ-linolenic acid on prostaglandin biosynthesis and platelet aggregation in the rabbit. *In* Advances in Prostaglandin and Thromboxane Research. B. Samuelsson & R. Paoletti, Eds. Vol. **2:** 787–790. Raven Press. New York, N.Y.
22. GLASS, D. B., J. M. GERRARD, J. G. WHITE & N. D. GOLDBERG. 1975. Cyclic GMP formation in human platelets aggregated by arachidonic acid. Presented 18th Ann. Mtg. Amer. Soc. Hematol. Dec. 6–9, 1975. Dallas. Texas. p. 79 (Abstr. 98).
23. HASLAM, R. J. & M. D. MCCLENAGHAN. 1974. Biochem. J. **138:** 317–320.
24. SALZMAN, E. W. 1976. Prostaglandins and platelet function. *In* Advances in Prostaglandin and Thromboxane Research. B. Samuelsson & R. Paoletti, Eds. Vol. **2:** 767–780. Raven Press. New York, N.Y.
25. SALZMAN, E. W. 1973. Prostaglandins in the function of blood platelets. Inserm Seminar on Prostaglandins : 347. Royaumont, France.
26. SALZMAN, E. W., P. C. KENSLER & L. LEVINE. 1972. Ann. N.Y. Acad. Sci. **201:** 61.
27. MARQUIS, N. R., R. L. VIGDAHL & P. A. TAVORMINA. 1971. Fed. Proc. 30–423.
28. SALZMAN, E. W. & H. WEISENBERGER. 1972. Adv. Cyclic Nucleotide Res. **1:** 231.
29. MASSINI, P. & E. F. LÜSCHER. 1974. Biochim. Biophys. Acta **372:** 109–121.
30. FEINMAN, R. D. & R. C. DETWILER. 1974. Nature **249:** 172–173.
31. MALMSTEN, C., E. GRANSTROM & B. SAMUELSSON. 1976. Biochem. Biophys. Res. Commun. **68:** 569–576.

32. Salzman, E. W., J. N. Lindon & R. Rodvien. 1976. J. Cyclic Nucleotide Res. **2:** 25–37.
33. Inceman, S. & Y. Tangun. 1969. J. Lab. Clin. Med. **74:** 174.
34. O'Brien, J. R. & M. A. Woodhouse. 1968. Exp. Biol. Med. **3:** 90.
35. Lüscher, E. F. & P. Massini. 1972. Thromb. Diath. Haemorrh. **27:** 121.
36. Salzman, E. W., E. B. Rubino & R. V. Sims. 1970. Ser. Haematol. **3:** 100.
37. Mills, D. C. B., I. A. Robb & G. C. K. Roberts. 1968. J. Physiol. **195:** 715–729.
37a. Izrael, V., K. Zawilska, R. Jaisson, S. Levy-Toledano & J. Caen. 1974. Effect of a fast removal of plasmatic ADP by the creatine phosphokinase system on human platelet function in vitro. *In* Platelets: Production, Function, Transfusion, and Storage. M. Baldini & S. Ebbe, Eds. : 187–196. Grune & Stratton, Inc. New York, N.Y.
38. Zucker, M. B. & J. Peterson. 1968. Proc. Soc. Exp. Biol. Med. **127:** 547.
39. Merrill, E. W. *et al.* In press.
40. Rodvien, R., D. Brier, J. N. Lindon, G. P. Clagett, E. W. Merrill & E. W. Salzman. In preparation.
41. Mills, D. C. B. & G. C. K. Roberts. 1967. Nature **213:** 35–38.
42. Zucker, M. B. & L. Vroman. 1969. Proc. Soc. Exp. Biol. Med. **131:** 318–320.
43. Salzman, E. W. 1971. Fed. Proc. **30:** 1503–1509.
44. Baier, R. E. & R. C. Dutton. 1969. J. Biomed. Mater. Res. **3:** 191–206.
45. Born, G. V. R., D. Bergqvist & K. E. Arfors. 1976. Nature **259:** 233–235.
46. Allen, J. E. & H. Rasmussen. 1971. Science **174:** 512–514.
47. Samuelsson, B. Personal communication.
48. Steiner, A. L., R. E. Wehmann, C. W. Parker & D. M. Kipnis. 1972. Radioimmunoassay for the measurement of cyclic nucleotides. *In* Advances in Cyclic Nucleotide Research. P. Greengard & G. A. Robison, Eds. Vol. **2:** 51–61. Raven Press. New York, N.Y.

REACTIONS OF PLATELETS NEAR SURFACES *IN VITRO*: LESSONS FROM THE PLATELET RETENTION TEST *

Marjorie B. Zucker and Jean McPherson †

Department of Pathology
New York University Medical Center
New York, New York 10016

Establishment of the role of blood platelets in the formation of the hemostatic platelet plug led to the development of *in vitro* tests of platelet adhesion and aggregation. Hellem developed the platelet adhesiveness test, in which he measured the number of platelets retained in a glass bead column through which blood was passed.[1] When the importance of aggregation within the column was recognized, it became clear that retention did not depend solely on adhesion. The test should therefore be called the platelet retention test.

The mechanisms by which platelet retention occurs are surprisingly complicated. Although not entirely understood, they have provided insights and information that must be kept in mind in studying the interaction of all biomaterials with blood.

Early Studies

The Role of Erythrocytes

Hellem examined the effect of pumping 1 ml of citrated blood from a syringe through a column of plastic tubing packed with glass beads.[1] Under standard conditions, about half the platelets were retained. Except for thrombasthenia, no striking abnormalities were noted in patients with various hemorrhagic disorders, including von Willebrand's disease. Erythrocytes were essential, however; retention was minimal when citrated platelet-rich plasma was passed through a column, and was restored when red cells were added prior to passage. Addition of an extract of boiled erythrocytes, so-called factor R, to platelet-rich plasma also restored retention. Factor R caused marked platelet aggregation as well,[1] and the finding soon afterward that its activity was due to adenosine diphosphate (ADP)[2] initiated a new era in the study of platelets.

The restoration of platelet retention in platelet-rich plasma with ADP, and the fact that erythrocytes contain ADP and restore retention, led to the assumption that red cells promote platelet retention by releasing ADP. Although release of ADP, adenosine triphosphate (ATP), and hemoglobin was demonstrated in ethylenediamine tetra-acetate (EDTA) blood passed through a glass bead column,[3] the relevance of this finding is doubtful, since retention as well as other platelet functions are abolished by EDTA.

One of Hellem's original observations—that red cell ghosts restore retention

* Supported in part by a research grant from the National Institutes of Health (HL-15596).

† Present address: Sydney Hospital, Sydney, Australia.

almost as effectively as whole red cells—was attributed to the presence of factor R in ghosts.[1] The effect of ghosts on retention has been confirmed.[4, 5] Stormorken showed that they do not contain ADP, however. To explain their effect, he suggested, without evidence, that they induce platelets to release ADP.[4] Goldsmith[6] showed that red cells or ghosts at the usual high concentration represented by a hematocrit of 40–45% cause platelets to collide with the walls of a tube or with each other with greatly increased frequency. This observation, which has been confirmed,[7-9] most likely explains why red cells are needed for normal platelet retention.

The Role of ADP

About 0.1 μM ADP was released into the plasma during passage of heparinized blood through a glass bead column, and a slightly higher concentration of ATP was also released.[10] The ATP/ADP ratio of 1.5 is much closer to that found in platelets (the electron-dense granules of which have an unusual pool of nonmetabolic but releasable ADP[11]) than to the ratio of about 10 in erythrocytes. Since the concentration of hemoglobin in the plasma of blood passed through a glass bead column was far too low for hemolysis to account for the concentration of ADP released, we suggested that platelets are the source of the adenine nucleotides released when heparinized blood passes through the column.[10]

Released ADP is essential for platelet retention. When creatine kinase and creatine phosphate are added to blood, ADP is converted to ATP and retention is virtually abolished.[12] With apyrase, an enzyme that degrades ATP to ADP and ADP to AMP, the situation is more complicated. Under certain circumstances, its addition actually enhances retention because most preparations degrade ATP more rapidly than ADP. Apyrase probably temporarily increases the plasma ADP concentration of blood passing through a glass bead column because the released ATP is converted to ADP more rapidly than the released ADP is destroyed. Evidence for this paradoxical effect is found in aggregation studies in which ATP, ADP, and apyrase were added together.[12] Inhibition induced by high concentrations of adenosine,[13] by EDTA,[1] and by PGE_1,[14] and the low retention of thrombasthenic platelets[1, 14] further attest the importance of ADP in platelet retention.

Reduced platelet retention in the blood of patients with storage pool disease[15] strongly suggests that the ADP required for normal retention is derived from the pool in the electron dense bodies.[11] The mechanism of release during the retention test is not known. In the most commonly studied mechanism in citrated platelet-rich plasma (the usual medium for investigating many platelet functions), serotonin is released with the adenine nucleotides during aggregation.[11, 16] None, however, was detected in the plasma of heparinized blood that had passed through the column, even when imipramine was added to prevent reincorporation of released serotonin.[12]

Another difference from release induced in citrated PRP by collagen, for example, is that retention is not inhibited by aspirin.[12, 17] This means that the breakdown of arachidonic acid to active products such as thromboxane A2 is not involved.[18] The possibility that platelets are retained by adhesion only, without the usual accompanying aggregation, was ruled out by our studies, revealing many aggregates in platelets fixed in a column after passing through it blood from an individual who had recently ingested aspirin. This is consistent with our earlier findings of a normal amount of released ADP during performance of the test after aspirin ingestion.[12]

Like aspirin, sulfinpyrazone inhibits the platelet release reaction.[19,20] Although unable to obtain inhibition at the low value we previously reported,[20] we have found consistent inhibition at a final concentration of 1 mM in citrated PRP (unpublished observations). Others have recently reported that sulfinpyrazone but not aspirin inhibits adhesion of platelets to aortic subendothelium.[21] Since this adhesion is also abnormal in blood from patients with von Willebrand's disease (vWD),[22] it seemed possible that sulfinpyrazone would inhibit platelet retention. We found no effect, however, when a final concentration of 1 mM was added to heparinized blood 20 minutes before it was passed through the glass bead column (FIGURE 1a).

The Role of the von Willebrand Factor

von Willebrand's disease is a hemorrhagic diathesis characterized by a prolonged bleeding time and low activity of all three aspects of factor VIII: the coagulant activity (antihemophilic factor or VIII-C), the activity required for agglutination of platelets by the antibiotic ristocetin (VIIIR-WF), and the activity that produces a precipitating antibody in rabbits (VIIIR-AG).[23] Hemophiliacs, with low VIII-C but normal VIIIR-WF and VIIIR-AG, have normal bleeding times and platelet retention.[23]

Since bleeding time is essentially a test of the platelets' ability to form hemostatic plugs, abnormal *in vitro* platelet function would be expected in blood from subjects with a prolonged bleeding time. Certain platelet aggregation tests are abnormal in patients with several congenital platelet abnormalities but not in vWD patients.[15,17] Under appropriate conditions, results of the platelet retention test on vWD blood are markedly abnormal.[24-29] However, the test is normal when heparinized blood is allowed to flow slowly through the glass bead column,[26] when ADP is added to citrated platelet-rich plasma,[29] and, except for one early study,[25] with citrated blood.[29] Since retention is abnormal only when blood is passed through the column rapidly,[26] another mechanism not requiring factor VIIIR-WF must be responsible when given adequate time.

If precautions are taken to minimize disturbance of the blood (see below), addition of partially purified factor VIII can correct the low retention noted in patients with vWD.[28,30,31] Addition of a very low concentration of antibody to factor VIII inhibits retention of normal blood,[14,32] so that plasma factor VIII seems necessary for normal retention.

Blood from patients with vWD releases less than the normal amount of adenine nucleotides when it is passed through a glass bead column, but reduced ADP release may be a secondary manifestation, since it occurs when retention is low for other reasons as well.[10]

ANALYSIS OF MECHANISM

The Effect of Column Condition

To obtain reproducible values for retention, the beads must be dry. In my laboratory, the columns are kept in a can of desiccant for at least 24 hours before use. Moisture may account for the low retention values in subjects with Hageman factor deficiency studied in The Netherlands.[33] We noted normal retention in one subject with this deficiency (unpublished observation), as did Salzman.[24]

Retention depends not only on the glass beads, but also on the type of plastic tubing in which they are placed.[34] Although the beads might appear to provide almost all of the surface to which the blood is exposed, the plastic tubing actually provides about 15%. Retention was higher in polyvinyl chloride tubing than in polyethylene or Teflon® tubing.[34] This finding was attributed to the release of an enhancing factor from the polyvinyl tubing, since retention was reduced in columns previously rinsed with saline.[34] To test this theory we prepared columns with tubing that had been well rinsed with distilled water; if they were kept overnight in a desiccator, retention was identical to that in control columns made with unwashed tubing. Thus it seems unlikely that polyvinyl chloride affects retention by leaching a plasticizer or other additive. Retention in citrated blood was found to be higher in columns prepared several weeks beforehand than in freshly prepared columns,[35] and retention occurred in citrated platelet-rich plasma passed through stored columns prepared with one batch of polyvinyl chloride tubing but not another.[36]

The first drop or two of EDTA blood clots after being passed through a column of unwashed beads, indicating that they carry calcium.[37] In recent experiments, we have therefore used beads thoroughly rinsed with distilled water.

Blood Factors

When blood is passed through the column and platelets are counted in successive ml emerging, the number retained increases progressively.[28] As did Bowie *et al.*, we have used conditions under which over 85% of the platelets in the fourth and fifth ml are usually retained. When blood flow is continued past 5 ml, platelets already retained begin to come through with the emerging blood, sometimes raising the count to levels even higher than in the entering blood.[13] If the beads are moistened with either saline or plasma before the blood is passed through the column, retention is lowered in all ml.[14] This result may be due to the time required for the blood cells to displace the fluid close to the beads and permit interaction with the glass.[38]

In recent studies,[14] we attempted to analyze the effects taking place during retention by passing a small volume of blood (termed blood A) through the column, washing it out with saline or plasma, and following it with the usual 5 ml of blood (termed blood B) on which retention was measured. Retention in the first few ml of blood B was markedly enhanced by passage of blood A if it contained normal platelets and fibrinogen. Washed platelets could substitute for blood A even without fibrinogen.[14] These findings agree with direct observations of adhesion of platelets to glass slides; fibrinogen is required in the presence of other plasma proteins[39-41] but not in their absence,[42] and thrombasthenic platelets fail to adhere even in the presence of fibrinogen.[40] Thus, the essential contribution of blood A toward enhancement in blood B is provision of platelets adherent to glass.

Factor VIIIR-WF is not necessary for platelet adhesion to glass, whether observed directly[40, 41] or deduced from the enhancing effect of blood A on

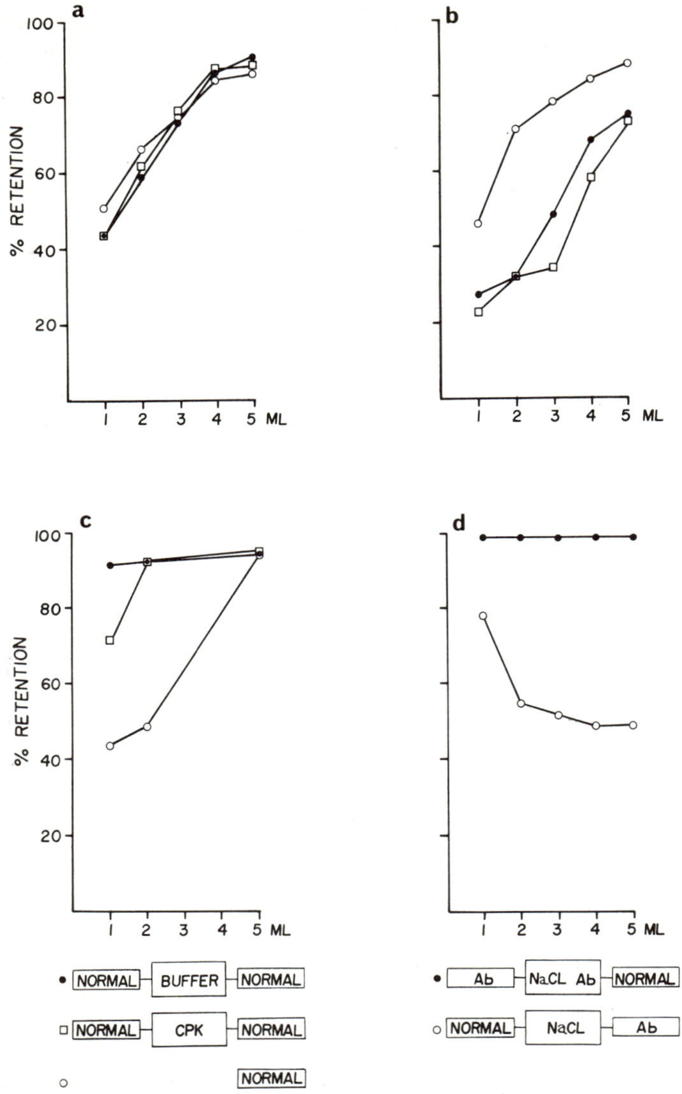

FIGURE 1. Platelet retention in successive ml of heparinized blood pumped through glass bead columns. a=No addition (● - - ●); 0.05 mM aspirin (○ - - ○); 1 mM sulfinpyrazone (Ciba-Geigy, Inc.); (□ - - □). b=5 ml saline (● - - ●), 5 ml fibrinogen solution (1.5 mg/ml, 92% clottable) (□ - - □) or nothing (○ - - ○) preceding blood. c=Retention in blood after passage of 1 ml normal heparinized blood followed by 5 ml imidazole buffered saline, pH 7.6 with 2 mM $MgCl_2$ with or without creatine phosphate plus creatine kinase (CPK) (final concentrations of 1 mM and 20 units/ml, respectively). d=Effect of antibody to factor VIII (Behring Diagnostics, Somerville, N.J.) on retention in blood after passage of 1 ml blood followed by 5 ml isotonic saline. Antibody added as shown, at final dilution of 1 in 100.

retention in blood B.[14] Diminished adhesion to glass is therefore not the cause of the abnormal retention found in vWD, and to state that platelet adhesiveness is abnormal in this disease is incorrect and misleading.

Poor adhesion is presumably responsible for the low retention in afibrinogenemic blood.[43] Passage of normal but not afibrinogenemic plasma through the column immediately prior to the blood corrects the abnormality.[14] With normal blood, an optimal amount of fibrinogen is apparently adsorbed to the glass during passage of blood through a dry column, inasmuch as platelet retention in blood following a fibrinogen solution is the same as that following its buffered saline vehicle (FIGURE 1b).

After the platelets in blood A have adhered to glass, they release ADP, which enhances retention in the first few ml of blood B; experiments such as that shown in FIGURE 1c show slightly less enhancement when the buffer used to flush the column between passage of blood A and blood B contains an enzyme system that rapidly destroys the released ADP.[14] Plasma VIIIR-WF does not play a role in enhancement, since it is very marked whether the column is flushed with saline or with plasma after passage of blood A.[14] Studies like that presented in FIGURE 1d show that the addition of antibody to VIII to the saline flushing solution, blood A, or both does not alter retention in blood B. However, when blood B contains antibody to factor VIII (FIGURE 1d) or is derived from a patient with vWD,[14] retention is low in all 5 ml. Thus, VIIIR-WF must be present *during* retention. The finding that passage of normal plasma immediately before vWD blood does not correct retention [14] reinforces this conclusion.

REDUCTION OF RETENTION BY DISTURBING BLOOD

Effect of ADP

When heparinized blood is disturbed by slow centrifugation, inversion in a tube, or by rapid passage from one syringe to another, retention is lowered but gradually returns toward the normal high value.[10, 44] We considered a low concentration of ADP released during disturbance to be responsible for the inhibition of retention,[5, 10] since retention was rapidly restored by adding apyrase and reduced by adding 0.1 μM ADP.[10] In view of the recent realization that apyrase can enhance retention by converting released ATP to ADP,[12] experiments using apyrase to provide evidence for the role of ADP in reducing retention during blood disturbance are of doubtful value. Yet, the addition of 10^{-7} M ADP has a marked inhibitory effect, strongly suggesting that released ADP is indeed responsible for reduced retention following disturbance. Retention measured with native blood is also reduced by disturbance. *In vivo* disturbance is probably responsible for the low retention in patients with abnormal cardiac valves,[45] and animal experiments have shown that ADP injection is followed by a reduction in platelet retention.[46] It is not clear whether the same mechanism governs ADP's inhibitory effect on both retention and aggregation,[47] or whether it is related to ADP-induced increase or decrease in electrophoretic mobility.[48]

Study of Centrifuged Blood

Salzman pointed out long ago that retention depends on aggregation as well as on adhesion within the column.[24] Since VIIIR-WF is not involved in adhesion, it presumably plays a role in the production of aggregates within the column, probably in combination with ADP. It would be very helpful to be able to study this synergism between ADP and VIIIR-WF in a more "visible" system than a glass bead column. Holdrinet *et al.*[49] counted the platelets in platelet-rich plasma separated by standard centrifugation of heparinized and EDTA blood and regarded the lower count in heparinized PRP as a result of the degree of aggregation taking place during centrifugation. They reported significantly lower aggregation in patients with vWD and their relatives than in the control group, although there was a great deal of overlap between the values. Since platelets appear to be exposed to ADP during preparation of platelet-rich plasma,[10, 48] this system might possibly provide the requisite "visible" interaction between ADP and vWF. Accordingly, we measured the platelet counts of platelet-rich plasma separated immediately after centrifugation. Ten ml of blood was collected in each of four syringes from seven normal subjects. The syringes contained either (a) 0.2 ml 0.135 M neutral EDTA, (b) and (c) 0.16 ml isotonic saline plus 0.04 ml heparin (1000 u/ml, Panheprin, Abbott Laboratories), or (d) 0.04 ml heparin plus 0.1 ml of creatine kinase (Sigma) and 0.1 ml of creatine phosphate with final concentrations in blood of 20 units/ml and 1 mM, respectively. The heparinized blood in syringe (c) was disturbed by rapid passage between two 50–ml syringes.[44] The contents of all the syringes were "twirled" at once,[44] transferred to 15–ml polypropylene tubes at speed 1 on a Harvard pump (Model 975) and left at room temperature for ten minutes before centrifugation for one minute at $2750 \times g$. The results are shown in TABLE 1. PRP from heparinized blood contained only 35% as many platelets/ml as PRP from EDTA blood. That is, 65% were lost, presumably

TABLE 1

EFFECT OF CENTRIFUGATION (1 MIN $2750 \times g$) OF BLOOD WITH VARIOUS ADDITIONS ON NUMBER OF PLATELETS IN PLATELET-RICH PLASMA

Subjects	No. Platelets in PRP of EDTA Blood $10^3/\mu l$	Percentage of Loss Compared to EDTA PRP				
		10-Min Delay Before Cent.			1-Min Delay Before Cent.	
		Heparin %	Heparin-CPK-CP %	Heparin-Disturb. %	Heparin %	Native %
7 normals	740±252 *	65±19	27±14	29±14	—	—
4 normals	661±80	56±26	—	—	28±22	23±19
J.B. (vWD)	908	70	—	—	22	22
Ma.M (vWD)	840	71	—	35	—	—

* S.D.

because they aggregated and sedimented with the erythrocytes. The loss of fewer platelets after CPK-CP was added or after the blood was disturbed indicated that the mechanism, like platelet retention, depended on ADP and was inhibited by disturbance.

In experiments on four other normal subjects, syringes (a) and (b) were collected as above, syringe (c) contained 0.2 ml saline with no anticoagulant, and syringe (d) the usual amount of heparin and saline. These were twirled and transferred to tubes. The tubes from syringes (c) and (d) were centrifuged 1 minute later, and the other two at ten minutes. Fewer platelets were lost in heparinized blood centrifuged at one minute than at ten minutes, and no difference was noted between native and heparinized PRP from blood centrifuged at one minute. Platelet loss during centrifugation of blood from two patients with severe von Willebrand's disease (J.B. and Ma.M.)[14] was entirely normal (TABLE 1). Thus, in our hands, VIIIR-WF was not essential for platelet aggregation during centrifugation of native or heparinized blood.

RELEVANCE FOR OTHER STUDIES

Investigation of the interaction of blood with biomaterials lies between Scylla and Charybdis. On the one hand, intact animals are expensive to purchase and maintain and are not always suitable for experimental studies. On the other hand, *in vitro* tests may introduce artifacts, some of which have been described here. Changes caused by disturbance of the blood must already have taken place in platelet-rich heparinized plasma, and perhaps never occur in citrated blood. Heparin permits or perhaps enhances release of ADP during centrifugation and probably other manipulations of blood;[48, 51] its anticoagulant action is not readily reversed to permit studies of coagulation, but citrate may obscure important reactions such as the role of VIIIR-WF in platelet retention. Although these problems cannot be avoided, awareness of them may lead investigators to design experiments with greater relevance to human health and disease.

REFERENCES

1. HELLEM, A. J. 1960. The adhesiveness of human blood platelets in vitro. Scand. J. Clin. Lab. Invest. **12**(Suppl. 51).
2. GAARDER, A., J. JONSEN, S. LALAND, A. HELLEM & P. A. OWREN. 1961. Adenosine diphosphate in red cells as a factor in the adhesiveness of human blood platelets. Nature **192:** 531–532.
3. RØRVIK, T. O., I. HOLMSEN & H. STORMORKEN. 1968. The release of ADP from red blood cells. Thromb. Diath. Haemorrh. **19:** 77–83.
4. STORMORKEN, H. 1971. Platelets, thrombosis and hemolysis. Fed. Proc. **30:** 1551–1555.
5. ZUCKER, M. B., P. L. RIFKIN, N. M. FRIEDBERG & B. S. COLLER. 1972. Mechanisms of platelet function as revealed by the retention of platelets in glass bead columns. Ann. N.Y. Acad. Sci. **201:** 138–144.
6. GOLDSMITH, H. L. 1971. Red cell motions and wall interactions in tube flow. Fed. Proc. **30:** 1578–1588.
7. TURITTO, V. T. & H. R. BAUMGARTNER. 1975. Platelet interaction with subendothelium in a perfusion system: physical role of red blood cells. Microvasc. Res. **9:** 335–344.

8. Grabowski, E. F., L. I. Friedman & E. F. Leonard. 1972. Effects of shear rate on the diffusion of blood platelets to a foreign surface. Industrial and Engineering Chemistry Fundamentals **11:** 224–232.
9. Robertson, C. R. & H. N. Chang. 1974. Platelet retention in columns packed with glass beads. Ann. Biomed. Eng. **2:** 361–391.
10. Friedberg, N. M. & M. B. Zucker. 1972. ADP as the cause of reversible inhibition of platelet retention in glass-bead columns. J. Lab. Clin. Med. **80:** 603–612.
11. Day, H. J. & H. Holmsen. 1971. Concepts of the blood platelet release reaction. Ser. Haematol. **4:** 3–27.
12. McPherson, V. J., M. B. Zucker, N. M. Friedberg & P. L. Rifkin. 1974. Platelet retention in glass bead columns: further evidence for the importance of ADP. Blood **44:** 411–425.
13. Rossi, E. C. & D. Green. 1972. A study of platelet retention by glass bead columns ("platelet adhesiveness" in normal subjects). Br. J. Haematol. **23:** 47–57.
14. McPherson, J. & M. B. Zucker. 1976. Platelet retention in glass bead columns: adhesion to glass and subsequent platelet-platelet interactions. Blood **47:** 55–67.
15. Weiss, H. J. & J. Rogers. 1972. Thrombocytopathia due to abnormalities in platelet release reaction—studies on six unrelated patients. Blood **39:** 187–196.
16. Zucker, M. B. 1972. Proteolytic inhibitors, contact and other variables in the release reaction of human platelets. Thromb. Diath. Haemorrh. **28:** 393–407.
17. Weiss, H. J. 1970. Aspirin ingestion compared with bleeding disorders—search for a useful platelet anti-aggregant. Blood **35:** 333–340.
18. Hamberg, M., J. Svensson & B. Samuelsson. 1975. Thromboxanes, a new group of biologically active compounds derived from prostaglandin endoperoxides. Proc. Nat. Acad. Sci. USA **72:** 2994–2998.
19. Packham, M. A. & J. F. Mustard. 1974. Drug-induced alteration of platelet function. *In* Platelets: Production, Function, Transfusion and Storage. M. G. Baldini & S. Ebbe, Eds. Chapt. **24:** 265–275. Grune & Stratton. New York, N.Y.
20. Zucker, M. B. & J. Peterson. 1970. Effect of acetylsalicylic acid, other nonsteroidal anti-inflammatory agents, and dipyridamole on human blood platelets. J. Lab. Clin. Med. **76:** 66–75.
21. Davies, J. A., E. Essien, R. L. Kinlough-Rathbone, J.-P. Cazenave & J. F. Mustard. 1975. Inhibitory effect of sulfinpyrazone and acetylsalicylic acid on platelet adhesion to damaged aorta. Blood **46**(6): 1003.
22. Tschopp, T. B., H. J. Weiss & H. R. Baumgartner. 1974. Decreased adhesion of platelets to subendothelium in von Willebrand's disease. J. Lab. Clin. Med. **83:** 296–300.
23. Holmberg, L. & I. M. Nilsson. 1975. von Willebrand's disease. Ann. Rev. Med. **26:** 33–44.
24. Salzman, E. W. 1963. Measurement of platelet adhesiveness: a simple in vitro technique demonstrating an abnormality in von Willebrand's disease. J. Lab. Clin. Med. **62:** 724–734.
25. Zucker, M. B. 1963. In vitro abnormality of the blood in von Willebrand's disease correctable by normal plasma. Nature **197:** 601–602.
26. O'Brien, J. R. & J. B. Heywood. 1967. Some interactions between human platelets and glass: von Willebrand's disease compared with normal. J. Clin. Pathol. **20:** 56–64.
27. Hellem, A. J. 1970. Platelet adhesiveness in von Willebrand's disease. A study with a new modification of the glass bead filter method. Scand. J. Haematol. **7:** 374–382.
28. Bowie, E. J. W., C. A. Owen, Jr., J. H. Thompson, Jr. & P. Didisheim. 1969.

Platelet adhesiveness in von Willebrand's disease. Am. J. Clin. Pathol. **52:** 69–77.
29. Cronberg, S., I. M. Nilsson & J. Silwer. 1966. Studies on the platelet adhesiveness in von Willebrand's disease. Acta Med. Scand. **180:** 43–54.
30. Meyer, D. & M.-J. Larrieu. 1970. von Willebrand factor and platelet adhesiveness. J. Clin. Pathol. **23:** 228–231.
31. Weiss, H. J. & J. Rogers. 1972. Correction of the platelet abnormality in von Willebrand's disease by cryoprecipitate. Am. J. Med. **53:** 734–738.
32. Meyer, D., C. S. P. Jenkins, M. Dreyfus & M.-J. Larrieu. 1973. Experimental model for von Willebrand's disease. Nature **243:** 293–294.
33. Walsh, P. N. 1970. Platelet adhesiveness in Hageman trait. Lancet **2:** 575.
34. Bowie, E. J. W. & C. A. Owen, Jr. 1971. Some factors influencing platelet retention in glass bead columns including the influence of plastics. Am. J. Clin. Pathol. **56:** 479–483.
35. Bennett, P. N. 1968. Observations on the measurement of platelet adhesiveness with the glass bead column technique. Scand. J. Haematol. **5:** 428–431.
36. Hellem, A. J. 1971. The effect of filter age in the platelet adhesiveness test. Scand. J. Haematol. **8:** 180–182.
37. Goldsmith, H. L., P. L. Rifkin & M. B. Zucker. 1975. Platelet retention test: accumulation of corpuscles at the advancing blood-air interface. Microvasc. Res. **9:** 304–309.
38. Butruille, Y. A., S. R. Savitz, E. F. Leonard & R. S. Litwak. 1976. Transient diffusion effects in the study of early platelet adhesion. J. Biomed. Mater. Res. **10:** 145–160.
39. Zucker, M. B. & L. Vroman. 1969. Platelet adhesion induced by fibrinogen adsorbed onto glass. Proc. Soc. Exp. Biol. Med. **131:** 318–320.
40. Mohammad, S. F., M. D. Hardison, C. H. Glenn, B. D. Morton, J. C. Bolan & R. G. Mason. 1974. Adhesion of human blood platelets to glass and polymer surfaces. Haemostasis **3:** 257–270.
41. George, J. N. 1972. Direct assessment of platelet adhesion to glass: a study of the forces of interaction and the effects of plasma and serum factors, platelet function, and modification of the glass surface. Blood **40:** 862–874.
42. Braunsteiner, H. & F. Pakesch. 1956. Thrombocytoasthenia and thrombocytopathia—old names and new diseases. Blood **11:** 965–976.
43. Weiss, H. J. & J. Rogers. 1971. Fibrinogen and platelets in the primary arrest of bleeding. N. Eng. J. Med. **285:** 369–374.
44. Coller, B. S. & M. B. Zucker. 1971. Reversible decrease in platelet retention by glass bead columns (adhesiveness) induced by disturbing the blood. Proc. Soc. Exp. Biol. Med. **136:** 769–771.
45. Rifkin, P. L., N. M. Friedberg & M. B. Zucker. 1973. The effect of apyrase on platelet retention in normal subjects and in patients with abnormal cardiac valves or with von Willebrand's disease. Thromb. Diath. Haemorrh. **30:** 215–220.
46. Busfield, D. & E. G. Tomich. 1967. Reduction of platelet adhesiveness by adenosine diphosphate and triphosphate. Nature **214:** 1360–1361.
47. Holme, S. & H. Holmsen. 1975. ADP-induced refractory state of platelets in vitro. I. Methodological studies on aggregation in platelet rich plasma. Scand. J. Haematol. **15:** 96–103.
48. Hampton, J. R. & J. R. A. Mitchell. 1966. Effect of glass contact on the electrophoretic mobility of human blood platelets. Nature **209:** 470–472.
49. Holdrinet, A., M. Ewals & C. Haanen. 1969. A simple test for measuring platelet aggregation. Results in von Willebrand's disease and uraemia. Thromb. Diath. Haemorrh. **22:** 174–191.
50. Zucker, M. B. 1975. Effect of heparin on platelet function. Thromb. Diath. Haemorrh. **33:** 63–65.
51. Zucker, M. B. Heparin and platelet function. Fed. Proc. In press.

PLATELET FUNCTION FOLLOWING SURFACE INJURY AND SHEAR STRESS: ADHESION, AGGREGATION, RELEASE, AND FACTOR 3 ACTIVITY *

Eugene F. Bernstein, Ulla Marzec, Michael D. Clayman,
Sherri Swanson, and G. Gilbert Johnston

Department of Surgery, School of Medicine
University of California/San Diego
La Jolla, California 92093

Introduction

Modern blood-handling, preservation, and transfusion techniques are concerned with delivering whole blood or blood components to patients with the least possible damage to blood elements. In the course of blood donation, preparation, storage and administration, the blood is exposed to a variety of artificial surface materials and fluid mechanical stresses. Newer extracorporeal devices for both assisted circulation and respiration result in even more intense surface and fluid stresses and more rapid and severe degrees of blood damage. Although a considerable body of information has accumulated concerning erythrocyte damage under many fluid mechanical and artificial surface exposure conditions,[1-3] relatively little is known of the functional effects of exposure of platelets to relatively well-defined fluid mechanical forces. The availability of two model damage systems, one for the selective imposition of variable shear stress and the second for the reproducible imposition of the surface injury, suggested the study of platelet function following both types of selective injury.

Methods

The general experimental plan involved the exposure of fresh human platelet-rich plasma to one of two cell-injury systems. One system, the Fleisch Hemoresistometer,[4] imposes a selective foreign surface type of cell injury. The other system utilizes the jet-stream injection device of Forstrom,[5] and produces well-controlled shear stress fields with minimal contact between cells and foreign surfaces. Measurements of various platelet functions were performed both before and after exposure to each form of trauma.

One hundred ml of blood were drawn into plastic syringes from fasted (at least 12 hours) human donors by venipuncture with a 19-gauge siliconized needle, and anticoagulated with 0.1 volume of 3.8% sodium citrate. Care was taken to use donors who were on no medication and had not ingested aspirin for 10 days prior to the time of donation. The blood was centrifuged in a PR-6 centrifuge at 170 *g* for 10 minutes at 24° C, to obtain platelet-rich plasma

* These studies have been supported by contract no. USA/DADA/17/73/C/3115 from the U.S. Army Medical Research and Development Command, Washington, D.C. 20314, and grant HL 18576, National Heart, Lung and Blood Institute, USPHS.

(PRP) with a high concentration of platelets for use in the jet shear stress device. The PRP was collected with polyethylene pipets; 1 ml was kept on ice for Platelet Factor 3 (PF-3) assay, and the remainder was stored at room temperature. PRP came into contact only with plastic tubes and siliconized glassware until the time of aggregation and PF-3 testing. For the Fleisch Hemoresistometer test of surface damage, the remaining blood was spun again at 280 *g* for 10 minutes at 24° C, and PRP was collected as above. Platelet concentrations for both samples were determined with use of the Coulter Counter, Model F (6).† To prepare platelet-poor plasma (PPP), the remaining blood was centrifuged at 1605 *g* for 10 minutes at 24° C. The PPP was collected with glass pipets and stored on ice.

Platelet damage was induced by exposure of PRP to either (1) the Fleisch Hemoresistometer for surface injury, or (2) the Forstrom jet injection device for shear stress damage. The Fleisch Hemoresistometer consists of a polymethyl methacrylate cup in which the PRP sample was placed, and a rotating polymethyl methacrylate cube, which was immersed into the PRP sample. The chamber was then sealed with a baffle (FIGURE 1). Ten ml of PRP at a concentration of 300,000 platelets/mm³ were placed in the Hemoresistometer cup. Previously collected PRP was diluted with PPP to this concentration when necessary. The cup was then sealed by closure with the baffle, eliminating the air-blood interface. The cube was rotated at 3600 rpm for 15 min at 24° C and the damaged PRP was collected in polystyrene tubes. One ml of damaged PRP was stored on ice for subsequent PF-3 testing; the remainder was stored at room temperature. At 3600 rpm, the Fleisch rotation cube has a tip speed of 456 cm/sec and a gap width of 0.15 cm. Therefore, the average shear rate was approximately 3040 sec^{-1}, and the shear stress was 44 dynes/cm^2.

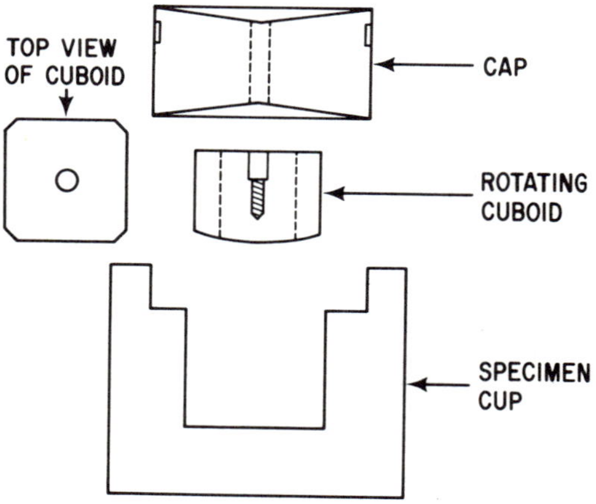

FIGURE 1. Diagram of the blood-handling components of the Fleisch Hemoresistometer. The PRP sample is placed in the cup, which is temperature controlled. The cuboidal rotor is then immersed into the sample. After the chamber is sealed by the cap, the rotor is turned at 3600 rpm for 15 min.

To impose shear stress selectively in the Forstrom jet injection device, 0.9% NaCl was injected through a small-bore needle into a stagnant pool of platelet-rich plasma (FIGURE 2). In this system, the efflux of fluid from the needle

† Coulter Electronics, Hialeah, Fla.

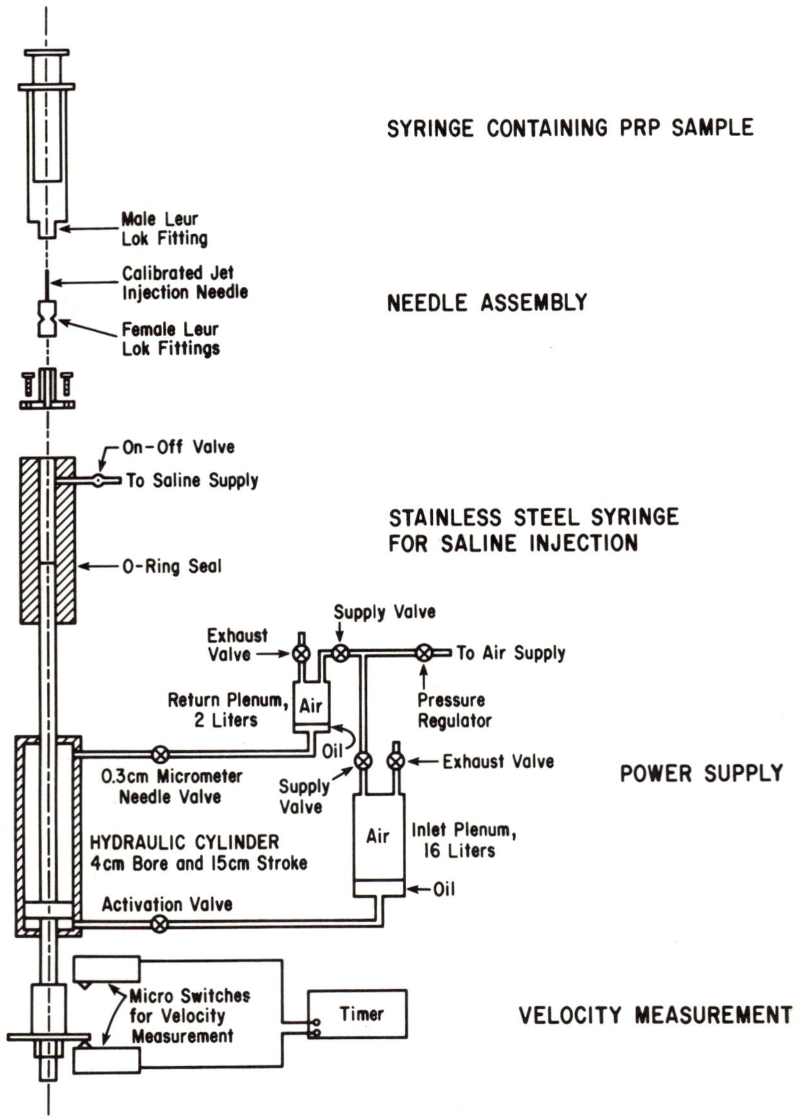

FIGURE 2. Scheme of the jet injection system used to impose high shear stresses in the bulk fluid of the PRP sample placed in the syringe. Rapid injection of saline through a calibrated needle is controlled by the micrometer valve, and the velocity of injection is measured by the two microswitches, with display on a digital timer.

orifice into another fluid is referred to as a submerged jet.[5] Upon leaving the nozzle, the fluid in the jet begins to entrain the surrounding quiescent fluid (PRP), and the width of the jet increases continuously downstream as the jet decreases in velocity (FIGURE 3A). The jet characteristics are dependent upon the exit Reynold's number, which is larger than 3000 in these experiments and therefore is turbulent. For about five jet diameters from the nozzle, the centerline jet velocity is essentially unaffected by mixing, and equal to the nozzle exit velocity. Then, the centerline velocity decreases as the reciprocal of the axial distance from the nozzle exit. Approximately 1% of the cells in suspension will be affected by 50% of the maximum centerline stress, 16% will be affected by 20% of the maximum, and more than 50% will be in the field of 5% or more of the maximum centerline stress (FIGURE 3B). This device

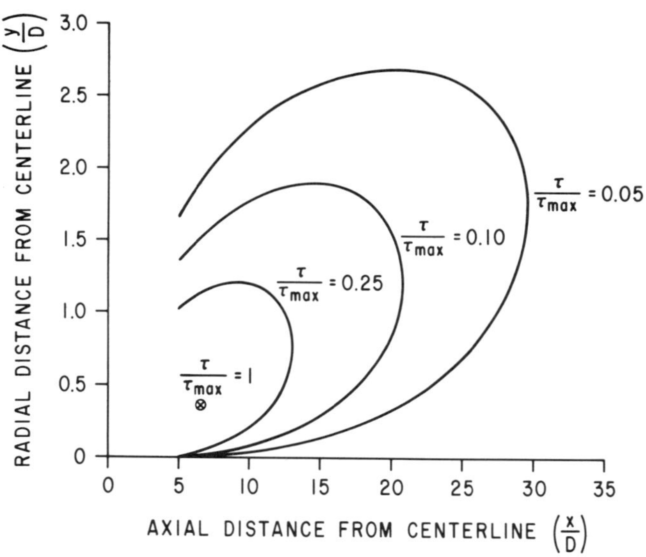

FIGURE 3A. Scheme of the stress pattern in the jet injection device where y=the radial axis from the injecting needle, x=the axial distance. D=the diameter of the needle. τ=the local shear stress, and τ_{max}=the maximum centerline shear stress.

is designed to produce damage by placing high shear forces on the cell membrane for a short time, and it tests membrane deformability and strength. The device includes a microswitch timing mechanism to permit measurements of the injection rate, which, when divided by the cross-sectional area of the needle (determined by microscopic measurement), permits calculation of the mean fluid velocity through the needle.

For shear stress injury, 2 ml of 0.9% NaCl were rapidly injected (approximately 0.5 seconds) at a constant rate at room temperature into a siliconized glass syringe holding 7.2 ml of PRP at a concentration of 380,000 platelets/mm^3. The jet of saline produced maximum centerline shear stresses of between 10^5 and 10^6 dynes/cm^2. The exposure time for individual platelets was in the order of milliseconds. The centerline velocity of injection was varied from 3000 to 10,000 cm/sec. Following the injection of normal saline, PRP was collected in polystyrene tubes and kept at room temperature.

For the platelet adhesion studies, initial efforts to utilize the glass bead techniques of Hellem [7] and Salzman [8] proved poorly reproducible. The present studies were performed with a modification of the method of George.[9, 10] Blood was collected from fasted human donors with plastic syringes and siliconized needles, and added to heparin for a final concentration of 2 I.U. heparin/ml blood. The blood was then centrifuged at 280 *g* for 10 min at 20° C and the platelet-rich plasma (PRP) was aspirated and saved. The remaining sample was centrifuged at 1605 *g* for 10 min and the platelet-poor plasma (PPP) was aspirated and saved. A 1:100 dilution of PRP in PPP was prepared. Chambers were prepared with brass plates and two Kimble Exax No. 1 cover glasses, 18 × 18 and 22 × 30 mm. Cleaning was performed by boiling twice in detergent, soaking overnight, rinsing 10× in deionized water, immersion in sulfuric acid overnight, rinsing 10× in deionized water, rinsing 2× in absolute alcohol and 2× in acetone. The slides were then air dried and stored in a dust-free container. The PRP-PPP solution was placed in a freshly prepared slide chamber, and the ends of the chamber were sealed with a drop of candle wax. The chambers were centrifuged to a maximal force of 860 *g* (the attaching force), and permitted to stand for 5 min (contact time). Then they were inverted and centrifuged to a maximal force of 560 *g* (the detaching force). The number of platelets adhering to both the top and the bottom of the chamber were counted with use of a Zeiss Ultraphot phase-contrast microscope. Five high-power fields (about 300 platelets) were counted for each chamber, and three chambers were

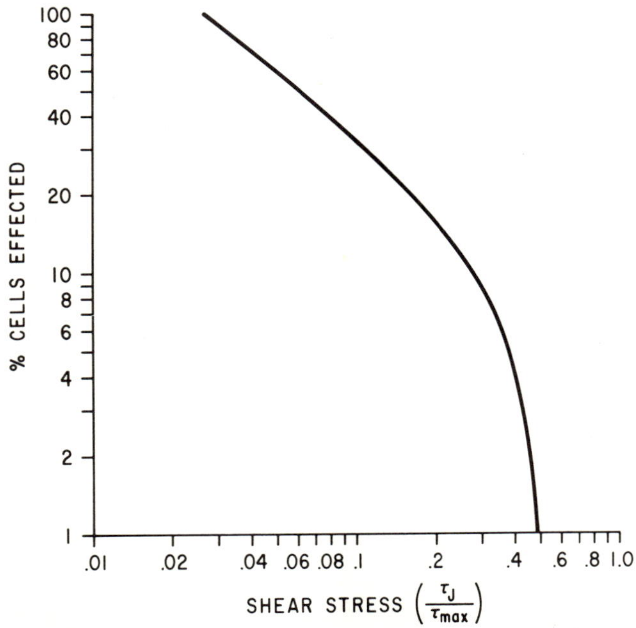

FIGURE 3B. Plot of the incidence of cell exposure to the degree of the maximum centerline shear stress in the jet injection device.

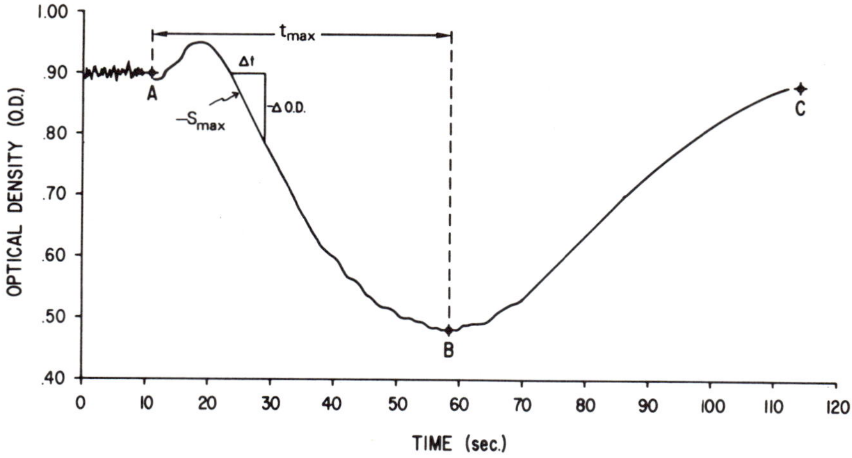

FIGURE 4. A schematic platelet aggregation response is illustrated to indicate the method of analysis employed. Measurements were made of the maximum OD change (A-B), the time for the maximum change (t_{max}) and the maximum negative slope of the aggregation optical density curve ($-S_{max}$).

prepared for each test sample. Platelet adhesion was calculated as the number of platelets remaining adherent to the top cover glass divided by the number on the bottom plus the top ×100, and was expressed as "% adhesion."

Platelet aggregation studies were performed by the method of Born [11] in a Gilford Model 2400S Spectrophotometer, with temperature controlled at 37° C by a Haake water bath and circulator. A magnetic mixing device (Gilford 2445 Spectro-Stir ‡) permitted constant mixing of the sample at 1000 rpm during the performance of the aggregation curve. Ten minutes prior to testing, the specific PRP sample was placed in a 37° C water bath. The degree of aggregation was recorded as the decrease in optical density (OD) of PRP at 620 nm. The PPP was assigned an optical density of 0, and the full scale of the recording was set to equal 1.5 OD units. In general, the recorder was operated at a paper speed of 0.1 in/sec prior to and for 2 min following the addition of each stimulant, and then at a speed of 1 in/min for 10 additional minutes.

Each platelet aggregation curve was analyzed for a variety of indices, as shown in FIGURE 4. Point A indicates the time of addition of the aggregation agent to the PRP, and B is the point of maximal change of OD, in a schematic reversible aggregation curve. Analyses of each curve included the initial optical density of the PRP (A), maximum OD change (A-B, or ΔOD_{max}), the maxi-inmum negative OD slope ($-\Delta OD/\Delta t$, or $-S_{max}$), and the time from the addition of the aggregating agent to the maximum OD change (t_{max}).

For the aggregation tests, solutions of adenosine diphosphate (ADP), thrombin, and collagen were prepared. A stock solution of 10 mg ADP §/ml distilled water was prepared, and stored at −20° C for not longer than one week prior to use. To prepare the working solution, a 1:80 dilution of stock

‡ Gilford Instrument Laboratories, Inc., Oberlin, Ohio.
§ Sigma Chemical Co., St. Louis, Missouri.

with 0.01 M Tris buffer in 0.9% saline (pH = 7.4) was performed to obtain a final ADP concentration of 125 μg/ml. Stock solution of thrombin was prepared by the addition of 2.5 ml sterile 0.9% saline and 2.5 ml glycerol to powdered thrombin ¶ to yield a concentration of 1000 units/ml, and was stored at —20° C until used. Stock solution was diluted 1:40 with 0.9% saline to obtain a final concentration of 25 units/ml. Two aggregation studies were performed, using different concentrations of ADP and thrombin and different collagen preparations. In Experiment 1, connective tissue was prepared from 20 g of human subcutaneous tissue from autopsy, washed three times in an equal volume of cold 0.9% saline. The tissue was homogenized with 200 ml of cold 0.9% saline for 3 minutes in a Waring® blender, and then centrifuged at 1605 *g* for 20 minutes. The turbid middle layer was removed, placed in a 1-ml aliquot and stored at —20° C until used. Either: (1) 25 λ of 125 μg/ml ADP (final concentration = 1.54 μg/ml) or (2) 100 λ of undiluted collagen solution (final concentration = 50 λ/ml) or (3) 50 λ of 25 units/ml thrombin (final concentration = 0.6 units/ml) were added to 2 ml of PRP in a glass cuvette.

In Experiment 2, collagen prepared from guinea pig skin by the method of Gross (12) was used.** Prior to the experiments, 4 mg of lyophilized guinea pig skin collagen was solubilized per ml of acid and then dialyzed against a buffer, as described by Gross. In Experiment 2, the concentration of ADP and thrombin was varied in each experiment, based on the aggregation response of the control PRP sample. The same concentrations of ADP, or thrombin, which produced an irreversible, or biphasic, response curve in the control sample were used in testing the damaged PRP.

Aggregation curves were performed within 30 min of exposure of PRP. In an effort to evaluate the duration of the observed responses, additional aggregation studies were performed at 1, 4, and 24 hours after injury.

To test for the ADP refractory state which is responsive to ADP hydrolysis, potato apyrase †† was added to samples of PRP in concentrations varying from 20 to 750 μg/ml prior to exposure to the Fleisch Hemoresistometer, according to the method of Ardlie.[13] The apyrase activity had been assayed by the supplier as: 1 Unit of apyrase will liberate 1 μM of inorganic P/minute at pH 6.5 at 30° C. To confirm continuing activity, ADP was exposed to the apyrase, and then used as an aggregation stimulant. Apyrase, 5 mg in 0.1 ml, was incubated with 125 μg ADP in 1 ml of buffer at pH 6.5 for 10 min at 30° C, and was then placed on ice. An ADP concentration of 3 μM was then used as an aggregation stimulant for normal PRP, in comparison with unaltered ADP. The apyrase-exposed material resulted in a reversible aggregation curve, in comparison to the irreversible curve seen following stimulation of PRP from the same donor with unaltered ADP. The previously described protocol was then followed for surface injury, and aggregation curves were performed following the addition of ADP, thrombin, and collagen as described under Experiment 2.

Platelet Factor 3 availability (PF-3A) was assayed by the Stypven time method of Spaet and Cintron.[14] Russell's Viper Venom (RVV) was diluted 1:100,000 and mixed with equal volumes of 0.035 M $CaCl_2$. This mixture was added to an equal volume (0.2 ml) of PPP or PRP, diluted 1:2 in refrigerated

¶ Parke-Davis Company, Detroit, Michigan.
** Generously supplied by Dr. E. J. Harper, Department of Chemistry, UCSD.
†† Potato apyrase (Grade One), Sigma Chemical Company, St. Louis, Missouri.

autologous plasma and the clot appearance time was measured in a Lanser Coagulyzer, Jr.

The platelet release reaction was studied by measuring the incorporation of [^{14}C]serotonin into platelets prior to and following injury, and measuring its release following injury by counting ^{14}C-activity in the plasma, according to the method of Jerushalmy and Zucker.[15] To 25 ml of PRP, 0.5 ml of [^{14}C] serotonin (2 μCi/ml, specific activity 48 mc/mMole) was added and the mixture incubated at room temperature for 60 min with intermittent inversion. In several experiments, imipramine (Tofranil, Geigy) was added, at a final concentration of 5 μM, to block reuptake of released serotonin by undamaged platelets. Appropriate quantities of this sample were removed and placed in the Fleisch Hemoresistometer or Forstrom's jet injection system, exposed to the function of these devices, and then immediately placed on ice to which 0.05 ml of 0.27 molar EDTA was added to block the release action. As a control, 0.05 ml of 0.27 molar EDTA was added to 2 ml of PRP [^{14}C]serotonin. Samples were centrifuged at 3000 rpm for 15 min to remove all platelets, and the clear plasma was collected. As a control for total ^{14}C-activity added to PRP, 40 λ of [^{14}C]serotonin were added to 2 ml of PPP and mixed. In other experiments, both control platelets and platelets exposed to the Fleisch surface injury device were incubated in [^{14}C]serotonin in a similar manner, to measure the serotonin uptake of the damaged cells.

Results

Platelet Adhesiveness

As studied with the modified George test, surface injury decreased platelet adhesion from 57.3 ± 14.6% (S.D.) in the control samples to 23.8 ± 12.8% ($p < 10^{-5}$) in 16 paired damaged specimens. Damaged specimens demonstrated less platelet adherence than controls in all but one of the 16 experiments. In the single exception, the control adhesiveness was unusually low. Following exposure to shear stresses, varying from 1.7×10^4 to 1.4×10^6 dynes/cm^2, there was relatively little effect on platelet adhesiveness (Table 1). Although the adhesiveness at 1.5×10^5 and 8.3×10^5 dynes/cm^2 decreased to means of 33.7% and 34.8% respectively, these values are of doubtful statistical significance ($0.01 < p < 0.1$).

Platelet Aggregation

The data from Experiment 1, in which standard concentrations of ADP, collagen, and thrombin were used to stimulate aggregation, are summarized in Table 2. These data demonstrate a marked reduction in platelet aggregation following exposure to surface injury. There was very little decrease, however, in the aggregation response after shear stress. Following surface injury and ADP stimulation, the maximum OD change averaged 0.178, in nine experiments, compared to 0.596 in the controls ($p < 0.001$). By comparison, following exposure to the magnitude of shear stress studied, ADP stimulation produced a maximum OD change of 0.518, which was not significantly different from the controls. In the surface-injury samples, the time for maximum change was significantly shortened, from 263 to 67 seconds, and the rate of change was significantly reduced, from 0.849 to 0.273 OD/minute. At the same ADP concentration, only 10% of the curves from damaged samples yielded an irreversible response in comparison to 64% of the controls. Ten percent of the damaged specimens did not respond at all, a finding never observed in the control group. By contrast, the samples exposed to shear stress were indistinguishable from controls when analyzed for each of these factors.

Following exposure to 50 λ/ml of human collagen, the surface-injured platelets failed to react in any detectable fashion in ten consecutive experiments. In marked distinction, the 15 control samples and ten shear stress samples demonstrated similar aggregation responses, both qualitatively and quantitatively, as they had to ADP.

The surface-injured samples also reacted far less actively following thrombin stimulation. The maximum OD change, and max neg slope were both significantly less ($p < 0.001$) than the controls, and the time for max change was decreased from a mean of 60 to 49 seconds.

TABLE 1

EFFECT OF SHEAR STRESS ON PLATELET ADHESIVENESS

		Shear Stress				
Jet Centerline Velocity (cm/sec)	Control	1000	3000	5000	7000	9000
Shear Stress ($\times 10^3$ dynes/cm^2)	0	17	153	425	833	1377
No. data points	30	5	12	3	6	25
Mean	51.1	41.1	33.7	53.3	34.8	58.7
Range	3.6–87.4	15.6–66.1	3.2–62.0	30.1–72.1	14–66.3	8.8–90.0
S.D.	17.8	8.8	22.0	21.3	17.7	20.0
Signif. vs. control (p)	—	.31	.02	.86	.07	.16

In Experiment 2, the concentration of ADP was varied in the control sample in an effort to identify the concentration required to obtain a biphasic and irreversible aggregation response, and that concentration of ADP was used to stimulate aggregation in the injured samples. The data from this experiment are presented in TABLE 3 and FIGURE 5, and confirm the results of Experiment 1. The max ΔOD of surface-injury samples was 0.178 as compared with 0.837 in the controls ($p < 0.01$). In addition, the time required to reach the minimum O.D. decreased from 362 to 76 sec, and the maximum negative slope of the aggregation curves decreased from 1.154 to 0.384 OD/min in the 18 paired samples. In this experiment, shear stresses of 1.4×10^6 dynes/cm^2, involving jet centerline velocities of 10,000 cm/sec, were employed. In response to this increased stress, the max OD change in 11 experiments was 0.432, compared with 0.837 in the matched controls. The time to reach minimum OD and

TABLE 2

EFFECT OF SURFACE INJURY AND SHEAR STRESS ON PLATELET AGGREGATION
EXPERIMENT 1

	ADP (2.96×10^{-6} M)			Collagen (50 λ/ml)			Thrombin (0.6 U/ml)		
	Control	Surface Injury	Shear Stress †	Control	Surface Injury	Shear Stress	Control	Surface Injury	Shear Stress
No. of samples	14	9	10	15	10	10	15	9	10
Mean max. O.D. change	.596	.178 *	.518	.574	0 *	.439	.558	.326 *	.607
Time for max. change (sec)	263	67	200	248	∞ *	259	60	49	65
Max. neg. slope (O.D./min)	.849	.273 *	.739	.450	0 *	.261	1.228	.725 *	1.286
Irreversible curves (%)	64	10	60	73	0	90	100 †	100 ‡	100 ‡
Curves with no response (%)	0	10	0	0	100	10	0	0	0
Significance (p)*	—	.001	NS	—	.001	NS	—	.001	NS

* Significant difference compared with control data at p value listed.
† 1.5×10^5 dynes/cm^2.
‡ Clotted.

TABLE 3

EFFECT OF SURFACE INJURY AND SHEAR STRESS ON PLATELET AGGREGATION
EXPERIMENT 2

	Control			Surface Injury			Shear Stress *		
Aggregation Stimulus	ΔOD_{max}	t_{max}	$-S_{max}$	ΔOD_{max}	t_{max}	$-S_{max}$	ΔOD_{max}	t_{max}	$-S_{max}$
ADP_1 3–12 μM									
Mean	.837	362	1.154	.178	76	.384	.432	271	.488
S.D.	.155	63	.234	.077	48	.180	.277	146	.341
p (vs. control)	—	—	—	<.01	<.01	<.01	<.01	<.01	<.01
n	24	—	—	18	—	—	11	—	—
Guinea pig collagen 50 μg/ml									
Mean	.996	548	.820	.689	1316	.201	.581	751	.261
S.D.	.126	133	.253	.244	287	.145	.298	336	.168
p (vs. control)	—	—	—	<.01	<.01	<.01	<.01	<.05	<.01
n	13	—	—	10	—	—	11	—	—
Thrombin									
Mean	.281	56	.782	.067	32	.348	.292	135	.663
S.D.	.204	61	.318	.091	14	.221	.246	219	.229
p (vs. control)	—	—	—	<.01	<.02	<.01	NS	NS	NS
n	13	—	—	9	—	—	10	—	—

* 1.4×10^3 dynes/cm^2.

maximum negative slope were also decreased when compared to the controls, but only about half as much as the surface-injured samples.

Highly purified guinea pig collagen (50 μg/ml) provoked a greater aggregation response in both the control and injured specimens than the human material used in Experiment 1. All control curves were irreversible, with an average max OD change of 0.996. By contrast, 4 of 14 surface-injury samples failed to respond at all to the collagen stimulus, and the average OD change

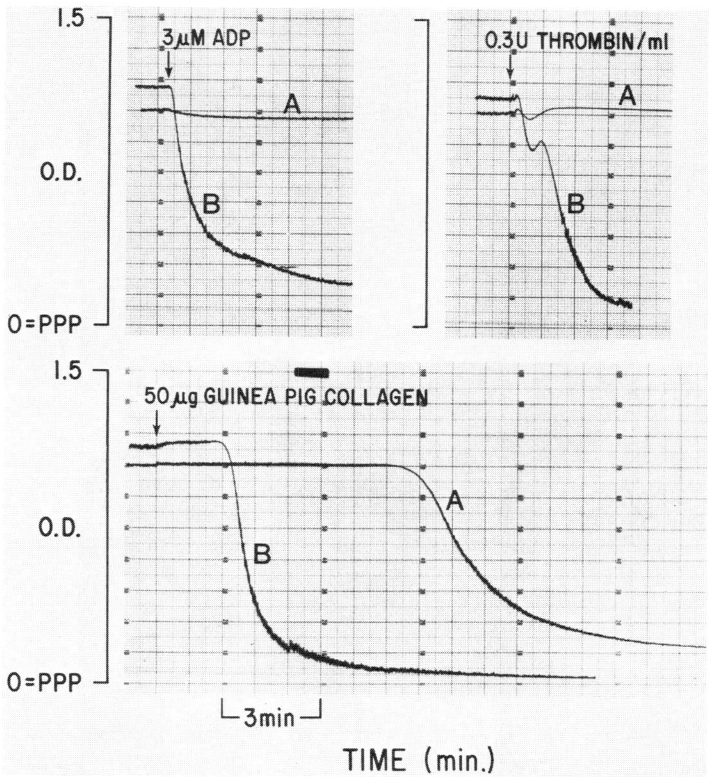

FIGURE 5. Typical platelet aggregation curves in response to ADP, thrombin, and collagen. A=after surface injury, and B=in control PRP samples. The marked depression of the aggregation response to all three stimuli may be noted.

of those responding was 0.689. The time for the max OD change was increased from 548 to 1316 sec and the max negative slope decreased from 0.820 to 0.201 OD/min. The shear stress samples were all less responsive to collagen stimulation than the controls, with a max OD change of 0.581, required a longer time to reach the max OD change 751 sec vs. 548 sec in controls), and had a greatly decreased maximum negative slope of OD 0.261 OD/min. The shear stress samples were more depressed in their response to collagen than those subjected to surface injury, in contrast to the ADP and thrombin responses, which were more depressed following surface injury.

The thrombin concentrations were similarly adjusted to produce a biphasic, irreversible aggregation curve in the control samples. Again, there was a striking decrease in the aggregation response of the surface injury samples, and a significant but substantially smaller decrease in responsiveness following shear stress (TABLE 3).

Duration of Effect

A group of control and surface-injured samples were incubated at room temperature for 4 and 24 hours, and retested for aggregation responsiveness to ADP, collagen, and thrombin. The data presented in TABLE 4 document persistent, severe depressions in the aggregation response noted to all three stimuli immediately following injury, without recovery for the observation periods studied (FIGURE 6).

Apyrase

The addition of potato apyrase failed to affect the diminished platelet aggregation response to ADP, collagen, and thrombin. The data in TABLE 5 summarizes six such experiments, one of which is also illustrated in FIGURE 6. This composite record demonstrates the normal platelet aggregation response to 3 μM ADP, and the decrease in responsiveness after two and four hours of incubation at room temperature. The addition of 20 or 40 μg/ml of potato apyrase had no detectable effect on this response. After surface injury, the aggregation response was markedly diminished. The effect persisted at two and four hours and was unaffected by the addition of 40 μg/ml of potato apyrase. In additional experiments (TABLE 5), up to 750 μg/ml of potato apyrase was added, with no detectable response.

Platelet Factor 3 Activity

The addition of RVV to surface-injured platelets resulted in a marked shortening of the Stypven time from a mean of 36.5 $\pm$ 5.5 sec in the controls to a mean of 16.6 $\pm$ 3.1 sec in eight paired experiments ($p < 0.01$).

Platelet Uptake and Release of [^{14}C]serotonin

Following exposure to the Fleisch surface-injury device, [^{14}C]serotonin uptake averaged 67.5 $\pm$ 16.7% S.D., in eight separate experiments, in comparison with 85.2 $\pm$ 2.6% in the control undamaged paired specimens ($p < 0.01$) in 17 experiments, platelet uptake of serotonin (^{14}C-5HT) averaged 91.3%. Following exposure to the surface-injury model, release of serotonin varied from 0 to 3.8% of the available 5HT pool, averaging 1.4%. In 11 additional experiments, serotonin uptake averaged 87.6%, and release following exposure to shear stress (1.4×10^6 dynes/cm^2) averaged 3.6%, varying from 0 to 7.3%.

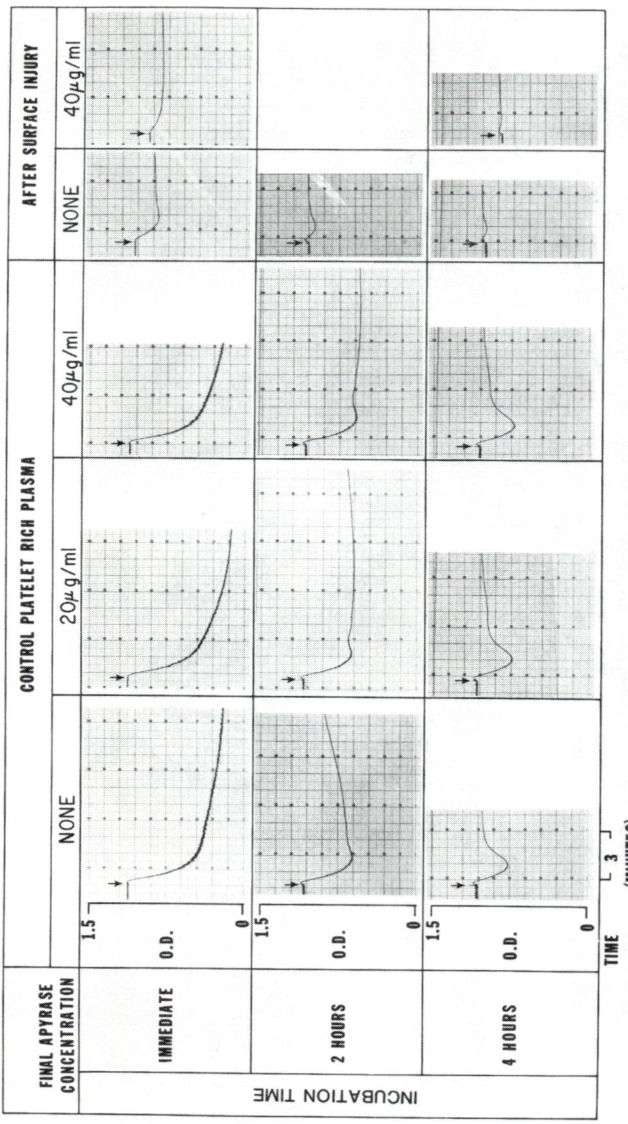

FIGURE 6. The addition of potato apyrase. and further observations at 2 and 4 hours after injury, indicate persistent damage to the surface-injured platelets. Three μM ADP were used in all experiments.

TABLE 4

EFFECT OF INCUBATION TIME ON THE PLATELET-AGGREGATION RESPONSE FOLLOWING SURFACE INJURY

Aggregation Stimulus (Conc.)		Initial Observation						Incub.	Following Incubation					
		Control			Surface Injury			Time	Control			Surface Injury		
		ΔOD_{max}	t_{max}	$-S_{max}$	ΔOD_{max}	t_{max}	$-S_{max}$	(hr)	ΔOD_{max}	t_{max}	$-S_{max}$	ΔOD_{max}	t_{max}	$-S_{max}$
ADP	3 μM	.870	360	.996	.125	108	.180	4	.295	40	.696	.070	56	.150
	12 μM	.850	280	1.200	.275	52	.600	4	.735	260	1.120	.195	44	.540
	12 μM	.900	504	1.270	.265	64	.450	5	.620	264	.822	.200	104	.396
	3 μM	.925	388	1.050	.135	48	.370	24	.255	48	.900	.030	28	.198
	3 μM	.750	332	1.572	.150	44	.276	24	.180	40	.558	.010	28	.066
Collagen	50 μg/ml	1.050	544	.822	.840	1508	.108	4	.985	660	.600	0	0	0
		1.120	500	.900	0	0	0	4	1.095	520	.900	0	0	0
		1.010	620	.750	.800	1508	.112	5	.845	700	.396	.210	1308	.012
		1.025	880	.636	.905	640	.396	24	.925	988	.546	.260	1140	.030
		.945	340	.672	.870	940	.192	24	.915	380	.450	0	0	0
Thrombin	0.13 μ/ml	.835	128	.636	.215	880	.696	24	.306	1028	.900	—	—	—
	0.24 μ/ml	.735	124	1.572	.240	612	.750	24	.090	24	.450	.015	32	.222

TABLE 5

EFFECT OF APYRASE ON THE PLATELET AGGREGATION RESPONSE FOLLOWING SURFACE INJURY

Aggregation Stimulus and Conc.		Initial Observation						Following Apyrase Addition			
		Control			Surface Injury			Apyrase Conc. (μg/ml)	Surface Injury		
		ΔOD_{max}	t_{max}	$-S_{max}$	ΔOD_{max}	t_{max}	$-S_{max}$		ΔOD_{max}	t_{max}	$-S_{max}$
ADP	3 μM	.920	396	1.200	.145	40	.555	75	.230	46	.750
	12 μM	.975	252	1.236	.270	52	.450	100	.210	48	.337
	1.8 μM	.790	336	1.350	.250	60	.747	750	.240	52	.671
	12 μM	.790	152	1.572	.205	44	.600	750	.430	54	.936
	12 μM	.630	64	1.050	.090	40	.330	750	.260	40	.672
	3 μM	1.175	624	1.296	.160	44	.510	750	.180	36	.600
Collagen	50 μg/ml	1.030	492	.998	.880	1380	.208	75	.730	1080	.169
		.790	600	.406	.490	1412	.103	750	.730	1298	.270
Thrombin	.25 U/ml	.130	22	.675	.010	24	.308	75	.030	28	.215
		.120	32	.514	.010	36	.192	750	0	∞	0

The addition of imipramine failed to significantly alter the serotonin-release results observed following exposure to the Fleisch surface-injury device, with release averaging 2.6% in 18 experiments. Following exposure to the jet device, there was a definite increase in serotonin release in the imipramine-treated samples averaging 13.3% in nine experiments (range 7.2–25.8%). To confirm that the serotonin remained within the damaged platelets, surface-injured cells were subjected to three freeze-thaw cycles (one series), and osmotic lysis (another series), and the mean recovery of serotonin was $86 \pm 12\%$.

Discussion

Previous efforts to characterize the injury to platelets from various forms of trauma have included a variety of *ex vivo* chambers and perfusion systems in which platelet adhesion to test surfaces was measured,[16–18] under circumstances of temporary extracorporeal circulation [19–22] and the permanent implantation of prosthetic valves.[23, 24] During cardiopulmonary bypass, thrombocytopenia and a depression of platelet adhesiveness have been reported by several authors,[19, 20] followed by a rebound platelet proliferation and a return of normal adhesiveness.

Following implantation of prosthetic heart valves, platelet life span is decreased, and thromboembolism may occur.[23] These complications were reduced or reversed by the addition of compounds that decrease platelet adhesiveness, particularly aspirin and dipyridamole,[23, 24] which were also effective in decreasing the loss of platelets from the circulation during cardiopulmonary bypass.[22]

The significance of the present experiments includes the development of a reproducible *in vitro* model of platelet membrane damage, the demonstrated usefulness of a technique for measuring platelet adhesiveness, and the findings of increased PF-3 activity following surface injury. In addition, the adhesion and aggregation inhibition resulting from surface injury, in comparison with the relatively modest effects of short exposures to high shear stresses in the bulk of the fluid, appears to be significant. In this way the platelet appears similar to the human erythrocyte, which is also far more susceptible to surface injury than to midstream fluid stresses. Previous studies from our laboratory [1–3] demonstrated the ready susceptibility of the human erythrocyte to surface injury in the Fleisch Hemoresistometer, an effect influenced by the lipid composition of the suspending media, temperature, and the species and sex of the erythrocyte donor. Shear stress damage to the erythrocyte, on the other hand, appeared to depend on both the magnitude of shear stress and the duration of exposure. This shear-time envelope of erythrocyte damage includes the range utilized in Experiment 1, in which no significant platelet injury was observed. Forstrom,[5] however, calculated that a maximum centerline jet velocity of 10,000 cm/sec would be necessary to injure the smaller platelet, and when this increased stress was applied in Experiment 2, evidence of a modest but definite decrease in platelet responsiveness to the aggregation stimuli employed was documented. In comparing the platelet and erythrocyte responses to these models of selective trauma, it must be noted that most measures of erythrocyte injury are based on hemolysis, implying disruption or leakage of the erythrocyte membrane. The platelet tests used in the present study are more varied, and perhaps more sensitive, measurements of platelet membrane dysfunction short of disruption, at least as judged by the measurements of almost negligible [^{14}C]serotonin losses, signifying little membrane leakage in the face of significant decreases in adhesion and aggregation.

The platelet adhesion data, which demonstrate a marked effect of surface injury, are also a confirmation of the method of George.[9, 10] This centrifugation-attachment approach, which was based on the earlier work of Fenn[25] and Hayry[26] with erythrocytes and cultured HeLa cells, measures adhesion without simultaneously causing aggregation, in contrast to the glass and plastic bead techniques. In addition, as modified by the heparin concentration used in the present experiments, the technique may be a clinically useful test of this important platelet function. It may also be useful in testing the relative platelet adhesion to various materials being considered for blood surface contact applications.

The second index of platelet damage in the present experiments was the diminished aggregation response to ADP, collagen, and thrombin. The ΔOD_{max}, t_{max} and $-S_{max}$ terms were developed in an effort to add quantitative parameters to the descriptive characterization of the platelet aggregation optical density tracings. Additional criteria initially used to assay the curves included measures of the positive slope of reversible curves and of the total time required to regain the initial OD under such circumstances. These terms, however, appeared to add little discriminative ability to the curve analysis. The three remaining parameters, which are used in TABLES 2–5 appear to characterize the major alterations of optical density, and permit the quantitation of degrees of deviation from the control tracings. Similar quantitative parameterization has recently been proposed by Frojmovic,[27] who showed the dependence of several features of the ADP-stimulated aggregation curve on platelet concentration, including the initial OD, the rate of OD change, and the maximum OD change. For this reason, all of our PRP specimens were adjusted to a platelet concentration of $300{,}000/mm^3 \pm 20{,}000$, by the addition of PPP. All control and surface-injured specimens had the same initial concentrations. The dilution of the shear stress samples (7.2 ml) by the jet injectate (2 ml) did not have significant effects on the aggregation curve parameters measured as indicated in TABLE 3. In addition, an earlier report by Born[28] showed no dependence of OD_{max} on platelet concentration. On the other hand, Frojmovic reported no platelet-concentration dependence for the oscillation amplitude, the initial OD change associated with ADP addition, or the time for the aggregation curve course, and suggested that these were more valuable parameters for detecting altered platelet responsiveness. However, only the last of these was measured in the present study, and appeared to vary in the same direction and degree as the OD_{max} and the $-S_{max}$ in the current experiments.

Previous work on the effect of trauma on platelet aggregation by Zucker and her associates (see References 29–31) demonstrated a transient decrease in the aggregation response of the injured platelets, which had been moved from one syringe to another. In Zucker's experiments, the platelet responses had returned to normal within an hour of injury. In the present experiments the marked inhibition of platelet responsiveness persisted for the 24-hour observation period. Although the degree of injury involved in the present experiments was considerably greater than in Zucker's experiments, the influence of multiple contacts between the platelets and the wall of the containing chamber might well be similar. It is therefore significant that the effects of injury in the current experiments persisted for the 24-hour period of observation.

Other factors have been described that can alter platelet responsiveness to aggregation stimulants such as ADP. The failure of potato apyrase in the aggregation suspension to restore the normal platelet response to ADP is evidence that simple ADP refractoriness is not involved. The possibility that other substances known to inhibit platelet aggregation were released during the course of the injuries produced is under continuing investigation. The possibility of some plasma factor interfering with or being responsible for these results was considered, and eliminated, by suspending surface-injured platelets in normal (undamaged) PPP with findings of decreased adhesion and aggregability.

The alterations in platelet factor 3 availability demonstrated in these experiments are consistent with other studies of platelet injury. Disruption of platelets by mechanical trauma[32] and freezing,[33] stimulation by the application of kaolin[34, 35] or brain phospholipid[36] and the washing of platelets[37-40] also result in increasing platelet clot-promoting activity or PF-3A. Subcellular platelet fractionation has demonstrated increased platelet procoagulant activity in the membrane and homogenaate fractions, in comparison with the granule fraction.[41] However, phospholipids extracted from each of these fractions were equally effective clot-promotors, leading Marcus et al. to suggest that the phospholipid of the platelet membrane may be more "available" for clotting activity than similar material present in the granules.

The relevance of these observations to whole blood, in which additional rheological and biochemical effects might be expected, was investigated in preliminary fashion by subjecting samples of whole blood to the Fleisch surface-injury device in the same fashion as described for the PRP in the present studies. When the damaged blood was then separated to provide PRP, as described in the protocol of these experiments, similar inhibition of aggregation was noted in the platelets.

Finally, the question of impaired serotonin release during the injury experiment was investigated as a possible explanation for the lack of platelet responsiveness observed following injury. The data indicate that serotonin release has not occurred to any significant degree and fail to adequately explain the mechanism of development of the unresponsive state observed.

Acknowledgments

The authors are particularly grateful to Dr. Richard J. Forstrom, Dr. Edwin W. Salzman, Dr. J. G. White, and Dr. M. B. Zucker for their helpful advice and thoughtful suggestions.

References

1. Bernstein, E. F., P. L. Blackshear, Jr. & K. H. Keller. 1967. Factors influencing erythrocyte destruction in artificial organs. Am. J. Surg. **114:** 126–138.
2. Indeglia, R. A., M. A. Shea, R. L. Varco & E. F. Bernstein. 1967. Mechanical and biological considerations in erythrocyte damage. Surgery **62:** 47–55.
3. Bernstein, E. F. 1971. Certain aspects of blood interfacial phenomena—Red blood cells. Fed. Proc. **30:** 1510–1515.
4. Fleisch, H. von & A. Fleisch. 1960. Der hamoresistometer. Schweiz. Med. Wschr. **90:** 186–190.
5. Forstrom, R. J. 1969. A new measure of erythrocyte membrane strength: The jet fragility test. Ph.D. Thesis. Univ. Minnesota. Minneapolis, Minn.

6. Bull, B. S., M. A. Schneiderman & G. Brecher. 1965. Platelet counts with the Coulter Counter. Am. J. Clin. Pathol. **44:** 678–688.
7. Hellem, A. J. 1960. The adhesiveness of human blood platelets in vitro. Scand. J. Clin. Lab. Invest. (Suppl. 12) **51:** 1–117.
8. Salzman, E. W. 1963. Measurement of platelet adhesiveness. J. Lab. Clin. Med. **62:** 724–735.
9. George, J. N., R. I. Weed & C. F. Reed. 1971. Adhesion of human erythrocytes to glass: The nature of the interaction and the effect of serum and plasma. Cell Physiol. **77:** 51–59.
10. George, J. N. 1972. Direct assessment of platelet adhesion to glass: A study of the forces of interaction and the effects of plasma and serum factors, platelet function, and modification of the glass surface. Blood **40:** 862–874.
11. Born, G. V. R. 1962. Aggregation of blood platelets by adenine diphosphate and its reversal. Nature (Lond.) **194:** 927–929.
12. Gross, J. 1958. Studies on the formation of collagen. Properties and fractionation of neutral salt extracts of normal guinea pig connective tissue. J. Exp. Med. **107:** 247–263.
13. Ardlie, N. G., D. W. Perry, R. A. Packham & J. F. Mustard. 1971. Influence of apyrase on stability of suspensions of washed rabbit platelets. Proc. Soc. Exp. Biol. Med. **136:** 1021–1023.
14. Spaet, T. H. & J. Cintron. 1965. Studies on platelet factor-3 availability. Brit. J. Haematol. **11:** 269–275.
15. Jerushalmy, Z. & M. B. Zucker. 1966. Some effects of fibrinogen degradation products (FDP) on blood platelets. Thromb. Diath. Haemorrh. **15:** 413–419.
16. Lyman, D. J., J. L. Brash, S. W. Chaikin, K. G. Klein & M. Carini. 1968. The effect of chemical structure and surface properties of synthetic polymers on the coagulation of blood. II. Protein and platelet interaction with polymer surfaces. Trans. Am. Soc. Artif. Int. Organs **14:** 250–255.
17. Friedman, L. I., H. Leim, E. F. Gradowski, E. F. Leonard & C. W. McCord. 1970. Inconsequentiality of surface properties for initial platelet adhesion. Trans. Am. Soc. Artif. Int. Organs **16:** 63–73.
18. Salzman, E. W. 1971. Role of platelets in blood-surface interactions. Fed. Proc. **30:** 1503–1509.
19. Nilsen, N. W. & A. Christensen. 1964. The influence of extracorporeal circulation combined with hypothermia on the thrombocytes. Acta Chir. Scand. **127:** 297–302.
20. Salzman, E. W. 1963. Blood platelets and extracorporeal circulation. Transfusion **3:** 274–277.
21. Sharp, A. A. & M. J. Eggleton. 1963. Haematology and the extracorporeal circulation. J. Clin. Pathol. **16:** 551–557.
22. Becker, R. M., M. R. Smith & A. R. C. Dobell. 1974. Effect of platelet inhibition on platelet phenomena in cardiopulmonary bypass in pigs. Ann. Surg. **179:** 52–57.
23. Harker, L. A. & S. J. Slichter. 1970. Studies of platelet and fibrinogen kinetics in patients with prosthetic heart valves. New Eng. J. Med. **283:** 1302–1305.
24. Sullivan, J. M., D. E. Harker & R. Gorlin. 1968. Pharmacologic control of thromboembolic complications of cardiac-valve replacement. New Eng. J. Med. **279:** 576–580.
25. Fenn, W. D. 1922. Hemolysis of erythrocytes in contact with glass. J. Exp. Med. **35:** 271–286.
26. Hayry, P. 1966. The role of factors in fresh serum in the attachment and growth of HeLa cells on glass. Ann. Med. Exp. & Biol. Fenniae **44:** (Suppl. 8) 1–47.
27. Frojmovic, M. M. 1973. Quantitative parameterization of the light-transmission properties of citrated, platelet-rich plasma as a function of platelet and adenosine diphosphate concentration and temperature. J. Lab. Clin. Med. **82:** 137–153.

28. Born, G. V. R. 1970. Observations on the change in shape of blood platelets brought about by adenosine diphosphate. J. Physiol. **209:** 487–511.
29. Friedberg, N. M., M. B. Zucker, R. A. Grant & S. J. Kim. 1971. Platelet retention in glass bead columns: Reversal of adenine nucleotide-induced inhibition by apyrase. Fed. Proc. **30:** 423.
30. Coller, B. S. & M. B. Zucker. 1971. Reversible decrease in platelet retention by glass bead columns (adhesiveness) induced by disturbing the blood. Proc. Soc. Exp. Biol. Med. **136:** 769–771.
31. Zucker, M. B., P. L. Rifkin, N. M. Friedberg & B. S. Coller. 1972. Mechanisms of platelet function as revealed by the retention of platelets in glass bead columns. Ann. N.Y. Acad. Sci. **201:** 138–144.
32. O'Brien, J. R. 1958. Phospholipids, proteins and platelet lipoid. Nature (Lond.) **181:** 420.
33. Fantl, P. & H. A. Ward. 1958. The thromboplastic component of intact blood platelets in present in marked form. Australian J. Exp. Biol. Med. Sci. **36:** 499–504.
34. Hardisty, R. M. & R. A. Hutton. 1965. The kaolin clotting time of platelet-rich-plasma: A test of platelet factor-3 availability. Brit. J. Haematol. **11:** 258–268.
35. Rabiner, S. F. & O. Hrodek. 1968. Platelet factor 3 in normal subjects and patients with renal failure. J. Clin. Invest. **47:** 901–912.
36. Bonin, J. A. & K. Cheney. 1961. The PTF test: An improved method for the estimation of platelet thromboplastic function. Brit. J. Haematol. **7:** 512–522.
37. Biggs, R. & A. S. Douglas. 1953. The thromboplastin generation test. J. Clin. Pathol. **6:** 23–29.
38. Hardisty, R. M. & H. H. Wolff. 1955. Hemorrhagic thrombocythaemia: A clinical and laboratory study. Brit. J. Haematol. **1:** 390–405.
39. Altschuler, G., A. J. Marcus & H. L. Ullman. 1960. Platelets and platelet phosphatides in uremia. Blood **16:** 1239–1446.
40. Weiss, H. J. & J. W. Eickelberger, Jr. 1962. The detection of platelet defects in patients with mild bleeding disorders. Am. J. Med. **32:** 872–883.
41. Marcus, A. J., D. Zucker-Franklin, L. B. Safier & H. L. Ullman. 1966. Studies on human platelet granules and membranes. J. Clin. Invest. **45:** 14–28.

DISCUSSION PAPER: HUMAN PLATELET PROTEIN KINASE PHOSPHORYLATION REACTION WITH PLATELET MEMBRANE AND CYTOPLASMIC ENZYMES AND CRYSTALLIZATION OF A CYCLIC AMP-INDEPENDENT PROTEIN KINASE *

Sáid A. Assaf †

University of Texas Medical School and
Graduate School of Biomedical Sciences
Houston, Texas 77025

The cyclic AMP (cAMP) ‡ level in human blood platelets decreases as a result of platelet interface reaction with collagen [1] as well as with surfaces coated with fibrinogen, kaolin, and other platelet-adhesive substances.[2, 3] On the other hand, an increase in intraplatelet cAMP concentration inhibits platelet aggregation and adhesiveness to various surfaces.[4-7] Since the first discovery that cAMP enhancement of glycogen breakdown in muscle occurs by stimulation of a phosphorylase kinase kinase,[8] later identified as protein kinase,[9] all of the physiological effects of cAMP in mammalian cells were found to be the result of the action of cAMP-dependent protein kinase.[10, 11] Protein kinase catalyzes the phosphorylation reaction of acceptor protein substrates as shown below: [11]

$$\text{protein} + n\text{ATP} \xrightarrow[\text{Mg}^{2+}]{\text{protein kinase}} \text{protein} - \text{P}n + n\text{ADP}.$$

The cAMP-induced dissociation of this enzyme to a catalytic and regulatory subunit is the mechanism by which it is activated by this cyclic nucleotide. The reverse enzymatic dephosphorylation reaction is catalyzed by phosphoprotein phosphatase:

$$\text{protein} - \text{P}n \xrightarrow{\text{phosphoprotein phosphatase}} \text{protein} + n\text{P}_i$$

This reaction was reported to be activated by Mg^{2+} [12] and inactivated by fluoride.[13] Because the phosphate in a phosphorylated protein is bound covalently, nonenzymatic cleavage of this bond is encountered only upon protein incubation in strong alkali but not in acid.[14]

The search for physiological substrates for protein kinase in platelets has not progressed as that in other tissues.[15-17] In 1973, however, two laborator-

* A review on this subject was recently reported by Assaf, S. A. Int. J. Biochem. 7: 1–8 (1976 in press).

† With the technical assistance of W. Grady Hicks, Joyce M. Liegel, and W. Timothy Woodward.

‡ Abbreviations: cAMP=cyclic adenosine 3′,5′-monophosphate; DTT=dithiothreitol; EGTA=ethyleneglycol-bis(2-aminoethylether)-N,N′-tetraacetic acid; ATPase=adenosine triphosphatase; PDE=cyclic AMP phosphodiesterase; NaK ATPase=$(Na^{+} + K^{+})$-stimulated adenosine triphosphatase.

ies[18, 19] and our own simultaneously reported§ success in phosphorylating components of the actomyosin complex. Adelstein and coworkers[20] pursued extensive phosphorylation studies using endogenous kinase; our approach entailed the purification and characterization of platelet protein kinase and some of its endogenous substrates, as has been briefly reported earlier[21-23] and is presented in detail in this manuscript. During the course of these studies we have, in addition to the "classical" cAMP-dependent protein kinase[10, 11, 17] isolated and crystallized a cAMP-independent protein kinase holoenzyme with a molecular weight similar to that of the cAMP-dependent enzyme from platelets and other tissues.[24-26] This finding suggests that, as in the case of muscle phosphorylase kinase,[27] the phosphorylation reaction is not directly the result of cAMP-dependent protein kinase. Various workers[28-33] have reported the phosphorylation of exogenous and endogenous proteins by a cAMP-independent kinase catalyzed reaction. These reports, however, did not include molecular weight studies which could rule out that the kinase in question is not simply a catalytic subunit of the cAMP-dependent protein kinase. Because of the possible effect of experimental conditions, neither the lack of stimulation by cAMP nor the lack of inhibition by the regulatory subunit and the heat-stable low molecular weight protein inhibitor[34, 35] are sufficient proof that the kinase in question is a cAMP-independent holoenzyme.

The phosphorylation-dephosphorylation of certain enzymes, e.g. glycogen phosphorylase, has been unequivocally shown to result in major modification changes, including net charge,[36] association-dissociation of subunits,[37-40] activation-inactivation[40, 41] and response to specific salt ions,[42, 43] reactivity of functional groups, and overall conformation.[40, 44] Changes in the structure and configuration of the surface platelet proteins and of the plasma proteins with which they are in contact were described by Vroman *et al.* as being essential for adhesiveness.[45] It is plausible, therefore, that the reversible changes in platelet adhesiveness occur as a result of physicochemical and catalytic alterations that occur following phosphorylation-dephosphorylation reactions of some platelet membrane and cytoplasmic surface enzymes. The synthesis of prostaglandins by various prostaglandin synthetases (especially of cyclo-oxygenase, an endoperoxide-producing enzyme) appears to be controlled by phosphorylation-dephosphorylation, inasmuch as Malmsten and colleagues[46] recently reported that cAMP turns off the production of prostaglandin endoperoxides which are now recognized[47-49] as physiological initiators of platelet adhesiveness and aggregation. A study of the phosphorylation of some of the easily purified and physiologically important substrates of platelet protein kinase is the subject of this paper.

Materials and Methods

γ-^{32}P was obtained from New England Nuclear and γ-^{32}P-ATP was prepared by a modification of the method of Walsh *et al.*[50] Whatman filter paper (3MM), 23 mm in diameter, used in the radioactive assay, was obtained from Arthur H. Thomas. Vitamin-free casein was dissolved according to Reimann *et al.*,[28] and unfractionated calf thymus histone was obtained from Dr. H. Hnilica, M. D.

§ An unpublished report was presented at the 2nd International Symposium on Thrombosis, Hemostasis and the Molecular Biology of the Platelet, May 1973, Chicago, Ill.

Anderson Hospital, Houston, Texas. DEAE-cellulose (Reeve Angel DE-52) was prepared according to Assaf and Graves.[51] The kinase-catalyzed incorporation of ^{32}P from γ-^{32}P–ATP into protein substrates was carried out essentially according to Wastila *et al.*[52] A 0.1 ml of reaction mixture contained 1 mM γ-^{32}P-ATP (specific activity 0.8–2.0 mCi/mmol), 10 mM $MgCl_2$, 0.5 mM DTT, 20 mM NaF, 1 mM EGTA, 2 mM theophylline, 0.002 mM cAMP (when present), 30 mM glycerophosphate, 30 mM potassium phosphate pH 6.5, protein substrate (2–10 mg/ml), and then 10–30 μg of protein kinase were added. Following incubation at 30° C for 10 minutes, 0.05 ml of the reaction mixture was spotted on filter paper disks which were immediately immersed in 10% TCA—0.01 M potassium phosphate, washed, dried, and counted according to Martelo *et al.*[53] Total counts per minute used in the assay were 300,000–500,000. The various blanks employed ranged from 100–400 cpm. A unit of enzyme activity was expressed as the number of picomoles of ^{32}P incorporated into protein substrate per minute per mg of protein kinase (pmol/min)/mg. Analytical ultracentrifugation and sucrose density gradient ultracentrifugation was done according to established methods.[54, 55]

Results and Discussion

Enzyme Purification and Partial Characterization

The overall purification of platelet enzymes from sonicated erythrocyte and leukocyte "free" platelet concentrates[56] was carried out as shown in Figure 1 and is discussed below.

Platelet Actomyosin and Membrane Enzymes

In contrast to that prepared by others,[57–61] the contractile actomyosin complex was not isolated along with the soluble cytoplasmic enzymes. We employed a low ionic strength buffer (0.002 M tris, 0.001 M EDTA, 0.001 M DTT, pH 7.5) during the platelet sonication and subsequent centrifugation at 20,000 *g* for 2½ hours, which resulted in the precipitation of the platelet actomyosin ATPase along with the membrane proteins. Solubilization of actomyosin was achieved at pH 7.5 with 1 M tris, 0.001 M DTT, or 0.6 M KCl–0.001 M tris-DTT. It was reprecipitated by overnight dialysis against 0.002 M tris or imidazole in 0.001 M EDTA, pH 6.2. Actomyosin solubilization and precipitation cycles were repeated at least twice before gel filtration on a Sepharose 6B column equilibrated with pH 7.5 buffer containing 0.6 M KCl.[58] ¶ The purified actomyosin preparation exhibited an SDS gel electrophoretic pattern, an activity for Mg-ATPase (0.03(μmole Pi/min)/mg) and Ca-ATPase (0.3 (μmol Pi/min)/mg) similar to that reported elsewhere.[59, 60] It sedimented in the analytical ultracentrifuge in a broad peak with an $S_{20,w}$ of 31S and a slow-moving sharper peak with an $S_{20,w}$ of approximately 7S. The other components of the contractile protein system actin and tropomyosin were obtained in crude form according to Spudich[61] and Cohen *et al.*[62] and were used as such in the phosphorylation studies.

¶ Assistance in some of the actomyosin experiments was provided by Mr. James Gum, Jr., student in the Graduate School of Biomedical Sciences.

Using platelet membranes** [63] and subjecting them to 5–25% sucrose density gradient ultracentrifugation, we collected fractions possessing the greatest activity for adenylate cyclase,[64] PDE,[65] and NaK-ATPase [66] (FIGURE 1) and

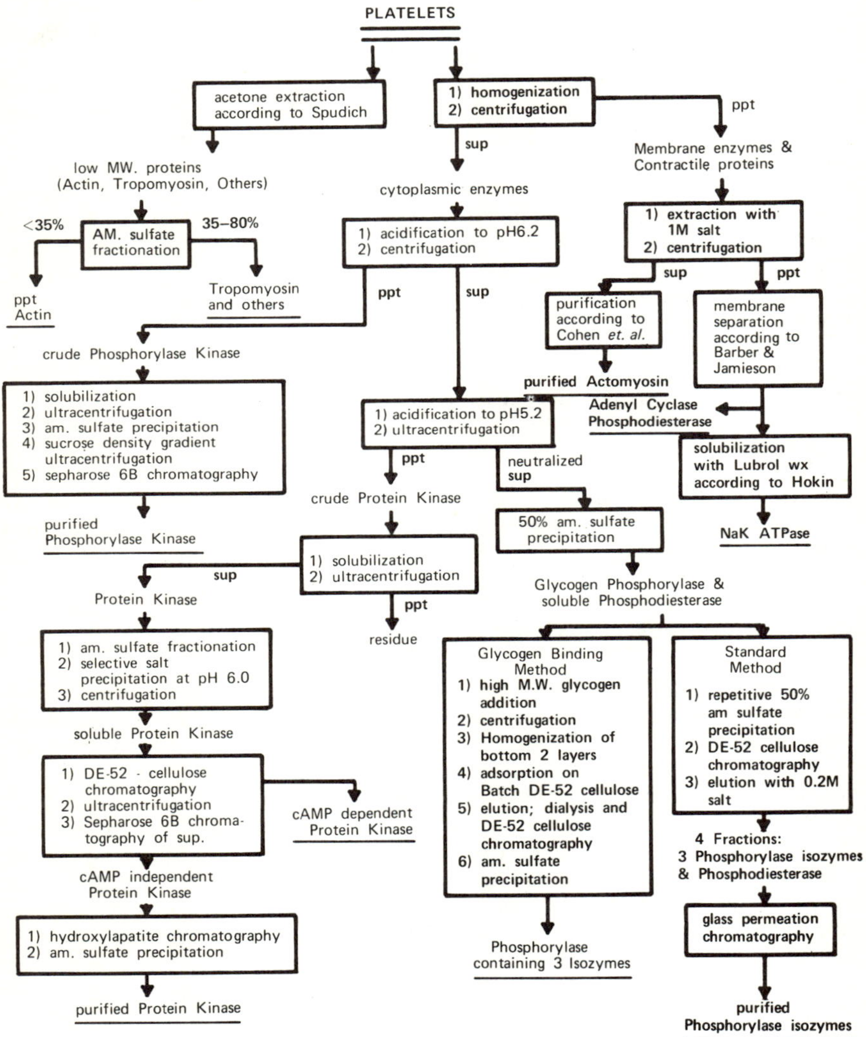

FIGURE 1. Procedure for the isloation of platelet enzymes.

employed them in the phosphorylation experiments. To identify the nature of the platelet membrane ATPase, it was separated away from other platelet membrane proteins by solubilization with Lubrol Wx and purification according to

** Assistance was provided by the research trainees Mr. Philip W. Mintz and Dr. Dolores M. Peterson.

the procedure of Hokin[67] for NaK ATPase of shark's rectal gland. A partially purified platelet NaK ATPase was found to resemble that of the shark in possessing electrophoretically separable catalytic and glycoprotein subunits[66] when incubated with SDS and stained according to Uesugi *et al.*[68] It differed from that of shark's rectal gland in being nearly two orders of magnitude lower in specific activity and in its apparent poor inhibition by ouabain.

Platelet Glycogen Phosphorylase and cAMP Phosphodiesterase

Glycogen phosphorylase was purified either as described[51] for that of lobster muscle or by the binding of the enzyme to glycogen with centrifugation at 20,000 *g* overnight and purification of the collected glycogen-enzyme layer by DE-52 cellulose column chromatography. Glycogen phosphorylase could be purified to a fraction with a specific activity of 20 (μmol/min)/mg with the glycogen binding method and to three chromatographically separate isozyme forms with specific activity of 0.5–4 (μmol Pi/min)/mg when the standard purification method was used (see FIGURE 1).

Cyclic AMP phosphodiesterase was obtained as the last peak eluted during the phosphorylase purification procedure of Assaf and Graves[51] and was employed in this form in the substrate phosphorylation experiments. Its specific activity when assayed at 1×10^{-4} M and 1×10^{-7} M cAMP according to Thompson and Appleman[65] was found to be 7200 and 3100 (pmol/min)/mg enzyme respectively. It sedimented in the analytical ultracentrifuge in two peaks with $S_{20,w}$ of 6.5–7.4 S and 1.8–3.2 S, similar to that encountered for the PDE purified from dog kidney (unpublished data by Thompson, Assaf, and Strada). Of potential interest in PDE purification is the finding that platelet PDE (dissolved at a concentration of 10–15 mg/ml in 0.005 M tris, 0.001 M EDTA-DTT, pH 7.5) could be precipitated at 22° C by the addition of 0.01 M magnesium acetate in the presence or absence of 1 mM cAMP. Disc gel electrophoresis of the resulting sparingly soluble amorphous precipitate exhibited one protein band possessing stainable PDE enzymatic activity when examined by the method of Goren *et al.*[69] Some platelet protein with PDE activity remained on top of the gel. Additionally, as indicated above, sucrose density gradient ultracentrifugation of the water-insoluble platelet membranes yielded a fraction with PDE activity.

Platelet Phosphorylase Kinase

This enzyme was purified following modification of the procedure outlined for its purification from aqueous muscle extracts.[70] When the precipitate of platelet phosphorylase kinase was collected in any given step, the ultracentrifugation time was increased to 1.5 times that used for the muscle enzyme. Additionally, 0.5 M glucose was included in the buffer system to increase enzyme solubility. The general properties of platelet phosphorylase kinase have been published by others,[71,72] and therefore this report will be restricted to that aspect of use of this enzyme as a substrate for platelet protein kinase.

Platelet Protein Kinase

Differing from that published recently[73,74] and originally employed in the purification of muscle protein kinase,[9,10] the pH 5.2 precipitate of platelet extract possessing a greater specific activity than the supernatant was used as the source of the platelet protein kinases employed in this study.

The standard purification steps are illustrated in TABLE 1 and FIGURE 1. The indicated ultracentrifugation steps were carried out at 50,000 *g* for 1½ hours. The DE-52 cellulose chromatography step was performed with a concave gradient of dilute buffer (0.002 M tris–0.001 M EDTA-DTT, pH 7.5) against the same with 1 M tris. The selective salt precipitation step (FIGURE 1) was

TABLE 1

PURIFICATION PROFILE OF HUMAN PLATELET PROTEIN KINASE *

Fraction	Volume ml	Conc. mg/ml	Specific Activity (pmol/min)/mg	Yield %
Platelet extract	2000	24	698	100
Supernatant of pH 6.2 precipitate	1850	14	980	76
Solubilized pH 5.2 precipitate	170	40	2100	43
Supernatant of glycerophosphate precipitation	160	21	3310	33
Dialyzed ammonium sulfate precipitate	80	25	3560	21
Supernatant after ultracentrifugation	60	15	4450	12
Concave gradient chromatography on DE-52 cellulose	6	30	14,000	8
Sepharose 6B chromatography				
Peak I	2	7	26,500	1
Peak II	2	11	58,000	4

* Approximately ½ kg of frozen packed platelets was used in a typical enzyme preparation such as the one shown here. The platelets were obtained from platelet concentrates approximately one week after plasmapheresis of healthy donors. Contaminating erythrocytes and leukocytes were removed by differential centrifugation.[56, 63] The platelets were freed of accompanying plasma proteins by centrifugation at 5000 *g* and washing in 0.004 M tris-EDTA, 0.85 M NaCl, pH 7.2. Packed platelets were then obtained by simply centrifuging at 10,000 *g* in the same buffer or after layering the cells on a 0–40% glycerol gradient in the buffer according to Barber and Jameison.[63] The protein kinase activities shown represent assays carried out at pH 6.5 in the presence of 0.002 mM cAMP with histone as a substrate, as indicated in MATERIALS AND METHODS. Peak I was stimulated at least threefold by cAMP. Peak II was not stimulated and was therefore referred to as cAMP-independent protein kinase. Re-assay of this enzyme in Dr. O. Martelo's laboratory at the University of Miami School of Medicine provided evidence that the enzyme was stable for at least 3 months of storage at −80° C.

employed before and after DE-52 cellulose chromatography in order to remove impurities. This step consisted of dialyzing the protein kinase enzyme solution against 0.05 M Na glycerophosphate, 0.001 M EDTA at pH 6.0, removing the resulting impurities by ultracentrifugation and then dialysis against 0.05 M tris, 0.001 M EDTA-DTT, pH 7.5, in which the enzyme is highly stabilized for several months if stored at −80° C.

Cyclic AMP-dependent and independent platelet protein kinase can be separated either by rechromatography on a DE-52 cellulose column with use of a linear gradient against 0.5 M tris buffer, pH 7.5, or following gel filtration on a Sepharose 6B column equilibrated with 0.05 M glucose dissolved in dilute buffer. The molecular weight (140,000 daltons) and dissociation behavior of the cAMP-dependent protein kinase by cAMP was found to be similar to protein kinase from other tissues.[23-26, 35] Other similarities were reported by various workers.[7, 16, 73, 74] The reported inactivation of this enzyme by DTT,[73] however, is in complete contradiction with our data. We found that platelet protein kinase required DTT (0.001–0.01 M) for protection against oxidation of its SH groups and that Ellman's reagent[75] used at 0.001 M completely abolished the kinase activity, an effect reversed upon enzyme incubation in 0.001 M DTT.

The cAMP-independent platelet protein kinase isolated in this work sedimented in the analytical ultracentrifuge in a peak with an $S_{20,w}$ of 7.4–8.0S. Its molecular weight (131,000 daltons), which is close to that of the dependent form, was found to be unaltered by cAMP (sucrose density gradient ultracentrifugation data not illustrated). Furthermore, the addition of the heat-stable cAMP-dependent protein kinase inhibitor[35] had no effect on the activity of this cAMP-independent kinase. These results suggest that the isolated cAMP-independent platelet protein is a holoenzyme and not a catalytic subunit of the cAMP-dependent form. In the latter stages of this work we found that the cAMP-independent protein kinase obtained following rechromatography on DEAE cellulose forms rhombohedral crystals (FIGURE 2) upon addition of 0.04 M magnesium acetate to a 10 mg/ml enzyme solution dissolved in 0.01 M tris, 0.001 M EDTA-DTT at pH 7.5. The resulting birefringent protein kinase crystals were sparingly soluble, and in order to enhance enzyme solubility, dilution as well as increasing the pH to approxiuately 9.0 was required, as encountered by us previously in the solubilization of crystalline glycogen muscle phosphorylase.[37-39] A further characterization of this enzyme and determination of its substrate specificity should aid our understanding of the regulation of phosphorylation of the various platelet proteins.

Substrate Phosphorylation

Since a study of phosphorylation of the isolated endogenous platelet protein substrates by protein kinase is the general aim of this work, the highly purified preparation of platelet protein kinase employed in these reactions was not fractionated into cAMP-dependent and independent forms. It is evident from TABLE 2 that in general, the endogenous platelet protein substrates were phosphorylated to a greater extent than nonplatelet protein substrates examined under similar experimental conditions. Platelet phosphorylase kinase, the physiological substrate for protein kinase[27 35, 70] served as a better substrate than calf thymus histone or casein, which are the most commonly employed substrates in the assay of protein kinase.[10, 11, 17, 35] Glycogen phosphorylase is a substrate for phosphorylase kinase[27, 35, 70] and not protein kinase unless it is denatured.[76]

The phosphorylation of platelet membranes (containing NaK ATPase, cAMP phosphodiesterase and adenylate cyclase) was generally higher than casein but fluctuated according to the activity of associated membrane protein kinase,[16, 31] i.e., endogenous kinase, in the various preparations. Our data on membrane proteins phosphorylation by endogenous kinase is consistent with

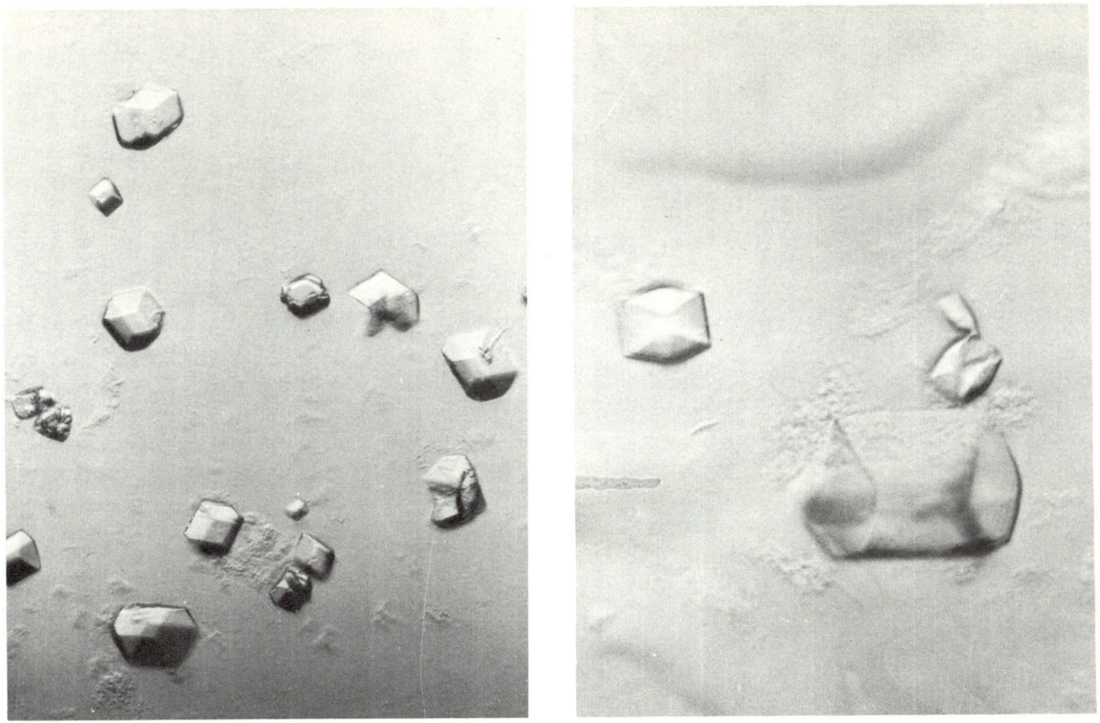

FIGURE 2. Crystals of platelet cAMP-independent protein kinase. The crystals were obtained from 10 mg/ml enzyme solution, 0.01 M tris, 0.001 M EDTA-DTT, pH 7.5, to which 0.04 M magnesium acetate was added to induce crystallization. Birefringence of the protein crystals was ascertained by Dr. F. A. Quiocho of the Department of Biochemistry, William Marsh Rice University, Houston, Texas. The photographs were taken by Dr. Charlene Moore of the Medical Cytogenetics Laboratory of the University of Texas Medical School, Houston, Texas, with a Zeiss Universal Photomicroscope. Phase contrast ×38 (left) and ×150 (right).

that published by Steiner[31] in that it is inhibited by calcium (5–10 mM) and by EDTA (1 mM) and can utilize casein as well as histones as substrate. Phosphorylation of the various proteins increased by only 1.5–2.0-fold in the presence of 2 mM cAMP, indicating that the endogenous cAMP-independent protein kinase present in these preparations is in the active form. It is possible that the cAMP-independent kinase could have been activated *in vivo* as a result of its phosphorylation by the catalytic subunit of the cAMP-dependent protein kinase utilizing intraplatelet ATP. This postulate remains to be investigated. The fact that cGMP at 3×10^{-2} mM was also found to stimulate phosphorylation of purified but unfractionated kinases of casein and histones by nearly 40% makes it difficult to understand the regulation of the platelet protein kinases without further characterization of the cAMP-independent kinase. Furthermore, it is interesting to note that calcium has been shown to stimulate cGMP but not cAMP-dependent phosphorylation.[77] As found with protein kinase from other tissues,[10, 11, 17, 35] calcium (0.005–0.10 M) was inhibitory to

TABLE 2

THE SUBSTRATE SPECIFICITY OF PURIFIED HUMAN PLATELET PROTEIN KINASE

Protein Substrate	(pmol ^{32}P/min)/mg	% Phosphorylation
Calf thymus histone	14,000	100
Platelet phosphorylase kinase	49,000	350
Platelet actomyosin	7,700	55
Platelet tropomyosin (crude)	8,400	60
Platelet actin (crude)	5,040	36
Platelet cAMP phosphodiesterase	5,600	40
Platelet membranes	4,200	30
Platelet phosphorylase	280	2
Human muscle phosphorylase	210	2
Rabbit troponin	3,500	25
Casein	3,500	25
Phosvitin †	3,000	21
Bovine serum albumin	120	1
Bovine thrombin	50	0
Bovine liver catalase	0	0
Horse myoglobin	0	0

* Substrate phosphorylation was carried out as indicated in MATERIALS AND METHODS. With the exception of actomyosin, which was dissolved in 0.25 M tris to induce solubility, all substrates were dissolved and dialyzed against 5×10^{-5} M EDTA, 1×10^{-3} M DTT, pH 6.7. The concentration of all substrates was adjusted to 2.0 mg/ml final concentration. Using unfractionated protein kinase (see text), the phosphorylation reactions were carried out at 30° C, pH 6.5, in the presence of 0.002 mM cAMP.

† The assay with phosvitin as substrate was kindly done in the summer of 1975 by Dr. O. Martelo and Dr. J. Hersch of the University of Miami School of Medicine and their assays were compared with those using casein and histone in the same experiment as performed by us.

platelet protein kinase when added to the phosphorylation reaction mixture in the presence or absence of 10 mM Mg^{2+} irrespective of the protein substrate used.

On the other hand, when studying the phosphorylation of platelet actomyosin, we found that this protein is best phosphorylated in the presence of 5×10^{-5} M Ca^{2+} and 0.01 M Mg^{2+} (conditions that better resemble this protein's physiological environment) [71, 72, 78] than without added calcium or in the total absence of calcium brought about by the addition of 0.002 M EGTA. These results vary from those of Daniel *et al.*,[79] who reported that the phosphorylation of platelet actomyosin by endogenous kinases was independent of Ca^{2+} concentration. Whereas the addition of 0.002 mM EDTA, which binds both magnesium and calcium, completely blocked any protein kinase-catalyzed phosphorylation of actomyosin, EGTA, which binds primarily calcium, did not inhibit this kinase reaction even when used at a concentration of up to 2 mM. Gross and Mayer [80] reported that the addition of EGTA does not completely inhibit endogenous phosphorylase kinase activity in skeletal muscle, and Assaf and Bratzler [81] found that more than half the calcium in aqueous extracts of muscle is in the bound state. As in muscle,[80, 82] platelet phosphorylase kinase was also found to phosphorylate actomyosin. The presence of phosphorylase kinase as an endogenous kinase in the actomyosin preparations along with protein kinase may therefore account for the increase in phosphorylation in the presence of 5×10^{-5} M calcium, a concentration known to activate phosphorylase kinase isolated from platelets and other tissues.[70–72, 78, 80, 83] It should also be noted that phosphorylation of purified platelet actomyosin by endogenous kinases was not significantly increased upon addition of cAMP under the assay conditions described in TABLE 2.

Effect of Phosphorylation on Enzyme Activity

The cytoplasmic cAMP phosphodiesterase purified as shown in FIGURE 1 was found to possess an endogenous kinase which, as illustrated in TABLE 3, catalyzed the incorporation of ^{32}P from added $AT^{32}P$ in the presence of the kinase activator, 0.01 Mg^{2+}, and the phosphoprotein phosphatase inhibitor, 0.02 M NaF. Complete dephosphorylation occurred when NaF was dialyzed overnight out of the incubation mixture. As expected, no loss in the ^{32}P label was observed when the dialysis was done in presence of fluoride or when the phosphorylated PDE was subjected to 1 M acid treatment. Incubation and washing in 0.3 M NaOH at 40° C completely removed the label, suggesting that the ^{32}P was covalently bound, as expected for a protein kinase catalyzed reaction.[14]

An assay of phosphorylated vs. dephosphorylated and unphosphorylated PDE, i.e., samples not subjected to phosphorylation but handled in the same manner, is summarized in TABLE 3. Under identical assay conditions, the phosphorylated enzyme exhibited a doubling in activity over the dephosphorylated form and a 67% increase over the unphosphorylated enzyme. The fact that we demonstrated that the phosphorylation and concomitant activation of a PDE preparation was reversible suggests that this reaction is physiological. Furthermore, our finding, when taken along with that of the report of Najjar and Constantopolous,[84] indicates that the activation of cAMP phosphodiesterase and inactivation of adenylate cyclase upon phosphorylation [75] may serve *in vivo* as a feedback inhibitory mechanism for a superactive cAMP-stimulated protein kinase. Determination of the exact site of phosphorylation in these enzymes can be achieved only once phosphorylation studies are made with the purified enzymes. These studies are planned with a large preparation of purified PDE.

O'Dea *et al.*[85] reported that inhibition of brain PDE resulted when protein kinase was added to the PDE assay mixture because the cAMP which complexed with the added protein kinase became unavailable for hydrolysis by PDE. These workers, however, did not undertake a phosphorylation study in the presence of ATP and NaF. On the other hand, we carried out this type of experiment using $AT^{32}P$-Mg and unfractionated protein kinase, which exhibited an approximately twofold cAMP dependence. We found that although the PDE preparations studied were phosphorylated, they exhibited either an inhibition or

TABLE 3

RELATION BETWEEN ACTIVITY AND PHOSPHORYLATION OF PLATELET cAMP PHOSPHODIESTERASE (PDE) *

PDE in Presence of NaF		PDE after Dialysis in NaF-Free Buffer		PDE not Subjected to Phosphorylation Activity
Phosphorylation ^{32}P cpm/ml	PDE Activity H^3 cpm/ml	Phosphorylation ^{32}P cpm/ml	PDE Activity H^3 cpm/ml	H^3 cpm/ml
9000	6500 (167%)	700	3200 (80%)	3900 (100%)

* A cAMP phosphodiesterase preparation obtained as indicated in the text and illustrated in FIGURE 1 was incubated with 1 mM γ-^{32}P-ATP, 10 mM $MgCl_2$ with buffer containing 30 mM sodium glycerophosphate, 30 mM potassium phosphate, 0.5 mM DTT, 20 mM NaF, 1 mM EGTA, 2 mM theophylline, 0.002 mM cAMP at pH 6.5 ^{32}P incorporation into protein was measured as described under MATERIALS AND METHODS. Samples of the phosphorylated enzyme were dialyzed against buffer (0.05 M tris, 0.01 M $MgCl_2$, pH 7.5) in the presence or absence of 0.03 M NaF as indicated in the text. Assays of phosphorylated (samples incubated and dialyzed overnight against buffer with NaF), dephosphorylated (samples incubated with NaF but dialyzed against buffer not containing this salt) and unphosphorylated (samples not subjected to phosphorylation) were carried out using 0.5×10^{-4} mM cAMP final concentration in buffer containing 0.04 M tris, 0.5 mM $MgCl_2$, 0.001 M DTT, pH 8.0, according to Thompson and Appleman.[65] To prevent dephosphorylation during the assay incubation period, the phosphorylated samples were assayed with buffer containing 0.03 M NaF. Cpm/ml refers to the number of counts incorporated per min per ml of enzyme solution of a fixed protein concentration. The first column, center column, and last column represent values for phosphorylated, dephosphorylated, and unphosphorylated PDE.

no change in enzymatic activity as a result of phosphorylation. These results could be explained only in the light of the data of O'Dea *et al.*,[85] i.e., that the added cAMP-dependent protein kinase complexed the cAMP needed as substrate for PDE. This also indicated that our success in demonstrating phosphorylation and activation of phosphodiesterase is due to the catalysis of the phosphorylation reaction by an endogenous cAMP-independent kinase, which obviously does not bind cAMP.

The ^{32}P in phosphorylated platelet actomyosin was found to co-elute with this protein on a Sepharose 6B column. Approximately one-half of the ^{32}P

label was found to meet the criteria of covalency as found above for PDE, i.e., stable to acid and labile to base, the rest being presumably bound to the active site. When actomyosin was incubated with purified platelet protein kinase (in the presence of 0.003 M ATP, 0.01 M Mg^{2+}, and 0.15 M tris and the phosphorylated actomyosin activity was measured as a magnesium ATPase), its specific activity was zero compared to 0.03 (μmol Pi/min)/mg for unphosphorylated actomyosin samples, which were handled similarly except for the omission of protein kinase from the incubation mixture. However, when the phosphorylated actomyosin was assayed as a Ca-ATPase, its specific activity compared to unphosphorylated actomyosin remained essentially the same (0.3 (μmol Pi/min)/mg) or increased slightly. Blanks for protein kinase assayed as a Mg-ATPase and as a Ca-ATPase were used in these experiments. It should be noted that Adelstein and Conti [86] recently reported an actin-induced stimulation of platelet actomyosin ATPase upon its phosphorylation by endogenous kinase. The difference from our results may be due to the manner in which actomyosin ATPase activity was evaluated and not in the phosphorylation. Our phosphorylated actomyosin preparations also showed the ^{32}P label to be mainly in the myosin light molecular chain as demonstrated by Booyse *et al.*[18] and Adelstein *et al.*[19, 20] In addition, Adelstein (personal communication) indicated that since their phosphorylation did not require cAMP, the cAMP-independent kinase which we have isolated may be the kinase responsible for the phosphorylation of their actomyosin preparations. This will certainly be explored in future studies.

The fact that agents which increase cAMP level result in an inhibition of clot retraction [87] supports the conclusion which may be derived from our data that a phosphorylated platelet actomyosin ATPase is enzymatically inactive at the *in vivo* cytoplasmic concentration of magnesium and calcium.

Based on the data in this paper and that of the literature, a model illucidating the control of blood platelet aggregation by cAMP-mediated phosphorylation was recently published.[88]

Acknowledgments

Human platelet concentrates were kindly provided by Dr. Benjamin Lichtiger, Acting Director of the Institute of Hemotherapy, Texas Medical Center, Houston, Texas. Mr. Joseph Troll, on an undergraduate work-study program from the University of Houston, assisted in the isolation of human blood platelets from platelet concentrates.

References

1. Salzman, E. W. & L. Levine. 1971. Cyclic 3′,5′-adenosine monophosphate in human blood platelets. II. Effect of N^6-2′-0 dibutyryl cyclic 3′,5′-adenosine monophosphate on platelet function. J. Clin. Invest. **50:** 131–141.
2. Lee, R. G. & S. W. Kim. 1976. Cyclic AMP and platelet adhesion to silastic surfaces. Thrombosis Res: **8:** 111–114.
3. Salzmann, E. W., J. N. Lindon & R. Rodvien. 1976. Cyclic AMP in human blood platelets: Relation to platelet prostaglandin synthesis induced by centrifugation or surface contact. J. Cycl. Nucl. Res. **2:** 25–37.
4. Jenkins, C. S., M. A. Packham & M. A. Guccione. 1973. Modification of platelet adherence to protein-coated surfaces. J. Lab. Clin. Med. **81:** 280–290.

5. Marcus, W. J. & M. B. Zucker. 1965. The Physiology of Blood Platelets : 49–56. Grune & Stratton. New York. N.Y.
6. Weiss, H. J. 1975. Platelet physiology and abnormalities of platelet function. New Engl. J. Med. **293:** 531–588.
7. Salzman, E. W. 1972. Cyclic AMP and platelet function. New Engl. J. Med. **286:** 358–363.
8. Krebs, E. G., D. J. Graves & E. H. Fischer. 1959. Factors affecting the activity of muscle phosphorylase *b* kinase. J. Biol. Chem. **234:** 2867–2873.
9. Walsh, D. A., J. P. Perkins & E. G. Krebs. 1968. An adenosine 3′-5′-monophosphate-dependent protein kinase from rabbit skeletal muscle. J. Biol. Chem. **243:** 3763–3774.
10. Kuo, J. F. & P. Greengard. 1969. Cyclic nucleotide-dependent protein kinases. IV. Widespread occurrence of adenosine 3′,5′-monophosphate-dependent protein kinase in various tissues and phyla of the animal kingdom. Proc. Nat. Acad. Sci. USA **64:** 1349–1355.
11. Krebs, E. G. 1972. Protein kinases. *In* Current Topics of Cell Regulation. B. L. Horecker & E. R. Stadtman, Eds. Vol. **5:** 99–133. Academic Press. New York, N.Y.
12. Assaf, S. A. & A. A. Yunis. 1971. Identification of a third form of glycogen synthetase in rat chloroma tumors. FEBS Letters **19:** 22–26.
13. Danforth, W. H., E. Helmreich & C. F. Cori. 1962. The effect of contraction and of epinephrine on the phosphorylase activity of frog sartorius muscle. Proc. Nat. Acad. Sci. USA **48:** 1191–1199.
14. Riley, W. D., R. I. DeLange, G. E. Bratvold & E. G. Krebs. 1968. Reversal of phosphorylase kinase activation. J. Biol. Chem. **243:** 2209–2215.
15. Salzmann, E. W., J. Lindon, D. Brier & E. W. Merrill. This volume.
16. Bishop, G. A. & M. C. Rozenberg. 1975. The effect of ADP, calcium and some inhibitors of platelet aggregation on protein phosphokinases from human blood platelets. Biochem. Biophys. Acta **384:** 112–119.
17. Langan, T. A. 1973. Protein kinases and protein kinase substrates. Adv. Cyc. Nuc. Res. **3:** 99–153.
18. Booyse, F. M., D. Guiliani, J. J. Marr & M. E. Rafelson. 1973. Cyclic adenosine 3′,5′-monophosphate dependent protein kinase of human platelets: Membrane phosphorylation and regulation of platelet function. Ser. Haematol. **6:** 351–366.
19. Adelstein, R. S., M. A. Conti & W. Anderson. 1973. Phosphorylation of platelet myosin. Ser. Haematol. **6:** 403–409.
20. Adelstein, R. S., M. A. Conti & W. Anderson. 1973. Phosphorylation of human platelet myosin. Proc. Nat. Acad. Sci. USA **70:** 3115–3119.
21. Assaf, S. A. 1974. Phosphorylation-dephosphorylation by human platelet protein kinase and phosphatase. Fed. Proc. **33:** 1346.
22. Assaf, S. A. 1974. Protein kinase and its role in the regulation of human platelet enzymes. Int. Symp. Blood Platelets. Istanbul, Turkey. Excerpta Medica : 3.
23. Assaf, S. A., W. G. Hicks & J. M. Liegel. 1975. Crystallization and properties of human platelet protein kinase. ACS Abstr. **170:** 160.
24. Tao, M., M. L. Salas & F. Lipmann. 1970. Mechanism of activation by adenosine 3′,5′-cyclic monophosphate of a protein phosphokinase from rabbit reticulocytes. Proc. Nat. Acad. Sci. USA **67:** 408–414.
25. Gill, G. N. & L. D. Garren. 1971. Role of the receptor in the mechanism of action of adenosine 3′,5′-cyclic monophosphate. Proc. Nat. Acad. Sci. USA **68:** 786–790.
26. Corbin, J. D., C. O. Brostrom, C. A. King & E. G. Krebs. 1972. Studies on the adenosine 3′,5′-monophosphate-dependent protein kinases of rabbit skeletal muscle. J. Biol. Chem. **247:** 7790–7798.

27. Yeaman, S. J. & P. Cohen. 1975. The hormonal control of activity of skeletal muscle phosphorylase kinase. Phosphorylation of the enzyme at two sites *in vivo* in response to adrenalin. Eur. J. Biochem. **51:** 93–104.
28. Reimann, E. M., D. A. Walsh & E. G. Krebs. 1971. Purification and properties of rabbit muscle adenosine 3′,5′-monophosphate-dependent protein kinases. J. Biol. Chem. **246:** 1986–1995.
29. Traugh, J. A. & R. R. Traut. 1974. Characterization of protein kinases from rabbit reticulocytes. J. Biol. Chem. **249:** 1207–1212.
30. Cenatiempo, Y., P. Maugeat & G. Marchis-Moureu. 1975. Purification and properties of cyclic AMP-dependent and independent protein kinases from rat pancreas. Biochimie **57:** 865–873.
31. Steiner, M. 1975. Endogenous phosphorylation of platelet membrane proteins. Arch. Biochem. Biophys. **171:** 245–254.
32. Lyons, R. M., N. Stanford & P. W. Majerus. 1975. Thrombin-induced protein phosphorylation in human platelets. J. Clin. Invest. **56:** 924–936.
33. Reimann, E. M. & K. K. Schlender. 1976. Multiple forms of glycogen synthase kinase: Isolation of forms which are independent of cyclic AMP. J. Cycl. Nuc. Res. **2:** 39–46.
34. Haddox, M. K., N. E. Newton, D. K. Hartle & N. D. Goldberg. 1972. ATP(Mg^{2+}) induced inhibition of cyclic AMP and reactivity with a skeletal muscle protein kinase. Biochem. Biophys. Res. Commun. **47:** 653–661.
35. Walsh, D. A. & C. D. Ashby. 1973. Protein kinases: aspects of their regulation and diversity. Rec. Prog. Horm. Res. **29:** 329–359.
36. Daile, P., P. R. Carnegie & J. D. Young. 1975. Synthetic substrate for cyclic AMP-dependent protein kinase. Nature [New Biol.] **257:** 416–418.
37. Assaf, S. A. & A. A. Yunis. 1973. Physicochemical and catalytic properties of crystallized human muscle glycogen phosphorylase. Ann. N.Y. Acad. Sci. **210:** 139–152.
38. Assaf, S. A. & A. A. Yunis. 1973. Subunit structure and amino acid composition of crystallized human muscle glycogen phosphorylase. Eur. J. Biochem. **35:** 282–292.
39. Assaf, S .A. & A. A. Yunis. 1973. Structural and catalytic properties of crystalline shark muscle glycogen phosphorylase. Biochemistry **12:** 1423–1433.
40. Graves, D. J. & J. H. Wang. 1972. α-glucan phosphorylases—chemical and physical basis of catalysis and regulation. Enzymes **7:** 435–482.
41. Segal, H. L. 1973. Enzymatic interconversion of active and inactive forms of enzymes. Science **180:** 25–32.
42. Appleman, M., E. H. Fischer & E. G. Krebs. 1966. Purification and properties of inactive liver phosphorylase. Biochemistry **5:** 2101–2108.
43. Yunis, A. A. & S. A. Assaf. 1970. Purification and properties of glycogen phosphorylase from bovine corpus luteum. Kinetics of salt activation. Biochemistry **9:** 4381–4388.
44. Madsen, N. B., O. Avarmovic-Zikic & K. O. Honikel. 1973. Structure-function relationships in glycogen phosphorylase with respect to its control characteristics. Ann. N.Y. Acad. Sci. **210:** 222–237.
45. Vroman, L., A. L. Adams, M. Klings & G. Fischer. 1975. Fibrinogen, globulins. albumin and plasma at interfaces. Adv. Chem. **145:** 255–289.
46. Malmsten, C. E., Granstrom & B. Samuelsson. 1976. Cyclic AMP inhibits synthesis of prostaglandin endoperoxides (PGG_2) in human platelets. Biochem. Biophys. Res. Commun. **68:** 569–576.
47. Gerrard, J. M. & J. G. White. 1975. The influence of prostaglandin endoperoxides on platelet ultrastructure. Am. J. Pathol. **80:** 189–202.
48. Flower, R. J. 1975. Aspirin, prostaglandins, endoperoxides and platelets. [New Biol.] **253:** 88–90.
49. Gorman, R. R. 1975. Prostaglandin endoperoxides: possible new regulators of cyclic nucleotides. J. Cycl. Nucl. Res. **1:** 1–9.

50. WALSH, D. A., J. P. PERKINS, C. O. BROSTROM, E. S. HO & E. G. KREBS. 1971. Catalysis of the phosphorylase kinase activation reaction. J. Biol. Chem. **246:** 1968–1976.

51. ASSAF, S. A. & D. J. GRAVES. 1969. Structural and catalytic properties of lobster muscle glycogen phosphorylase. J. Biol. Chem. **244:** 5544–5555.

52. WASTILA, W. B., J. T. STULL, S. E. MAYER & D. A. WALSH. 1971. Measurement of cyclic 3′,5′-adenosine monophosphate by the activation of skeletal muscle protein kinase. J. Biol. Chem. **246:** 1996–2003.

53. MARTELO, O. J., S. L. WOO, E. M. REIMANN & E. DAVIE. 1970. Effect of protein kinase on ribonucleic acid polymerase. Biochemistry **9:** 4807–4813.

54. SCHACHMAN, H. K. 1959. Ultracentrifugation in Biochemistry. Academic Press. New York, N.Y.

55. ASSAF, K. & S. A. ASSAF. 1974. Handbook of Mathematical Calculations for Science Students and Researchers : 166–171. Iowa State University Press. Ames, Iowa.

56. BAENZIGER, N. L. & P. W. MAJERUS. 1974. Isolation of human platelets and platelet surface membranes. Meth. Enzymol. **31:** 149–155.

57. BETTEX-GALLAND, M. & E. F. LUSCHER. 1961. Thrombosthenin. a contractile protein from thrombocytes. Its extraction from human blood platelets and some of its properties. Biochim. Biophys. Acta **49:** 536–547.

58. GANGULY, P. 1969. Studies on platelet proteins. IV. Some physical and chemical properties of thrombosthenin. Blood **34:** 511–520.

59. ADELSTEIN, R. S., T. W. POLLARD & M. W. KUEHL. 1971. Isolation and characterization of myosin and two myosin fragments from human blood platelets. Proc. Nat. Acad. Sci. USA **68:** 2703–2707.

60. ADELSTEIN, R. S. & M. A. CONTI. 1972. The characterization of contractile proteins from platelets and fibroblasts. Cold Spring Harbor Symp. Quant. Biol. **37:** 599–606.

61. COHEN, I., E. KAMINSKI & A. DEVRIES. 1973. Actin-linked regulation of the human platelet contractile system. FEBS Letters **34:** 315–317.

62. SPUDICH, J. A. 1972. Effects of cytochalasin B on actin filaments. Cold Spring Harbor Symp. Quant. Biol. **37:** 585–593.

63. BARBER, A. J. & G. A. JAMIESON. 1970. Isolation and characterization of plasma membranes from human blood platelets. J. Biol. Chem. **245:** 6357–6365.

64. THOMPSON, W. J., R. H. WILLIAMS & S. A. LITTLE. 1973. Activation of guanyl cyclase and adenyl cyclase by secretion. Biochim. Biophys. Acta **302:** 329–333.

65. THOMPSON, W. J. & M. M. APPLEMAN. 1971. Multiple cyclic nucleotide phosphodiesterase activities from rat brain. Biochemistry **10:** 311–316.

66. HOKIN, L. E., J. L. DAHL, J. D. DEUPREE, J. F. DIXON, J. F. HACKNEY & J. F. PERDUE. 1973. Studies on the characterization of sodium-potassium transport adenosine triphosphatase. Purification of the enzyme from the rectal gland of *Squalus acanthias*. J. Biol. Chem. **248:** 2593–2605.

67. HOKIN, L. E. 1974. Purification and properties of the (sodium + potassium)-activated adenosinetriphosphatase and reconstitution of sodium transport. Ann. N.Y. Acad. Sci. **242:** 12–23.

68. UESUGI, S., N. C. DULAK, J. F. DIXON, T. D. HEXUM, J. L. DAHL, J. F. PERDUE & L. E. HOKIN. 1971. Studies on the characterization of the sodium-potassium transport adenosine triphosphatase. Large scale partial purification and properties of lubrol-solubilized bovine enzyme. J. Biol. Chem. **246:** 531–543.

69. GOREN, E. N., A. H. HIRSCH & O. M. ROSEN. 1971. Activity stain for the detection of cyclic nucleotide phosphodiesterase separated by polyacrylamide gel electrophoresis and its application to the cyclic nucleotide phosphodiesterase of beef heart. Anal. Biochem. **43:** 156–161.

70. BROSTROM, M. A., F. L. HUNKELER & E. G. KREBS. 1971. The regulation of skeletal muscle phosphorylase kinase. J. Biol. Chem. **246:** 1961–1967.

71. GEAR, A. R. & W. SCHNEIDER. 1975. Control of platelet glycogenolysis. Activation of phosphorylase kinase by calcium. Biochim. Biophys. Acta **392:** 111–120.
72. CHAIKEN, R., D. PAGANO & T. C. DETWILER. 1975. Regulation of platelet phosphorylase. Biochem. Biophys. Acta **403:** 315–525.
73. KAULEN, H. D. & R. GROSS. 1974. Purification and properties of a soluble cyclic AMP-dependent protein kinase from human platelets. Hoppe-Seylers Z. Physiol. Chem. **355:** 471–480.
74. BOOYSE, F. M., J. MARR, D. C. YANG, D. GULLIANI & M. E. RAFELSON. 1976. Adenosine cyclic 3′,5′-monophosphate-dependent protein kinase from human platelets. Biochem. Biophys. Acta **422:** 60–72.
75. ELLMAN, G. L. 1958. A colorimetric method for determining low concentrations of mercaptans. Arch. Biochem. Biophys. **74:** 443–450.
76. BYLUND, D. B. & E. G. KREBS. 1975. Effect of denaturation on the susceptibility of proteins to enzymic phosphorylation. J. Biol. Chem. **250:** 6355–6361.
77. MALKINSON, A. M. 1975. Effect of calcium on cyclic AMP-dependent and cyclic GMP-dependent endogenous protein phosphorylation in mouse brain cytosol. Biochem. Biophys. Res. Commun. **67:** 752–759.
78. ALEDORT, L. M., S. PUSZKIN, E. PUSZKIN, J. HANSON & A. M. KATZ. 1973. Control of platelet contraction. Ser. Haematol. **6:** 410–417.
79. DANIEL, J., R. S. ADELSTEIN & M. A. CONTI. 1974. Platelet myosin phosphorylation. Studies on the kinase and phosphatase light chains. Fed. Proc. **24:** 1579.
80. GROSS, S. R. & S. E. MAYER. 1975. Phosphorylase kinase mediating the effects of cAMP in muscle. Metabolism **24:** 369–380.
81. ASSAF, S. A. & L. J. BRATZLER. 1966. Inorganic elements in beef muscle and their relative degree of binding in aqueous beef muscle extracts. J. Agr. Food Chem. **14:** 487–489.
82. PERRIE, W. T., L. B. SMILLIE & S. V. PERRY. 1974. A phosphorylated light-chain component of myosin from skeletal muscle. Biochem. J. **135:** 151–164.
83. KHOO, J. C. 1976. Ca^{2+}-dependent activation of phosphorylase kinase in adipose tissue. Biochem. Biophys. Acta **422:** 87–97.
84. NAJJAR, V. A. & A. CONSTANTOPOULOS. 1973. The activation of adenylate cyclase. 1. A postulated mechanism of fluoride and hormone activation of adenylate cyclase. Molec. Cell Biochem. **2:** 87–93.
85. O'DEA, R. F., M. K. HADDOX & N. D. GOLDBERG. 1971. Interaction with phosphodiesterase of free and kinase-complexed cyclic adenosine 3′,5′-monophosphate. J. Biol. Chem. **246:** 6183–6190.
86. ADELSTIN, R. S. & M. A. CONTI. 1975. Phosphorylation of platelet myosin increases actin-activated myosin ATPase activity. Nature [New Biol.] **256:** 597–598.
87. MÜRER, E. H. 1971. Compounds known to affect the cyclic adenosine monophosphate level in blood platelets. Effect on thrombin-induced clot retraction and platelet release. Biochim. Biophys. Acta **237:** 310–315.
88. ASSAF, S. A. 1976. Cyclic AMP-mediated phosphorylation reactions in the regulation of blood platelet aggregation. Int. J. Biochem. **7:** 1–8.

DISCUSSION

DR. BLACKSHEAR: I wanted to ask the bead-test people if they could tell us something about the relative flow rates of red cells and platelets through the bead column. Is there any tendency of the platelets to be in low-flow regions and red cells to be in high-flow regions?

DR. SALZMAN: I can't tell you anything about the relative flow rates of red cells and platelets in our system, but the flow rate of whole blood was .9 ml per minute. In response to Dr. Zucker's comment about the liberation of nucleotides by red cells, I don't think there really is a great area of dispute. I have no quarrel with the idea that the principal action of red cells in influencing platelet retention in these systems is a mechanical function. Whether red cells also serve as a source of nucleotides in the plasma is, I think, the point that's at issue; our system was not one involving glass beads, but rather organic polymers in which the flow rate was much slower than in her system, and in which the anticoagulant was different. I think it is very difficult to compare the two experimental models.

DR. WEISS: Dr. Zucker, do you have something to add?

DR. ZUCKER: With Dr. Harry Goldsmith (who I thought might answer Dr. Blackshear's question), we did measure the hematocrit and platelet count in the first few drops of blood that came through the glass-bead column, using EDTA. Obviously, if you don't use EDTA you get platelet retention, and that confuses life. There is a transient concentration of red cells in the first few drops which, I understand, is caused by the leading edge of blood. After a few drops the hematocrit was perfectly normal.

DR. FROJMOVIC: If one centrifuges through a density gradient carefully, so that one minimizes cell/cell contact, what is the effect, for example, on platelet retention? And, if one is dealing here in terms of retention and in terms of adhesion, if this is a physical/chemical property, what is the adhesion of aldehyde-fixed cells in different states?

DR. SALZMAN: I can't really answer that from experimental data. We have tried various methods of separating platelets from their plasma. We have not centrifuged through a density gradient. We have used separation by filtration through a gel. In that instance there is activation of platelets to the extent that they are stimulated to form prostaglandins. But, as Dr. Lindon has shown, if they are passed through gel in the company of their own plasma (that is, the gel had previously been incubated with plasma so that the platelets are never out of their own plasma), prostaglandin synthesis is the only effect that can be demonstrated. They are otherwise intact functionally, biochemically, as far as can be shown, and morphologically.

DR. ZUCKER: Using an albumin density gradient, I think that Peter Walsh found it necessary to add apyrase to obtain platelets that were normally responsive to aggregating agents. Formalin-fixed platelets do not adhere to glass at all. I would also like to mention that the release reaction produced in citrated platelet-rich plasma by high concentrations of collagen and most concentrations of thrombin is not inhibited by aspirin. Thus, aspirin does not block all release but only prostaglandin-related release.

DR. PACKHAM: While you are there, Dr. Zucker, perhaps you can answer my question. I'm intrigued with the source of the ADP in platelets passing through the glass bead columns. You have ruled out the red cells, which means that it either has to be the platelet cytoplasm or the platelet granules. Do you have any evidence—and this would be a question for Dr. Bernstein as well—about how much lysis the platelets undergo during passage through the column or during the injury which you caused? Because the cytoplasmic pool is, of course, a source of adenosine nucleotides as well.

DR. ZUCKER: That is a good question. Blood from patients with storage pool disease shows subnormal platelet retention, suggesting that the storage pool is the source of the ADP. It would be helpful to determine the source of the nucleotides by using radioactively labeled platelets, but separating platelet-rich plasma affects retention, and erythrocytes will take up the nucleotides if whole blood is used. I have not measured release of lactic dehydrogenase (LDH), but I doubt that it would be helpful, since there would be too few lysed platelets to increase the plasma level of LDH appreciably. We expected to find released ^{14}C-serotonin but didn't. So we do not know how to devise experiments to answer the question.

DR. BERNSTEIN: We have just begun to look at ADP/ATP release from these injured platelets; it is of a very modest order of magnitude, perhaps in the same order of magnitude as the percentage of serotonin release. That differs from what one would expect: a large fraction of the platelets looks structurally impaired, yet there isn't evidence of chemical release of either 5HT or ADP or ATP to significant levels.

DR. WEISS: I would like to ask Dr. Packham whether she studied the platelet retention in her thrombin-depleted platelets. Is it normal or abnormal?

DR. PACKHAM: We haven't studied the glass-bead columns, no.

DR. KELLER: On this question of centrifugation, we have recently made measurements on simple pressure applied to red blood cells and found profound changes in active transport and in sodium and potassium transport, at even as little as 100 atmospheres of pressure, which is well within the range of what one sees, certainly in ultracentrifugation experiments. If the platelets were more sensitive to that sort of effect, one might be seeing nothing other than the pressure effects on the metabolic processes of the membrane, and, in fact, on the chemical potential of materials in the membrane which would have an effect on transport. About the glass-bead tests, as a chemical engineer I thought the most information would be at what is called the break-through curve; that is, as the column becomes saturated with platelets at a point of the column retaining platelets and past it to a point where the column no longer retains platelets. I'm wondering if anyone using the glass-bead test has examined that part of the spectrum. It seems that the data reported were on the initial part of the spectrum on the initial outflow when the column is far from saturated, and it's difficult to tell very much about the kinetics of the actual transfer process between the flow and the beads at that point.

DR. WEISS: That sounds like a very simple question. Would you like to take that up, Dr. Salzman?

DR. SALZMAN: We haven't done any experiments in which we reached such a saturation point, and I'm not sure one can, because some aggregates of platelets form in the column and are washed out. Some aggregates that form in the bulk fluid phase, passing through the column, are retained mechanically, so that it would be a very difficult experiment to do.

DR. HOFFMAN: Most of your surfaces, at least in those pictures, looked very smooth. What is the effect of surface composition on the differences in retention and release?

DR. SALZMAN: We have not specifically studied surface texture in that respect. All the materials that we have studied have been prepared by Professor Merrill.

DR. MERRILL: The preparation of beads for these columns from organic polymers requires free-radical bead polymerization. Therefore, one is limited to a narrow choice of material, such as the classical polystyrene, methyl methacrylate, methyl acrylate, vinyl acetate, and so on. One is specifically forbidden from making the polyamides because they cannot be made by bead polymerization. It's very tedious to grind little ball bearings of nylon, and if you did, you would still worry about the grinding material on the surface. So only part of our story has been accomplished thus far, and our next task is to coat the spheres with crystallizable polymers like nylon, polyethylene, and polypropylene by solution-deposition techniques. But, in answer to Professor Hoffman's question, those beads that we have studied are always of the glassy or rubbery type, and never of the spherolitic crystalline type. The compositional differences ranged from the very glassy polystyrene to the rubbery polymethylacrylate, and polyvinvylacetate, the glass transition of which is way down to about 6° C, and our tentative conclusion, based on very limited evidence, is that the more rubbery the material, the more liquid-like the molecules in the surface layer of the bead, and the less the retention. Polymethyl methacrylate poses a curious problem, because its beta transition is probably well below the temperature of the test, +37° C. Furthermore, all of us involved in polymers are confounded by the general fact that the classical transition temperatures, the alpha transition and the beta transition, are drastically modified by small amounts of adsorbed water. For example, while polymethylacrylate will adsorb out of blood 2% of its volume in water, polyvinylacetate will pick up 20% by volume water, thereby greatly reducing its glass transition from the usually quoted value of 30° C down to about 5° C.

UNIDENTIFIED SPEAKER: Perhaps we are not necessarily limited to this type of polymers, as Professor Merrill said. For instance, polymers that crystallize could be precipitated as very, very small-sized single crystals. Was any work ever done on this?

DR. MERRILL: As far as I know, it has not. One of the difficulties would be with single crystals. The thickness would be of the order of 100–200 angstrom units, whereas the surface dimensions would be in the micron scale. In other words, the thickness of the crystal would be comparable to the diameter of a protein molecule. If you have spheres all of the same diameter, they can be packed well into columns, so that one could avoid the classical problems of channeling, whereas it is very difficult to pack plates or needle-like materials without then raising questions of the total amount of effective surface exposed to flow. And as long as one is driven to spheres, one is driven usually to the classical free radical *bead* polymerization.

DR. GOLDSMITH: I speak for the Society for the Prevention of Cruelty to Platelets. Dr. Bernstein is knocking the hell out of those poor little particles when he spins them at 3600 RPM. Events happen in the opposite direction, with an enhancement of platelet aggregation and of release at much lower shear stress—in fact, shear rates in whole blood of the order of 50–75 reciprocal seconds. They also occur in cone-and-plate viscometers at shear rates in whole blood or platelet-rich plasma of 50–75 reciprocal seconds—that is to say, shear stresses below one dyne per square centimeter—and they occur only in citrated blood, as far as I'm aware. If you shear a platelet suspension in citrated plasma in one of these viscometers, you get formation of aggregates, and when you test this platelet suspension in the aggregometer afterwards, there is enhanced activity. At much lower shear stresses than in Dr. Bernstein's work you can also get enhanced platelet aggregation, and I am wondering whether this range of shear rate isn't really much more typical of the kind of conditions that you find in the circulation, rather than where you are exceeding the conditions that you find even, perhaps, in some artificial organs.

DR. BERNSTEIN: With the jet test we did tests down to 100 dynes per cm^2, but not down to the level of one dyne, or less than one, which Harry Goldsmith mentioned. In our tests, under those conditions we were not able to elicit any changes in the platelet-function studies that we described here. With the rotation device we went down to a sixth of the rate I described, and one does not begin to see changes except for the platelet factor 3 activity and factor 4 release, which occur at 600 RPM. But otherwise, one does not see the same changes that I described until one gets up to 1800 RPM; they flourish at 3600 RPM. Also, there is a remarkable absence of histologic evidence of aggregation in the damaged cells that have been exposed to the rotation device. We begin to see aggregates with the jet test or the shift stress test only when the rates are at a peak level that we have used for testing, that is to say 10^6 per cm square, where we also begin to see functional change. Finally, in an attempt to answer Dr. Goldsmith's last question as I interpret it (of what significance are our studies to the normally expected circulatory conditions), they probably are not of any significance, but our goal was rather to define the conditions against which one could design devices for artificial purposes such as pumps and valves. We therefore tried to study the limitations in design concepts of such devices, not really the situation in normal circulation.

DR. TURITTO: Dr. Bernstein, you defined two types of injury to the cells. The second one you called "surface injury," I assume because you are operating shear stresses of some four orders of magnitude smaller than the shear stresses in the jet test. Are you assuming that the platelets are contacting the surface and are being removed, and is there any loss of cells in this test?

DR. BERNSTEIN: We are unable to detect a difference in the platelet count following these tests, and no difference at all in the surface-injury device. The reason we call it "surface injury" is that we don't have a better explanation for what it does. In the red cell, with this device there were profound effects from coating the surface of the device with various materials. For example if you coated the surface of the device with albumin, there was a marked decrease in the amount of hemolysis you would see under otherwise similar circumstances; that was not true if you simply added albumin to the solution. Similar effects were obtained by using other surface-coating materials with the same device. For that reason, in working with red cells, we began to feel that there was, in fact, some effect of the red cell approaching or touching the surface that was very important. In trying to study the same kinds of coatings with the platelet, also using albumin and fibrinogen, we have been unable to detect any differences to date in any of the parameters that we have measured. This may be simply due to some physical force within the chamber, although we tend to think that the physical force has to do with moving the platelets against the wall of the chamber. This is a device with a very large surface and a very small volume, compared with the other device.

PART V. INTERFACIAL REACTIONS OF RED AND WHITE CELLS

THE ADHESION OF LEUKOCYTES, ERYTHROCYTES, AND NONCELLULAR MATERIAL TO THE LUMINAL SURFACE OF NATURAL AND ARTIFICIAL BLOOD VESSELS *IN VIVO*

Gwendolyn J. Stewart, Peter R. Lynch, Frederick A. Reichle, William G. M. Ritchie, Allen Smith, and Robert G. Schaub

Specialized Center for Thrombosis Research
Temple University Health Science Center
Philadelphia, Pennsylvania 19140

INTRODUCTION

The accumulation of thrombotic material on veins, arteries, and artificial bypasses has been extensively studied from three different approaches: the characteristics of the luminal surface of the vessel or bypass; the adhesiveness of blood platelets; and the activation of the clotting and fibrinolytic mechanisms. The significance of flow is frequently mentioned but has not been studied as much as the factors just mentioned, especially *in vivo*. The interaction of these factors in the thrombosis of natural vessels has been appreciated since the days of Virchow (1860)[1] and Welsh (1899).[2] Of these factors, only the blood (platelets, components of clotting and fibrinolytic systems) remains fairly constant on the arterial and venous side of the circulation. The characteristics of venous and arterial walls are very different with respect to composition and type of junction between endothelial cells;[3] also, the blood flow is different with respect to pressure, velocity, and pattern. In arteries and artificial arterial bypasses only the characteristics of the conducting vessels are radically different. Thus, it might be anticipated that the kind, rate, and pattern of deposition of material would vary from vein to artery to bypass.

Until recently the study of the early events in the deposition of cells and fibrin on vessel walls was severely limited by the lack of a suitable means of examining vessels. The amount of sectioned material that could be examined by light microscopy was very limited, whereas the amount that could be examined by transmission electron microscopy was miniscule. Furthermore, neither provided an *en face* view of the luminal surface of the vessel. Small areas of endothelium could be removed and examined *en face* but this was also limited since it was not possible to obtain large, uninterrupted expanses of surface.[4-6] Furthermore, the magnification and especially the resolution were inadequate for identification of many details of structure.

The scanning electron microscope (SEM), which became widely available in the late nineteen sixties provided a means of examining the entire luminal surface of blood vessels over a wide range of magnification and with a resolution of 100–200 Å. In addition, sample preparation was easy and sure, if a few essential precautions were observed (for review, see Stewart et al.[7]). Samples up to 2 cm long can be examined in some scopes. The surface characteristics of the endothelium were well visualized, with such changes as pseudopod and crater formation on individual cells being evident. Additionally, blood cells could be identified as erythrocytes, leukocytes, or platelets. The periodicity of fibrin could not be distinguished, but it is quite safe to assume that fibrous strands formed on vessels containing blood are fibrin (when the basement membrane and the vessel were intact, so that there was no means for the exposure of collagen fibers). The granular or amorphous noncellular material cannot be identified with certainty, but it is reasonable to suspect that it may be insoluble derivatives of fibrinogen resulting from thrombin action and limited plasmin action. Such insoluble derivatives lack the well-ordered structure of fibrin.[8] In addition, the frequency of deposition of cells and fibrin could be shown at low and intermediate magnifications.

In this communication we 1) present new observations on a canine model that resembles the situation in clinical postoperative deep venous thrombosis; 2) review our observations on models resembling clinical situations in the construction of autogenous venous bypasses for peripheral and myocardial revascularization and replacement of segments of diseased aortas with artificial material; and 3) integrate our observations with those of other investigators and use the information to try to understand better the early events in the deposition of cells and fibrin on blood vessel walls.

Presentation of New Material

Materials and Methods

Experimental Model

Preconditioned female dogs weighing 15–17 kg were anesthetized with intravenous (i.v.) sodium pentobarbital (32.5 mg/kg). Four experiments were done with two dogs each, one control and one operated (hysterectomy), in which the procedures were carried out on the same day with the same reagents. The other six operated dogs were done by exactly the same procedures. The hysterectomy was performed, and after 60 minutes one jugular vein was occluded for seven minutes by percutaneous pressure just above the brachial notch. Blood flow was allowed to return and both the occluded and nonoccluded veins were exposed by blunt dissection. Great care was taken to avoid accidental occlusion of the vein during dissection, since this would cause massive leukocyte adhesion and invasion. The control dog was held under anesthesia for approximately the same length of time as the hysterectomized dog. The veins were exposed in the same manner in all dogs. Except for a slightly longer period of anesthesia, the control dogs were the same as those described by us previously;[9] we therefore elected to limit the number of controls in this study.

The treatment of veins was:

Control (no hysterectomy, 4 dogs)

1. one vein not occluded at any time;
2. one vein occluded before dissection for removal of vein.

Operated (hysterectomy, 10 dogs)

1. one vein not occluded at any time
2. one vein occluded for 7 minutes, starting 60 minutes after hysterectomy, but *before* dissection for removal of vein; i.e., there was occlusion after remote trauma but no occlusion after adjacent trauma.

Surgical Exposure and Perfusion of Veins

These procedures were performed as previously described,[9] with care being taken to avoid even brief stasis in the vein during dissection.

The Preparation of Veins for Scanning and Transmission Electron Microscopy

Veins for scanning electron microscopy were prepared according to the procedure previously described by us.[9] Samples for transmission electron microscopy were taken from the veins and processed according to conventional methods.

Human Veins

At the time of constructing arteriovenous fistulas, segments of cephalic veins were perfused with lactated Ringer's solution with 5% dextrose, tied off under normal pressure, removed, and immediately submerged in 1% glutaraldehyde.

At the time of amputation, segments of veins containing mural thrombi were exposed, perfused with lactated Ringer's solution with 5% dextrose, tied off under normal pressure, removed, and immediately submerged in 1% glutaraldehyde.

Both normal and thrombosed veins were further processed in the same way as the canine veins.[9]

Results

The association of the luminal surface of veins with leukocytes, erythrocytes, and amorphous and/or fibrous material was studied by scanning electron microscopy. The results are summarized in Tables 1–3. Details of these associations and of the appearance of the endothelial sheet are provided in the following text and in the figure descriptions.

Control: No Surgical Trauma

In this model, one vein was not occluded at any time, and one vein was occluded prior to starting dissection in the neck. This enabled us to assess the effects of occlusion in the absence of trauma as well as the effects of the necessary dissection. In the absence of occlusion there was limited adhesion of leukocytes to the luminal surface of the vessel (Figures 1A & 1B). Occlusion prior to dissection increased this somewhat. The vessels were free of red cells and amorphous material except for one occluded vein that had many red cells and a moderate amount of fibrous material (Table 2).

Surgical Trauma: Hysterectomy

There were ten dogs in this group.: In each case one of the jugular veins was occluded continuously for seven minutes, starting 60 minutes postopera-

TABLE 1

DESCRIPTION OF LUMINAL SURFACE OF JUGULAR VEINS

	Type of Association	Extent of Association	Arrangement of Adhering or Invading WBCs
Leukocytes (WBCs)	adhesion—on surface only—many "ruffling" invasion—forcing endothelial intercellular junctions or between endothelium and basement membrane	rare sparse moderate heavy	patchy uniform
	Occurrence	Frequency	
Erythrocytes (RBCs)	single cells clumps of cells	rare sparse moderate heavy microthrombi	
	Distribution	Frequency	
Amorphous Material	patchy uniform	sparse moderate frequent	

tively but *before* any dissection in the neck region. After occlusion of one vein, both veins were exposed, perfused, and removed for further processing. The results are shown in TABLE 3. The association of leukocytes, red cells, and fibrous and/or amorphous material with the vessel wall was greater in these animals than in the control group. While there was variation in the extent of leukocyte adhesion and invasion from one animal to another, the occluded vessel always showed more leukocyte association than the contralateral, nonoccluded vessel. There was also more red cell adhesion and the occluded vessels contained microthrombi composed of leukocytes, erythrocytes, and fibrin, while one contained a large thrombus composed of erythrocytes and fibrin anchored by leukocytes (see FIGURE 3). Amorphous or fibrous material was deposited on the walls of seven of the 10 occluded veins (FIGURES 1C, 1D, 2, 3, 4A & 4B).

The emigration of leukocytes across endothelial cell junctions was inevitably associated with at least temporary opening of the junction, but when the emigration was sparse with only a single leukocyte in an area it appeared that the junction reclosed (FIGURE 4C). However, scanning microscopy provided no evidence of restoration of the permeability characteristics of the junction. In cases of massive leukocyte emigration and accumulation, numerous wide gaps between endothelial cells were present. In some instances there were obvious disturbances of the intercellular junction some distance from even single-cell leukocyte invasion (FIGURE 4C).

Human Veins

The appearance of the vascular endothelium, leukocyte emigration, and deposition of thrombotic material were indistinguishable from canine veins.

COMMENTS

In this study the control and experimental dogs were treated the same, except that those in the experimental group were subjected to surgical trauma in the form of hysterectomy. The veins in each group were treated identically with respect to occlusion, exposure, and perfusion. Thus the difference in the control and experimental groups of veins could be taken as an indication of the influence of surgery on the deposition of cells and noncellular material on veins in another part of the body. Control veins without occlusion were compared with experimental veins without occlusion while occluded veins from each group were compared.

The data on leukocyte invasion given in TABLES 2 and 3 are summarized in FIGURE 5. It appears that three of the dogs subjected to hysterectomy were

TABLE 2

DOGS SUBJECTED TO NO TRAUMA PRIOR TO EXPOSURE OF VEINS (4 ANIMALS)*

Dog No. and Treatment	WBCs	RBCs	Amorphous Material or Fibers
71477			
not occluded	adhesion, sparse, patchy invasion, sparse, patchy	sparse, single cells	none
occluded	adhesion, moderate, patchy invasion, sparse, patchy	sparse, single cells	sparse amorphous material
76905			
not occluded	adhesion, sparse, patchy invasion, sparse, patchy	rare, single cells	sparse amorphous material
occluded	adhesion, moderate, patchy invasion, sparse, patchy	rare, single cells	sparse amorphous material
76042			
not occluded	adhesion, sparse, patchy invasion, sparse, patchy	sparse, single cells	sparse amorphous material
occluded	adhesion, moderate, patchy invasion, sparse, patchy	many single cells and clumps	moderate amorphous material
81948			
not occluded	adhesion, rare invasion, rare	rare, single	sparse amorphous material
occluded	adhesion, sparse, patchy invasion, sparse, patchy	rare, single	sparse amorphous material

* One vein not occluded, contralateral vein occluded 7 minutes predissection.

TABLE 3

DOGS SUBJECTED TO HYSTERECTOMY 60 MINUTES PRIOR TO CONTINUOUS OCCLUSION OF ONE JUGULAR VEIN FOR 7 MINUTES (10 ANIMALS)

Dog No. and Treatment	WBCs	RBCs	Amorphous Material or Fibers
40241–1			
Not occluded	adhesion, moderate, uniform invasion, sparse, uniform	sparse single cells	none
Occluded	adhesion, moderate, patchy invasion, heavy, patchy	sparse single cells	none
65574–2			
Not occluded	adhesion, sparse, patchy invasion, rare	sparse single cells	none
Occluded	adhesion, sparse, uniform invasion, heavy, patchy	many microthrombi	fibers associated with WBCs and RBCs
61348–3			
Not occluded	adhesion, sparse, uniform invasion, rare	sparse single cells	none
Occluded	adhesion, moderate, uniform invasion, moderate, uniform	moderate single cells	none
66642–4			
Not occluded	adhesion, rare invasion, rare	sparse single cells	none
Occluded	adhesion, heavy, patchy invasion, heavy, patchy	single cells and microthrombi	fibers associated with RBCs
66055–5			
Not occluded	adhesion, rare invasion, rare	sparse single cells	none
Occluded	adhesion, moderate, patchy invasion, sparse, patchy	sparse single cells	none

TABLE 3 (*continued*)

Dog No. and Treatment	WBCs	RBCs	Amorphous Material or Fibers
68345–6			
Not occluded	adhesion, sparse, uniform invasion, rare	sparse single cells	none
Occluded	adhesion, sparse, patchy invasion, sparse, patchy	many microthrombi	amorphous associated with clumps
69565–7			
Not occluded	adhesion, moderate, patchy invasion, sparse, patchy	rare aggregates & sparse single cells	none
Occluded	adhesion, moderate, patchy invasion, moderate, patchy	many aggregates	none
67314–8			
Not occluded	adhesion, moderate, patchy invasion, rare	moderate single cells patchy	sparse amorphous material
Occluded	adhesion, heavy, patchy invasion, sparse, patchy	moderate uniform single cells	moderate amorphous material
78049–9			
Not occluded	adhesion, moderate, patchy invasion, rare	microthrombi	dense amorphous material
Occluded	adhesion, heavy, patchy invasion, moderate, patchy	large thrombus, rest, moderate, single cells, clumps	much, fibers and amorphous
79170–10			
Not occluded	adhesion, moderate, patchy invasion, rare	sparse single cells	sparse, patchy amorphous material
Occluded	adhesion, heavy, patchy invasion, moderate, patchy	many microthrombi	amorphous and fibrous material in thrombi

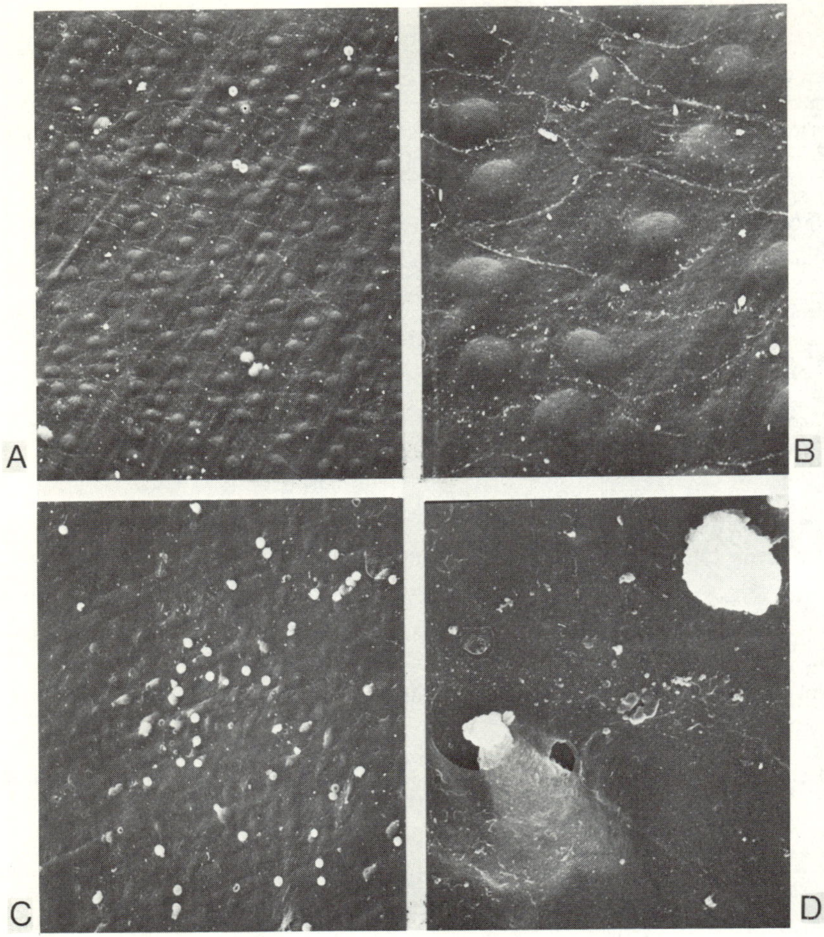

FIGURE 1. A and B. Scanning electron micrographs showing a survey and details of the limited adhesion of leukocytes (L) and red cells (RBC) to the luminal surface of veins from a control (nonoperated) dog. This vein was not occluded. The endothelial cells are quite uniform in size and shape and form a flat layer. The nuclei (N) and intercellular junction (arrows) are just discernable. A: × 300; B: × 2250. C and D: Scanning electron micrographs of a vein that was occluded continuously for seven minutes, starting one hour posthysterectomy. The occlusion was completed before there was any dissection in the neck. Frame C shows cells (white spheres) distributed in patches over the surface. × 175. D shows that the adhering cells were mostly leukocytes (L), some of which were in the process of emigrating between the endothelial cells (arrows). There were a number of craters (C) and pseudopods, especially along the intercellular junctions (double arrows). × 1500.

no different from the controls, whereas seven showed a higher extent of leukocyte invasion. A similar situation was observed when the permeability of veins to [^{131}I]-labeled fibrinogen was studied.[10] The lack of increase in permeability in some dogs could be causally related to the low level of leukocyte invasion; i.e., it could account for the lack of generation of messenger, as will be discussed shortly. The leukocyte invasion is possibly more important than leukocyte adhesion, since entrapped leukocytes can be expected to release the contents of their lysosomal granules in a short time. Collagenase and elastase and cytotoxins that are released could easily cause a small area of necrosis and serve as a nidus for the deposition of other leukocytes and fibrin.

The adherence of erythrocytes to the occluded vein in operated (experimental) dogs was prominent, yet there had been no erythrocytes on the occluded vein in the previous study, even though leukocyte invasion was massive (FIGURES 6 & 7). Also, there appeared to be little fibrin in many of the microthrombi or the mural thrombus on these veins. This could be the result of the high molecular weight derivative of fibrinogen that were formed intravascularly in response to hysterectomy. The significance of fibrinogen and its derivatives in erythrocyte-erythrocyte interaction will be considered in DISCUSSION.

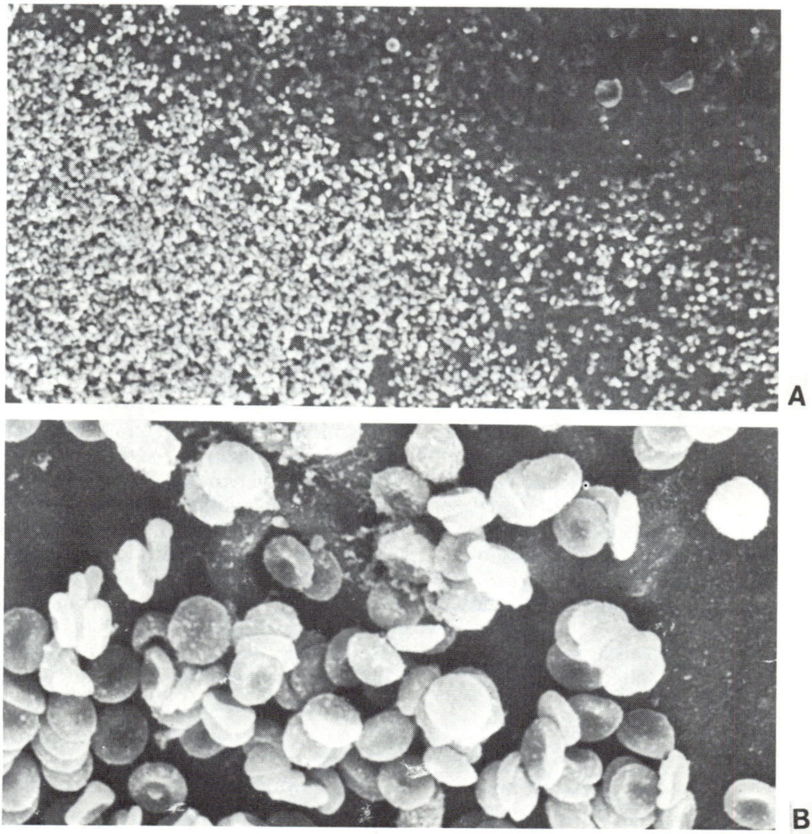

FIGURE 2. A and B: Scanning electron micrographs showing a vein that was occluded for seven minutes, starting one hour posthysterectomy. Frame A shows the massive accumulation of cells (white spheres) on the vessel wall. B shows that both leukocytes (L) and red cells (RBC) were adherent, with red cells being more numerous. The cell surfaces were coated with finely granular material that in places (arrows) formed rough fibrils. A: × 390; B: × 1900.

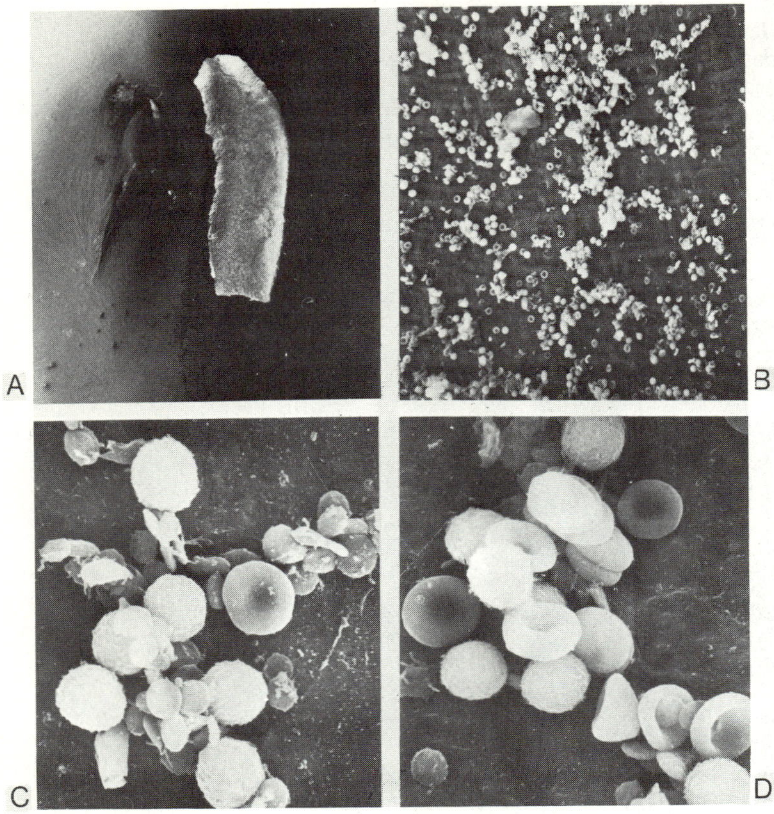

FIGURE 3. A. B, C and D: Scanning electron micrographs of the luminal surface of a vein with part of an attached thrombus. After glutaraldehyde fixation, part of the thrombus was gently lifted off to reveal the vessel underneath. The part of the thrombus that was removed was fractured after critical point drying to reveal the interior structure. A is a survey showing the thrombus (arrow) attached to the vessel wall in the vicinity of the inlet of a feeder vessel (double arrows). None of the thrombi originated in a valve pocket. × 16. B is a survey showing the vessel wall from which the thrombus was removed. There are numerous aggregates composed of leukocytes and red cells. Fibrin is not visible at this magnification. × 200. C and D show details of a cell aggregate shown in B. Leukocytes (L) and red cells (RBC) are prominent, some platelets (P) are present. There is only a small amount of fibrin here. ×2000.

The observations on canine veins appear to contribute directly to our understanding of events in patients, since the endothelium of normal veins, the leukocyte emigration, and deposition of thrombotic material in human and canine veins was indistinguishable.

Review of Previous Work

During the past few years we have used a combination of transmission and scanning electron microscopy to examine veins, aorta, and artificial bypasses from canine models that closely resemble common clinical situations. During these studies we have been impressed with the prominent interaction of leukocytes, erythrocytes, and fibrin with the vessel wall or bypass during the initial deposition of thrombotic material. Platelets were rarely observed on veins. On the damaged area of the aorta immediately adjacent to the anastomoses with the bypass they were limited to a discontinuous layer, usually only one platelet thick. Masses of platelets, however, accumulated on woven Dacron® bypasses in the thoracic aorta, starting at the junction of aorta and bypass and

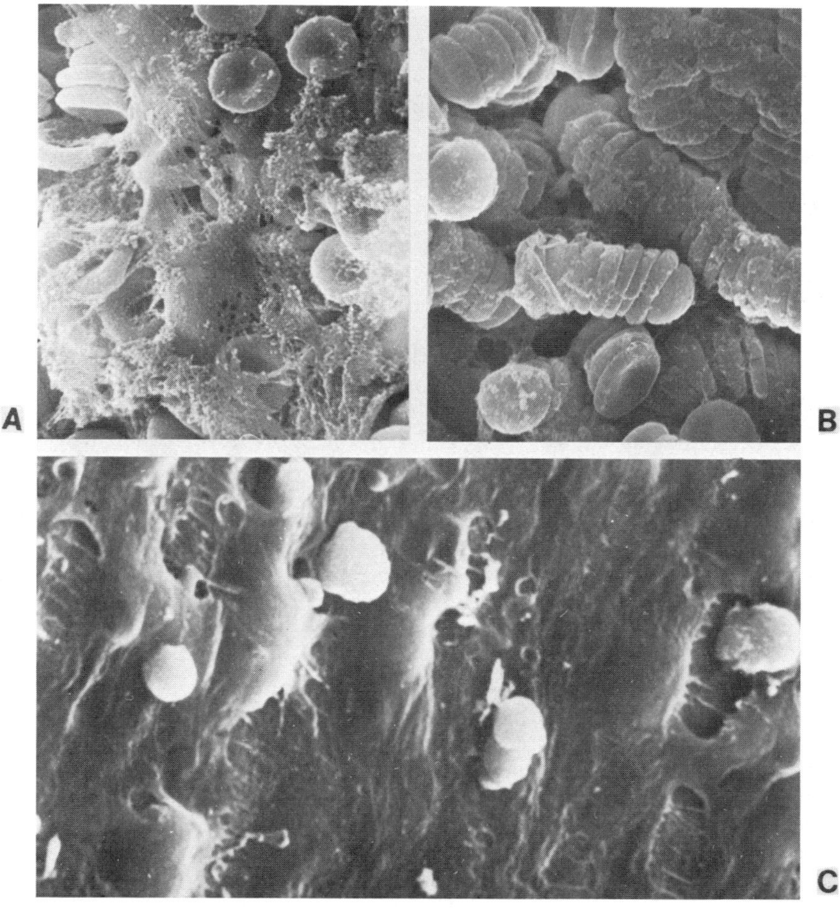

FIGURE 4. A, B, and C: Scanning electron micrographs. A shows the surface of a recently formed thrombus that was composed mostly of red cells held together by fibrin. These recently formed thrombi were extremely fragile, and it was possible that there was a continuous turnover of cells and fibrin at the surface; however. the thrombus was stable enough to withstand perfusion with Tyrode's solution and glutaraldehyde. × 2100. B shows the interior of the same thrombus to be composed mostly of rouleaux of red cells with surprisingly little fibrin. × 2100. C shows endothelial cell separation that occurred both in association with leukocyte emigration (arrow) and independently of, or at least some distance from, leukocyte emigration. × 1500.

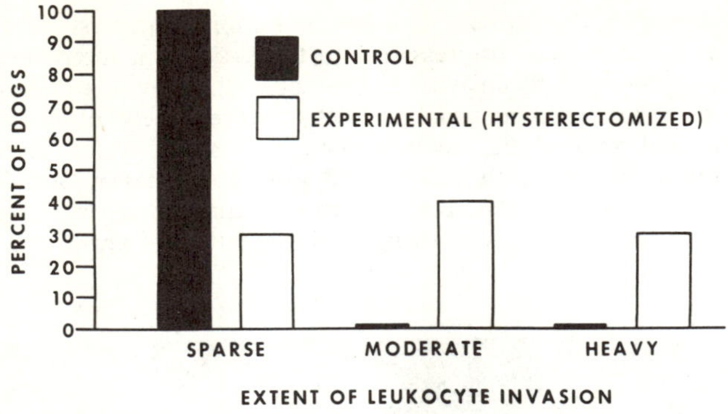

FIGURE 5. The extent of leukocyte invasion occurring in control (nonoperated) and experimental (hysterectomized) dogs. The dogs in both groups were held under anesthesia for approximately the same length of time and the veins were exposed, perfused, and processed by the same methods. The only variable was the surgery performed on the experimental group.

covering the entire surface of the bypasses removed after 10 and 40 minutes of blood flow.

Venous Endothelial Damage Produced by Massive Sticking and Emigration of Leukocytes

In our studies of canine veins, the veins were exposed, cannulated, and perfused with Tyrode's solution followed by 1.0% glutaraldehyde in the same solution at less than 20 cm water pressure. The veins were tied off under pressure, removed, and, still under pressure, immersed in 1.0% glutaraldehyde, postosmicated, the critical point dried, and coated with carbon and gold. Samples of the same veins were processed conventionally for transmission electron microscopy (TEM).

Spontaneous Disease in Mongrels

In normal vessels SEM examination revealed continuous cell sheets with regularly spaced, slightly raised nuclei. Underlying cords of fibers were sometimes visible. Cell junctions were easily identifiable. In four out of a series of ten mongrel dogs, one vein was grossly abnormal, being small, rigid, and grey in comparison with the contralateral vein. Examination of these veins by scanning and transmission electron microscopy revealed 1) abnormal adhesion of polymorphonuclear neutrophils (PMN) to the endothelium; 2) excessive migration of PMN across the endothelial sheet; 3) accumulation of PMN between the endothelium and basement membrane; 4) discontinuities, apparently between cells in areas of excessive PMN emigration; 5) desquamation of endothelial cells; 6) denuded areas in which the basement membrane was exposed; 7) fibrin formation and entrapment of platelets and red cells; 8) loss of intracellular contents from the endothelial cells, leaving them rather transparent ghosts.[11] The appearance of the affected veins indicated that the condition was of long duration but the basic cause remains unknown, since the history of the dogs is unknown.

Leukocyte Invasion In Healthy Dogs and In Patients

In the dog the occlusion of a jugular or femoral vein for as short a time as one minute following exposure by blunt dissection resulted in large numbers of leukocytes adhering to the luminal surface of the vessel and passing through the endothelial intercellular junction, where they accumulated in pockets be-

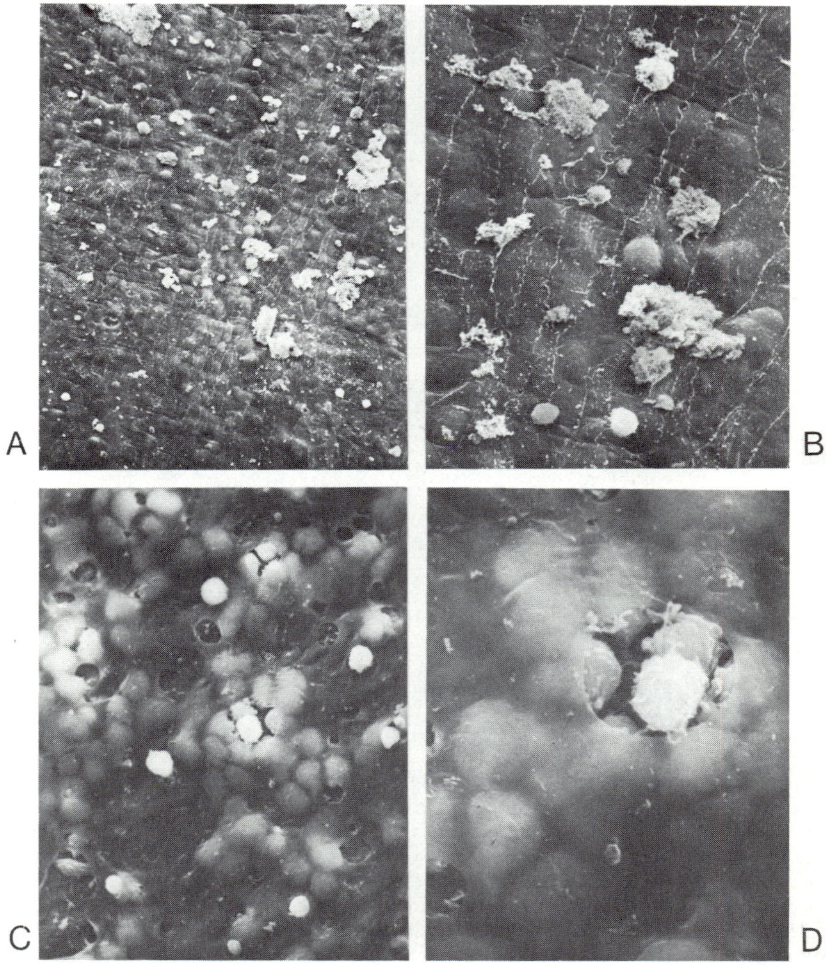

FIGURE 6. A, B, C, and D. Scanning electron micrographs showing the range of leukocyte invasion observed in veins that were occluded for one minute *after* the dissection that was required for exposure and ligation of side branches. These dogs had been exposed to no experimental procedures prior to exposure of the veins. A and B show the limited leukocyte adhesion and emigration that was only occasionally observed in these veins. A: × 225; B: × 750. C and D show the massive leukocyte emigration that was commonly observed. The accumulation of pockets of leukocytes between the basement membrane and endothelium separated the endothelial cells from the basement membrane and from each other. C: ×225; D: ×2250.

tween the endothelium and the basement membrane. This leads to extensive separation and desquamation of endothelial cells with exposure of subendothelial structures in many areas.[9, 12]

A

B

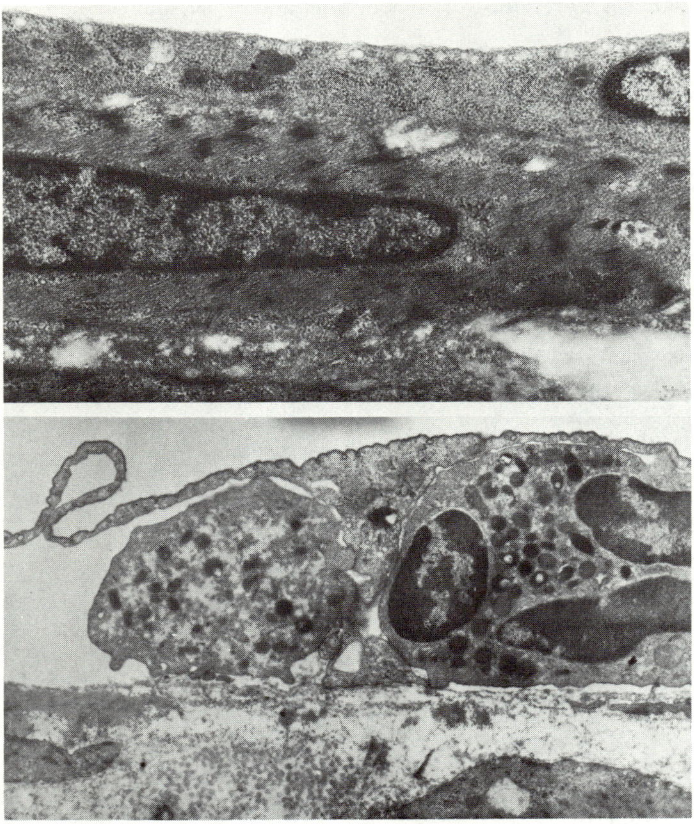

FIGURE 7. Transmission electron micrographs showing jugular veins with and without occlusion. The dogs were subjected to no experimental procedures prior to exposure of the veins. A shows a vein that was not occluded at any time. The endothelial cells (E) have typical caveolae and a long intercellular junction (IJ). There is a thin basement membrane (BM) separating the endothelium from the underlying smooth muscle (SM). The myofilaments (M) and dense bodies (DB) are well preserved. × 18,000. B shows a vein that was occluded for one minute after dissection and ligation of side branches. Two leukocytes (L) are located between the endothelium (E) and basement membrane (BM). Part of the detached endothelial cell (arrows) is separated from the basement membrane by several microns.

Endothelial damage and desquamation appeared to be a direct consequence of the massive leukocyte invasion that resulted in multiple forcings of intracellular junctions and accumulation of pockets of white cells between the endothelial sheet and basement membrane. It appeared that patches of these loosened cells were swept away by the flowing blood. If they had been swept away by the perfusion fluid, there would have been no association of blood cells or fibrin strands with the damaged areas (FIGURES 6 & 7).

The role of leukocytes in producing endothelial damage was further indicated by the observation that lidocaine, which is known to inhibit white cell sticking *in vivo,*[13] prevented both white cell invasion and endothelial damage. That the protection of the vessel was due to action on leukocytes rather than the vessel wall was shown by the invasion of veins from lidocaine-treated animals by leukocytes that had not been exposed to lidocaine and by the failure of leukocytes in lidocaine-exposed blood to invade veins that had not been exposed to lidocaine.[9]

Further evidence for the role of leukocytes in producing vascular damage was provided by the experiments with dogs made neutropenic with vinblastin. When the white cell count was reduced to 500–1000/mm^3 and the veins were occluded after surgery, there was minimal white cell sticking and emigration. This was in contrast to the consistent massive leukocyte invasion produced in untreated dogs. The protection of the vein was associated with the absence of leukocytes rather than a change in the vessel or surrounding tissues. This was shown by the fact that when the vein from a vinblastin-treated animal was perfused with normal blood, leukocyte invasion was as extensive as it was in the untreated dogs.[9]

Taken together, these three groups of experiments provide strong support for the concept that massive leukocyte invasion was the means of producing extensive endothelial separation and desquamation in response to trauma to adjacent tissue followed by even brief stasis. The normal ultrastructural detail of endothelium and leukocytes in thin sections suggests that the damage was partly, perhaps largely, due to physical separation of endothelial cells from each other and the basement membrane rather than to release of lysosomal enzymes with accompanying necrosis. If the leukocytes had released their enzymes, there would have been ultrastructural evidence of degranulation,[14] and this was not present. Furthermore, the basement membrane and limiting membrane of endothelial cells showed no evidence of lysis as would be expected if they had been acted upon by hydrolytic enzymes.

At construction of arteriovenous shunts, small segments of human veins were perfused *in situ* with lactated Ringer's solution with 5% dextrose, tied off under physiologic pressure, and removed. The segments of veins, still under pressure, were immediately submerged in 1% glutaraldehyde and further processed by the method used in preparing canine veins. Despite care to avoid accidental occlusion of these veins during dissection, there were some areas of leukocyte adhesion and emigration, similar to that observed in the dog (FIGURE 8).[15–17]

Since it is well established that *in vitro* [15–17] and, most likely, *in vivo,*[18-20] leukocytes emigrate in response to an increasing gradient of leukotactic agent, these results led to the conclusion that the source of the leukotactic agent was external to the endothelium. The location could be either within the vessel wall, or in this case, in the damaged tissue surrounding the vessel. The site of generation, and therefore the highest concentration, could not be intraluminal. Local stasis allowed the leukotactic agents that reached the lumen, probably by diffusion, to accumulate and thereby attract leukocytes to and across the endothelial sheet.

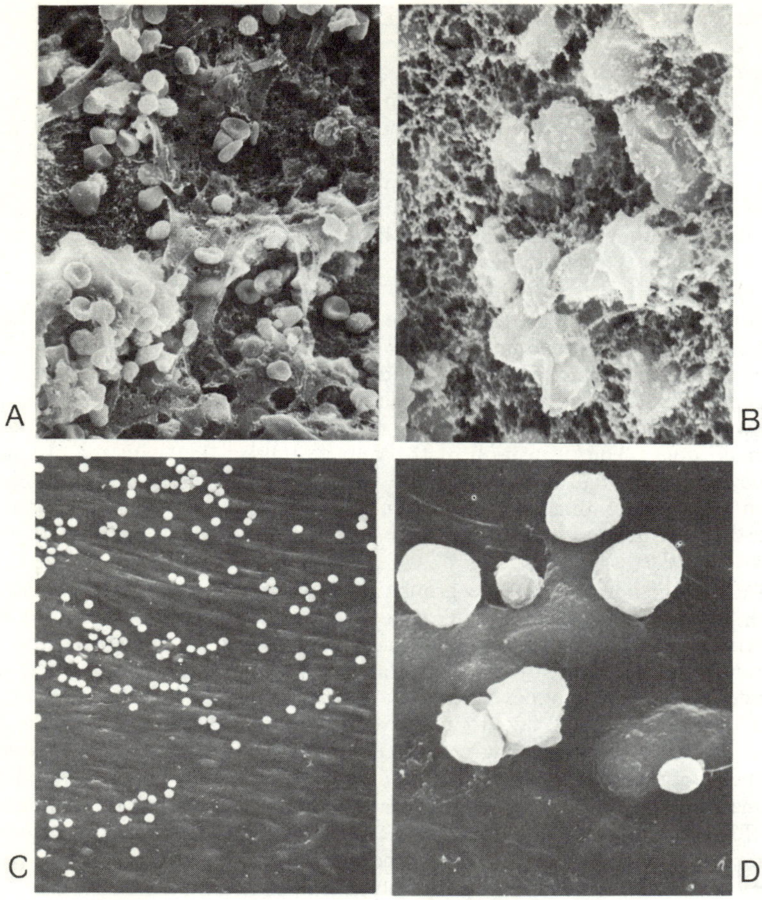

FIGURE 8. Scanning electron micrographs of two human veins, one thrombosed and the other not. A shows a thrombosed vein that was removed from a leg at amputation. In this frame it appears that only ragged remnants of the endothelium remains (arrows). Distorted erythrocytes and noncellular material were deposited on the subendothelial structures. × 650. B shows the interior of the thrombus in this vein. It was composed primarily of erythrocytes, many of which were distorted or pinocytotic, and fibrin. The uneven, fuzzy appearance of the fibrils may be a result of fracturing the fibrin net at many orientations to individual fibrils; i.e., the line of fracture ran parallel to some, perpendicular to others, and at angles to still others. Erythrocyte distortion and lysis set in soon after formation of a thrombus. ×1950. C and D show a segment of vein that was taken at the time of construction of an arterio-venous fistula for arterialization of a vein to be used subsequently as a bypass. The vein was exposed, and after ligation of side branches, were perfused locally with lactated Ringer's solution with 5% dextrose. After tying off under pressure, it was excised and submerged in 1% glutaraldehyde for initial fixation. Despite great care to avoid occlusion, adhering and invading leukocytes were found on some of these vessels. The characteristics of the endothelium, leukocytes, and leukocyte adhesion and emigration were indistinguishable from those of the canine model. C: × 195; D: × 1900.

Effect of Contrast Media on Normal and Inflamed Canine Veins

Contrast media are commonly used in diagnosis of both venous and arterial pathology and are reported to have adverse effects on the endothelial lining of vessels. In our study the luminal surface of canine jugular and femoral veins was exposed to Hypaque 50% or Conray 60 under three different conditions.[12] In Group I the contrast media were administered as a slow flow through injection via a side branch. In Group II contrast media were injected via a side branch and venous stasis was induced by percutaneous compression of the downstream end of the external jugular vein for 7 minutes prior to local dissection for exposing the vein. In Group III the local dissection for exposing the vein was performed before injection of contrast media and introduction of stasis. Controls for each group consisted of similar procedures in the absence of contrast media. In Group I, contrast media caused little or moderate adhesion of leukocytes in 5 of 6 cases, but heavy leukocyte invasion in one vein. In Group II, contrast media caused an increase in the extent of leukocyte adhesion and invasion of 2 of 6 veins of paired sets. In Group III, contrast media increased the extent of leukocyte adhesion and invasion in 6 of 13 veins of paired sets. In the other sets the control and contrast-exposed veins were similar. These findings suggest that contrast media may exaggerate the adhesion to and invasion of the venous wall by leukocytes when surrounding tissues are damaged and stasis of several minutes' duration is induced.

Deposition of Leukocytes and Platelets on Bypasses

Woven Dacron grafts 10 cm in length and 10 mm in diameter were anastomosed to the thoracic aorta end-to-end proximally and end-to-side distally. The dogs were given antibiotics postoperatively and fed routine rations for periods ranging from one day to 27 months. At the time the graft was to be removed, the animal was anesthetized with i.v. Nembutal® and systemically heparinized (1.5 mg/kg, i.v. injection). Thoracotomy was rapidly performed and the graft carefully removed so as to avoid mechanical trauma. Immediately after removal the graft was gently rinsed with saline, opened longitudinally along the greater curvature, and fixed overnight in 2.5% glutaraldehyde.[21]

The sequence of events occurring in a woven Dacron bypass in the canine thoracic aorta was followed from the first exposure to flowing blood for a period of 27 months. After 10 or 40 minutes exposure to flowing blood, the surface was covered with masses of leukocytes, platelets, red cells, and some fibrin (FIGURES 9A & 9B). By 24 and 48 hours most of the leukocytes had disappeared, leaving the two end areas of the bypass covered with a thick film composed of red cells entrapped in a fibrin net (FIGURES 9C & 9D). In the central portion of the bypass the Dacron fibers were covered by a rough film of particulate material and some fibrin strands reaching between widely spaced clumps of platelets and occasional leukocytes. At 6 and 7 days the surface covering consisted primarily of red cells and fibrin. Between 2 and 8 weeks this was replaced by a matrix that was composed mostly of cells resembling fibroblasts or transition forms between these and smooth muscle cells. Some typical smooth muscle cells were observed in grafts 4 months or older. A sheet of flat cells had grown a few millimeters below the anastomoses at 7, 12, and 14 months (FIGURES 10A & 10B). By 27 months the entire length of the graft

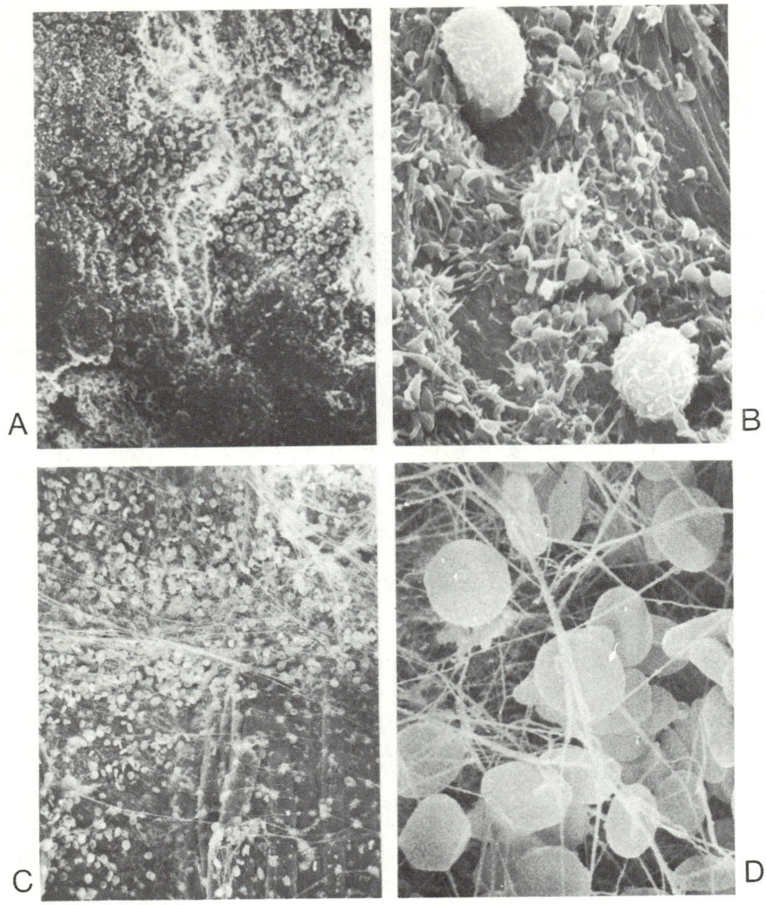

FIGURE 9. Scanning electron micrographs of woven Dacron bypasses that had been exposed to flowing blood for varying periods after insertion. A and B show massive deposition of platelets and leukocytes on a bypass after 10 minutes of blood flow. The platelets had rounded up and sent out one or at most a few pseudopods. Leukocytes adhered to the surface and emigrated into the bypass. A: × 195; B: × 1900. C and D show the appearance of bypasses after 24 hours of blood flow. The platelet and leukocyte deposition was largely replaced by fibrin and erythrocytes; however, scattered clumps of platelets remained. C: × 195; D: × 1900.

had a patchy covering of endothelium. Only occasional isolated platelets were stuck to the exposed collagen. Thickening of the intraprosthetic lining was associated with infiltration of the cell-fiber matrix by masses of red cells. Thus it appears that the lining of a limited number of human woven Dacron bypasses had similar ultrastructural characteristics and behaved similarly with respect to deposition of platelets and fibrin (FIGURES 10C & 10D). From these observations it may be concluded that collagen can be "conditioned" to become nonthrombogenic in high-flow systems.[10, 21] In distal vessel bypasses, the early partial endothelial lining and the eventual complete reendothelialization of an autogenous vein graft may be necessary for low-flow graft function, possibly to supply plasminogen activator to initiate lysis of deposited fibrin.[22]

Discussion

These morphological observations reflect the net results of a number of complex events that were initiated by the various experimental procedures and

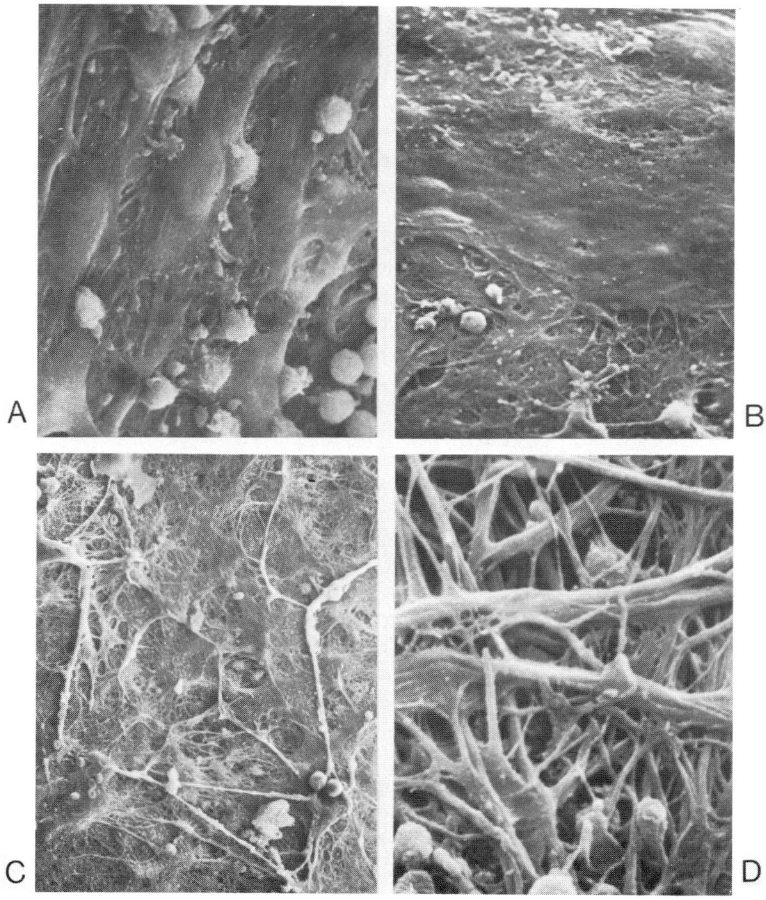

FIGURE 10. Scanning electron micrographs of long-term canine and human bypasses that were functioning at the time of removal from the living animal or patient. A and B show the surface of a 14-month bypass. The surface was composed of a fibrous matrix, presumably collagen, and scattered, irregulary shaped cells that resemble fibroblasts. There was little accumulation of cells or noncellular material on these surfaces. A: × 780; B: × 2700. C and D show the surface from a human femoropopliteal bypass, that was and had been functional for 4 years. A segment was removed at reconstruction for a bypass to the other leg. The appearance of the surface was very similar to that of the canine bypasses. Again, there was no endothelial lining and only limited deposition of thrombotic material. C: × 200. D: × 6,500.

had continued up to the time of removal of blood and fixation of the vessel. The composition of the material that was deposited on the luminal surface of both natural and artificial vessels provided a clear indication of some of the events and helpful clues to others. This is so because there is already a large body of information on how cells and fibrinogen or its derivatives come to be deposited on the vessel wall. For example, the generation of leukotaxins and thrombin was indicated by leukocyte emigration and fibrin formation. The deposition of amorphous noncellular material provided a clue that plasmin as well as thrombin had been acting on fibrinogen.

In most instances the accumulation of blood elements (cellular and fibrin) on veins in patients occurs in response to tissue destruction somewhere in the body. In the case of deep venous thrombosis, the site of injury is frequently a considerable distance from the veins that thrombose, but in construction of autogenous bypasses for revascularization of low extremities or heart muscle, the tissue injury is adjacent to the vein that is being transplanted, and indeed, to the vein itself. Thus, a consideration of the consequences of tissue injury may contribute to an understanding of the deposition of thrombotic material on veins.

The response of tissues to injury is similar regardless of the kind of cell or injury.[23-27] Among the products that have been found in the lymph following tissue injury are intracellular enzymes (cytoplasmic, mitochondrial, lysosomal), histamine, components of the kinin system, and Prostaglandin E.[24, 27-32] Some of these substances influence blood vessel permeability and diameter, leukocytes (leukotaxins), and platelets (inhibit or promote aggregation). Released substances (histamine, kinins, prostaglandins, other?) find their way into the circulation and influence blood vessels throughout the body, as indicated by generalized vasodilation (shock). Evidence of this is provided experimentally by cross-circulation experiments in which one dog was traumatized by many blows to the hind legs while the other dog was not traumatized. The nontraumatized dog went into shock and died a few minutes before the traumatized one.[33] Tourniquet shock is another example of a generalized vascular response to localized tissue destruction. In this case the products from ischemic tissue destruction enter the general circulation and cause circulatory collapse.[34] The crushed-limb syndrome first described in World War II has some features of tourniquet shock.[35, 36] Additionally, patients may suffer serious hypotension following severe injury with no evidence of hemorrhage.[37]

In trauma there is an increase in the total amount of plasma protein passing into the lymph, indicating increased permeability.[24, 38-40] Furthermore, it was shown experimentally that topically applied histamine, serotonin, and kinins increased the permeability of venular endothelium to markers and presumably to plasma proteins.[41-43] Thus it is reasonable to expect that these substances produce the same effects when released or generated endogenously. Since there is no evidence that the endothelial cells or junctions in veins are different from those in venules, one result of tissue injury anywhere in the body may be a generalized increase in the permeability of venous endothelium to plasma protein. The increase may be small compared with that observed in response to topical application of permeability agents. Furthermore, the thickness of the vessel wall in veins as compared to venules likely restricts the amount of plasma that passes from intra- to extravascular spaces. Still, one may inquire as to what is "enough."

Since the leukocyte emigration observed in jugular and femoral veins appears to be basically the same as leukocyte emigration from small vessels in response to local tissue destruction (i.e., it is one aspect of the inflammatory response), this knowledge can contribute to our understanding of leukocyte emigration in medium-sized veins. In the normal healthy animal, leukocytes in the blood flow freely, with little attraction to the vessel wall; however, under various pathological conditions many leukocytes are attracted to the vessel wall. In small vessels, especially venules, this is expressed by the sticking of leukocytes to the walls and their subsequent migration across the endothelium and into the surrounding tissues. This has been recognized as part of the response of tissues to sublethal injury since the inflammatory process was described in the nineteenth century.[44] However, there is no evidence that white cell passage *per se* causes serious damage to small vessels.[45] In many instances of the inflammatory response, the attraction of leukocytes to the wall of small vessels appears to be the result of injury to adjacent tissue rather than to the vessel itself.[17]

The directional movement of leukocytes in response to chemotactic stimulation has been extensively studied *in vitro* for a number of years.[16, 44, 46] Although it was assumed that the direction of cell movement was determined by the concentration of the chemotactic agent, this has been clarified and firmly established only since the development of the Boyden chamber.[15] It is now generally accepted that *in vitro* leukocytes move from a lower to higher concentration of chemotactic substance. Furthermore, leukocyte accumulation may result from chemotactic trapping (the leukocytes reach and remain in the area of maximum concentration of chemotactic gradient).[17]

The directed movement of leukocytes *in vivo* has been much more difficult to establish with a reasonable degree of confidence. There are, however, two models that appear to be adequate for demonstrating directed leukocyte movement *in vivo*. In one model Buckley [18] showed the directional movement of leukocytes toward small, discrete heat injuries produced under aseptic conditions while in another, Loosli and Baker [19] showed the emigration of leukocytes from the lumen of sinusoids to the lumen of alveoli. The leukocytes passed through junctions between endothelial cells, "dissected" between the endothelium and basement membrane, possibly toward epithelial cell junctions. In the case of trauma to adjacent tissue [9, 11, 12] there was ample opportunity for the generation of leukotactic agents external to the vessel wall via the contact of plasma from disrupted veins with the collagen in the vessel wall and surrounding connective tissue. "Minced tissue in serum" was described as highly leukotactic by Hurley.[47]

In the study of the response of jugular veins to hysterectomy there was no destruction of adjacent tissue prior to stasis; therefore another mechanism must have been responsible for the generation of leukotaxins. One possibility is that there was an increase in permeability of the endothelial sheet that allowed the unselective passage of unusually large amounts of plasma into the vessel wall where factor XII was activated by collagen. This could give rise to kallikrein and possibly other leukotaxins. Leukotaxins generated within the vessel wall would be expected to diffuse in all directions and to reach the luminal surface by diffusion across the disturbed intercellular junctions. In this system, the endothelial sheet would function as the millipore filter in the Boyden chamber, i.e., as the perforated membrane across which leukotaxins diffuse and across which leukocytes emigrate.

Several groups of investigators have provided information that suggests a mechanism whereby the extravasation of plasma may lead to the generation of leukotaxins. The extensive work of Niewiarowski et al.,[48] Wilner et al.,[49] and Cochrane et al.[50] has shown that factor XII is activated by contact with collagen *in vitro*. Furthermore, activated factor XIII leads to generation of kallikrein and plasmin. Kallikrein has been reported to be selectively chemotactic for neutrophils from a mixed leukocyte population.[51] Also, plasmin acts on complement component, C3 by direct proteolytic cleavage to give 3Ca, which is highly leukotactic [51a] (FIGURE 11).

The leukocyte emigration in response to trauma to adjacent tissue was much greater than it was in response to trauma to a remote site. This could be the

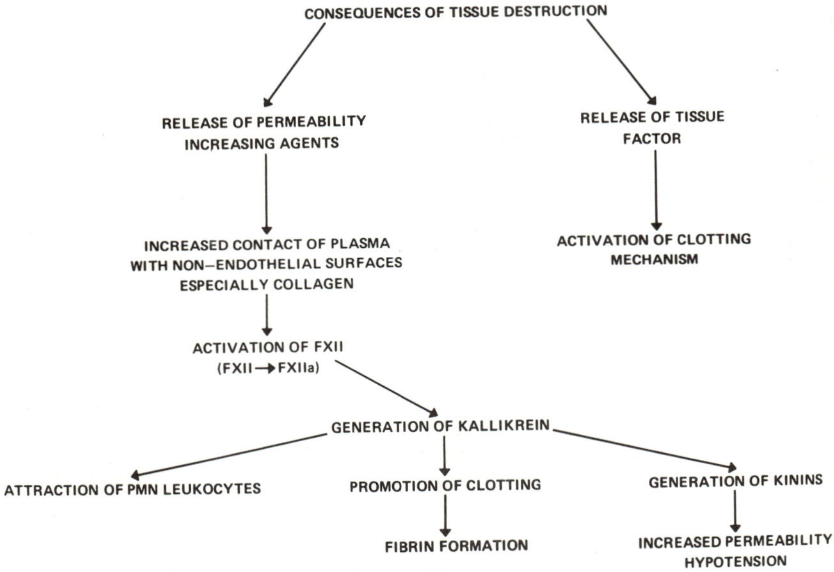

FIGURE 11. Summary of consequences of tissue destruction. The deposition of blood elements, cellular, and molecular, on both veins and arteries, is usually secondary to tissue destruction at some site in the body. In veins, the site is usually remote from the veins on which the material is deposited, whereas in arteries vessel-wall lesions are involved. The sequence of events that accompany tissue destruction provide valuable insight into the mechanisms by which blood cells and fibrin are deposited on vessel walls. With the exception of the release of tissue factor into the general circulation, all of the steps in this sequence have been well documented by investigators in a number of laboratories. (References are contained in the text.)

result of a difference in the amount of leukotaxin generated in the two models. Dissection in the neck or groin released considerable plasma into extravascular space, but increased permeability could be expected to result in only a low level of plasma extravasation.

While there was no endothelial desquamation in veins with low or moderate invasion by single leukocytes, their potential for producing vessel-wall damage should not be disregarded. It is to be expected that the leukocytes will soon release their cyotoxic substances, thereby producing numerous foci of damage.[53] These foci of damage may well serve as points for the attraction of more leukocytes and for the local activation of the clotting system with the resultant formation of microthrombi.

Leukocytes also appeared to help anchor mural thrombi to the vessel wall, as indicated by the leukocytes that were present in microthrombi and in remaining remnants when a segment of mural thrombus was removed from the vessel wall (FIGURES 3C & 3D). We have previously seen evidence that leukocytes are involved in the attachment of a thrombus to the vessel wall.[12] It appeared that fibrin strands were attached to leukocytes that had emigrated across the endothelial sheet. Leukocytes have been shown to interact with polymerizing fibrin.[54]

The accumulation of leukocytes on the 10–40 minute bypasses could also be a consequence of the extravascular generation of leukotaxins and their diffusion across the woven Dacron. This possibility is supported by two observations. First, leukocytes do not accumulate on the damaged but relatively impervious aorta that abuts the porous bypass. From this we may conclude that neither the leukocytes themselves, the messengers generated intravascularly, nor the flow are responsible. On the other hand, the porous Dacron allowed relatively free passage of materials, whereas the impervious aorta retained most substances, as indicated by the necessity for a vaso vasorum. Second, the leukocytes had disappeared by the end of 24 hours. This could be a reflection of the decreased porosity of the bypass (due to clotting and platelet fusion) or to the sequential nature of events following injury, in this case, surgery. One might postulate that leukocyte adhesion was caused by the release of leukotactic agents from platelets if platelets were not still present to some extent (at 24 hours) after the leukocytes had disappeared.[21]

Leukocyte accumulation on bypasses during the period immediately after institution of blood flow could be very greatly reduced by preoperative low-dose heparin,[55] an agent that has no known effects on leukocytes but is a potent cofactor in the inhibition of activated Hageman factor. Inhibition of activated Hageman factor could prevent the generation of kallikrein and thereby inhibit leukocyte attraction.

In the early bypasses the accumulation of leukocytes was reminiscent of leukocyte margination and sticking observed in small vessels in response to local tissue injury. In small vessels the adhesion of leukocytes has been attributed to changes that make the endothelium sticky for the leukocytes. However, this cannot be the case in early bypasses, since there is no endothelium.

In our studies the generation of thrombin was indicated by the observation of fibrous material (likely fibrin) on veins and bypasses. Fibrin was observed on four of ten veins following hysterectomy and stasis (TABLE 3). While activation of the clotting mechanism might have occurred either systemically or locally, circulating fibrin monomer was deposited on medium and large blood veins only to a very limited extent when dogs were infused with canine brain thromboplastin in the absence of injury of any kind.[56] Thus, the local generation of thrombin appears to be required for the accumulation of bothersome deposits of fibrin such as those observed in jugular veins in our studies. In bypasses the amount of fibrin was very limited at the end of one hour of blood flow but was massive at 24 hours. It should be recalled that at one hour the bypasses were covered with leukocytes and platelets, but at 24 hours essentially all leukocytes and most platelets had disappeared.

Thus, in both veins and bypasses there were three obvious possibilities for triggering clotting. These were 1) leukocytes or platelets that adhered to the luminal surface; 2) collagen in the vessel wall or Dacron in the bypass; and 3) cells and collagen in extravascular space.

Leukocytes generate tissue factor activity in response to endotoxin[57] and after adhesion and emigration in veins.[58] The platelets might have triggered clotting in the bypasses via one or more of the platelet coagulant activities described by Walsh.[59-61] Vessel-wall and connective-tissue collagen could have contributed to the generation of thrombin through activation of Hageman factor with subsequent activation of other clotting factors (that reached the luminal surface of the vessel by diffusion). Tissue factor could have been released from smooth muscle or other cells in or around the blood vessel. At present we have no evidence to indicate which of these were responsible, but our guess would be that all contributed to some extent.

The rather granular, amorphous material that was observed on four of ten veins following hysterectomy and occlusion could have resulted from the combined action of thrombin and plasmin. As mentioned earlier, Bang[8] showed that the combined action of thrombin and plasmin resulted in the formation of masses of material that was insoluble but lacked the highly ordered structure of typical fibrin. We, however, have no proof that this occurred in our model.

It is generally accepted that erythrocytes play a passive role in thrombosis, that they are simply physically entrapped in the fibrin net and, at most, release procoagulant phospholipid. Two observations made during our studies suggest that this may not be entirely correct. First, numerous erythrocytes, both singly and in clumps, adhered to the luminal surface of jugular veins after hysterectomy and stasis. With all single cells and many clumps there was no visible fibrin or other means of attaching the erythrocytes to the endothelium. Therefore, either one or both had become sticky. This could have come about by absorption of a sticky substance (fibrin monomer) from the plasma or by changes of the cells themselves. A low level of interaction of erythrocytes and polymerizing fibrin was recently shown by Brown and Niewiarowski.[60]

In mural thrombi observed during this study and in a previous study[12] the amount of fibrin appeared hardly sufficient to prevent the erythrocytes on the surface from being washed away by the flowing blood. Additionally, masses of rouleux with little fibrin were observed in the center of the thrombus. Erythrocytes were also observed on the surface of the fibrin net in 24-hour bypasses despite the high blood flow.[21] It is known that fibrinogen influences erythrocyte-erythrocyte interaction as expressed in blood viscosity.[61-63] According to Wells,[64] erythrocyte aggregation is principally a function of fibrinogen. The integrity of the erythrocyte aggregate is increased in disease or following trauma (sludged blood of Knisley),[65] even in the presence of normal fibrinogen levels.[66, 67] After correction for hematocrit and fibrinogen level, blood viscosity at low shear rates was positively related to the percentage of high molecular weight fibrinogen complexes.[68] In our studies we have found no fibrin monomer in preoperative samples, but easily demonstrated strands (fibrin monomer) when we[69] tested postoperative plasma samples by the serial dilution protamine sulfate test.[70] Taken together, these observations suggest that the adhesion of erythrocytes to the endothelium and to each other in our postoperative dogs, especially in the occluded vein, may depend on the presence of high molecular weight fibrinogen derivatives.

In view of the emphasis placed on platelet adhesion to subendothelial structures, we were initially surprised to find no platelets on areas of exposed basement membrane in canine veins and only very limited adhesion and accumulation on the basement membrane of the canine aorta. The latter was in sharp contrast to the massive platelet accumulation on the Dacron bypass that joined the aorta. At one time we had thought that the lack of platelets on venous basement membrane was due to the low blood flow in these vessels, since the adhesion of platelets to various surfaces increases with flow up to a point.[71–74] However, this could not be the explanation for the limited adhesion to the basement membrane in the aorta.

In recent studies on the adhesion of platelets to vessel walls denuded of endothelium other investigators have also found a limited accumulation of platelets. Baumgartner described any platelet accumulation of as much as five μ in thickness as a thrombus. Cazenave et al.[75] found a discontinuous layer of platelets on the scarified surface of an everted rabbit aorta after rotating it in plasma *in vitro*. An examination of the scanning electron micrograph of their control aorta indicates that it too was denuded of endothelium, yet it had even more limited platelet adhesion than the scarified surface. These observations suggest that the rapid accumulation of platelets on pierced, ruptured, or severed blood vessels differs from the accumulation of platelets on vessels from which only the endothelium has been removed. Although there may be "collagenic elements" in the basement membrane, they are very different from the collagen fibers that are exposed when the entire thickness of a blood vessel is disrupted. Simmons et al.[76] have recently shown that the degree of polymerization (multimerization) of collagen is an important factor in its ability to aggregate platelets. Massive platelet adhesion to early bypasses could result from the fact that Dacron is a "foreign surface" and from the extravascular generation and ingress of platelet aggregating agents such as thrombin and plasmin that adsorbed to the Dacron.

The scattered clumps of platelets that remained on the bypasses at 24 and 48 hours appeared to serve as attachment sites for fibrin strands, an observation consistent with the interaction of platelets with polymerizing fibrin *in vitro*.[77]

Summary

In conclusion, we suggest that the deposition of thrombotic material (blood cells, fibrinogen derivatives) on the luminal surface of blood veins is the result of a complex series of reactions set in motion by extensive tissue destruction at some site in the body. The site of tissue destruction may be adjacent to or remote from the veins. Tissue injury results in the release or generation of histamines, kinins, and probably other permeability-increasing agents that enter the general circulation via lymph draining from the injured area. As a result of this, the permeability of endothelium is increased throughout the venous system (medium-sized veins have junctions similar to venules which are known to be "leaky"). This means that an abnormally large amount of plasma protein passes from the intravascular to extravascular space, where contact with collagen is inevitable. If, *in vivo* as *in vitro*, Hageman factor is activated by contact with collagen, activated products of the clotting, plasma kinin, and fibrinolytic systems are generated within the collagen-cell matrix of the venous wall as well as in the loose connective tissue surrounding the veins and venules. Among these substances we may expect to find kallikrein, thrombin, and plasmin. Once formed, these active substances diffuse in all directions, including toward the luminal surface of the veins. As these substances reach the luminal surface, they could cause several responses. Kallikrein could activate leukocytes to follow up its (kallikrein) gradient and thereby emigrate across the endothelial sheet. Thrombin could act on the fibrinogen in the plasma layer adjacent to the vessel wall, thereby causing the deposition of fibrin on the vessel wall. A combination of thrombin and plasmin could act on fibrinogen and form insoluble but amorphous material at the vessel wall-plasma interface. The microthrombi resulting from these events could either resolve, probably by plasmin digestion of fibrinogen derivatives, or serve as nidi for further deposition of thrombotic material. This concept is summarized schematically in FIGURE 11.

The accumulation of leukocytes on bypasses after 10 or 40 minutes of blood flow could also have been a consequence of the ingress of products of tissue injury, and their disappearance by 24 hours could reflect the sequential nature of tissue response to injury, in this case surgical injury at the operative site. Platelet accumulation could be a consequence of these products and also of the "foreign surface" of the Dacron. Thrombin generation (as indicated by fibrin) could have been via either the extrinsic or intrinsic pathway or both.

This concept involves two original observations: 1) substances such as leukotactic agents reach the luminal surface of medium-sized veins from an extraendothelial source (back diffusion across open endothelial gaps, patent channels across endothelial cells, vesicular transport) and 2) the permeability of the endothelium of medium-sized veins is increased in response to tissue injury in a remote part of the body.

REFERENCES

1. VIRCHOW, R. 1860. Lecture in cellular pathology. *In* Metastatical Dyscrasiae: 196–229. Churchill. London, England.
2. WELCH, W. H. 1899. Thrombosis and Embolism. *In* A System of Medicine. T. C. Allbutt, Ed. Vol. **VI:** 155–285. Macmillan. London, England.
3. SIMIONESCU, M., N. SIMIONESCU & G. E. PALADE. 1975. Segmental differentiations of cell junctions in the vascular endothelium. The microvasculature. J. Cell Biol. **67:** 863–885.
4. O'NEILL, J. F. 1947. Effects on venous endothelium of alterations in blood flow through vessels in vein walls, and possible relation to thrombosis. Ann. Surg. **126:** 270–288.
5. MCGOVERN, V. J. 1955. Reactions to injury of vascular endothelium with special reference to problems of thrombosis. J. Pathol. Bacteriol. **69:** 283–293.
6. MCGRATH, J. M. & G. J. STEWART. 1969. The effects of endotoxin on vascular endothelium. J. Exp. Med. **129:** 833–848.
7. STEWART, G. J., P. R. LYNCH & R. G. SCHAUB. Scanning electron microscopy as a means of studying blood vessel pathology: A review and critique. Submitted for publication.
8. BANG, N. U. 1967. Ultrastructure of the fibrin clot. *In* Blood Clotting Enzymology. W. H. Seegers, Ed. : 476–550. Academic Press, Inc. New York, N.Y.
9. STEWART, G. J., W. G. M. RITCHIE & P. R. LYNCH. 1974. Venous endothelial damage produced by massive sticking and emigration of leukocytes. Am. J. Pathol. **74:** 507–532.
10. STEWART, G., P. LYNCH, H. STERN & L. MALMUD. 1975. Plasma protein within canine venous walls. (abstr.) Circulation **51**, **52:** 576.
11. STEWART, G. J., W. G. M. RITCHIE & P. R. LYNCH. 1973. A scanning and transmission electron microscopic study of canine jugular veins. Scanning electron microscopy (Part III). Proceedings of the workshop on Scanning Electron Microscopy in Pathology: 473–480. ITT Research Institute. Chicago, Ill. April 25–27.
12. RITCHIE, W. G. W., P. R. LYNCH & G. J. STEWART. 1974. The effect of contrast

media on normal and inflamed canine veins: A scanning and transmission electron microscopic study. Invest. Radiol. **9:** 444–455.
13. GIDDON, D. B. & J. LINDHE. 1972. *In vivo* quantitation of local anesthetic suppression of leukocyte adherence. Am. J. Pathol. **68:** 327–338.
14. HORN, R. G. & R. D. COLLINS. 1968. Fragmentation of granulocytes in pulmonary capillaries during development of the generalized Schwartzman reaction. Lab. Invest. **19:** 451–459.
15. BOYDEN, S. 1962. The chemotactic effect of mixtures of antibody and antigen on polymorphonuclear leukocytes. J. Exp. Med. **115:** 453–466.
16. KELLER, H. N. & E. SORKIN. 1968. Chemotaxis of leucocytes. Experientia **24:** 641–652.
17. SORKIN, E., V. J. STECKER & J. F. BOREL. 1970. Chemotaxis of leucocytes and inflammation. Ser. Haematol. III: 131–162.
18. BUCKLEY, I. K. 1963. Delayed secondary damage and leucoyte chemotaxis following focal aseptic heat injury *in vivo*. Exp. Mol. Pathol. **2:** 402–417.
19. LOOSLI, C. G. & R. F. BAKER. 1963. Acute experimental pneumococcal (Type I) pneumonia in the mouse: The migration of leukocytes from the pulmonary capillaries into the alveolar spaces as revealed by the electron microscope. Trans. Am. Clin. Climatol. Assoc. **74:** 15–28.
20. GRANT, L. 1973. The sticking and emigration of white blood cells in inflammation. *In* The Inflammatory Process. B. W. Zweifach, L. Grant & R. T. McCluskey, Eds. 2nd edit. Vol. **II**, Chap **7:** 205–250. Academic Press. New York, N.Y.
21. STEWART, G. J., W. ESSA, K. H. Y. CHANG & F. A. REICHLE. 1975. A scanning and transmission electron microscope study of the luminal coating on Dacron prosthesis in the canine thoracic aorta. J. Lab. Clin. Med. **85:** 208–226.
22. REICHLE, F. A. & G. J. STEWART. 1973. A transmission and scanning electron microscopic study of luminal surfaces in Dacron and autogenous vein bypasses in man and dog. Surgery **74:** 945–960.
23. LEWIS, G. P. 1967. Intracellular enzymes in local lymph as a measure of cellular injury. J. Physiol. (London) **191:** 591–607.
24. LEWIS, G. P. 1969. Changes in composition of rabbit hind limb lymph after thermal injury. J. Physiol. (London) **205:** 619–634.
25. MORITZ, A. R. & L. ADELSON. 1971. Physical agents in causation of injury and disease. *In* Pathology. W. A. D. Anderson. Ed.: 152–158. C. V. Mosby Co. St. Louis, Mo.
26. EBERT, R. H. & L. GRANT. 1974. The experimental approach to the study of inflammation. *In* The Inflammatory Process. B. W. Zweifach, L. Grant & R. T. McCluskey, Eds. 2nd edit. Vol. I: 4–51. Academic Press. New York. N.Y.
27. LEWIS, G. P. 1975. A lymphatic approach to tissue injury. New Eng. J. Med. **293:** 287–291.
28. HAYNES, F. W. 1932. Factors which influence flow and protein content of subcutaneous lymph in dog. II. The effect of certain substances which alter the capillary circulation. J. Physiol. (London) **101:** 612–620.
29. EDORY, H. & G. P. LEWIS. 1963. Kinin-forming activity and histamine in lymph after tissue injury. J. Physiol. (London) **169:** 568–582.
30. BOYLES, S., G. P. LEWIS & B. WESTCOTT. 1970. Intracellular enzymes in local lymph after chemical injury. Br. J. Pharmacol. **39:** 798–808.
31. LEWIS, G. P. & W. A. WAWRETSCHEK. 1971. Effect of thermal injury on the system in rabbit hind limb lymph. Br. J. Pharmacol. **43:** 127–139.
32. COLMAN, R. W. 1974. Formation of human plasma kinin. New England J. Med. **291:** 509–515.
33. LIU, C. T. 1971. Traumatic shock: Evidence for chemical release from traumatized tissue in dogs. Aerospace Med. **42:** 403–407.
34. MYLON, E. & M. C. WINTERNITZ. 1946. The differentiation of potassium from other agents associated with the toxic effects of tourniquet shock. Am. J. Physiol. **146:** 254–261.

35. Bywaters, E. G. L. & D. Beall. 1941. Crash injuries with impairment of renal function. Br. Med. J. **1:** 425–435.
36. Mayon-White, R. & O. M. Solandt. 1941. A case of limb compression ending in uraemia. Br. Med. J. **1:** 434–435.
37. Shoemaker, W. C., L. Lim, D. R. Boyd, R. S. Corley, J. M. Reinhard, D. A. Dreiling & A. E. Kark. 1971. Sequential hemodynamic events after trauma to the unanesthetized patient. Surg. Gynecol. Obst. **132:** 651–656.
38. Sevitt, S. 1958. Early and delayed edema and increase in capillary permeability after burns of the skin. J. Pathol. Bacteriol. **75:** 27–37.
39. Lewis, G. P. & N. P. Winsey. 1970. The action of pharmacologically active substances on the flow and composition of cat hind limb lymph. Br. J. Pharmacol. **40:** 446–460.
40. Bach, C. & G. P. Lewis. 1974. Lymph flow and lymph protein concentration in the skin and muscle of the rabbit hind limb. J. Physiol. (London) **235:** 477–492.
41. Majno, G. & G. E. Palade. 1961. Studies on inflammation. I. The effect of histamine and serotonin on vascular permeability: an electron microscope study. J. Biophy. Biochem. Cytol. **11:** 571–605 .
42. Buckley, I. K. & G. B. Ryan. 1969. Increased vascular permeability: The effect of histamine and serotonin on rat mesenteric blood vessels *in vivo*. Am. J. Pathol. **55:** 329–347.
43. Majno, G., S. M. Shea & M. Leventhal. 1969. Endothelial contraction induced by histamine type mediators. An electron microscopic study. J. Cell Biol. **42:** 647–672.
44. Grant, L. 1965. The sticking and emigration of white blood cells in inflammation. *In* The Inflammatory Process: 197–244. B. W. Zweifach, L. Grant & R. T. McCluskey, Eds. Academic Press. New York, N.Y.
45. Hurley, J. V. 1964. Substances promoting leukocyte emigration. Ann. N.Y. Acad. Sci. **116:** 918–935.
46. McCutcheon. M. 1946. Chemotaxis in leucocytes. Physiol. Rev. **26:** 319–336.
47. Hurley, J. V. 1963. Incubation of serum with tissue extracts as a cause of chemotaxis of granulocytes. Nature **198:** 1212–1213.
48. Niewiarowski, S., E. Bankowski & I. Rogowicka. 1965. Studies on the adsorption and activation of the Hageman factor (factor XII) by collagen and elastin. Thromb. Diath. Haemorrh. **14:** 387–400.
49. Wilner, G. D., H. L. Nossel & E. C. LeRoy. 1968. Activation of Hageman factor by collagen. J. Clin. Invest. **47:** 2608–2615.
50. Cochrane, C. G., S. D. Revak, B. S. Aiken & K. D. Wuepper. 1972. The structural characteristics and activation of Hageman factor. *In* Inflammation: Mechanism and Control. I. H. Lepow & P. A. Ward, Eds. : 119–138. Academic Press. New York, N.Y.
51. Kaplan, A. P., A. B. Kay & K. F. Austen. 1972. A prealbumin activator of prekallikrein. III. Appearance of chemotactic activity for human neutrophils by the conversion of human prekallikrein to kallikrein. J. Exp. Med. **135:** 81–97.
51a. Ward, P. A. 1967. A plasmin-split fragment of C3 as a new chemotactic factor. J. Exp. Med. **126:** 189–206.
52. Zachariae, H., J. Malmquist, J. A. Oates & W. Pettinger. 1967. Studies on the mechanism of kinin formation in inflammation. J. Physiol. **190:** 81–90.
53. Janoff, A. 1970. Mediators of tissue damage in human polymorphonuclear neutrophils. Ser. Haematol. **3:** 96–130.
54. Niewiarowski, S. E. Regoecz & J. F. Mustard. 1972. Platelet interaction with fibrinogen and fibrin: Comparison of the interaction of platelets with that of fibroblasts, leukocytes and erythrocytes. Ann. N.Y. Acad. Sci. **201:** 72–83.
55. Reichle, F. A., G. J. Stewart & H. S. S. Sue. 1967. Unpublished observation.
56. Stewart, G. J. & P. R. Lynch. 1976. In preparation.

57. Niemetz, J. & K. Fani. 1973. Thrombogenic activity of leukocytes. Blood **42:** 47–59.
58. Lerner, R. G. 1974. Private communication.
59. Walsh, P. N. 1972. The role of platelets in the contact phase of blood coagulation. Br. J. Haematol. **22:** 237–254.
60. Brown, R. S. & S. Niewiarowski. 1976. Measurements of human platelet and red cell interaction with polymorizing fibrin by a double isotope technique. Fed. Proc. **35:** 648.
61. Wells, R. E. Jr. & E. W. Merrill. 1962. Influence of flow properties of blood upon viscosity-hematocrit relationships. J. Clin. Invest. **41:** 1591–1598.
62. Merrill, E. W., G. C. Cokelet, A. Britten & R. E. Wells, Jr. 1963. Non-Newtonian rheology of human blood—effect of fibrinogen deduced by "subtraction." Circ. Res. **13:** 48–55.
63. Merrill, E. W., E. R. Gilliland, T-S Lee & E. W. Salzman. 1966. Blood Rheology: Effect of fibrinogen deduced by addition. Circ. Res. **18:** 437–446.
64. Wells, R. E. 1969. Rheologic aspects of stasis in thrombus formation. *In* Thrombosis. : 469–476. S. Sherry, K. Brinkhous, E. Genton, & J. Stengle, Eds. National Academy of Science USA. Washington. D.C.
65. Knisley, M. N. 1965. Intravascular erythroycte aggregation (blood sludge). *In* Handbook of Physiology, Circulation **III:** 2249–2292. Am. Physiological Soc. Washington. D.C.
66. Gelin, L. E. 1962. Rheologic disturbances and the use of low viscosity dextron in surgery. Rev. Surg. **19:** 385–400.
67. Ham, T. H. & F. C. Curtis. 1938. Sedimentation rate of erythrocytes; influence of technical, erythrocyte and plasma factors and quantitative comparison of 5 commonly used sedimentation methods. Medicine **17:** 447–517.
68. Bemis, A. M. 1968. A simple low shear capillary viscometer for blood. Bio-Rheol. **5:** 263–270.
69. Schaub, R. G., G. J. Stewart & P. R. Lynch. 1975. Unpublished observation.
70. Niewiarowski, S. & V. Gurewich. 1971. Laboratory identification of intravascular coagulation. The serial dilution protamine sulfate test for the detection of fibrin monomer and fibrin degradation products. J. Lab. Clin. Med. **77:** 665–676.
71. Friedman, L. I., H. Liem, E. F. Grabowski, E. F. Leonard & C. W. McCord. 1970. Inconsequentiality of surface properties for initial platelet adhesion. Trans. Am. Soc. Artif. Intern. Organs. **16:** 63–73.
72. Friedman, L. I. & E. F. Leonard. 1971. Platelet adhesion to artificial surfaces: Consequences of flow, exposure time, blood condition and surface nature. Fed. Proc. **30:** 1641–1646.
73. Begent, N. & G. V. R. Born. 1970. Growth rate *in vivo* of platelet thrombi, produced by iontophoresis of ADP, as a function of mean blood flow velocity. Nature **227:** 926–930.
74. Baumgartner, H. R. 1973. The role of blood flow in platelet adhesion fibrin deposition and formation of mural thrombi. Microvasc. Res. **5:** 167–179.
75. Cazenave, J-P, M. A. Packham, M. A. Guccione & J. F. Mustard. 1975. Inhibition of platelet adherence to damaged surface of rabbit aorta. J. Lab. Clin. Med. **86:** 551–563.
76. Simons, E. R., C. McI. Chesney, R. W. Colman, E. Harper & E. Samberg. 1975. The effect of the conformation of collagen on its ability to aggregate platelets. Thromb. Res. **7:** 123–140.
77. Niewiarowski, S., E. Regoeczi, G. J. Stewart, H. F. Senyi & F. M. Mustard. 1972. Platelet interaction with polymerizing fibrin. J. Clin. Invest. **51:** 685–700.
78. Gottlob, R., G. Blumel, F. Piza, P. Brucke & H. J. Bohmig. 1968. Studies on thrombolysis with streptokinase. II. The influence of changes due to age in thrombi and whole blood clots. Thromb. Diath. Haemorrh. **19:** 516–525.

PROCOAGULANT ACTIVITY OF LEUKOCYTES *

J. Niemetz, T. Muhlfelder, M. E. Chierego, and B. Troy

Veterans Administration Hospital
The Bronx, New York 10468
Mt. Sinai Medical School
New York, New York 10029

INTRODUCTION

A few years ago, a talk about the procoagulant activity of leukocytes might have generated mild amusement even if given to an audience of experienced clotters. There are, however, bits of evidence suggesting that leukocytes may indeed play a role in intravascular clotting and thrombosis. One such bit of evidence is the generalized Shwartzman reaction. The generalized Shwartzman reaction which is provoked in rabbits by two appropriately spaced sublethal doses of endotoxin is a thrombohemorrhagic reaction [1-4] due to clotting because it is preventable by either oral anticoagulants such as warfarin [5] or heparin.[1] Furthermore, it is prevented by pretreatment of the animal with fibrinolytic enzymes.[6] It was suggested almost a quarter of a century ago that leukocytes may have been involved in the generalized Shwartzman reaction,[2, 4] because rabbits rendered severely neutropenic with rather high doses of nitrogen mustard are protected from the generalized Shwartzman reaction caused by two doses of endotoxin but not by an infusion of thrombin.[7]

Another bit of evidence is that patients with acute leukemias often develop defribrination as well as arterial and venous thrombosis,[8-14] which is all the more striking because these patients are often thrombocytopenic and young.[14]

The third bit of evidence is the procoagulant activity of leukocytes themselves. Occasionally, in some patients with acute leukemia, procoagulant activity of the leukocytes has been demonstrated along with some fibrinolytic overtones.[15-18] In our experience, however, patients having leukocytes with a significant procoagulant activity have a rather shortened survival, and further studies of their leukocytes become difficult. Thus it became desirable to have an animal model in which leukocytes could be depended on at will to produce a procoagulant activity. Indeed, in normal conditions neither circulating nor peritoneal leukocytes have any significant procoagulant activity. It is of interest that this very weak procoagulant activity has been correctly assessed as being a tissue factor (thromboplastic) activity.[19]

It is also noteworthy that leukocytes have phospholipids (besides the tissue factor activity) which may play a role in clotting via the intrinsic pathway; [20] of further interest but beyond the scope of this review are the presence in leukocytes of an inhibitor of clotting,[21] an antiheparin activity,[22-24] and lytic and, in particular, fibrinolytic [25-27] activities.

Leukocytes can be obtained from the peritoneal cavity of rabbits after stimulation with starch [28] (or from peripheral blood after differential sedimentation in the presence of aggregating agents such as high molecular weight Dextran [29]).

* Supported in part by Veterans' Administration funds and NIH grant HL 13155.

TABLE 1

EFFECT OF LEUKOCYTES ON PLASMA CLOTTING TIME (IN SECONDS) *

	Control Leukocytes	E. Leuko-cytes	Buffers
Human plasma	100	53	200
Human plasma and cephalin	80	48	115
Celite-exhausted plasma and cephalin	105	52	134
Rabbit plasma	65	28	120

* Leukocytes were tested at a concentration of 60,000 mm^3. 0.1 ml of leukocyte suspension was added to 0.1 ml of CaCl2 0.05 M and the clotting time recorded after addition of 0.1 ml of plasma. E. leukocytes=peritoneal rabbit leukocytes obtained after endotoxin. Control=peritoneal leukocytes without endotoxin.

If, in addition to the starch, these rabbits are given endotoxin,[30, 31] their leukocytes are stimulated to generate an important procoagulant activity evidenced by the shortening of clotting time of a normal plasma (TABLE 1). The effect is best observed if the plasma is from the same species. This clotting activity is best qualified as tissue factor (tissue thromplastic) activity, because it is demonstrable even in the presence of optimal amounts of phospholipids and surface activation or on plasma deficient in factors of the intrinsic pathway, but not when plasma-deficient in factors of the extrinsic pathway (factor VII-deficient) are tested.[31-33] Furthermore, activity is developed when leukocytes are incubated with a plasma fraction containing factor VII and X activities[19, 31] which is used in the two-stage assay (FIGURE 1).[34] Another argument in favor of tissue factor activity is that the activity is lost on delipidition but recovered when relipidated.[34, 35]

The activity is also generated *in vitro,* and the endotoxin-stimulated leukocyte is committed to it within one hour, as indicated by experiments with protein, synthesis inhibitors.[36] After about two to three hours, almost maximum activity is made available within the cell as evidenced by testing leukocytes after disruption, most of the activity being localized in a light microsomal fraction.[37] The activity becomes available on the surface of the cell a little later, and it may be possible that *in vivo,* a second dose of endotoxin will enhance this process. Part of the activity is also released in the surrounding milieu if this milieu contains

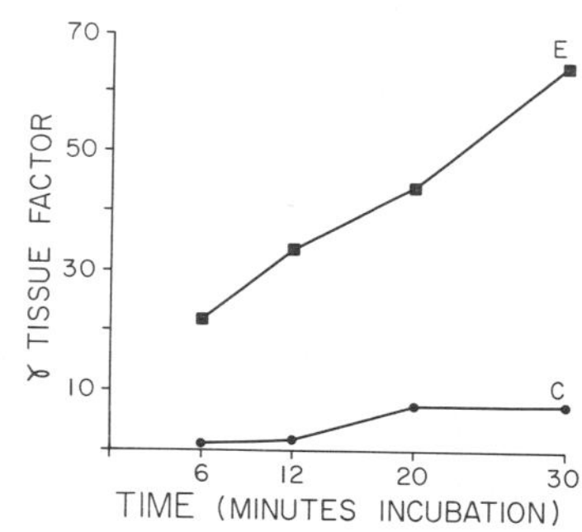

FIGURE 1. Tissue factor (thromboplastic) activity of leukocytes. Leukocyte suspensions were incubated with factor VII–X fraction and CaCl2. At the indicated intervals, 0.1 ml of the mixture was assayed, by its ability to clot a VII–X-deficient plasma, in the presence of optimal amounts of cephalin and CaCl2. C=control peritoneal leukocytes, E=peritoneal leukocytes after two doses of endotoxin. (By permission of the publishers of Nature [New Biol.][56]).

calcium (2.5 mM being optimal) has a neutral pH and the temperature is 37° C. Tissue-factor activity release is inhibited by Velban but not by some other agents which also inhibit microtubular structures.[38] Most of the findings reported heretofore apply to human and rabbit leukocytes. Human leukocytes (*in vitro*) generated less activity than rabbit leukocytes; at low cell concentrations, generation of activity by human leukocytes required the presence of human serum.[33, 36, 39]

The effects of endotoxin on mammals have been studied extensively, but the mode of action remains unclear. Labeled endotoxin injected intravenously into rabbits rapidly disappears from the plasma, with a significant amount localizing in the buffy coat.[40] Leukocytes pinocytize endotoxin, and while polymorphonuclears inactivate endotoxin within three hours, monocytes appear incapable of doing so.[41, 42] It is not obvious at the present time that endotoxin must be internalized to cause generation of the procoagulant activity. Indeed, the findings that some modified endotoxins, with low stimulatory effect, can inhibit the stimulating effect of active endotoxin suggests that competition for a binding "site" on the surface of leukocytes may occur.[43]

Experiments designed to determine which part of the endotoxin molecule has the stimulatory effect strongly suggest that most of the polysaccharide (O side chains and central core) are inactive, but the lipid part—lipid A—possesses the stimulatory capacity.[43, 44]

Agents other than Endotoxin—Stimulating the Procoagulant Activity of Leukocytes

This is a chapter of considerable interest because it shows that leukocytes may be stimulated by agents other than endotoxin. It should, however, be approached with great caution, because endotoxin is ubiquitous and it has been demonstrated that nanogram amounts of endotoxin are sufficient to activate leukocytes.[43, 44] Rickles *et al.*[45] have shown that hemagglutinins presumably free of endotoxin are capable of stimulating lymphocytes to produce procoagulant activity.

Platelets have also been shown to have a stimulatory effect on the leukocytes, as follows: platelets or platelet membranes and granules obtained from freshly harvested platelets stimulate the leukocytes to produce procoagulant activity even in the absence of endotoxin. Furthermore, platelets greatly enhance the stimulatory effect of endotoxin. However, for the enhancement of human leukocytes to occur, a human serum fraction is necessary.[46]

Leukocytes adhere to artificial membranes,[47, 48] and it appeared interesting to investigate if these leukocytes generated any procoagulant activity. Leukocytes were obtained from Gambro® filters immediately at the end of hemodialysis of patients with chronic renal disease. These patients had received 1.5 mg of heparin per kg of body weight during the six hours of the procedure. After the filter was opened, leukocytes were rinsed off the membranes with cold citrated saline, washed three times in citrate saline, concentrated to 60,000 per mm 3, and tested for procoagulant activity, which was easily detected (Table 2). It has been reported that in some experimental conditions, leukocytes have a tendency to adhere to the endothelium and even burrow under the endothelial cells.[49] Lerner *et al.*[50] have reported that dog leukocytes collected on vascular surfaces in similar experiments do indeed have a procoagulant activity. It has also been reported that peritoneal leukocytes may develop procoagulant activity after incubation at 37° C without the addition of endotoxin.[51, 52] It is not certain, however, that contamination with endotoxin did not occur.

Thrombogenic Effect of Leukocytes

Interest in the procoagulant activity of leukocytes is sustained by their marked thrombogenic effect. Leukocytes have been suspected of having this effect in the generalized Shwartzman reaction,[2, 4] and infusion of leukocyte fractions and only one dose of endotoxin[54] or infusion of leukocytes after thorotrast[55] have produced thrombohemorrhagic lesions. Infusion of endotoxin-stimulated leukocytes into normal rabbits caused pulmonary thrombi when given intravenously and much more widespread thrombi (heart, lung, GI tract, and kidney) when given into the arterial circulation.[24, 56, 57] The kidney lesions in particular resemble lesions observed in the generalized Shwartzman reaction (Figure 2).

Table 2

Coagulant Activity of Cells from Hemodialysis Membranes (clotting times in seconds)*

Substrate	Leukocytes	Cephalin	Buffer
Human plasma	40	83	183
Human plasma and cephalin	44	—	88
Fibrinogen	600+	—	—
VII-Deficient plasma	150	134	275
Two-Stage Assay: Tissue factor activity=31 u.			

Type of Leukocytes Capable of Generating Procoagulant Activity

Polymorphonuclear leukocytes, lymphocytes (but not lymphocytes from patients with chronic lymphocytic leukemia) and macrophages (human and rabbit)[39, 37] are capable of generating procoagulant activity. Macrophages appeared severalfold more active than polymorphonuclear cells.[39] Other reports propose that only polymorphonuclear leukocytes[32, 51] or monocytes[53] are capable of generating this activity.

Localization and Characterization of Procoagulant Activity

When the specific activity of subcellular particles of rabbit leukocytes with tissue factor activity are studied, most of the activity is not sedimentable at 8,000 × *g* for 10 minutes but sediments at 150,000 × *g* for 20 minutes. When these microsomal particles are put on a sucrose gradient, the highest specific activity is found in the very light fractions.[37] The activity is tightly bound to particles and can be solubilized only after extraction with detergent such as sodium deoxycholate. When the extracted activity is applied and eluted on a Sepharose 6B column equilibrated with sodium deoxycholate, optical density at 280 nanometers shows three peaks (FIGURE 3) which, tested separately, are devoid of the procoagulant activity. However, the recombination of peak II and III restores the activity.[35] Furthermore, the activity can also be restituted if

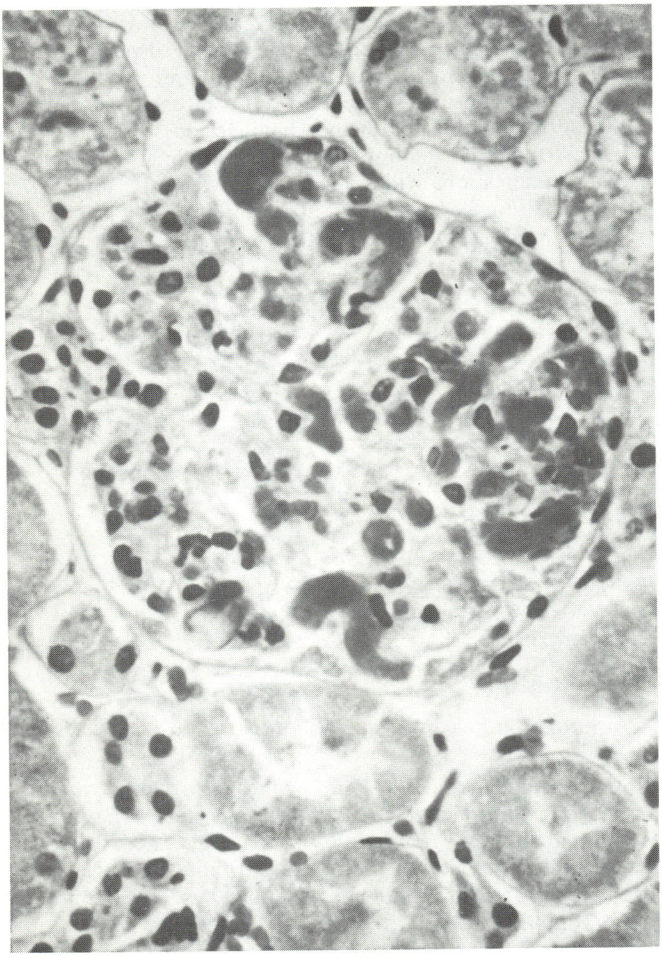

FIGURE 2. Fibrinoid necrosis of a glomerulus after infusion into the aorta of endotoxin-stimulated leukocytes. Fibrin deposits are homogeneous and dark.

peak II is relipidated with phospholipids obtained from sources other than leukocytes.[35] Thus leukocyte tissue factor activity is not unlike tissue factor activity from some other tissues such as brain and lung, which also are lipoproteins, the delipidated protein of which is inactive.[58] If advantage is taken of the relatively high binding affinity of tissue factor activity to subcellular particles, removal of

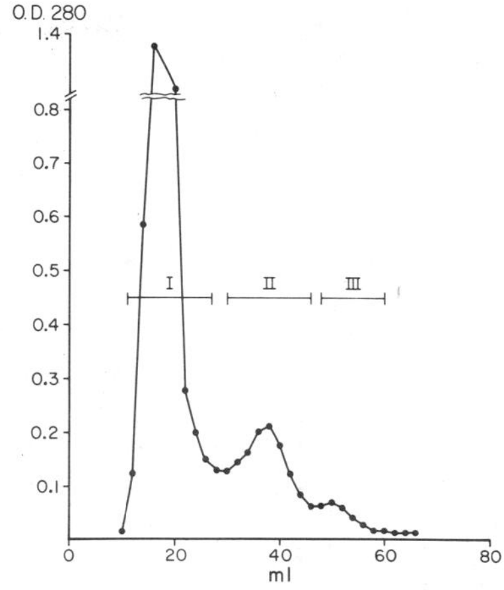

FIGURE 3. Gel chromatography of leukocyte tissue factor. The subcellular fraction which did not sediment at 8000 × *g* but sedimented at 150,000 × *g* was extracted with Na deoxycholate and applied on a Sepharose 6B Column 50 × 1.5 cm, equilibrated with 0.5% Na deoxycholate in 0.05 M barbital buffer pH 8.3. Peak I contained little protein and had no activity. Peak II was active only if relipidated. Peak III contained phospholipids.

some unwanted proteins can be done by successive extraction with 0.5 m NaCl, bicarbonate (pH 9.5, 0.2 M), and 0.5 M KCL, followed by Na-deoxycholate extraction and adsorption with QUSO.[35]

Further similarity between tissue factor from leukocytes and other tissues is shown by the study of antibodies. Antibodies to rabbit lung tissue factor inactivate leukocyte tissue factor,[39] but antibody to leukocyte tissue factor from humans is active against human brain tissue factor.[59]

LEUKOCYTE TISSUE FACTOR ACTIVITY AND C-6 DEFICIENCY

It has been proposed that complement may play a role in the generalized Shwartzman reaction, because rabbits pretreated with cobra venom factor and "decomplemented" are protected against the generalized Shwartzman reaction.[60] Furthermore, it has been shown that rabbits deficient in the 6th component of complement (C-6-deficient) had a peculiar clotting defect.[61] To study the role of complement, C-6-deficient rabbits were tested, as shown in TABLE 3, leu-

TABLE 3

EFFECT OF ENDOTOXIN ON THE PROCOAGULANT ACTIVITY OF NORMAL AND C-6-DEFICIENT RABBIT LEUKOCYTES *

		One-Stage Test (Sec)	Two-Stage Test (U)
C-6-deficient WBC	no endotoxin	142	1.2
C-6-deficient WBC	10 μg endotoxin	46	30
Control WBC	no endotoxin	120	1.1
Control WBC	10 μg endotoxin	39	45

* Peripheral blood leukocytes were incubated with or without endotoxin in medium 199 for 18 hours, then tested.

kocytes from C-6-deficient rabbits developed a significant procoagulant activity when compared to control rabbits. Experiments showing that the deficient rabbits are in fact susceptible to the generalized Shwartzman reaction have been reported,[62, 63] keeping alive the hypothesis that leukocyte tissue factor activity plays a role in this reaction.

Prostaglandins and Inhibitors of Tissue Factor Activity

Prostaglandins were studied for their effect on the procoagulant activity. As shown (Table 4), many prostaglandin compounds, when added to the leukocyte incubation mixtures, were without any appreciable effect. However, PgA and PgA2, admittedly at very high concentrations, were capable of inhibiting generation of procoagulant activity but had no effect on the already generated activity.

The effect of polymyxin B is quite different. Polymyxin B binds with lipid A,[64] thus inhibiting the stimulatory effect of endotoxin.[43] Furthermore, polymyxin B is capable of inhibiting the procoagulant activity generated via the intrinsic or extinsic pathway,[65] and leukocytes in particular.[31]

Table 4

Effect of Prostaglandins on the Procoagulant Activity of Leukocytes

WBC incubated with PgE1, E2, F1α, F2α, B2 (0.01–40 μg/ml) without endotoxin = O or very mild stimulation with endotoxin = no effect
WBC incubated with PgA (20–40 μg/ml) with endotoxin = 90% inhibition no effect on preformed tissue factor activity

A base hydrolyzed lipopolysaccharide from *E. coli* 0111B4 (BHLpsII) had an inhibitory effect on active lipopolysaccharide, suppressing generation of procoagulant activity by rabbit leukocytes, possibly by acting as an endotoxin analog.[43]

References

1. Good, R. A. & L. Thomas. 1953. Studies on the generalized Shwartzman reaction. II Prevention of the local and generalized Shwartzman reactions with heparin. J. Exp. Med. **97:** 871.
2. Thomas, L. & R. A. Good. 1952. Studies on the generalized Shwartzman reaction. I. General observations concerning the phenomenon. J. Exp. Med. **96:** 605.
3. Levin, J. & E. Beck. 1966. A Re-appraisal of the role of blood coagulation and platelets in the generalized Shwartzman phenomenon. Thromb. Diath. Haemorr. **15:** 519 No. 3/4 1966.
4. Stetson, C. A. & R. A. Good. 1951. Studies on the mechanism of the Shwartzman phenomenon: Evidence for the participation of polymorphonuclear leukocytes in the phenomenon. J. Exp. Med. **93:** 49.

5. SHAPIRO, S. S. & D. A. MCKAY. 1958. The prevention of the generalized Shwartzman reaction with sodium warfarin. J. Exp. Med. **107:** 377.
6. CONDIE, R. M., C. Y. HONG & R. A. GOOD. 1957. Reversal of the lesions of the generalized Shwartzman phenomenon by treatment of rabbits with streptokinase. J. Clin. Lab. Med. **50:** 803.
7. HJORT, P. F., W. MCGHEE & S. I. RAPAPORT. 1964. Studies of the effect of granulocytes in the generalized Shwartzman reaction. (Abstr. XII) Congr. Int. Soc. Hematology. Stockholm paper G:1.
8. BAKER, W. A., N. U. BANG, R. NACHMAN, F. RAAFAT & H. I. HOROWITZ. 1964. Hypofibrinogenemic hemorrhage in acute myelogenous leukemia treated with heparin with autopsy findings of widespread intravascular clotting. Ann. Intern. Med. **61:** 116.
9. HIRSH, J., J. G. BUCHANAN, G. C. DE GROUCHY & A. G. BAIKIE. 1967. Hypofibrinogenemia without increased fibrinolysis in leukemia. Lancet **1:** 418.
10. DIDISHEM, P., J. S. TROMBOLD, R. L. E. VANDEVOORT & R. S. MIBASHAN. 1964. Acute promyelocytic leukemia with fibrinogen and factor V deficiencies. Blood **23:** 716.
11. ROSENTHAL, R. L. 1963. Acute promyelocytic leukemia associated with hypofibrinogenemia. Blood **21:** 495.
12. DIDISHEM, P., J. S. TROMBOLD, R. L. E. VANDEVOORT & R. S. MIBASHAN. 1964. Acute promyelocytic leukemia with fibrinogen and factor V deficiencies. Blood **23:** 716.
13. NIEMETZ, J. & H. L. NOSSEL. 1969. Activated coagulation factors: *In vivo* and *in vitro* studies. Br. J. Haematol. **16:** 337.
14. RICHTER, P., M. DANA & J. NIEMETZ. Unpublished.
15. MARTIN, M. & L. ROKA. 1951. Beinflussung der Blutgerrinung durch Leukocyten. Klin. Wochenschr. **29:** 510.
16. EISMAN, A. & M. STEFANINI. 1954. Thromboplastic activity of leukemic white cells. Proc. Soc. Exp. Biol. Med. **86:** 763.
17. CATTAN, A., L. SCHWARZENBERG, J. L. AMIEL, M. SCHNEIDER, J. R. SCHLUMBERGER & G. MATHÉ. 1966. Syndrome de fibrinogenopenie au cours de leucemies aigues rôle determinant des cellules leucemiques: Etude *in vitro* de leur pourvoir fibrinolytique. Rev. Fr. Etudes Clin. Biol. **11:** 155.
18. GRALNICK, H. R. & E. ABRELL. 1973. Studies on the procoagulant and fibrinolytic activity of promyelocytes in acute promyelocytic leukemia. Br. J. Haematol. **24:** 89.
19. RAPAPORT, S. I. & P. F. HJORT. 1967. The blood blotting properties of rabbit peritoneal leukocytes *in vitro*. Thromb. Diath. Haemorrh. **17:** 222.
20. LISIEWIEZ, J. 1969. Studies on the influence of normal and leukemic leukocytes on blood coagulation. Ann. Med. Sec. Pol. Acad. Sci. **XIII:** 234.
21. SABA, H. I., H. R. ROBERTS & J. C. HERION. 1967. The anticoagulant activity of lysosomal cationic proteins from polymorphonuclear leukocytes. J. Clin. Invest. **46:** 580.
22. SABA, H. I., H. R. ROBERTS & J. C. HERION. 1968. Antiheparin activity of lysosomal cationic protein from polymorphonuclear leukocytes. Blood **31:** 369.
23. POPLAWSKI, A., J. PROKOPOWIEZ & S. NIEWIAROWKI. 1969. Antiheparin activity in subcellular fractions of human granulocytes. Thromb. Diath. Haemorrh. **21:** 170.
24. NIEMETZ, J. & K. FANI. 1973. Thrombogenic actiivty of leukocytes. Blood **42**(1): 47–59.
25. JANOFF, A. & J. SCHEZER. 1968. Mediators in inflammation in leukocyte lysosomes IX elastindytic activity in granules of human polymorphonuclear leukocytes. J. Exp. Med. **128:** 1137.
26. PLOW, E. F. & T. S. EDGINGTON. 1975. An alternative pathway for fibrinolysis in the cleavage of fibrinogen by leukocyte proteases at physiologic pH. J. Clin. Invest. **56:** 30.

27. BILEZIKIAN, S. 1976. Unique pattern of fibrinogen cleavage by human leukocyte proteases. N.Y. Acad. Sci. In Press.
28. HIRSCH, J. G. 1956. Phagocytin: A bactericidal substance from polymorphonuclear leukocytes. J. Exp. Med. **103:** 589.
29. BOYUM, A. 1968. Isolation of leukocytes from human blood. Scand J. Clin. Lab. Invest. (Suppl.) **97.**
30. NIEMETZ, J. 1969. Thromboplastic activity of leukocytes from rabbits receiving endotoxin. Fed. Proc. (abstr.) **28**(2): 448.
31. NIEMETZ, J. 1972. Coagulant activity of leukocytes tissue factor activity. J. Clin. Invest. **51:** 307.
32. LERNER, R. G., R. GOLDSTEIN & G. CUMMINGS. 1971. The generation of coagulant activity by leukocytes. Fed. Proc. **30:** 479 (abstr.).
33. LERNER, R., G. R. GOLDSTEIN & G. CUMMINGS. 1971. Stimulation of human leukocyte thromboplastic activity by endotoxin. Proc. Soc. Exp. Biol. Med. **138:** 145.
34. NEMERSON, Y. 1966. The reaction between bovine brain tissue factor and factors VII and X. Biochemistry **5:** 601.
35. NIEMETZ, J. 1974. Separation and characterization of leukocyte tissue factor (tissue thromboplastic) activity. (abstr.) Proc. XV Congr. Int. Soc. Hematol. : 141.
36. NIEMETZ, J. 1972. The role of protein synthesis on the generation of tissue factor activity by leukocytes. Proc. Soc. Exp. Biol. Med. **139:** 1276.
37. NIEMETZ, J. Unpublished results.
38. MUHLFELDER, T., I. KHAN & J. NIEMETZ. 1975. The role of calcium on the release of tissue factor (thromboplastic) activity from leukocytes. (abstr.) Vth Congress I.S.T.H. : 424.
39. GARG, S. K. & J. NIEMETZ. 1973. Tissue factor activity of normal and leukemic cells. Blood **42:** 729.
40. BRAUDE, A. I., F. J. CAREY & M. ZALESKY. 1955. Studies with radioactive endotoxin. II. Correlation of physiologic effect with distribution of radioactivity in rabbits injected with lethal doses of *E. Coli* endotoxin labelled with sodium chromate. J. Clin. Invest. **55:** 858.
41. MESROBEANU, L., I. MESROBEANU, C. BONA & D. VRANIALICI. 1969. Le destin des endotoxines thermostables pinocytées par les leucocytes: 429–445. *In* La Structure et les Effets Biologiques des Produits Bactetriens Provenant de Germes Gram Negatifs, H. L. Chedid, Ed.: 429–445. Editions du CNRS Colloque 194.
42. BONA, C. A. 1973. Fate of endotoxin in macrophages biological and ultrastructural aspects. *In* Bacterial Lipopolysaccharides. E. H. Kass and S. M. Wolf, Eds. : 66. Univ. Chicago Press. Chicago, Ill.
43. NIEMETZ, J. & D. C. MORRISON. 1976. Role of lipid A on the procoagulant activity of leukocytes. Fed. Proc. (abstr.) **35:** 804.
44. RICKLES, F. R. & P. D. RICK. 1976. Structural features of S. typhimurium lipopolysaccharide (LPS) required for activation of monocyte tissue factor. Fed. Proc. (abstr.) **35:** 804.
45. RICKLES, F. R., J. A. HARDIN, F. A. PITLICK, L. W. HOYER & M. E. CONRAD. 1973. Tissue factor activity in lymphocyte cultures from normal individuals and patients with hemophilia. J. Clin. Invest. **52:** 1427.
46. NIEMETZ, J. & A. J. MARUS. 1974. The stimulatory effect of platelets and platelet membranes on the procoagulant effect of leukocytes. J. Clin. Invest. **54:** 1437.
47. SCHWARTZ, A., K. M. STENZEL, I. KOHNO, D. AST, T. MIYATA & A. L. RUBIN. 1975. Deposition of blood cells on collagen and cuprophane membranes. J. Bio. Med. Mater. Res. **9:** 453.
48. VROMANN, L. Personal communication.
49. STEWART, G. This volume.
50. LERNER, R. G., R. GOLDSTEIN & G. CUMMINGS. 1975. Granulocyte thrombo-

plastin as a mechanisum of thrombosis in venous hemostsis. Clin. Research **23**(3) (abstr.) 277A.

51. Saba, H. I., J. C. Herion, R. I. Walker & H. R. Roberts. 1973. The procoagulant activity of granulocytes. Proc. Soc. Exp. Biol. Med. **142:** 614.
52. Kociba, G. J., W. F. Loeb & R. F. Wall. 1972. Development of procoagulant (tissue thromboplastin) activity in cultured leukocytes. J. Lab. Clin. Med. **79:** 778.
53. Rivers, R. P. A., W. E. Hathaway & W. L. Weston. 1975. The endotoxin-induced coagulant activity of human monocytes. Br. J. Haematol. **30:** 311.
54. Horn, R. G. & R. D. Collins. 1968. Studies on the pathogenesis of the generalized Shwartzman reaction. Lab. Invest. **18**(2): 101.
55. Forman, E. N., C. F. Abildgaard, J. F. Bolger, C. A. Johnson & I. Schulman. 1969. Generalized Shwartzman reaction: Role of the granulocytes in intravascular coagulation and renal cortical necrosis. Br. J. Haematol. **16**(5): 507.
56. Niemetz, J. & K. Fani. 1971. Role of leukocytes in blood coagulation and the generalized Shwartzman reaction. Nature [New Biol.] **232:** 247.
57. Kociba, G. & R. A. Griesmer. 1972. Disseminated intravascular coagulation induced with leukocyte procoagulant. Am. J. Pathol. **69:** 407.
58. Nemerson, Y. 1969. Characteristics and lipid requirements of coagulant proteins extracted from lung and brain. The specificity of the protein component of tissue factor. J. Clin. Invest. **48**(2): 322.
59. Gouault-Heilmann, M., E. Chardon, C. Sultan & F. Josso. 1975. The procoagulant factor of leukaemic promyelocytes. Demonstration of immunologic cross reactivity with human brain tissue factor. Br. J. Haematol. **30:** 151.
60. Fong, J. S. C. & R. A. Good. 1971. Prevention of the localized and generalized Shwartzman reaction by an anticomplementary agent, cobra venom factor. J. Exp. Med. **134:** 642.
61. Zimmerman, T. S., C. M. Arroyave & H. J. Muller-Eberhard. 1971. A blood coagulation abnormality in rabbits deficient in the sixth component of complement (C6) and its correction by purified C6. J. Exp. Med. **134:** 1591.
62. Muller-Berghans, G. & E. Lohmann. 1974. The role of complement in endotoxin-induced disseminated intravascular coagulation studies in congenitally C6 deficient rabbits. Br. J. Haematol. **28:** 403.
63. Stafford, B. T., S. I. Rapaport & S. M. C. Shen. 1976. Effects of endotoxin in cortisone-treated rabbits with a hereditary deficiency of the sixth component of complement (C6 Deficiency) Thromb. Hemostasis **35:** 460.
64. Morrison, D. C., P. M. Henson & L. F. Kline. 1976. Lipopolysaccharide (LPS) initiated lipid A independent (alternative) and lipid A dependent (classical) activation of complement in plasma mediated platelet lysis. Fed. Proc. **35:** 3, 2476 (abstr.).
65. Ottolenghi, A. C. 1967. Cationic antibiotics and phospholipase C as tools in the study of phospholipid structure and function. Can. J. Biochem. **45:** 239.

CONTRACTILE PROTEINS IN PLATELET ACTIVATION AND CONTRACTION *

Thomas D. Pollard,† Keigi Fujiwara,† Robert Handin,‡
and Gary Weiss †

† Department of Anatomy
Harvard Medical School
‡ Division of Hematology
Department of Medicine
Peter Bent Brigham Hospital
Harvard Medical School
Boston, Massachusetts 02115

Our role in this annal is to review recent progress in characterizing platelet contractile proteins and to suggest how contractile proteins may participate in platelet activation and clot retraction. There has been a rapid expansion of knowledge about the molecular basis of cell motility since 1970, and platelets have been one of the important model systems. Readers interested in the exciting advances made in other aspects of the motility question can refer to recent books and reviews [1–3] on the subject.

Properties of Platelet Contractile Proteins

It has now been 17 years since Bettex-Galland and Lüscher [4] isolated from human platelets a mixture of proteins with some properties similar to muscle actomyosin, the unfractionated mixture of muscle contractile proteins including actin, myosin, and associated proteins. Unfortunately, perhaps, they chose to call this platelet material "thrombosthenin," which tended to obscure the fact that they were dealing with actin and myosin. In subsequent experiments [5] they separated a crude actin fraction from a crude myosin fraction and showed that reconstituted mixtures of these two fractions would undergo a test tube analogue of contraction called "super-precipitation." Still, there was some skepticism about the meaning of this work, because the components of the system had not been purified.

Now there are methods to purify the contractile proteins actin,[6, 7] myosin,[8, 9] tropomyosin,[10] and troponin [11] from platelets. These isolated proteins are similar to their muscle counterparts, so it is generally believed that they are the motile force generating system of platelets, although there are no experiments which prove this point directly.

Platelet actin is a globular protein of which the most important property is its ability to polymerize into 6 nm-wide filaments under physiological conditions

* Supported by NIH research grant GM–19654 and NIH research Career Development Award GM–70755 to Dr. Pollard, a Postdoctoral Fellowship from the Muscular Dystrophy Association, Inc. to Dr. Fujiwara, and NIH research grant HL–17513 to Dr. Handin. Dr. Handin is a Cancer Research Scholar, Massachusetts Division of the American Cancer Society.

(FIGURE 1A). It has a molecular weight of 43,000 daltons, like all other actins, and limited amino acid sequence data [12] indicate that platelet actin is very similar, but not identical, to muscle actin. Accordingly, platelet actin filaments are indistinguishable from muscle actin filaments.

Two types of platelet actin filament-myosin interaction provide important circumstantial evidence that platelet actin filaments can interact with myosin to generate and transmit motile force. Like all actins that have been studied,

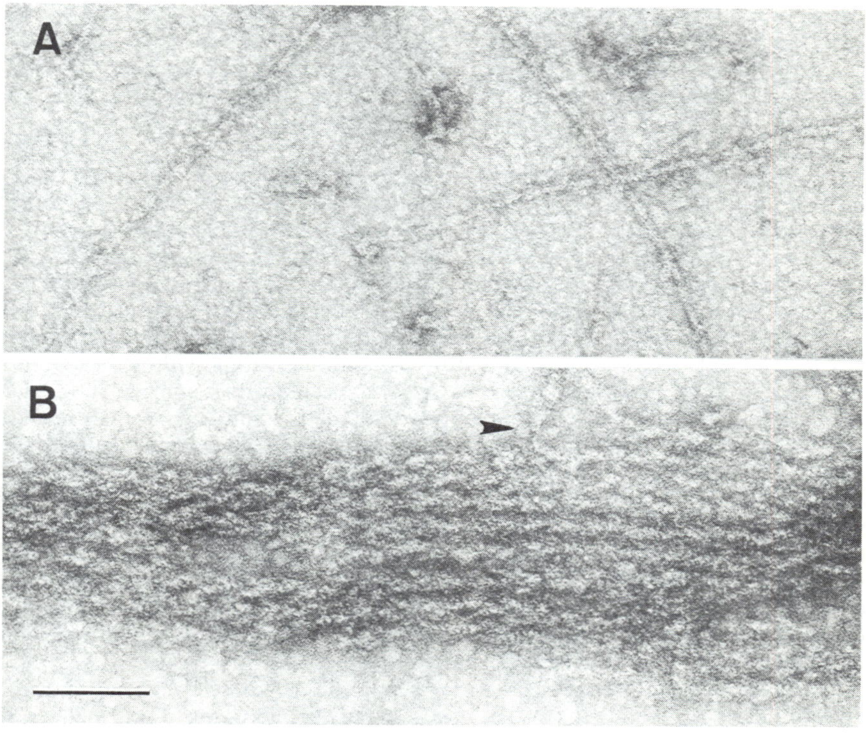

FIGURE 1. Electron micrographs of platelet actin filaments negatively stained with 1% uranyl acetate. A. Bare 6 nm-wide actin filaments in a sample of actomyosin treated with ATP to dissociate myosin from the actin. B. A bundle of actin filaments decorated with the head fragments of platelet myosin. The arrowhead-shaped complexes spaced periodically along the filaments can be appreciated most readily by viewing from the side. $\times$150,000. Bar is 0.1 μm.

platelet actin filaments bind myosin to form arrowhead-shaped complexes [8] (FIGURE 1B), due to the helical structure of the actin filament and the rigidity of the actin-myosin bond. In addition, platelet actin filaments stimulate the ATPase activity of myosin.[13] This actin-activated ATPase activity is thought to be the energy-transducing reaction in muscle contraction.

In platelets, actin is the major contractile protein, comprising about 10% of the total platelet protein (TABLE 1). In fact, there is more actin than any

TABLE 1

CONCENTRATIONS OF ACTIN AND MYOSIN *

	Percentage TotalProtein	Concentration (μmoles/kg)	Molar Ratio Actin: Myosin
Actin			
Platelet	10	240	109
Skeletal muscle	19	900	6
Myosin			
Platelet	1	2.2	
Skeletal muscle	35	144	

* The data in this table is taken from Ref. 3, p. 260, and from Ref. 9.

other protein in platelets. Since actin is present in vast molar excess over myosin (TABLE 1), it may have other functions in platelets besides motile force generation. One suggestion is that actin filaments are cytoskeletal elements. For example, morphological evidence indicates that they provide internal support for platelet filopodia.[14-16] In addition, platelet actin filaments may also participate in controlling cytoplasmic consistency, as suggested for other cells.[17]

Platelet myosin is a fibrous protein with the multiple functions of forming bipolar filaments, catalyzing ATP hydrolysis, and interacting with actin to generate motile force. It is a large asymmetrical molecule with a molecular weight of about 460,000 daltons,[9] composed of two 200,000 dalton "heavy chains" and two pairs of "light chains" with molecular weights of 19,000 and 16,000 daltons[9, 13] (FIGURE 2A). The molecule has two domains: a long (150 nm) tail and two globular heads.[8] As in muscle myosin, the light chains are associated with the heads of the platelet myosin molecule.[9] The heads are the business end of the molecule, each posessing an actin-binding site and an active site for catalyzing ATP hydrolysis.[8] The function of the tails is to form the backbone of bipolar filaments from which the heads project (FIGURE 2B, 2C).[8, 18] During the storage of platelets in blood banks,[19] part of the myosin is cleaved into heads and tails which can be isolated separately.[8, 9]

Although there are many superficial similarities to muscle myosin, platelet myosin differs from muscle myosin in a number of interesting ways, including amino acid sequence, filament structure, interaction with actin and concentration *in vivo*. No direct sequence comparisons have been made, but the absence of immunological cross-reactions indicates that platelet and muscle myosins from the same species have different primary structures. Antibodies against human platelet, skeletal muscle, and smooth muscle myosins react only with the myosin type used to elicite them.[20]

Muscle myosin forms 1.5 μm long, 15–30 nm wide, thick filaments, whereas platelet myosin forms much smaller filaments under conditions similar to those which might be found intracellularly (FIGURE 2B, C).[18] The filaments formed from purified platelet myosin in 0.1 M KCl, 1 mM Mg at pH 7, are about 325 nm long and 10.7 nm wide in the center of the bare zone. They have bipolar symmetry, with rows of myosin heads projecting from the filament backbone on either side of the central bare zone. Since the heads are the location of the actin-binding sites, the bipolar arrangement of heads in these filaments makes it possible for the filaments to cross-link oppositely polarized actin filaments to form a structure topologically identical to a muscle sarcomere (FIGURES 3 & 4). Thus, although the platelet myosin does not form thick filaments, the short, thin platelet myosin filaments combine with actin filaments in a way that is *structurally* equivalent to the force-generating systems in muscle. This suggests that platelets may use a sliding filament mechanism like striated muscle.

Muscle myosin alone interacts with actin and ATP in a cyclic reaction in which ATP hydrolysis is coupled to force generation,[21] but platelet myosin,[20] and some other nonmuscle myosins,[22, 23] require a "cofactor" protein for this vital enzymatic reaction. Cofactor has not been isolated from platelets, but we found that highly purified platelet myosin is activated little by actin unless other protein fractions are present.[20]

The myosin concentration is very high in muscle and very low in platelets (TABLE 1, FIGURE 4). Because myosin is the energy-transducing enzyme responsible for catalyzing the conversion of chemical energy stored in ATP into force for movement, the maximum force developed by the platelet contractile

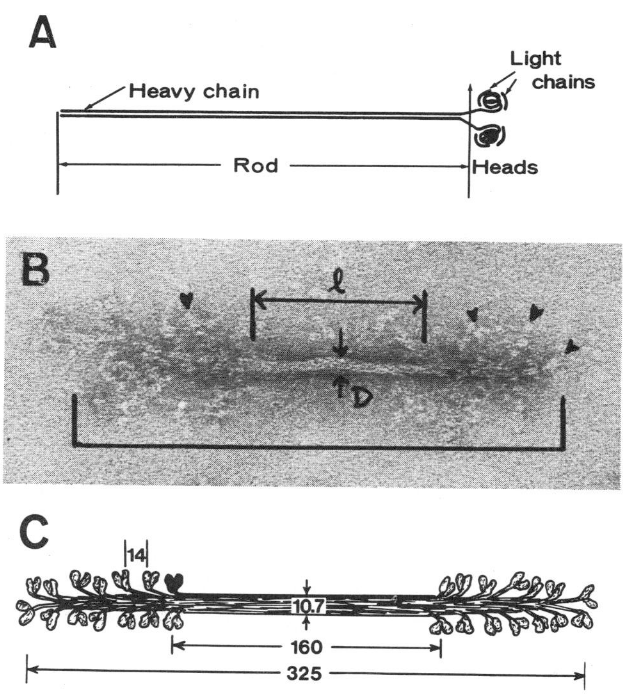

FIGURE 2. A. A drawing of the platelet myosin molecule. The vertical arrow between rod and heads marks the site where the molecule can be split in two. (By permission of the publishers of Ref. 3). B. An electron micrograph of a filament formed in 0.1 M KCl, 1 mM $MgCl_2$ at pH7 from purified human platelet myosin, negatively stained with uranyl acetate. Arrowheads mark some of the myosin heads. which are connected to the backbone of the filament by a flexible portion of the rod; ℓ marks the length of the bare zone; D marks the diameter of the shaft; and the brackets mark the filament length. ×150,000. C. A two-dimensional model of the platelet myosin filament. (B and C by permission of the publishers of J. Cell Biol.[18])

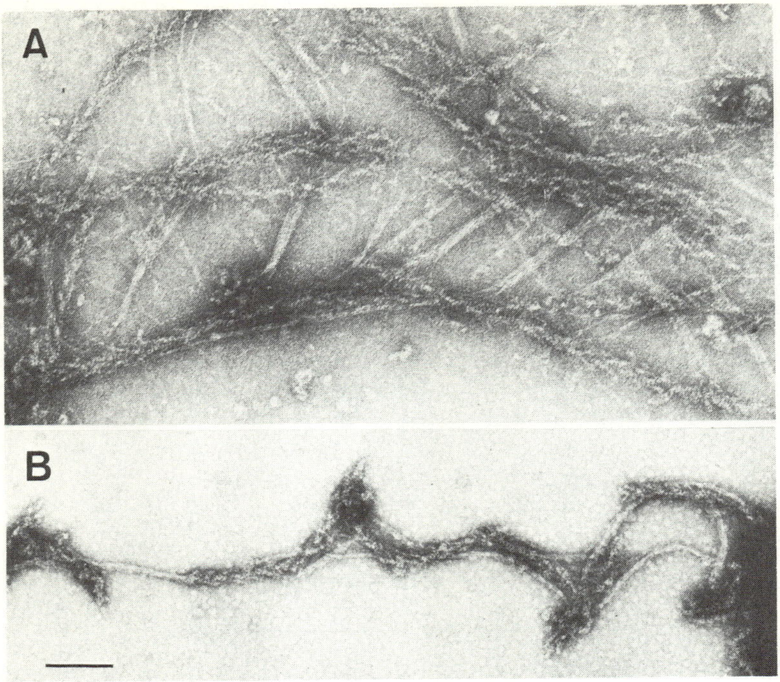

FIGURE 3. A and B. Electron micrographs of platelet actomyosin in 0.1 M KCl, negatively stained with 1% uranyl acetate. In A the short myosin filaments cross-link decorated actin filaments like the rungs on a ladder. In B myosin filaments link a series of short actin filaments, forming a actin-myosin-actin-myosin, etc. chain. To do this without Z lines to reverse the actin polarity, some of the myosin filaments are doubled back on themselves. ×90,000. Bar is 0.1 μm. (A is reproduced by permission of the publishers of J. Cell Biol.[18])

system must be far less than that developed by muscle. On the other hand, the high concentration of actin suggests that the contractile apparatus may be capable of extreme shortening (FIGURE 4).

The mechanisms controlling contractile activity in platelets are not well understood. Since three different mechanisms have been suggested, there is a good chance that the situation in platelets is more complex than in vertebrate striated muscle, where there is a simple calcium-activated on-off switch composed of the proteins tropomyosin and troponin attached to the actin filaments.[24] The three mechanisms proposed for platelets are a tropomyosin-troponin system, reversible phosphorylation of myosin light chains, and cofactor.

Both tropomyosin [10] and troponin [11] have been isolated from platelets. The tropomyosin is much like muscle tropomyosin, except that it is about 1/7 smaller. Troponin components have been isolated by virtue of their affinity for actin. Extensive characterization has not been done, but platelet troponin seems to be composed of subunit polypeptides similar to their counterparts in muscle.[25] Based on their properties, these proteins are reasonable candidates for calcium-modulated regulators of the platelet contractile system, providing that their concentration in platelets is high enough. Unfortunately there is no information about the quantity of platelet tropomyosin-troponin. This is a crucial issue, because in muscle tropomyosin and troponin form a negative regulatory system that blocks the myosin binding site on the actin filaments. To be effective, all of the myosin binding sites on all of the actin filaments must be regulated. It is not yet clear whether there is enough tropomyosin and troponin in platelets to regulate the vast number of actins. It would require about 2–2.5 mg/ml of both tropomyosin and troponin, so that together they would have to be about 5% of total platelet protein. If there is insufficient tropomyosin-troponin, other complementary regulatory systems may be present.

The reversible phosphorylation of platelet myosin light chains may represent such a complementary regulatory system, which is positive rather than negative, like tropomyosin-troponin. Adelstein et al.[26] and Adelstein and Conti[57] have shown that platelets possess a protein kinase which phosphorylates one of the platelet myosin light chains. The actin-stimulated ATPase of phosphorylated platelet myosin is about five times higher than that of the dephosphorylated platelet myosin.[27]

Since protein fractions distinct from actin or myosin can stimulate the actin-stimulated platelet myosin ATPase by 10–20 fold,[20] proteins with this cofactor-like activity could be a second positive regulator of contractile activity in platelets. In addition, platelets may have means to control the assembly and disassembly of the actin and myosin filaments and their disposition in the cytoplasm. The overall picture of the regulatory mechanisms is far from complete, although one can tentatively conclude that multiple factors are involved.

Localization of Platelet Contractile Proteins

There is clear electron microscopic evidence that the platelet actin is located in the cytoplasm,[16] but there is a controversy about the location of the myosin. There are a number of reports[28–30] in the literature describing the binding of antibodies against more or less purified platelet myosin to the outer surface of platelets, in addition to their binding to the cytoplasm. This has led to the concept that part of the myosin is on the surface of platelets (surface actomyosin). We have been unable to confirm these claims, using two immunological approaches and surface-labeling techniques. Rather, we find all of the myosin in the cytoplasm.

Our immunological studies[20, 31] have been carried out with antisera raised

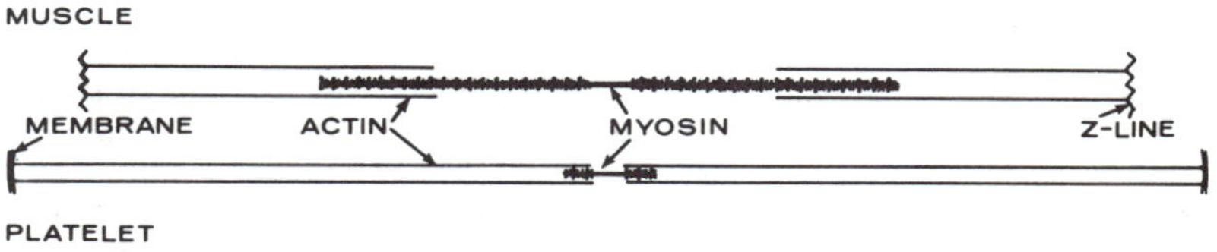

FIGURE 4. Scale drawings comparing the relative amounts of actin and myosin in a muscle sarcomere and a platelet. The actin-myosin associations shown here for platelets have been observed by electron microscopy of the isolated proteins but have been proved to exist *in vivo*.

in rabbits immunized with highly purified human platelet myosin or the rod fragment of the platelet myosin. These antigen preparations are greater than 95% pure. In particular, our KI-gel filtration procedure separates the myosin from all of the *plasma membrane fragments* that we have found in conventional platelet actomyosin preparations. The rabbits were given a primary injection of about 200 μg of myosin in complete Freund's adjuvant and boosted a single time after one month with a similar preparation of antigen. Serum was collected during the second week after the boost, and eight of eight rabbits had positive sera following this regimen. All of these sera reacted with intact platelet myosin and the rod portion of the myosin by double diffusion in agar (FIGURE 5), immunoelectrophoresis or crossed-immunoelectrophoresis. Myosin is the only antigen in platelet homogenates that reacts with the antisera. Isolated platelet myosin head does not react with the antibodies.

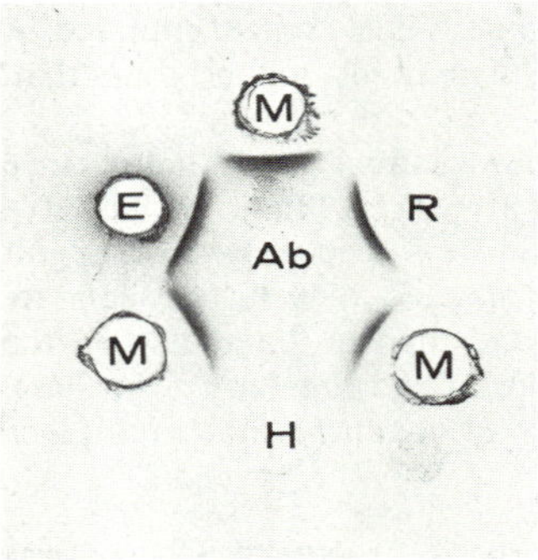

FIGURE 5. Reactivity of rabbit antiserum against human platelet myosin. Double diffusion analysis in 1% agarose containing 20 mM sodium pyrophosphate pH 8.6 buffer. The antibody (Ab) forms a single precipitin line against purified human platelet myosin (M), purified human platelet myosin rod (R), and a 20 mM pyrophosphate extract of whole human platelets (E). The antiserum does not react with the head fragment of human platelet myosin (H), which is also contaminated with actin and tropomyosin.

For immunofluoresence staining, we coupled immunoglobulin-G isolated from these sera with tetramethylrhodamine isothiocyanate. Those immunoglobulins coupled with either excess or insufficient fluorochromes were separated from the ideal conjugates by ion exchange chromatography.[32] For intracellular staining, smears of human blood were freeze substituted in —20° C acetone, air dried, stained with the labeled antibody, and washed extensively. For surface-staining, undried human blood smears were fixed with 3% formalin in phosphate buffered saline, washed with saline, and then stained with labeled antibody.

The antibodies against platelet myosin stained the cytoplasm very brightly (FIGURE 6). The cytoplasm of the leukocytes also stained brightly, but there is little or no detectable staining of the erythrocytes. When smears of intact platelets are stained with antimyosin antibody, no surface staining of the platelets is detectable (FIGURE 6). The cytoplasm of a few of the platelets in these smears is stained, presumably because they were lysed during the preparation of the specimen.

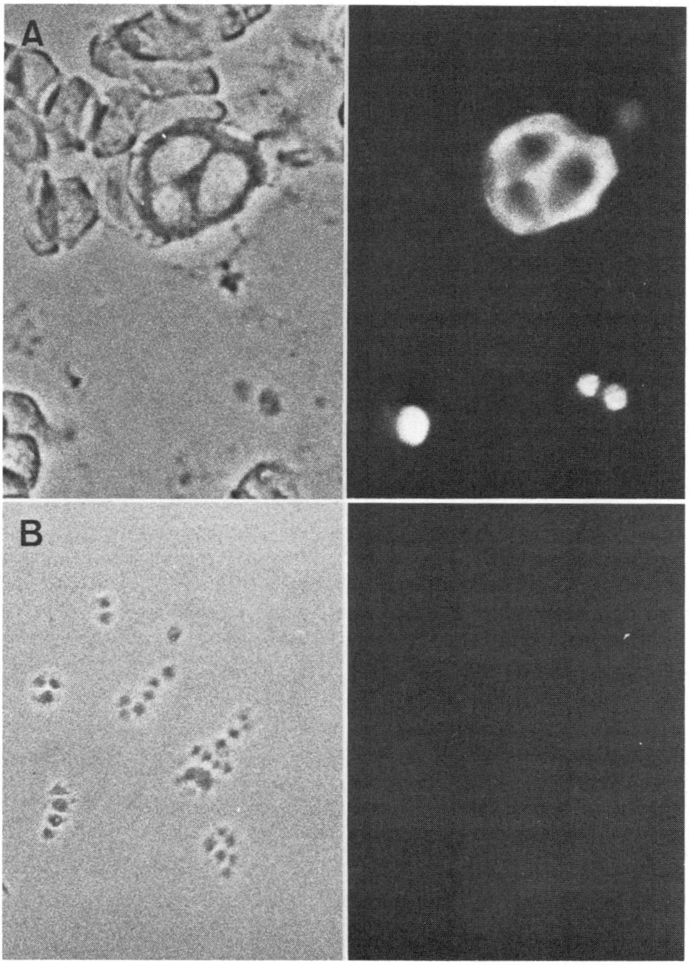

FIGURE 6. Staining of platelets with fluorescent antibodies against platelet myosin. The antibodies were directly conjugated with tetramethyl rhodamine and purified by ion exchange chromatography. A. Phase contrast and fluorescence micrographs of the same area of a human blood smear, treated with cold acetone and then stained with the fluorescent antimyosin. This example illustrates the bright staining of the platelet and leukocyte cytoplasm and the absence of erythrocyte and nuclear staining. B. Phase contrast and fluorescence micrographs of platelets from a smear fixed with 3% formalin in phosphaste-buffered saline and then stained with fluorescent antimyosin without acetone treatment to lyse the membranes. This illustrates the absence of detectable staining on the external surface of intact platelets with these antibodies against myosin.

We have also looked at the influence of these antisera on platelet function. Platelet-dense bodies were labeled by incubating platelet-rich plasma with [^{14}C]serotonin.[33] The platelets were then separated from the majority of plasma proteins by gel filtration[34] and the washed platelets were incubated with rabbit antimyosin serum that had previously been heated at 56° C for thirty minutes. As shown in TABLE 2, incubation with the rabbit antimyosin serum did not stimulate the release of intraplatelet [^{14}C]serotonin. For comparison, the effect of similar amounts of antiserum prepared against platelet membranes[35] is also tabulated. As little as 10 μl of antimembrane serum/10^8 platelets caused release of [^{14}C]serotonin, and maximum amounts were released by incubation with 50 μl of antiserum. Moreover, exposure to the serum containing antimyosin did not prevent the release of serotonin following subsequent activation with ADP (TABLE 2).

To determine if antimyosin might interfere with normal platelet responses to aggregating stimuli, we measured spectrophotometrically platelet aggregation with adenosine diphosphate (ADP) after incubation of the washed platelets with the antisera. As shown in FIGURE 7, the rate and degree of aggregation was not affected by antimyosin serum. In addition, incubation of platelets with this antiserum did not induce aggregation, whereas the antiplatelet membrane serum caused spontaneous platelet aggregation during five minutes of incubation (FIGURE 7).

TABLE 2

RELEASE OF [^{14}C] SEROTONIN (%)*

Addition	Antibody	Antibody and ADP
Antiplatelet myosin (5–2)	3	38
Antiplatelet myosin (5–3)	4	40
Antiplatelet myosin (4–2)	2	22
Antiplatelet myosin (3–5)	1	25
Antiplatelet myosin (6–2)	1	21
Antimyosin rod (8–2)	1	23
Antimyosin rod (9–2)	0	28
Antismooth muscle (12–2)	<1	27
Antiskeletal muscle (10–2)	<1	25
Anticardiac (11–2)	<1	32
Control serum (8–2)	<1	27
Antiplatelet membrane	89	—

* In these experiments, 2.0×10^8 platelets in 0.4 cc modified Tyrode's albumin buffer (0.15 M NaCl, 5×10^{-3} M KCl, 5×10^{-5} M $CaCl_2$ 2.9×10^{-4} M $MgCl_2$, 1.1×10^{-2} M Tris HCl pH 7.4, 10 mg/ml albumin, and 10 mg/ml glucose) were incubated with 0.1 ml of rabbit antiserum for 30 minutes at 37° C. The antisera had been heated at 56° C for 30 minutes. Where indicated, a second 10-minute incubation was carried out with 2.5 μM ADP. The reactions were stopped by the addition of 0.2 ml ice-cold 0.15 M NaCl, 0.02 M EDTA followed by centrifugation at 1000 xg for 15 minutes at 4° C. A portion of the supernatant was then removed for determination of released radioactivity by liquid scintillation counting. The percentage of release of [^{14}C]-serotonin due to incubation of antiserum or antiserum and ADP is compared to the % release induced by addition of 0.15 NaCl alone. The numbers in parentheses identify the rabbit from which the serum came and the number of immunizations; e.g. 5–2 is rabbit no. 5, immunized by myosin injections on two occasions.

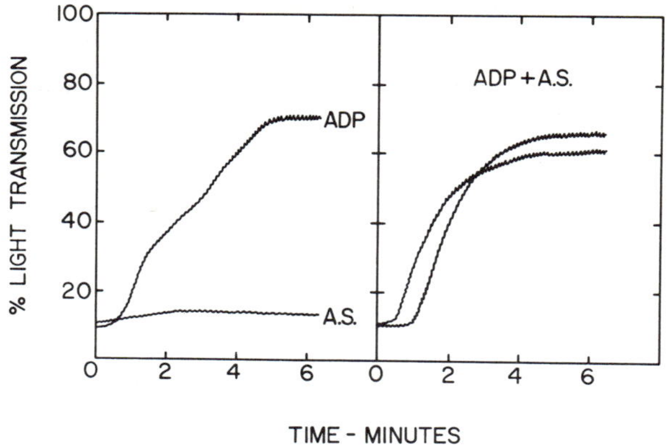

FIGURE 7. Photometric determination of platelet aggregation in response to rabbit antimyosin serum and ADP is depicted. For these studies, 2.0×10^8 platelets in 0.4 cc of modified Tyrode's albumin buffer (see footnote for TABLE 2) were incubated, with stirring, at 37°C in a spectrophotometer. At time zero, rabbit antimyosin serum (A.S.) or 2.5 μM ADP were added, as indicated, and the change in light transmission recorded. On the right are two examples of platelets first treated with antimyosin and then ADP to show that antibody does not interfere with ADP-induced aggregation.

The possibility that antimyosin antibody might bind to the platelet surface, but not affect platelet aggregation or release, was examined with use of an assay in which phagocytic cells recognize and ingest antibody-coated platelets.[35] Rabbit antiserum was added to platelet-rich plasma and the platelets were sedimented and resuspended in Krebs Ringer phosphate buffer. The washed platelets were then incubated with a suspension of granulocytes, prepared from the same donor, in the presence of 0.2% nitroblue tetrazolium dye (NBT). As shown in FIGURE 8, following sensitization with antiplatelet membrane antibody, there was an increase in the rate of NBT reduction by the granulocytes indicative of injestion of platelets. In contrast, incubation with antimyosin serum had no effect on NBT reduction.

These functional studies suggest that externally applied antimyosin antibody neither binds to the platelet surface nor stimulates nor inhibits platelet reactions in which contractile proteins may participate; however, the results obtained with antiplatelet membrane antibody suggest that binding to surface antigens can indirectly influence several platelet functions that may involve the contractile protein system.

In addition to these two immunological approaches, our colleague Richard Niederman has repeated the ^{125}I-lactoperoxidase surface-labeling experiments reported earlier by Nachman et al.,[36] with special emphasis on detecting any surface labeling of the myosin. He confirmed their finding that a glycoprotein with a molecular weight of about 100,000 daltons is the major surface component labeled with ^{125}I but was unable to detect any myosin labeling. This suggests that a large portion of the myosin is not exposed on the outer surface. The experiment must be interpreted cautiously, because the tail of the myosin has only a few tyrosine residues. Significant portions of the tail could be exposed and still escape labeling by this technique.

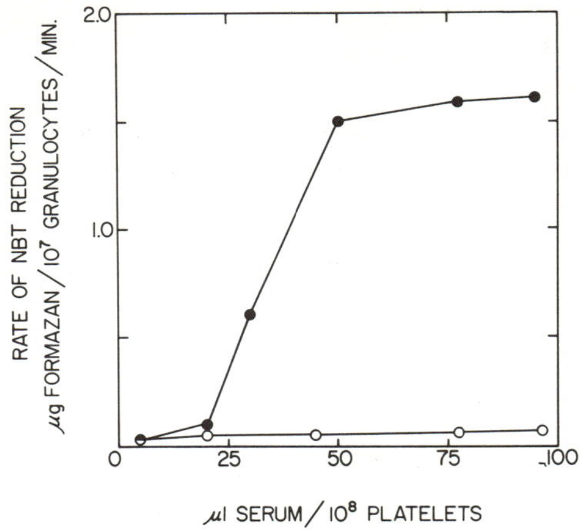

FIGURE 8. The rate of reduction of NBT dye by granulocytes incubated with platelets. In these studies, 2.0×10^8 platelets in 1 ml plasma were incubated with various quantities of rabbit antiserum for 30 minutes at 37°C, centrifuged at $1000 \times g$ for 10 minutes and resuspended in Krebs Ringer phosphate buffer. The washed platelets were then incubated in KRP buffer containing 0.2% NBT dye with 2.0×10^7 granulocytes prepared from the same donor by dextran sedimentation differential centrifugation. Following five minutes of incubation, the reaction was terminated with 0.2 M EDTA in 0.15 M NaCl followed by centrifugation at $500 \times g$ for 10 minutes. The leukocyte pellet was then extracted with dioxane and the absorbance at 550 nm determined. (●—●) = antimyosin serum; (-○—○-) = antiplatelet membrane serum.

On the basis of these results we feel that whole myosin molecules are not exposed on the surface of platelets. It remains possible that a small part of this large molecule may poke through the membrane to the outside world, but we suspect that most of the previously published claims for surface myosin can be attributed to contamination of the antigen preparations by membrane fragments that gave rise to antibodies against membrane components in addition to antibodies against myosin.

Participation of Contractile Protein in Shape Changes during Platelet Activation

During activation, there is a considerable redistribution of platelet cytoplasm and it seems likely that the contractile proteins are involved with these changes, particularly the formation of long filopodia. The shape changes are illustrated in FIGURE 9. Three things are seen to happen within 30 seconds. Platelet shape changes from discoid to spherical, the body of the platelet is reduced in size, and numerous long filopodia form. Filopod formation during platelet activation was previously deduced from physiological measurements [37] and has been documented in several scanning electron microscope studies.[38-40] It would be interesting to have detailed measurements of the size change that occurs after ADP activation, because our casual observations by scanning electron microscopy and light microscopy suggest that the diameter of the spherical activated platelets is less than half of the diameter of the discoid resting platelets. If this is true, and the platelets do not change volume during activation, as others have suggested,[37] then more than half the platelet cytoplasm is somewhere else beside the spherical body of the platelet. This large fraction of the total mass must be used to form the filopodia. Since these filopodia are only about 0.1 μm wide, hundreds of micrometers of these filopodia can be formed from the redistributed cytoplasm. Such a large quantity of filopodia is, in fact, what is seen in scanning electron micrographs of carefully prepared, ADP-activated platelets (FIGURE 9).

When the activated platelets are collected on a porous surface such as a millipore filter (FIGURE 9), the filopodia are seen to form nets over the holes in the filters. We have no evidence that similar nets are formed *in vivo,* but if they are, they may play a role in hemostasis. Filopodial nets across small defects in the microvasculature might limit the extravasation of formed elements from injured vessels.

We have not studied the redistribution of actin during filopod formation, but others have reported that the filopodia are nothing more than a bundle of

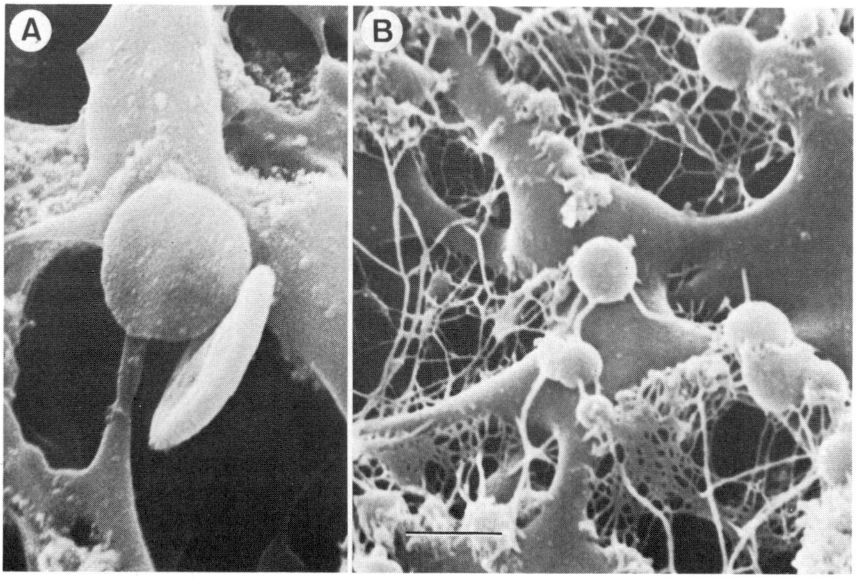

FIGURE 9. Scanning electron micrographs of resting and ADP-activated human platelets supported by a Teflon® millipore filters. Left, a pair of resting platelets fixed at 37°C by dilution of warm platelet-rich plasma into buffered 2% glutaraldehyde. Right, platelets activated with 12 μm ADP for 4 minutes in platelet-rich plasma at 37° C, prior to fixation and processing for electron microscopy on the millipore filter. $\times$12,600. Bar is 1 μm.

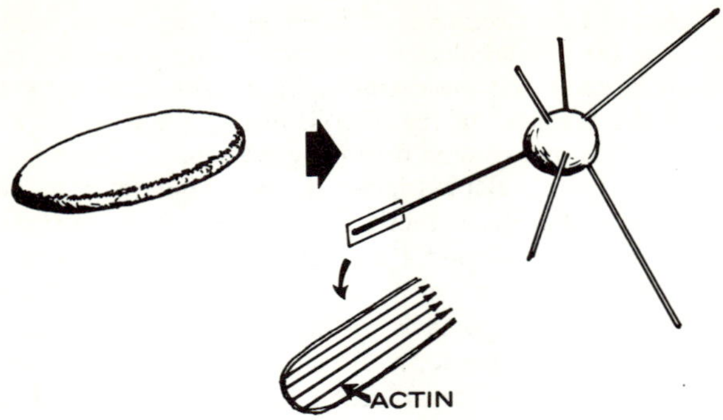

FIGURE 10. A drawing interpreting the scanning electron micrographs of events during platelet activation by ADP. The detail shows the probable arrangement of actin filaments and their attachment at the tip of a filopod.

parallel actin filaments surrounded by a closely fitting membrane.[14–16] There are some reports of microtubules in filopodia, but most filopodia we have observed in thin sections of activated platelets contain only thin filaments. Asch et al.[41] have found that all of the actin filaments in each filopod have the same polarity (FIGURE 10). If these filopodia are similar to other microvilli, such as the intestinal brush border,[42] then the actin polarity will be such that the tip of the filopodia will be an actin filament anchoring site equivalent to the Z-line in striated muscle. This arrangement has important functional implications, described below.

The mechanism of platelet filopod formation is not known, but two general models can be considered. In one, small bundles of preformed actin filaments are pushed out of the cell body. In the other, actin polymerization at specific sites at the periphery of the platelet drives the growth of the filopod. Both types of mechanism have been found in sperm which extend a thin filopod during the acrosomal reaction.[43] It might be possible to distinguish between these two alternatives, if one could rule out the presence of actin filaments in resting platelets, but unfortunately, actin filaments are much more difficult to preserve for electron microscopy than previously appreciated.[17, 20] Thus, the apparent absence of actin filaments in resting platelets does not mean that the filopodial actin filaments polymerize during activation.

We have used immunofluorescence staining to show that much of the platelet myosin remains in the body of the platelet after activation by ADP (FIGURE 11). We find antimyosin staining extending out a short distance into a few filopodia, but the small central body of the activated platelet continues to stain intensely. Since most of the filopodia are below the limit of resolution of the phase-contrast microscope, we cannot be sure that the filopodia survived the preparation for antibody staining. If they did survive and contained significant amounts of myosin, we should have been able to detect them by fluorescence microscopy.

Some of the events taking place during platelet activation are summarized in FIGURE 10. For the present discussion, the most important aspects of the transformation are that a significant fraction of the platelet mass is converted into filopodia containing bundles of unipolar actin filaments, whereas the bulk of the platelet myosin remains in the spherical body. As suggested in the next section, this relationship provides some hints about the mechanism of clot retraction.

Participation of Contractile Proteins in Clot Retraction

At first glance it seems unlikely that the platelets, which constitute roughly 0.2% of the blood volume, could cause a clot to retract by 40–50%. One solution to this paradox would be to use fibrin strands as levers to amplify contractions of the small platelets, as suggested in the mechanism of clot retraction proposed by Cohen and deVries.[44] We are skeptical that either fibrin or platelet filopodia are rigid enough to act as levers, so we favor a mechanism in which flexible fibrin strands are pulled toward platelets by the traction of filopodia (Figure 12). A contractile clot retraction mechanism of this general type was suggested years ago by Budtz-Olsen.[45] For a filopodial contraction mechanism to work, the filopodia must fill a volume equal to the volume of serum displaced, the filopodia must bind to fibrin strands, and the contractile proteins must be arranged in a way to pull the filopodia into the body of the platelet. Evidence for each of these conditions is discussed in the paragraphs that follow.

First consider the volume problem. Since the volume decrease during clot retraction is many times the volume of the active components, the platelets, the effective volume of each platelet must be considerably larger than its real size. For each platelet, with a volume of about 7 μm^3, about 2000 μm^3 of serum is squeezed from a clot during retraction. Since this remarkable feat is clearly impossible for a 7 μm^3 discoid platelet, and since platelet volume does not

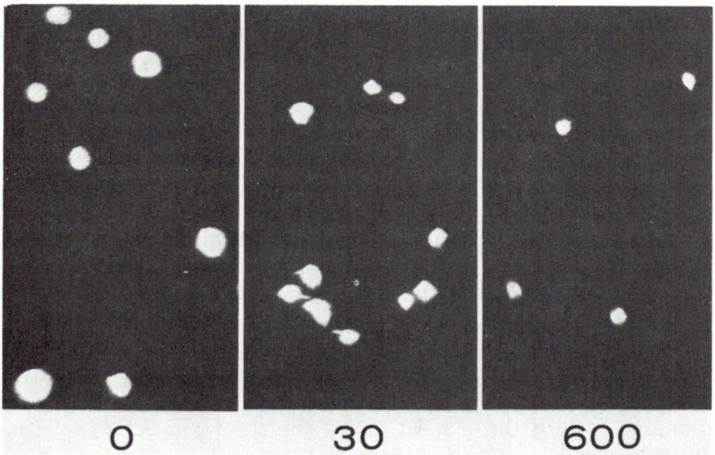

Figure 11. Fluorescence light micrographs of platelets stained with rhodamine-antimyosin rod at rest in platelet-rich plasma (0), and after 30 seconds or 600 seconds in 12 μm ADP. The proximal part of several filopodia are stained, but most of the staining remains in the central body of the platelet. Also note the decrease in size of the platelets after activation.

change appreciably with activation, the platelets *must* change shape. An isovolumetric transformation from a disc to a spiny sphere as shown in FIGURES 9 and 10 could easily increase the effective volume of each platelet an appropriate amount. Filopodia only 7 μm long, extending in all directions from the platelet surface, would penetrate a volume of 2000 μm^3. Since the erythrocytes comprise about 40% of the blood volume, the effective platelet volume must actually be about 4000 μm^3. Filopodia 9 μm long would penetrate this volume. Formation of such filopodia should present no problem for the platelet. As discussed above, the mass redistribution taking place during platelet activation could generate more than 200 μm of filopodia. An independent calculation based on the data in TABLE 1 shows that there is enough actin in a platelet to form 140 μm of filopodia containing a bundle of 20 actin filaments.

Second, consider platelet-fibrin interactions. There is both physiological and morphological evidence for platelet-fibrin interactions,[46-48] including the close

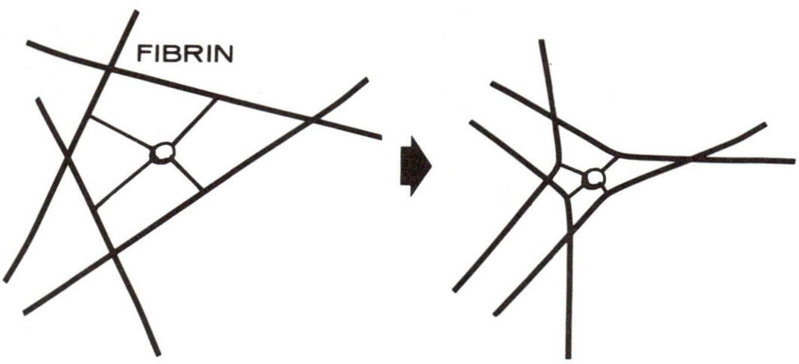

FIGURE 12. A drawing depicting a contractile mechanism for clot retraction, showing how the shortening of filopodia attached to fibrin strands could pull them together. Similar activity by other platelets would reduce the volume of the clot and squeeze out serum. For simplicity only one platelet is shown, although it is realized that the concerted action of many platelets is necessary for such a mechanism to work. It is likely that the platelet filopodia are attached to each other in addition to fibrin.

associations seen in electron micrographs (FIGURE 13). The physiological data indicate that platelets interact with polymerizing fibrin, so that it is possible that the interactions depicted in FIGURE 13 could be established during clot formation. The details of this binding have yet to be established. The relation of the platelets and fibrin in contracted clots suggests that the fibrin has been pulled toward the platelets (FIGURE 13). The fibrin strands tend to be radially oriented around individual platelets and clumps of platelets. Moreover, some fibrin strands associated with the platelets are bent to acute angles, with the vertex pointing toward the platelet and a finger of platelet cytoplasm in the crook of the bend.

Finally, consider the arrangement of actin and myosin in activated platelets. As discussed above, the filopodia are filled with a bundle of actin filaments, all of which have the same polarity [41] and which are likely to be oriented in a way that makes the tip of the filopodia comparable to the Z-line in muscle. We also noted that platelet myosin forms bipolar filaments and that the bulk of the

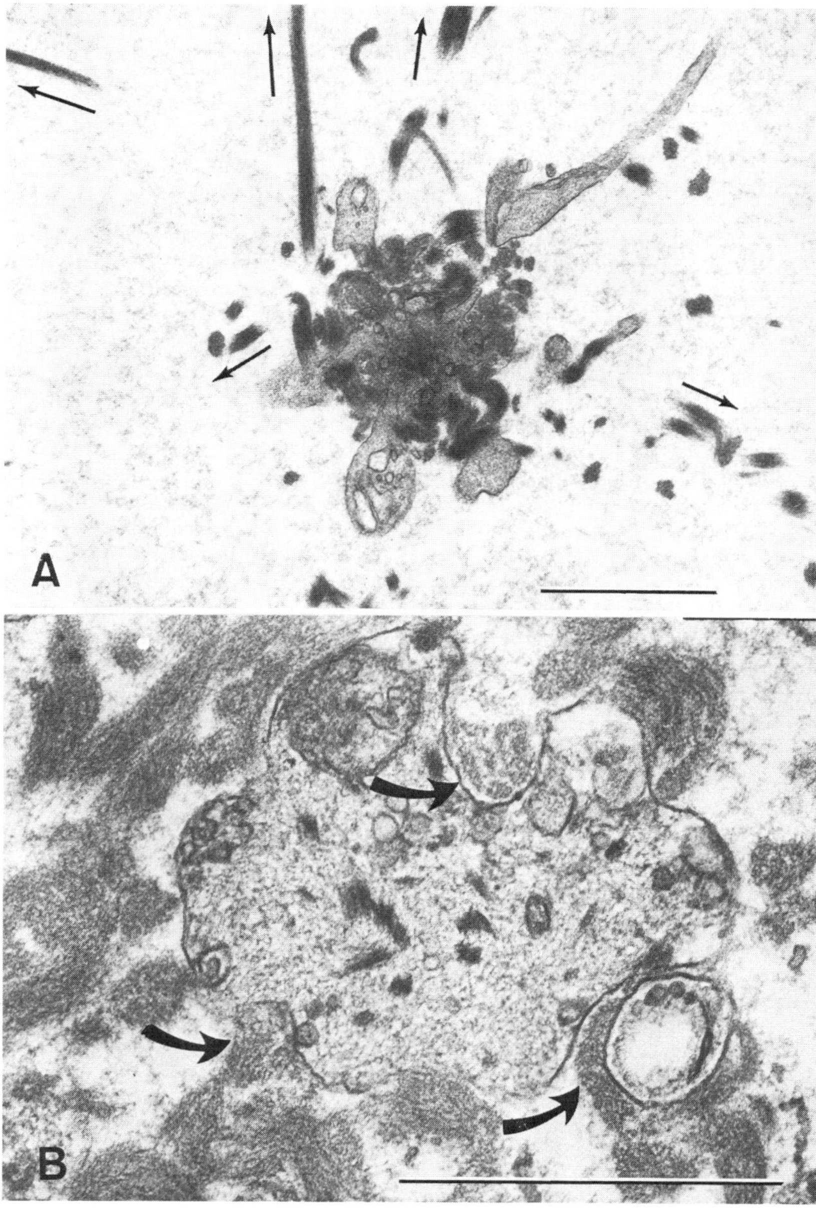

FIGURE 13. Transmission electron micrographs of platelets and fibrin in a retracted clot of platelet-rich plasma. Citrated platelet-rich plasma was clotted by recalcification with 20 mM $CaCl_2$ and allowed to retract. After retraction, platelets were surrounded by a concentration of fibrin strands, many of which extended radially from the platelet (arrows). Many of the fibrin strands were closely applied to the platelet surface (arrows in B). A = ×23,000; B = ×51,000. Bars are 1 μm.

myosin seems to remain in the spherical body of the activated platelet. This arrangement of actin and myosin would make it possible for bipolar myosin filaments to cross-link antiparallel actin filaments directed toward the center of the platelet from filopodia on opposite sides. This would form a contractile unit within the platelet with the same geometrical features as a muscle sarcomere (FIGURE 4). The contractile unit would consist of a bundle of actin filaments in one filopod and a centrally located bipolar myosin filament cross-linking these actin filaments to an oppositely polarized bundle of actin filaments from a filopod on the opposite side of the platelet. Presumably the interaction of the actin filaments with the myosin and ATP in the center of the platelet would develop a force pulling the actin filaments, the filopodia, and any attached fibrin strands toward the center of the platelet. Although the proportions are different, this mechanism is exactly the same as the actin-myosin arrangement that pulls the Z-lines toward the center of the sarcomere in striated muscle (FIGURE 4).

This filopodial contractile mechanism of clot retraction is compatible with the available evidence but needs further experimental verification. We and others familiar with platelet contractile proteins[49] find it attractive, because it uses very conventional actin-myosin interactions to generate the force. Similar mechanisms have been proposed for thrombocyte activity[50] and for microvillar actin-myosin interactions in the intestinal brush border.[42] The proposed mechanism suggests that the platelet uses filopodia filled with actin filaments to solve two problems at once: expansion of its effective volume to at least 50% of the blood volume and transmission of forces generated in the central body of the platelet to far-flung sites of attachment to fibrin and other platelets. Since platelet filopodia are likely to attach to each other as well as fibrin, filopodial contraction would also draw the platelets together in clumps, as observed in contracted clots.

REFERENCES

1. HUXLEY, H. E. 1973. Muscular contraction and cell motility. Nature **343:** 445.
2. POLLARD, T. D. & R. R. WEIHING. 1974. Actin and myosin and cell movement. CRC Crit. Rev. Biochem. **2:** 1–65.
3. INOUE, S. & R. E. STEPHENS, Eds. 1975. Molecules and Cell movement. Raven Press. New York, N.Y.
4. BETTEX-GALLAND, M. & E. F. LÜSCHER. 1959. Extraction of an actomyosin-like protein from human platelets. Nature **184:** 276.
5. BETTEX-GALLAND, M. & E. F. LÜSCHER. 1965. Thrombosthenin, the contractile protein from blood platelets and its relation to other contractile proteins. Adv. Prot. Chem. **20:** 1.
6. PROBST, E. & F. LÜSCHER. 1972. Studies on thrombosthenin-A, the actin-like moiety of the contractile protein from blood platelets. I. Isolation, characterization and evidence for two forms of thrombostenin-A. Biochim. Biophys. Acta **278:** 577–584.
7. BOOYSE, F. M., T. P. HOVEKE & M. E. RAFELSON. 1973. Human platelet actin. Isolation and properties. J. Biol. Chem. **248:** 4083.
8. ADELSTEIN, R. S., T. D. POLLARD & W. M. KUEHL. 1971. Isolation and characterization of myosin and two myosin fragments from human blood platelets. Proc. Nat. Acad. Sci. USA **68:** 2703.
9. POLLARD, T. D., S. M. THOMAS & R. NIEDERMAN. 1974. Human platelet myosin. I. Purification by a rapid method applicable to other non-muscle cells. Anal. Biochem. **60:** 258–266.

10. COHEN, I. & C. COHEN. 1972. A tropomyosin-like protein from platelets. J. Mol. Biol. **68:** 383.
11. PUSZKIN, S., S. KOCHWA & R. E. ROSENFIELD. 1975. Regulatory complex of human platelet actomysin. J. Cell Biol. **67:** 346a.
12. ELZINGA, M., B. J. MARON & R. S. ADELSTEIN. 1976. Human heart and platelet actins are products of different genes. Science **191:** 94–95.
13. ADELSTEIN, R. S. & M. S. CONTI. 1973. The characterization of contractile proteins from platelets and fibroblasts. Cold Spring Harbor Symp. Quant. Biol. **37:** 599.
14. ZUCKER-FRANKLIN, D., R. L. NACHMAN & A. J. MARCUS. 1967. Ultrastructure of thrombosthenin, the contractile protein of human platelets. Science **157:** 945–946.
15. WHITE, J. G. 1968. Fine structural alterations in platelets by ADP. Blood **31:** 604–622.
16. BEHNKE, O., B. I. KRISTENSEN & L. E. NIELSEN. 1971. Electron microscopical observations on actinoid and myosinoid filaments in blood platelets. J. Ultrastruct. Res. **37:** 351.
17. POLLARD, T. D. 1976. The role of actin in the temperature dependent gelation and contraction of extracts of *Acanthamoeba.* J. Cell Biol. **68:** 579.
18. NIEDERMAN, R. & T. D. POLLARD. 1975. Human platelet myosin II. In vitro assembly and structure of myosin filaments. J. Cell Biol. **67:** 72–92.
19. ABRAMOWITZ, J., STRACHER & T. C. DETWILER. 1974. Proteolysis of myosin during platelet storage. J. Clin. Invest. **53:** 1493–1496.
20. POLLARD, T. D., K. FUJIWARA, R. NIEDERMAN & P. M. SZAMIER. 1976. The importance of cytoplasmic actin and myosin for cellular structure and motility. *In* Cell Motility. R. Goldman, T. D. Pollard & J. Rosenbaum, Eds. Cold Spring Harbor Press. Cold Spring Harbor, N.Y. In press.
21. TAYLOR, E. W. 1972. Chemistry of muscle contraction. Ann. Rev. Biochem. **41:** 577.
22. POLLARD, T. D. & E. D. KORN. 1973. Acanthamoeba myosin. II. Interaction with actin and with a new cofactor protein required for actin activation of Mg-ATPase activity. J. Biol. Chem. **248:** 4691–4697.
23. STOSSEL, T. P. & J. H. HARTWIG. 1975. Interactions between actin, myosin and an actin-binding protein from rabbit alveolar macrophages. Alveolar macrophage myosin Mg^{++} ATPase requires a cofactor for activation by actin. J. Biol. Chem. **250:** 5706–5712.
24. WEBER, A. & J. M. MURRAY. 1973. Molecular control mechanisms in muscle contraction. Physiol. Rev. **53:** 612–673.
25. COHEN, I., E. KAMINSKI & A. DE VRIES. 1973. Actin-linked regulation of the human platelet contractile system. FEBS Lett. **34:** 315–317.
26. ADELSTEIN, R. S., M. A. CONTI & W. ANDERSON. 1973. Phosphorylation of human platelet myosin. Proc. Nat. Acad. Sci. USA **70:** 3115–3119.
27. ADELSTEIN, R. S. & M. A. CONTI. 1975. Phosphorylation of platelet myosin increases actin-activated myosin ATPase activity. Nature **256:** 597–598.
28. NACHMAN, R. L., A. J. MARCUS & L. B. SATIER. 1967. Platelet thrombosthenin: subcellular localization and function. J. Clin. Invest. **46:** 1380.
29. BOOYSE, F. M., L. A. STERNBERGER, D. ZSCHOCKE & M. E. RAFELSON. 1971. Ultrastructural localization of contractile protein (thrombosthenin) in human platelets using an unlabeled anti-body peroxidase staining technique. J. Histochem. Cytochem. **19:** 540–550.
30. PUSZKIN, E. G., M. B. ZUCKER & T. H. SPAET. 1975. Effect of antibody to platelet rod myosin on platelet function. Blood **46:** 1031 (abstr.).
31. FUJIWARA, K. & T. D. POLLARD. 1976. Fluorescent antibody localization of myosin in the cytoplasm, cleavage furrow and mitotic spindle of human cells. J. Cell Biol. **71.** In press.
32. CEBRA, J. & G. GOLDSTEIN. 1965. Chromatographic purification of tetramethyl-

rhodamine-immune globulin conjugates and their use in the cellular localization of rabbit α-globulin polypeptide chains. J. Immunol. **95:** 230.
33. HARADA, K. & M. B. ZUCKER. 1971. Simultaneous development of platelet factor four activity and release of ^{14}C serotonin. Thromb. Diath. Haem. **25:** 41.
34. TANGEN, O., H. J. BERMAN & P. MURFEY. 1971. Gel filtration: a new technique for separation of blood platelets from plasma. Thromb. Diath. Haem. **25:** 208.
35. HANDIN, R. I. & T. P. STROSSEL. 1974. Phagocytosis of antibody-coated platelets by human granulocytes. New Eng. J. Med. **290:** 989.
36. NACHMAN, R. L., A. HUBBARD & B. FERRIS. 1973. Iodination of the human platelet membrane. Studies of the major surface glycoprotein. J. Biol. Chem. **248:** 2928–2936.
37. BORN, G. V. R. 1970. Observations on the changes in shape of blood platelets brought about by ADP. J. Physiol. **209:** 487.
38. HATTORI, A., J. TOKUNAGA, T. FUJITA & M. MATSUOKA. 1969. Scanning electron microscope observations on human blood platelets and their alterations induced by thrombin. Arch. Histol. Jap. **31:** 37–54.
39. BARNHART, M. L., R. T. WALSH & J. A. ROBINSON. 1972. A three-dimensional view of platelet responses to chemical stimuli. Ann. N.Y. Acad. Sci. **201:** 360–390.
40. KAY, M. M. & H. H. FUNDENBERG. 1973. Inhibition and reversal of platelet activation by cytochalasin B or colcemid. Nature **244:** 288–289.
31. ASCH, A., E. S. ELGART & V. T. NACHMIAS. 1975. Relationship of microfilaments to membrane in human blood platelets. J. Cell Biol. **67:** 12a.
42. MOOSEKER, M. S. & L. G. TILNEY. 1975. Organization of an actin filament-membrane complex. Filament polarity and membrane attachment in microvilli of intestinal epithelial cells. J. Cell Biol. **67:** 725–743.
43. TILNEY, L. G. 1975. The role of actin in nonmuscle cell motility. *In* Molecules and Cell Movements. S. Inoue & R. E. Stephens, Eds. Raven Press, New York, N.Y.
44. COHEN, I. & A. DE VRIES. 1973. Platelet contractile regulation in an isometric system. Nature **246:** 36–37.
45. BUDTZ-OLSEN, O. E. 1951. Clot Retraction. Blackwell Scientific Pub. Oxford, England.
46. WHITE, J. G., W. KRIVIT & R. L. VERNIER. 1965. The platelet-fibrin relationship in human blood clots: an ultrastructural study utilizing ferritin-conjugated anti-human fibrinogen antibody. Blood **25:** 241.
47. NIEWIAROSKI, S., E. REGOECZI & G. J. STEWART. 1972. Platelet interaction with polymerizing fibrin. J. Clin. Invest. **51:** 685–700.
48. COHEN, I., J. GABBAY, T. GLASER & A. OPLATKA. 1975. Fibrin blood platelet interaction in a contracting clot. Brit. J. Haemataol. **31:** 45.
49. LÜSCHER, E. F., E. PROBST & M. BETTEX-GALLAND. 1972. Thrombosthenin: structure and function. Ann. N.Y. Acad. Sci. **201:** 122–130.
50. SHEPRO, D., F. A. BELAMARICH, F. B. MERK & F. C. CHAO. 1969. Changes in thrombocyte ultrastructure during clot retraction. J. Cell Sci. **4:** 763.

DISCUSSION

DR. BAIER: Dr. Stewart, in light of all we have heard from Dr. Ratnoff and Dr. Kaplan about Hageman factor, I was wondering if there was any role in your system with regard to chemotaxis and leukocytes for Hageman factor?

DR. STEWART: I was very distressed yesterday to see that after so many years Dr. Ratnoff is becoming disenchanted with Hageman factor, just when we need it. I would suggest that in the normal person the Hageman factor does function, and it seems that there really must be a bypass for activation of the intrinsic coagulation system, if our whole concept of the clotting is correct. In leukotaxis, I think that kallikrein would certainly be one of the major candidates as a messenger, and of course this would suggest that Hageman factor is very much involved here.

DR. BAIER: Dr. Pollard, about ten years ago I did some experiments with model membranes of muscle myosin showing that the "A" band of filaments of myosin aggregates could persist at the gas/liquid interface, and with just a tiny excess beyond the amounts required for a monolayer there was retention of enzymatic activity. Rather than the myosin filaments being exposed to the cell exterior where you could be staining them with their antibodies, if they are slightly inside they could provide the other half of the link you need in your sarcomere without invoking any peculiar additional structure, in the platelet membrane.

DR. POLLARD: Nothing, as far as I'm concerned, is known about the detailed localization of myosin inside of platelets. It could very well be near plasma membranes. There are published reports showing where myosin is in the platelets, but I'm critical of them for technical reasons. They could be misleading.

DR. E. PUSZKIN (*Dept. of Hematology, Montefiore Hospital, Bronx, N.Y.*): I have a question for Dr. Pollard. We have used prepared antibodies against rod myosin and we confirmed the question that was just asked. Also you said that your antibody did not induce the platelets to do anything. What kind of inducers did you use for clot retraction and for testing aggregating? Did the antibody, by itself, do anything?

DR. POLLARD: The question should really be addressed to somebody who isn't here—Bob Handen, who works at the Peter Brigham Hospital in Boston. But as I understand what he's done with our antisera, he's tested to see whether the antibody against myosin will activate platelets or whether they will interfere with activation of clot retraction due to normal stimuli. He has tested our ADP and collagen, and they just don't seem to do anything to the platelets. This is consistent with our other results. The difference between us and the majority view may be that our antibodies are different. That's the simplest explanation, and we've discussed this in great detail; certainly we make our antibodies in different ways, and that might help account for some of the differences.

DR. PUSZKIN: It is quite possible that you broke the molecule into pieces. You inject whole myosin and you obtain only an antibody against the rod, and not against the head. Now in our experience, we find no difficulty in obtaining antibodies against the head. Possibly you broke your molecules and will obtain an antibody against a specific fragment of the rod which is not exposed in the membrane.

DR. KELLER: When one uses an immunofluorescent technique, what type of preparation or smearing or fixation results in staining the outside of the platelet, the cytoplasm of the platelet, and internal granules of the platelet?

DR. POLLARD: We haven't succeeded in staining the outside of the platelet. But in order to stain the inside of the platelet or any other cell you have to render the membrane permeable, and for this we use acetone, which is a terrible but time-honored procedure. It is good for myosin, I believe, because myosin is completely insolubilized by acetone, so that after we treat cells with acetone we can be reasonably sure that it isn't wandering off to some place where it shouldn't be. The cells look remarkably good and almost lifelike even after this acetone treatment, providing you do it the right way. Some of the platelets stain on the outside and some of the platelets stain in the cytoplasm. Most of the platelets, even after air-drying, appear to be intact and don't stain at all. That's where the preparation came from. I showed two slides of the same preparation. One had a whole bunch of platelets that were completely unstained; those were air dried. It isn't clear to us that the granules in the platelets stain particularly, but it's difficult to tell because they are not very big.

DR. P. KRONICK (*University of Pennsylvania, Philadelphia, Pa.*): Dr. Stewart, how do you know the fibers on Dacron grafts are collagen, in view of the last slide shown by Dr. Niemetz? Where are the platelets?

DR. STEWART: Just from the scanning microscope, we wouldn't have known that the fibers were collagen. We had to confirm this, of course, by the periodicity of the collagen with transmission electron microscopy. While we had massive platelet adhesion to these bypasses early, in as short a time as 24 hours, most of the platelet adhesion had disappeared; and thereafter, for months or longer, the endothelial surface is rich in collagen but does not bear any platelets.

DR. WEISS: I have two questions for Dr. Pollard. First, Dr. Behnke earlier reported that there was no structural relationship between the actin and myosin. Do you have any explanation for your discrepant findings which show an ordered relationship between actin and myosin, and which can account for some kind of contractile mechanism? The other question is: Contractile mechanisms have been implicated in the platelet-release reaction. Could you tell us how platelet contractile activity might play a role in this secretory mechanism?

DR. POLLARD: Dr. Behnke's interpretation of his electron micrographs is probably correct. The difference between his work and our work is that he wasn't sure what he was looking at, and we are. He was working with whole platelets or whole homogenates of platelets, and we are working with purified proteins, so we know exactly what we've got in the test tube. What he observed was that there were some thin filaments which he could decorate with myosin from muscle. There were some filaments which would not decorate with myosin, suggesting that they were something else and that these other filaments tended to cross-link the decorated filaments, and he suggested that the undecorated filaments were myosin or myosin-like. He called them "myosinoid," which I think is a very regrettable term. But it would seem that his observations are entirely consistent with the sort of thing you can see with the purified proteins where the myosin seems to cross-link the actin. What our contractile proteins have to do with secretion is a question that a great many cell biologists are looking at, and as far as I know, there is minimal hard data on any connection between contractile proteins and secretory processes, but there is an enormous amount of speculation. Part of this is generated by drug studies, which are difficult to interpret, using drugs that definitely inhibit some secretory systems and that are supposed to interact with contractile proteins but have never been proved to do it. I think it is very attractive to think about how secretory mechanisms might be triggered, or powered, or so on, by contractile proteins, but I'd say that the data has yet to be produced to prove that point.

DR. ASSAF: My question is to Dr. Pollard. Could you comment on the differences between muscle and platelet with respect to their magnesium-to-calcium ATP-ase activities of platelet actomyosin and muscle myosin?

DR. POLLARD: The audience may not appreciate how difficult that question is to answer, because a great many experimental variables have to be taken into consideration. But in general, I can say that the ATP-ase activity of the contractile proteins from platelets and other nonmuscle cells is less than the activity of the contractile proteins from muscle. The pattern of activation by calcium, magnesium, EDTA, and potassium, and so on, is similar, but in general it is about an order of magnitude less at the same temperature and under the same ionic conditions.

PART VI. TRANSPORT TO AND FROM THE BLOOD-MATERIAL INTERFACE

INTRODUCTION

DR. KELLER: The very natural flow of this conference takes us now to a consideration of how particles get to and from interfaces. When people discovered the vastly different behavior of a test section of synthetic material in arteries and veins, they began to understand the very important questions that relate to the physical environment and the flow factors and what happens at a biomaterial. The fluid mechanical factors affect particle behavior in several ways: before they ever get to a surface, how they are transported to and from that surface, and then what happens to them when they get to the surface. The same diffusional and hydrodynamic or fluid mechanical forces will affect all particles whether they be microscopic or cellular elements or inorganic molecules. As we move from the small inorganic molecule to a cell, there is a continuum of change in which the relative importance of different factors changes. With very small inorganic molecules the fluid mechanical effect may be somewhat less, and diffusional effects predominate; to larger and larger particles, fluid mechanical effects become somewhat more important than diffusion.

DR. TURITTO: The speakers today will be dealing, in large part, with physical models, and in an attempt to understand some of the physical mechanisms that govern cell attachment, cell adhesion, and the complex processes that occur in, say, thrombus formation. A combination of physical and chemical steps occur in complex blood flow situations.

MICROSCOPIC CONSIDERATIONS: THE MOTIONS OF INDIVIDUAL PARTICLES *

Harry L. Goldsmith and Takeshi Karino

McGill University Medical Clinic
Montreal General Hospital
Montreal, Quebec, Canada H3G 1A4

INTRODUCTION

This paper is concerned with the events occurring at the blood-vessel wall interface and how they are affected by the flow patterns and fluid mechanical stresses existing in the circulation and in artificial organs. It seeks to understand the phenomena at the level of the individual corpuscle and surrounding plasma because it is at the microscopic level that the processes of thrombosis and hemostasis begin. However, the cellular and fluid motions within the blood are rather complex, since there are millions of red cells suspended in every μl of plasma, and these continually interact with each other during flow. Thus, any attempt to give a quantitative description of the mechanics of the flow becomes very difficult. Nevertheless, it has proved possible, by observing particle and suspending fluid motion through a microscope in the interior of red cell suspensions, to obtain an understanding of the overall flow behavior of the system. This microrheological approach to the problem of suspension flow has been described previously, both in model systems [1-3] and in suspensions of red cells.[3-5] In the present context interest centers on the interactions between the erythrocytes, which constitute 99% by volume of the cellular phase in whole blood, and how these affect the paths of the far less numerous platelets, especially those close to the vessel wall. In addition, the paper will deal with blood cell behavior in a region of separated flow where a vortex exists. There is considerable evidence that bifurcations, T-branches, bends, and changes in vessel diameter in the arterial circulation, where flow separation can occur, are associated with the formation of early atheroma and that subsequent interactions of blood cells with the altered vessel wall can result in the adhesion of platelets and platelet aggregates.

The work represents a series of *in vitro* studies in which human red cell and platelet suspensions were subjected to steady or pulsatile flow in rigid glass tubes of diameters from 60 to 1000 μm.[4-6] The technique involves observing and photographing individual cells and other small model particles through a high-power microscope and tracking them in the flow by mechanically or hydraulically moving a stage on which the flow tube and infusion syringe are mounted.[3-5] The principle of the method is illustrated in FIGURE 1. In the case of red cells, these *in vitro* studies have demonstrated the rotation, deformation, and inward radial migration of the corpuscles, phenomena that are essentially similar to those observed in high-speed cine microphotometric studies of living vessels.[7-9]

* This work was supported by grant MT 1835 from the Medical Research Council of Canada, and by a grant from the Quebec Heart Foundation.

Suspensions of Blood Cells in Straight Tubes

Behavior at Very Low Concentrations

In the absence of particle interactions, isolated red cells and platelets suspended in plasma or in Tyrodes-albumin solution undergoing Poiseuille flow (Figure 1) at mean linear velocities <3 tube diameters/second rotate with periodically varying angular velocities disturbed only by Brownian rotational diffusion.[5, 10] The cells move along paths parallel to the tube wall, except for some inward radial drift, which, as previously found with emulsion droplets,[1, 2] is related to the shear deformation of the particles and the proximity of the vessel wall. Thus, at a given flow rate, the rate of inward migration of red cells markedly increases if the plasma viscosity is raised through the addition of low

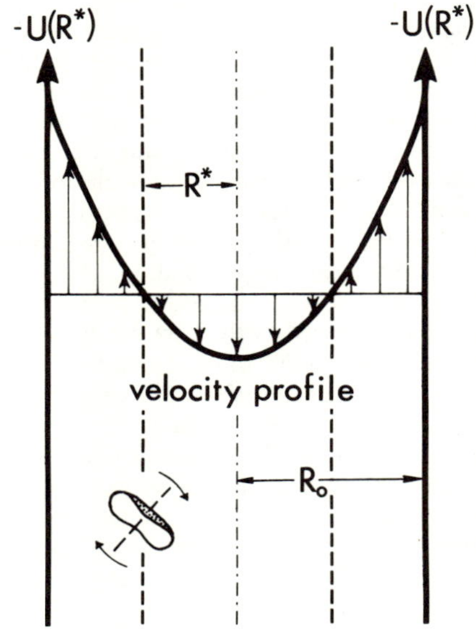

Figure 1. Tracking particles in Poiseuille flow through a tube-schematic. A downward flowing red cell, situated in the median (diametrical) plane of the tube with its center at a radial distance R* from the tube axis, is rendered stationary by moving the tube of radius R_0 upward with a velocity $-U(R^*)$, equal but opposite to that of the cell. The parabolic velocity profile in the tube is given by a modified form of Equation 5:

$$U(R) - U(R^*) = \frac{2Q}{\pi R_0^4}(R^{*2} - R^2). \quad \textbf{(5A)}$$

The red cell rotates in the direction shown during flow. (By permission of the publisher of Platelets, Drugs and Thrombosis.[44])

molecular weight Dextran,[11] which increases the fluid stresses acting on the cells. There is then a pronounced deformation of the corpuscles into ellipsoid-like shapes, which are carried at a constant orientation to the direction of flow while the membrane rotates about the cell interior.[5, 12, 13] Thus also, in a given suspension and tube, the rate of migration decreases rapidly with increasing distance from the wall; one never observes red blood cells or platelets in apparent contact with the vessel boundary, an experimental finding which holds true at all flow rates, even when the mean linear velocity is much greater than three tube diameters per second. At the higher velocities, inward radial migration due to inertia of the fluid and the proximity of the vessel wall has to be considered, a phenomenon that occurs with rigid particles.[1, 14–16] Whether due to particle deformation or fluid inertia, the rate of migration away from the tube wall is greatly dependent on the ratio of particle to tube diameter (to the fourth and third power, respectively), and except for particles in the immediate vicinity of the wall, is not likely to be important for blood cells in vessels having diameters larger than ~500 μm.

Hence, in *dilute* suspensions of blood cells, in the absence of other effects such as sedimentation in a horizontal vessel, or the chemotaxis of polymorphonuclear leukocytes, forces arising from an interaction of the flow field around a particle with the vessel wall [2, 16] would act to prevent the cells from reaching the vascular endothelium. One therefore has to look for factors that oppose the inward drift of corpuscles, the most important of which is a dispersive process arising from continual collisions between the cells during flow.

Dispersion of Cells in Flow Due to Collisions

When the number of blood cells per unit volume becomes appreciable (e.g. already at ½% hematocrit there are $\sim 7 \times 10^4$ RBC/μl), corpuscles traveling along adjacent streamlines at different velocities (see FIGURE 1) will be carried into close proximity to each other and collide during flow through the tube. The frequency at which these interactions occur depends on the velocity gradient G, the number of cells, n, per unit volume of suspension and their size—the larger their diameter the greater the distance from their center of rotation over which they interact with each other.

In the geometrically simpler case of interactions between two small spherical particles of radius b, the number of two-body collisions per second experienced by a sphere, the center of which is situated at a radial distance R in a tube of radius R_0, has been shown to be: [1]

$$f = \frac{32}{3} G(R) b^3 n, \tag{1}$$

$$= \frac{8}{\pi} G(R) c. \tag{2}$$

Here, G(R) is the velocity gradient, a function of R, and given by

$$G(R) = \frac{dU(R)}{dR} \tag{3}$$

$$= \frac{4Q}{\pi R_0^4} R, \tag{4}$$

U(R) being the undisturbed fluid velocity at R (which, providing $b/R_0 \ll 1$ is identical with the particle velocity [1, 16])

$$U(R) = \frac{2Q}{\pi R_0^4}(R_0^2 - R^2), \tag{5}$$

Q the volume flow rate, and c the volume fraction of spheres ($=4\pi b^3 n/3$). At a given Q, the highest collision rates therefore occur close to the wall; moreover, at a given number concentration, the rate would be 11× greater for a sphere having the volume of a red cell (b = 2.78 μm) than that of a platelet (b = 1.24 μm).

More important for the subject of platelet-wall interactions is the fact that, while colliding, the trajectories of the particles are radially displaced: the smaller the radial distance between the streamlines of the approaching particles the greater the displacement as they move around each other during the period of closest approach, when they form a "doublet" which rotates for a time before the participants in the collision again separate.[1] The effect of a series of such collisions on the observed particle paths is shown in panel (a) of FIGURE 2 for the case of a 2% suspension of 320-μm spheres flowing through an 8-mm diameter tube. It is evident that the radial displacements (in a direction normal to that of the flow) are small compared to the particle diameter; the time average radial displacement is found to be only 3.5–5.0% of the sphere diameter.[17] However, this increases appreciably as the concentration is increased, as more 3-, 4-, and multibody collisions, involving much greater particle radial displacements, occur.[17] In fact, even at volume concentrations as low as 15%, it can be shown on the basis of two-body collisions alone (Equation 1), that all spheres at a given instant will be in the process of colliding.[1] Therefore, at hematocrits of 20% and above it is impossible to conceive of the red cells having any lifetime separate from each other. Continuous interactions result in appreciable radial dispersion of cells which, at the periphery of the tube, lead to wall collisions. This, in turn, affects the movements of the smaller and less numerous platelets that otherwise would be estimated to spend only 2 or 3% of their time as collision doublets.

Flow Behavior at Normal Hematocrits

To probe into the movements of particles in the interior of a crowded suspension one has to make it transparent to light, since otherwise the rays are reflected and refracted in all directions and no detail can be discerned under the microscope. In blood this can be achieved by use of reconstituted biconcave ghost cells in plasma[18, 19] to which trace amounts of normal blood cells from the same donor, or latex spheres, can be added and used to follow particle motions in the interior of the tube.

The tracer red cell movements in a ghost cell suspension at volume concentrations ≥40% are strikingly different from those described in very dilute systems. The cell no longer rotates as a biconcave disc with periodically varying angular velocity,[5] but instead is continually deformed into a variety of shapes that suggest that the membrane is rotating about the cell interior.[19, 20] The degree of deformation and the alignment of the cells in the direction of flow increases with increasing ghost-cell concentration. Only in the core of the tube, where the velocity gradient is close to zero, are biconcave tracer red cells observed.

At the same time, as illustrated in FIGURE 3, the paths of the cells in the tube are subjected to continuous erratic radial displacements, whose magnitude at a given concentration is greatest at radial distances between 0.5 R_0 and 0.8 R_0. Closer to the tube wall, the amplitude in radial displacement is reduced; e.g. the root mean square radial distance moved in one second was 5.6 and 7.1% of the tube radius, respectively, for the RBC in curves 1 and 2 of FIGURE 3. The amplitude is also less near the tube center, where the velocity gradients are very low. In a given tube, the magnitude of the displacements increases with increasing ghost-cell concentration, reaching a maximum between 30 and 45%.[19] At very high concentrations (>60%), the crowding of ghost cells in the system, while leading to increased particle deformation, limits the amplitude of the radial excursions of the red cells.

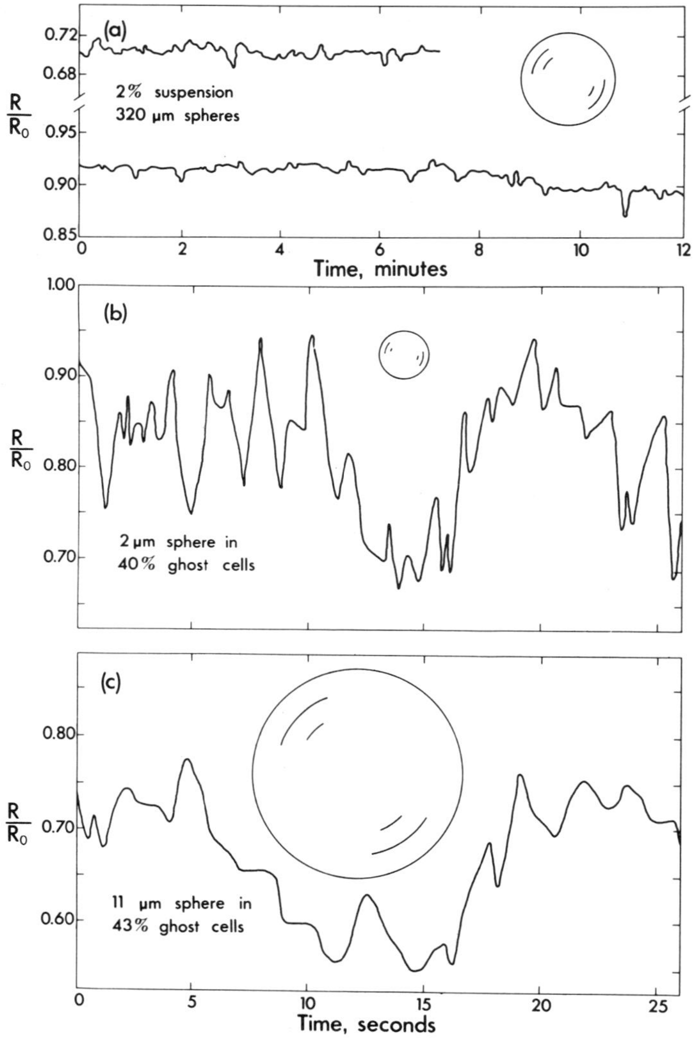

FIGURE 2. The radial position R (relative to the tube radius R_0) of rigid spheres with time in (a) a very dilute suspension of particles in an oil in which the small displacements were due to two body collisions [17] ($R_0 = 4$ mm); (b) and (c) in concentrated ghost-cell suspensions where the displacements are much larger, both relative to the sphere diameter (shown in each panel) and to the tube radius, $R_0 = 38$ μm. The effect of size on the particle movements is illustrated in panels (b) and (c).

The effect of tracer particle size on the radial displacements is illustrated for the case of rigid spheres in FIGURE 2 (which also shows the pronounced increase of the displacements in going from the two-body collisions in panel (a), to the interactions in concentrated suspensions in panels (b) and (c)).

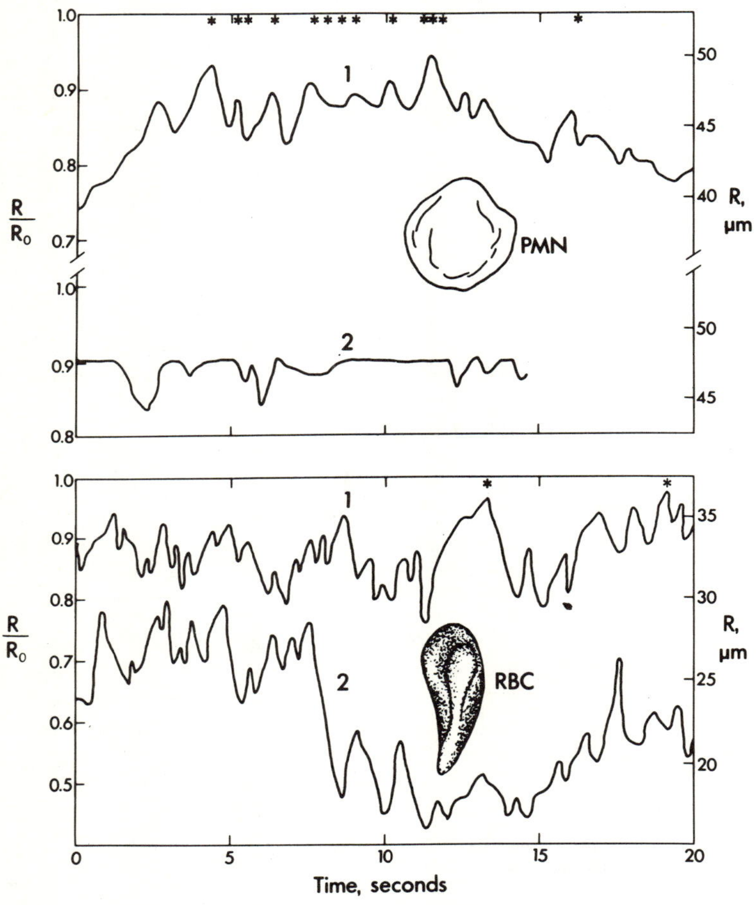

FIGURE 3. The radial position with time (as in FIGURE 2) of a tracer human polymorphonuclear leukocyte (PMN) and a red cell (RBC) in a 40%-ghost-cell suspension; $R_0 = 53$ μm (upper) and 38 μm (lower). The particles which were tracked along paths 1 in the periphery of the tube collided with the wall at times indicated with an asterisk. The slightly deformed PMN and the considerably deformed RBC were drawn from actual cinemicrographs and are typical of the shapes seen during flow.

It is evident that the increase in sphere diameter results both in a lower amplitude and frequency of radial movement. Thus the root mean square radial displacements for the 2- and 11-μm particles were 6.9 and 4.5% of the tube radius over a period of one second. The behavior of the 2-μm sphere may be expected to imitate that of a platelet in blood flow. Similar, though not so striking, differences are observed between human RBC and polymorphonuclear leukocytes (PMN), as shown in FIGURE 3. The PMN undergoes some deformation from the spherical shape in the ghost-cell suspension, but this is not as drastic as that of the RBC, as illustrated by the shapes drawn in the figure from cinemicrographs.

Cell-Wall Interactions

One of the earliest questions raised by researchers in blood rheology,[21, 22] and still debated today, is to what extent is there a reduction in red cell concentration near the endothelial wall of vessels and how deep into the interior does the cell-depleted zone extend. Since visual observations can be made only in smaller arteries and veins,[9] the only *in vivo* measurements stem from examination of sections of quick-frozen rabbit femoral arteries.[23] This work, and the *in vitro* analysis of cine films of blood flow in glass tubes [24] as well as measurements of the reduction in ghost-cell concentration at the vessel periphery [25] makes it appear unlikely that at hematocrits of 40–45% and normal flow rates, the plasma-rich zone can be much larger than 4 μm in vessels whose diameters exceed 100 μm. The resistance to crowding by the particles at these high-volume concentrations will oppose any appreciable inward migration from the wall, such as would have occurred in more dilute suspensions.

Such resistance to crowding is seen at the microscopic level as the continuous interactions between the cells which produce the marked radial displacements illustrated in FIGURES 2 and 3. For particles at radial distances $>0.9\ R_0$, as shown in FIGURE 3 by the asterisks, this leads to collisions with the tube wall. In the case of the 2-μm spheres, it has been shown that the large amplitude of the radial excursions can bring the smaller particles all the way from the core of the tube to the wall. Certainly the increased radial dispersion of platelets due to the presence of red cells in blood flow is well established,[26, 27] a dispersion which leads to an increased adhesion of platelets to surfaces with increasing hematocrit [28, 29] and results in an increased frequency of collision between platelets and the glass beads in the platelet retention test.[30] Recently, it has also been suggested that the increase in platelet momentum induced by the red cell motions might result in platelet-surface collisions of higher energy.[29]

It remains now to consider platelet and red blood cell behavior in channels where there are eddies in a region of separated flow.

BLOOD CELLS IN AN ANNULAR VORTEX

Thus far, we have described the flow of human red cells in straight, rigid, unbranched tubes, whereas the circulation consists of distensible vessels of continually changing diameter. There are also innumerable bifurcations, T-branches, and bends, where it is known that early atherosclerotic changes in the vessel wall occur more often than elsewhere in the arterial tree,[31, 32] and there is evidence that platelet aggregates accumulate and are deposited onto the wall at these sites.[33] Blood flow through channels of the above geometry can result in a separation of the streamlines from the vessel wall with backflow and the formation of a vortex between the forward flowing mainstream and the wall. The work outlined below was motivated by our interest in the contribution made by fluid mechanical factors to the formation of platelet aggregates in a region of flow separation. We had previously investigated the flow of blood cells and rigid spheres in a vortex formed distal to an asymmetric spherical obstruction in a tube [6] and had shown that particle aggregates could accumulate in a flow region associated with the vortex. Recently, Morton *et al.*[34] have shown that platelet aggregates form and grow in the vortex situated in the corner of a forward-facing step surrounding a stagnation point flow chamber. We have used an idealized model of flow at an arterial constriction consisting of an abrupt axisymmetric expansion of a 150-μm tube opening squarely into a 500-μm tube.[35, 36] *In vitro* studies using constrictions and abrupt expansions,[37–39] as well as *in vivo* experiments with implanted orifice rings,[40] have previously demonstrated that platelet thrombus formation and adhesion to the wall occur in the region of the vortex. Such work was mostly used to test the compatibility of biomaterials on the surface of the flow channel to blood, rather than to study the relation between the flow regime and platelet aggregation. Hence, we carried out microscopic observations of the detailed motions of red blood cells, platelets, and latex spheres of 2.6–50 μm diameter in the annular vortex formed at the corner of the tubular expansion [36] (FIGURE 4).

Particle Size and Flow in the Vortex: Dilute Suspensions

The paths and orientations of normal and gluteraldehyde-hardened human red cells (HBC) in dilute suspensions within the vortex were determined at Reynolds numbers Re (based on the upstream tube radius) from 0 to 75:

$$\mathrm{Re} = \frac{2R_0\bar{U}\rho}{\eta}, \qquad \textbf{(6)}$$

$\bar{U}$ being the mean linear (steady) fluid velocity, ρ and η the respective fluid density and viscosity. As illustrated in FIGURE 4, in steady flow a triangular-shaped vortex formed at the corner of the expansion the length of which increased with increasing Re. At the lower Re, and in the almost circular orbits close to the vortex center, the cells traveled with virtually constant linear velocities, whereas in the outer, more elliptical orbits, the velocities varied considerably, being high in the forward flowing portion of the vortex, low in the reverse flow region, and remaining low until forward motion was resumed.

The orbits traced out by the HBC shown in FIGURE 4 were in good agreement with theory [41] that predicts that fluid in the vortex circulates in closed streamlines. It was observed, however, that at low Reynolds numbers (<15) HBC, RBC, platelets, and latex spheres <20-μm diameter migrated spirally outward across the fluid streamlines and rejoined the mainstream. By contrast, the larger latex spheres and aggregates of HBC > 30-μm diameter remained in the vortex at all Re and were situated close to or at the center of the vortex. Measurements of the residence times of cells and spheres in the vortex (defined as the interval between the onset of flow with the vortex filled with particles and the last sphere rejoining the mainstream) showed that there existed a critical Re at which one or two particles remained indefinitely in the vortex circulating in an equilibrium orbit. Results obtained for three sizes of latex spheres are given in TABLE 1. As Re was further increased, more and more spheres remained within the annular vortex and there were frequent collisions, some of which resulted in the formation of nonseparating doublets of spheres which, because of the increase in particle size, migrated into the center; others resulted in the elimination of one or both of the spheres from the vortex.

Thus, at sufficiently low Reynolds numbers, the vortex in steady flow acted as a region in which larger particles and aggregates could accumulate, while

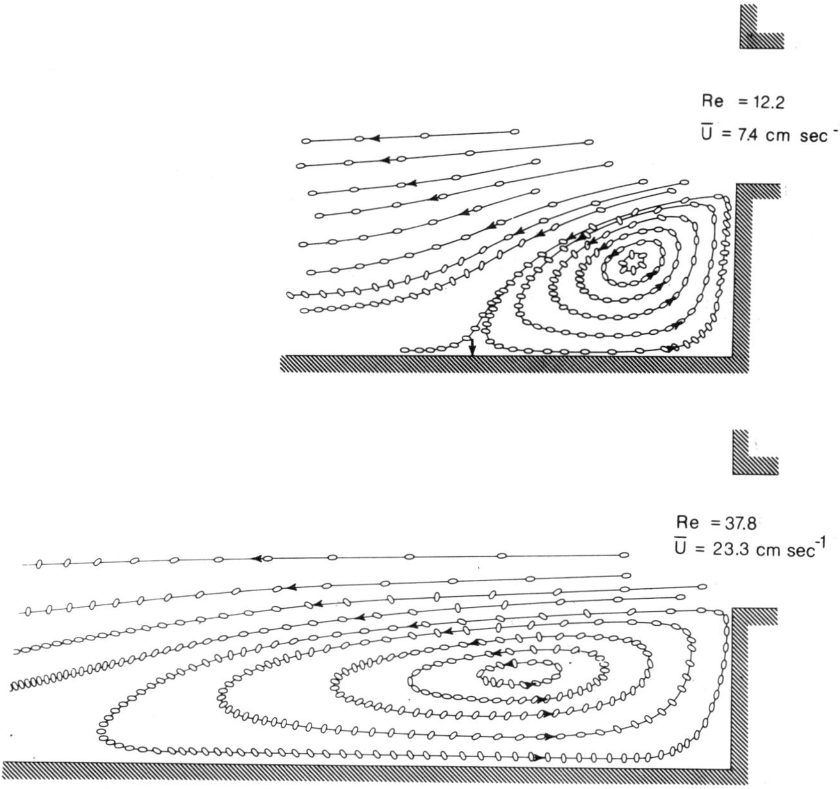

FIGURE 4. The paths and orientations of human gluteraldehyde-hardened red cells in orbits of the annular vortex formed at the sudden, concentric entry of a 150-μm into a 500-μm diameter tube at two different Reynolds numbers; $\bar{U}$ is the mean linear velocity in the 150-μm tube. The arrow in the upper part indicates the point of re-attachment of the flow.

the smaller particles eventually rejoined the mainstream of the suspension. The same particle-size dependent migration (aggregates remaining in the vortex) was observed in pulsatile flow at frequencies of ½–3 cycles/second. The cells described spiral orbits of continually changing diameter, as illustrated in FIGURE 5, and the vortex moved in phase with the upstream fluid velocity.[36]

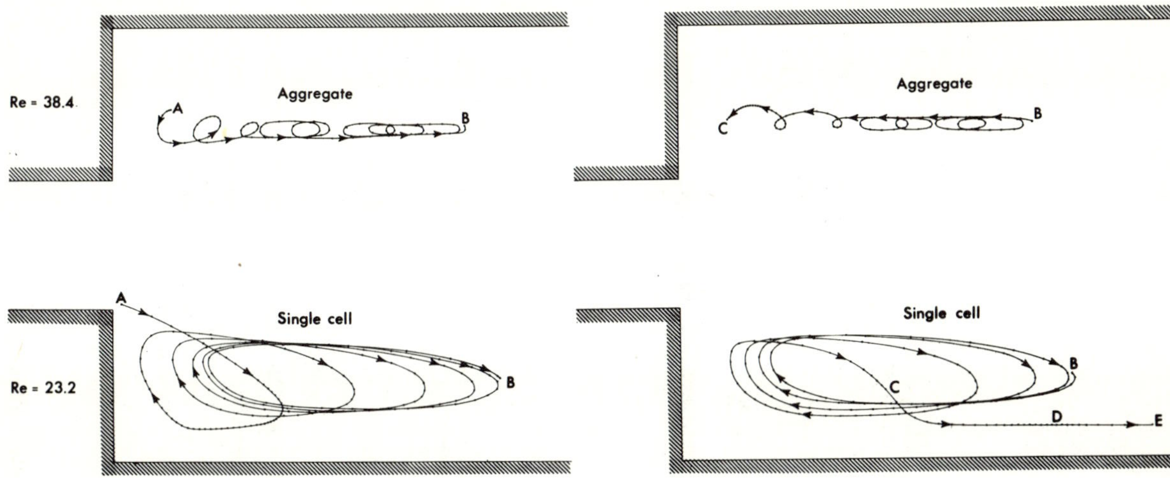

FIGURE 5. The spiral orbits followed by a single HBC (lower part) and a 55-μm aggregate of cells (upper part) in pulsatile flow during the advance (left) and recession (right) of the vortex during one cycle. The cell, initially at A (outside the vortex) was caught up in the advancing vortex and followed a series of expanding orbits reaching the furthest point B at the end of the forward part of the cycle. During the receding part, the cell executed a series of shrinking orbits, the last of which took it to a position outside the retreating vortex, and as flow changed direction again, the cell rejoined the mainstream along CDE. By contrast, the aggregate remained within the oscillating vortex along spiral orbits that took it from A to B and back again to C, close to its starting point. Pulsatile flow was obtained by superimposing a sinusoidal oscillatory flow at 1.5 cycles/second in parallel with a steady flow at Re=38 (upper) and Re=23 (lower). (By permission of the publishers of Phil. Trans. Roy. Soc.[36])

Concentrated Suspensions of Red Cells

Red cells in plasma at hematocrits from 15 to 45% were also observed to migrate out of the vortex in steady flow at low Reynolds numbers, sometimes resulting in a completely cell-free annular region, at other times leaving behind a few large rouleaux circulating in equilibrium orbits near the center. At higher Re, an equilibrium red cell concentration was established in the vortex, as cells both entered and left the annular region.

In pulsatile flow, the periodic changes in vortex size and intensity were here accompanied by variations in red cell concentration; the hematocrit was lower in the advancing than in the receding period of the flow, and at all times lower than that in the mainstream. At a given amplitude of the oscillatory flow, the concentration of red cells in the vortex increased with increasing frequency and reservoir hematocrit.

TABLE 1

RESIDENCE TIMES OF POLYSTYRENE SPHERES IN VORTEX

Reynolds Number	Residence Time, Seconds ± s.d. 9.8 μm	20 μm	32 μm
2.3	25.0 ± 7.0	26.1 ± 10.4	>600*
4.5	13.4 ± 5.2	23.1 ± 9.3	>600*
6.6	9.9 ± 1.9	15.2 ± 5.0	>600*
9.1	12.9 ± 3.4	25.2 ± 12.9	>600*
15	135 ± 83	>600*	>600*
24	>600*	>600†	>600*
45	>600†	>600†	>600*
110	>600‡	>600‡	>600‡

* 1–3 spheres remain in orbit.
† 5–15 remain in orbit.
‡ Large numbers remain in orbit.

Platelets in the Vortex

The aggregation of platelets in the vortex was studied at 37° C with use of platelet-rich plasma (PRP) or washed platelets suspended in Tyrodes-albumin solution containing apyrase.[42] It was found that in a given suspension the formation and growth of platelet thrombi could be observed only in a range of Reynolds numbers between 3 and 15, when, on the one hand, the particles spent sufficient time circulating in the vortex for frequent interactions to occur, and, on the other hand, the shear stresses acting on the particles in the orbits were low enough for an appreciable fraction of the collisions to result in the production of nonseparating doublets and higher order multiplets.

TABLE 2 gives a summary of the results obtained at Re = 10 in steady flow. It can be seen that in heparinized PRP (2 units heparin/ml blood), which contained a few small, loosely bound aggregates even before the suspension was subjected to flow, pronounced aggregation occurred. The events were recorded on cine film and the progressive formation of thrombi followed in detail. Initially, small aggregates (2–5 platelets) were formed through collisions between platelets circulating in orbits near the periphery of the vortex. These then migrated into smaller orbits near the center, where they grew in size as more aggregates arrived from the periphery. Eventually, one large aggregate was formed, and being about 600 μm long, stretched half-way around the annulus in the center of the vortex. It consisted of a large number of smaller platelet thrombi loosely held together in the flow, and broke up into its constituent parts if the flow was disturbed.

TABLE 2 shows that in citrated PRP the degree of aggregation was much reduced, a thrombus of about 20–30 μm diameter being formed that did not

TABLE 2

AGGREGATION OF HUMAN PLATELETS IN THE ANNULAR VORTEX

Suspension	Additive	Threshold Concentration in Aggregometer	Degree of Aggregation in Vortex
Heparinized PRP	none	2×10^{-6} M ADP	++++
	1mg/ml ASA	2×10^{-6} M ADP	++++
Citrated PRP	none	2×10^{-6} M ADP	++
	1mg/ml ASA	2×10^{-6} M ADP	++
	1.3×10^{-7} M ADP	2×10^{-6} M ADP †	++++
Washed platelets in Tyrodes-albumin (apyrase)	none	0.03 units/ml thrombin	0 to +
	0.5g/l fibrinogen		+ to ++
Washed platelets in Tyrodes-albumin (apyrase+fibrinogen)	none	0.025 units/ml thrombin †	+ to ++
	10^{-6} M ADP		++
	0.01 units/ml thrombin		+
	0.02 units/ml thrombin		++++

† Tests done on the original suspension.

grow further in size. However, when the PRP was activated with ADP at a concentration below the threshold required to produce a reaction in a Payton aggregometer, the large particle seen in the heparinized PRP was again formed. ASA, which suppressed the collagen-induced reaction in the aggregometer, had no effect on thrombus formation in the vortex.

The degree of aggregation observed in the washed platelet suspensions was less than that in the PRP, although the addition of fibrinogen (0.5 gm/l) to the Tyrodes-albumin increased the number of 10–20 μm diameter aggregates formed in the vortex. Here, the addition of subthreshold concentrations of thrombin [43] again resulted in the formation of one very large aggregate.

When the above suspensions were subjected to pulsatile flow in the tubular expansion, the formation of a single large aggregate was never observed. Presumably, the continuously changing orbits during the alternate expansion and contraction of the vortex (see FIGURE 5) did not permit the growth of one large thrombus. Nevertheless, single smaller platelet thrombi were observed in the heparinized and citrated PRP as well as in the washed platelet suspension containing fibrinogen.

A few experiments carried out with heparinized whole blood also revealed the formation and growth of platelet thrombi.

Applications to in Vivo *Blood Flow*

Stenoses produced by the growth of intravascular plaques are not uncommon in the arteries of mammals. Once formed, the subsequent development of the constriction will be affected by the flow condition at and downstream of the stenosis. It is suspected that among the effects of disturbed flow at a stenosis in an artery is the deposition of platelets and platelet aggregates in the region of flow separation.[11, 15, 31] Previous work in this laboratory has shown that aggregates of 2-μm spheres serving as models of blood platelets accumulate in the low flow rate region of a vortex formed downstream of an asymmetric, one-sided spherical obstruction in a tube.[6] Flow at the sudden expansion described above, which provided an idealized model of conditions downstream of an axisymmetric stenosis, demonstrated that platelet aggregates can accumulate and grow within the annular vortex. The effect was much more pronounced in platelet suspensions activated by ADP and thrombin. In this connection, the possibility that platelets may be activated by exposure to the high and variable shear stresses existing at the entry and within the region of the vortex should be raised.[6, 11, 20] Experiments have shown that platelet aggregation in plasma[45] and the release reaction in Tyrodes-albumin[43] are stimulated by exposure to high shear stresses.

Finally, the observed red cell migration out of the vortex, both in steady and pulsatile flow, make it probable that in the living system, the region of separated flow will be one of relatively low hematocrit. This would result in a lowered availability of oxygen for the artery wall, which, it has been claimed, might lead to an increased atherogenesis.[46]

ACKNOWLEDGMENTS

We thank Mary Pitteway and Jean Marlow for their excellent technical assistance, and Pamela Lilley for typing this manuscript.

REFERENCES

1. GOLDSMITH, H. L. & S. G. MASON. 1967. The microrheology of dispersions. *In* Rheology: Theory and Applications. Vol. IV. F. R. Eirich, Ed. : 85–250. Academic Press, New York, N.Y.
2. COX, R. G. & S. G. MASON. 1971. Suspended particles in fluid flow through tubes. Ann. Rev. Fluid. Mech. **3:** 291–316.
3. GOLDSMITH, H. L. & S. G. MASON. 1975. Some model experiments in hemodynamics—V. Microrheological techniques. Biorheology **12:** 181–192.
4. GOLDSMITH, H. L. 1971. Red cell motions and wall interactions in tube flow. Fed. Proc. **30:** 1578–1588.

5. Goldsmith, H. L. & J. Marlow. 1972. Flow behaviour of erythrocytes. I. Rotation and deformation in dilute suspensions. Proc. Roy. Soc. B **182:** 351–384.
6. Yu, S. K. & H. L. Goldsmith. 1973. Behavior of model particles and blood cells at spherical obstructions in tube flow. Microvas. Res. **6:** 5–31.
7. Bloch, E. H. 1962. A quantitative study of the hemodynamics in the living microvascular system. Amer. J. Anat. **110:** 125–153.
8. Brånemark, P.-I. 1966. Intravital microscopy. Its present status and potentialities. Med. Biol. Ill. **16:** 100.
9. Schmid-Schönbein, G. & B. W. Zweifach. 1975. RBC velocity profiles in arterioles and venules of the rabbit omentum. Microvas. Res. **10:** 153–164.
10. Frojmovic, M. M., M. Newton & H. L. Goldsmith. 1976. The microrheology of mammalian platelets: studies of rheo-optical transients and flow in tubes. Microvas. Res. **11:** 203–215.
11. Goldsmith, H. L. 1972. The flow of model particles and blood cells and its relation to thrombogenesis. *In* Progress in Hemostasis and Thrombosis. Vol. 1. T. H. Spaet, Ed. : 97–139. Grune and Stratton. New York, N.Y.
12. Schmid-Schönbein, H. & R. E. Wells, Jr. 1971. Rheological properties of human erythrocytes and their influence upon the "anomalous" viscosity of blood. Ergeb. Physiologie **63:** 146–219.
13. Schmid-Schönbein, H. 1975. Erythrocyte rheology and the optimization of mass transport in the microcirculation. Blood Cells **1:** 285–306.
14. Segré, G. & A. Silberberg. 1962. Behaviour of macroscopic rigid spheres in Poiseuille flow. II. Experimental results and interpretation. J. Fluid Mech. **14:** 136–157.
15. Goldsmith, H. L. & S. G. Mason. 1971. Some model experiments in hemodynamics IV. *In* Theoretical and Clinical Hemorheology. H. H. Hartert & A. L. Copley, Eds. : 47–59. Springer-Verlag. New York, N.Y.
16. Brenner, H. 1966. Hydrodynamic resistance of particles at small Reynolds numbers. *In* Advances in Chemical Engineering. Vol. 6. T. R. Drew, J. W. Hoopes, Jr. & T. Vermeulen, Eds. : 287–438. Academic Press. New York, N.Y.
17. Karnis, A., H. L. Goldsmith & S. G. Mason. 1966. The kinetics of flowing dispersions. I. Concentrated suspensions of rigid particles. J. Colloid Interface Sci. **22:** 531–553.
18. Goldsmith, H. L. 1967. The microscopic flow properties of red cells. Fed. Proc. **26:** 1813–1820.
19. Goldsmith, H. L. & J. Marlow. 1976. Flow behaviour of erythrocytes. II. Concentrated suspensions of ghost cells. To be submitted.
20. Goldsmith, H. L., S. S. K. Yu & J. Marlow. 1975. Fluid mechanical stress and the platelet. Thromb. Diath. Haemorrh. **34:** 32–41.
21. Fahraeus, R. & T. Lindqvist. 1931. The viscosity of blood in narrow capillary tubes. Amer. J. Physiol. **96:** 562–568.
22. Scott-Blair, G. W. 1959. An equation for the flow of blood, plasma and serum through glass capillaries. Nature **183:** 613–614.
23. Phibbs, R. H. 1969. Orientation and distribution of erythrocytes in blood flowing through medium-sized arteries. *In* Hemorheology. A. L. Copley, Ed. : 617–630. Pergamon Press. New York, N.Y.
24. Bugliarello, G. & J. Sevilla. 1971. Velocity distribution and other characteristics of steady and pulsatile flow in fine glass capillaries. Biorheology **7:** 85–107.
25. Blackshear, P. L., Jr., R. J. Forstrom, F. D. Dorman & G. O. Voss. 1971. Effect of flow on cells near walls. Fed. Proc. **30:** 1600–1609.
26. Turitto, V. T., A. M. Benis & E. F. Leonard. 1972. Platelet diffusion in flowing blood. Ind. Eng. Chem. Fund. **11:** 216–223.
27. Feuerstein, I. A., J. Brophy & J. L. Brash. 1975. Platelet transport and adhesion to reconstituted collagen and reconstituted surfaces. Trans. Amer. Soc. Art. Int. Organs. **21:** 427–435.

28. FRIEDMAN, L. I. & E. F. LEONARD. 1971. Platelet adhesion to artificial surfaces: consequences of flow, exposure time, blood condition, and surface nature. Fed. Proc. **30:** 1641–1646.
29. BRASH, J. L., J. M. BROPHY & I. A. FEUERSTEIN. 1976. Adhesion of platelets to artificial surfaces: Effect of red cells. J. Biomed. Mater. Res. **10:** 429–443.
30. ZUCKER, M. B., P. L. RIFKIN, N. M. FRIEDBERG & B. S. COLLER. 1972. Mechanism of platelet function as revealed by the retention of platelets in glass bead columns. Ann. N.Y. Acad. Sci. **201:** 138–144.
31. FOX, J. A. & A. E. HUGH. 1966. Localization of atheroma. A theory based on boundary layer separation. Brit. Heart J. **28:** 388–399.
32. CARO, C. G., J. M. FITZ-GERALD & R. C. SCHROTER. 1971. Atheroma and arterial wall shear. Observation, correlation and proposal of a shear dependent mass transfer mechanism for atherogenesis. Proc. Roy. Soc. B. **177:** 109–159.
33. PACKHAM, M. A., H. C. ROWSELL, L. JØRGENSEN & J. F. MUSTARD. 1967. Localized protein accumulation in the wall of the aorta. Exp. Mol. Pathol. **7:** 214–232.
34. MORTON, W. A., E. M. PARMENTIER & H. E. PETSCHEK. 1975. Study of aggregate formation in region of separated blood flow. Thromb. Diath. Haemorrh. **34:** 840–854.
35. GOLDSMITH, H. L. 1974. Blood flow and thrombosis. Thromb. Diath. Haemorrh. **32:** 35–48.
36. KARINO, T. & H. L. GOLDSMITH. 1976. Flow behaviour of blood cells and rigid spheres in an annular vortex. Phil. Trans. Roy. Soc. In press.
37. BLACKSHEAR, P. L., R. J. FORSTROM, M. LOBERBAUM, V. L. GOTT & R. SOVILJ. 1971. A role of flow separation and recirculation in thrombus formation on prosthetic surfaces. AIAA 9th Aerospace Sciences Meeting. Paper 71-103, New York, N.Y.
38. BENIS, A. M., H. L. NOSSEL, L. M. ALEDORT, R. M. KOFFSKY, J. F. STEVENSON, E. F. LEONARD, H. SHIANG & R. S. LITWAK. 1975. Extracorporeal model for study of factors affecting thrombus formation. Thromb. Diath. Haemorrh. **34:** 127–144.
39. SMITH, R. L., E. F. BLICK, J. COALSON & P. D. STEIN. 1972. Thrombus production by turbulence. J. Appl. Physiol. **32:** 261–264.
40. FOSTER, E. D. & A. R. C. DOBELL. 1971. Evaluation of rigid prosthetic rings as *in vivo* intravascular thrombogenic models. J. Surg. Res. **11:** 550–558.
41. MACAGNO, E. O. & T.-K. HUNG. 1967. Computational and experimental study of a captive annular eddy. J. Fluid Mech. **28:** 43–64.
42. MUSTARD, J. F., D. W. PERRY, N. G. ARDLIE & M. A. PACKHAM. 1972. Preparation of suspensions of washed platelets from humans. Brit. J. Haematol. **22:** 193–204.
43. GOLDSMITH, H. L., J. C. MARLOW & S. K. YU. 1976. The effect of oscillatory flow on the release reaction and aggregation of human platelets. Microvas. Res. **11:** 335–359.
44. YU, S. K. & H. L. GOLDSMITH. 1975. Some rheological aspects of platelet thrombosis. *In* Platelets, Drugs and Thrombosis. J. Hirsch, Ed. : 78–93. Karger. Basel, Switzerland.
45. BROWN, C. H., L. B. LEVERETT, C. W. LEWIS, C. P. ALFREY, JR., & J. D. HELLUMS. 1975. Morphological, biochemical and functional changes in human platelets subjected to shear stress. J. Lab. Clin. Med. **86:** 462–471.
46. BACK, L. H. 1975. Theoretical investigation of mass transport to arterial walls in various blood flow regions. II. Oxygen transport and its relationship to lipoprotein accumulation. Math. Biosciences **27:** 263–285.

BLOOD ELEMENTS AT FOREIGN SURFACES: ANALYSIS OF INHOMOGENEITIES IN ADSORBED LAYERS OF PROTEINS AND PLATELETS *

Edward F. Leonard and Yves Butrille

Artificial Organs Research Laboratory
School of Engineering
Columbia University
New York, New York 10027

Saul Puszkin and Shaul Kochwa

Mt. Sinai School of Medicine
New York, New York 10029

INTRODUCTION

Thrombus initiation does not usually occur uniformly over a surface. This paper is concerned with how *patterns* of nonuniformity in surface chemical reactions thought to be part of the thrombus-forming process may be described and analyzed.

Some patterns are essentially *deterministic:* they can be seen to occur in relation to a reference locus on a surface in accord with an analytical relationship. A germane example is the adhesion of blood platelets downstream from the leading edge of a glass disc over which blood is flowing. Grabowski *et al.*[1] showed that for such a case the platelet density follows the Leveque equation:

$$\bar{\rho} = 2/3 \ (2 \ \beta/\bar{x})^{1/3} \ \bar{t}$$

where $\bar{x}$ and $\bar{t}$ are proportional to axial distance and time respectively, β is a physical constant, and $\bar{\rho}$ is proportional to the local platelet density. The relationship predicts that $\bar{\rho}$ varies with the cube root of distance from the leading edge; it is thus *essentially* deterministic.

However, some patterns are essentially *stochastic:* dense and sparse areas can be predicted from those starting conditions that are known only in a probabilistic sense; repetition of such experiments will produce the same result only in the sense that the patterns will be samples from a definite population of all such patterns and this population will have large variability.

Analysis of deterministic patterns is straightforward. The distribution is experimentally measured, often along special loci dictated by the available analytical relationship, and compared with that relationship, often in such a manner as to identify its unspecified parameters. On the other hand, analysis of stochastic patterns (*pattern recognition*) is not straightforward, as will be shown repeatedly in subsequent parts of this paper. Such analysis, however, can be fruitful, particularly when used to test specific hypotheses about the behavior of the system of interest. Experiments described in previous [6] and contemporaneous [9] papers from our group demonstrate several kinds of stochastic patterns that suggest: (1) features of the mechanism of platelet-platelet

* Supported in part by Contract NO1–HB–3–2910 from the National Heart, Lung, and Blood Institutes, NIH.

interactions on surfaces; (2) macroscopic variations in protein adsorption on surfaces (apparently similar in a stochastic sense among samples of the same material, from the same batch and identically treated but apparently different among batches, materials, and methods of treatment); (3) correlation between patterns of protein adsorption and platelet adhesion. In this paper consideration is given to these situations in which stochastic patterns related to thrombus formation are generated, and attention is directed as to how information about the roles of material, blood condition, and fluid mechanics can be inferred from these patterns.

From published descriptions of studies by Baier and Dutton,[12] Dutton *et al.*,[13] Petschek and colleagues,[14] and Vroman *et al.*,[7] in all of which stochastic patterns of cell or protein adhesion were at least sometimes found, it appears that such pattern analysis may be applicable to other situations related to thrombogenesis.

Principles of Pattern Recognition

The essence of the pattern-recognition problem as it pertains to thrombogenesis can be described by an example. In 1967 two of our colleagues † disagreed regarding whether a surface that was some 30% covered with adherent canine platelets showed a meaningful pattern, such as streaking or clustering, or whether the picture could have arisen purely on the basis of equal *a priori* probability of a particle adhering to any empty position. Using a simple computer program randomly to assign occupancy to each site in a matrix, we generated a pattern like that of Figure 1. (For details, see legend.) If such a pattern were to be produced by exposure of a surface to platelets, the areas labeled 1 suggest streaking, those labeled 2 suggest clustering, and those labeled 3 a refractory zone, but, in fact, this mathematically generated pattern is random. Such pictures show that recognizing nonrandom clustering is not easy.

Testing actual surface patterns to demonstrate significant features can be done by two basic methods: scanning the surface for defined subpatterns, much as a modern bank check might be scanned for characters printed with magnetic ink, after which the subpatterns are examined in detail to determine their nature. Techniques such as template matching, common properties (example: only the number 8 has two closed loops), or clustering can be used. With the clustering technique, each subpattern is somehow described as a set of N numerical values and correspondingly assigned a point in N-dimensional "pattern space"; it is hoped that this point will be in a part of the space that is unique for one of the characters to be recognized.

In some instances, separation of subpatterns is difficult or undesirable, and "scene analysis" is employed. A two-dimensional black and white picture can be considered to be a mathematical function $q(i,j)$ that can be obtained digitally and variously processed to enhance the clarity of edges, smooth out noise, find a prescribed shape in the picture, identify connected regions in which the density is constant, and trace contours. A fundamental technique for scene analysis is the two-dimensional Fourier transform, which can be efficiently calculated digitally or can be obtained directly, in analog form, by optical means. Fourier

† The conversation was between L. I. Friedman (Columbia University), who prepared the original random diagram, and Leo Vroman (Brooklyn V.A. Hospital) at an early meeting of the Columbia University Seminar on Biomaterials (1967).

FIGURE 1. 264 of 900 squares (29.3%) in a 30×30 array are filled according to the value of a random number N ($0 \leq N \leq 99$) assigned each square. For the filled squares, $N \leq 30$. To many observers such arrays incorrectly suggest nonrandom clustering.

transformation gives both theoretical meaning and operational convenience to most of the processes enumerated in the last sentence.

Much of pattern recognition is made tractable by foreknowledge of what is important in a picture. Special procedures exist for line description, shape description, and descriptions dependent upon metric properties (actual dimensions). These procedures are utilized to recognize suspected or desired aspects of a picture. Thus, because the overall field of pattern recognition is not governed by a universal theory, approaches to information retrieval are largely intuitive and influenced by the observer's expectations. While the form of questioning is thus biased, the answers can be statistically objectivized. In the balance of this paper three specific approaches to analysis of patterns of adhered blood platelet and adsorbed radiolabeled plasma proteins on artificial surfaces are described; results are given and interpretations made. Emphasis is placed on the formulation and testing of hypotheses that relate to current, useful concepts of the problem rather than to more abstract and general statistical concepts.

Application of Pattern-Recognition Theory to Platelet Adhesion on Surfaces Exposed as Spinning Discs: Microscopic Patterns

Most artificial surfaces, when spun as discs in stationary pools of fresh, heparinized canine blood, acquire a monolayer of adhered platelets. The platelet density may vary radially in a deterministic manner; it may also vary macroscopically in a random manner ("blotching," see below). In this section, however, attention is confined to patterns in pictures of small area (of diameter ca. 0.1 mm) in which only a few hundred platelets appear, whence large-scale variations are not apparent. The key questions are: Do the platelets adhere randomly or is the adherence of one platelet affected by the previous adherence of other platelets? Is the pattern isotropic (i.e., independent of the angular orientation at which the picture is viewed)? FIGURE 2A shows a typical photomicrograph of the sort under consideration; FIGURE 2B shows a digitized version of the same picture in which the symbol "1" marks the center of each platelet in the original picture. FIGURE 3 gives the "annular distribution function" of the digitized picture, FIGURE 2b. This function reports the probable platelet density (i.e., platelets per unit area) at various radii measured from a central, reference platelet. The annular distribution function should remain at unity for a random distribution. The picture of FIGURES 2a and 2b and others obtained under similar conditions show statistically significant variations from unity in two different radius ranges: For radii less than twice that of a platelet (i.e., 2 μm) the normalized density function is much less than unity, indicating that platelets do not adhere to other platelets to form multilayers; in fact, an incomplete monolayer forms under the conditions of this experiment. In the radius range 4–16 μm the normalized density function is significantly greater than unity, indicating a tendency toward clustering during formation of platelet monolayers.

Pictures taken at high spinning rates and analyzed in this manner appeared anisotropic: different clusters appeared similarly elongated, in a direction close to that of the gradient of shear rate on a spinning-disc surface, an angle of —0.880 radians with respect to the radius vector. (See FIGURE 4a.) In an attempt to quantify this observation, opposite sectors of included angle $\pi/8$

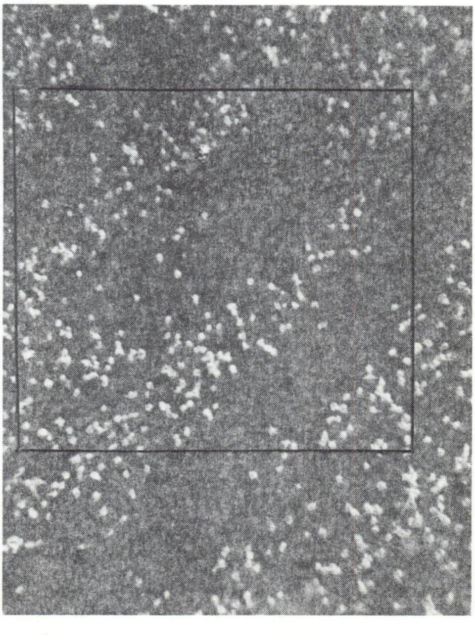

FIGURE 2A. Photomicrograph ($\times$364) of platelets adhered to Type A polyurethane, Stanford Research Institute. Note the appearance of anisotropic clusters.

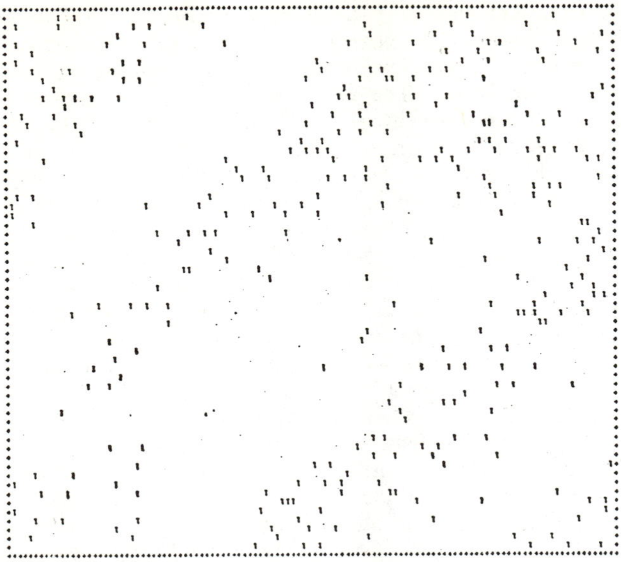

FIGURE 2B. Digitized picture corresponding to the area in FIGURE 2A enclosed by a rectangle. Each symbol "1" represents the center of one platelet. No other detail has been translated. (See FIGURE 2A).

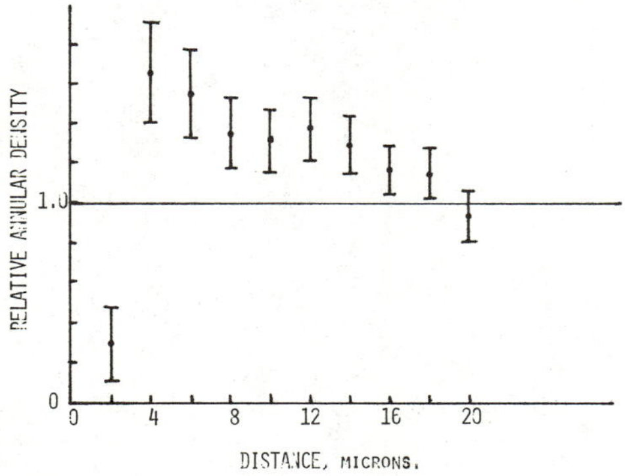

FIGURE 3. Relative annular density plotted versus distance from the center of a reference platelet. To obtain this function each platelet center in the original picture is taken, in its turn, as a reference point, and the number of platelets in an annulus of radii r, $r+\Delta r$ are counted. The count is divided by the area of the annulus, $2\pi r\Delta r$. The results for all reference points are averaged and then divided by the average density (platelets/area) to obtain the ordinate that is plotted. For a random pattern the ordinate should be a horizontal line with value 1. For details, including corrections for centers near the edges of the picture, see reference 6.

radians (see FIGURE 4b) were analyzed separately to produce 8 annular distribution functions, FIGURE 5. In these the direction of elongation is inferred as that in which the statistically significant elevation of the annular distribution function extends to the largest radius. According to this criterion the direction of maximum clustering is near to but not coincident with the gradient of shear rate on the surface.

The utility of establishing patterns of platelet adhesion can be demonstrated by the following line of reasoning, principally supported by pattern analysis:

1. Platelet adhesion rates from heparinized canine blood show a dependence on axial distance in lineal flow over a flat plate and on speed of rotation in axisymmetric flow near a spinning disc. These observations suggest that the process is dependent on platelet arrival rate, i.e., that it is "diffusion limited." [1]

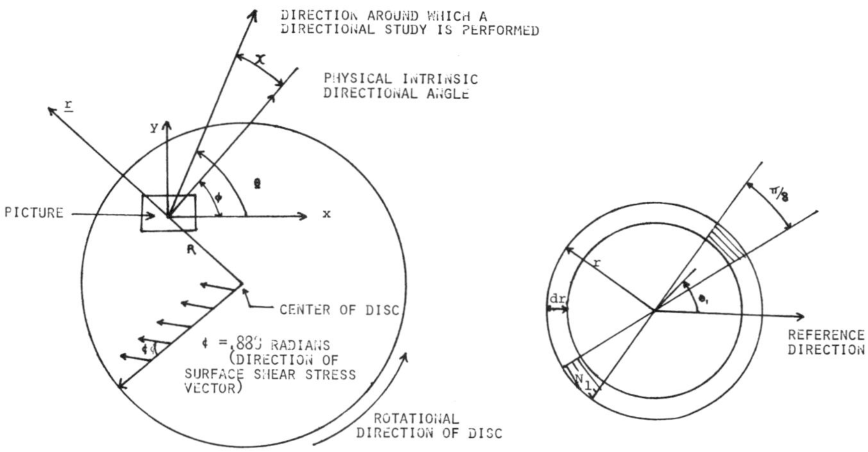

FIGURE 4. *Left:* Definition of two coordinate systems necessary for picture analysis. Points over the disc including that which locates the picture's center are located from the disc center ($r=R$ at picture center). Three angles plus x and y coordinates are used on the picture: x and y as shown, parallel to the edges of the picture, ϕ relating the x-axis to the tangent line (labeled physical intrinsic directional angle); χ relating an angle θ measured on the picture to the tangent line. Lines representing the shear stress vector on the surface are also shown.
Right: Definition of sector pairs for analysis of anisotropic pictures.

2. The fact that platelets cluster must mean, however, that rates of adhesion are perceptibly faster at some points on the surface (e.g. near where platelets have already adhered) than at others (e.g. far from other platelets or onto adhered platelets). Since the rate can nowhere be greater than the arrival rate, which is hard to imagine as other than uniform, many platelets must arrive in sparsely populated or unpopulated areas without subsequently adhering.

3. Arrival without adherence has the effect of causing platelets to accumulate near the surface and thus seemingly to make the reaction independent of how fast additional platelets arrive, contrary to the dependence on arrival rate that

is actually observed. The conundrum is solved if one postulates that *all* platelets arriving at a surface react, *some* to adhere and *some,* perhaps reacting less violently, to become at least temporarily passive to adhesion. That

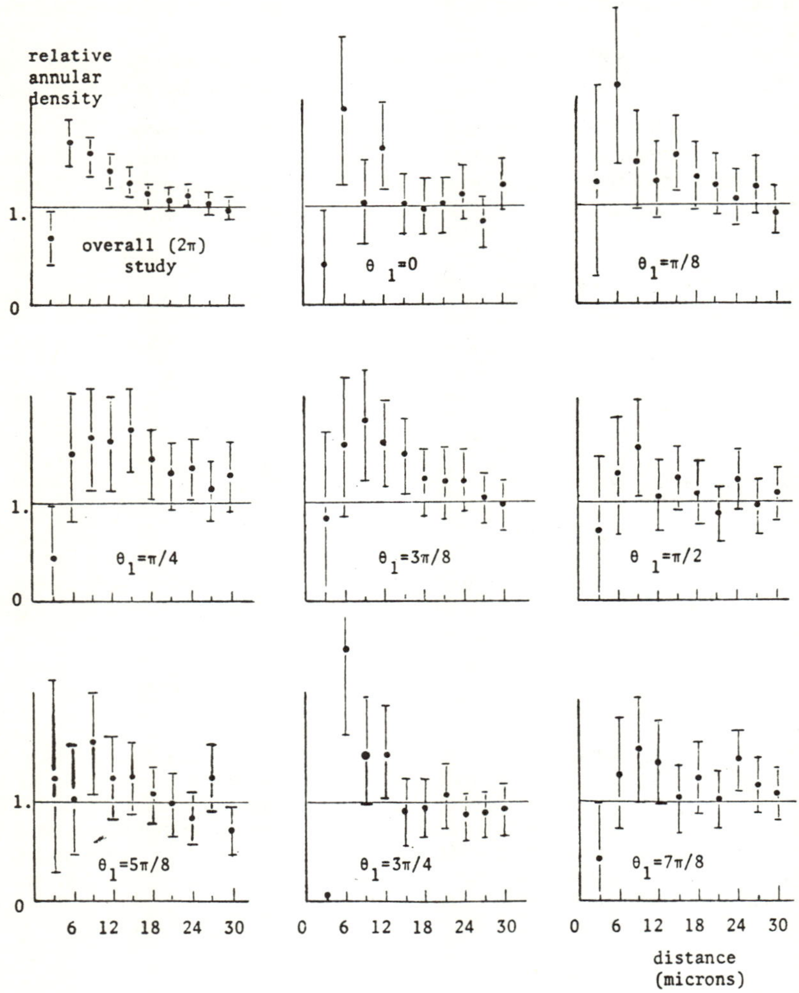

FIGURE 5. Angular annular distribution functions for the picture of FIGURE 2. Note that for angles θ of $\pi/4$ and $3\pi/8$, close to that on which the surface shear vector is pointed, the significant elevation of the relative annular density persists over the longest distance.

is, since some of the arriving platelets do not adhere and since the observed dependence on arrival rate proscribes the possibility of accumulating adherable platelets, all approaching platelets must react—some to adhere and some (whatever else they do) to become at least temporarily passive to adhesion.

The adherence reaction is more probable at a radius of 4–15 μm from an already adhered platelet than at other radii.

4. The dimensions of the clusters and increased anisotropy of adhesion with surface shear rate on the disc can be shown to be consistent with preadhered platelets serving as a source of an adhesion-potentiating metabolite of low molecular weight (i.e., with a molecular diffusion coefficient equal to about 10^{-5} cm^2/sec), and to be inconsistent with platelets serving as flow disturbances on the surface.

Although these studies strongly indicate that platelet adhesion in canine blood is strongly affected by prior adhesion, that the spreading of the effect from the adhered platelet is consistent with diffusive spreading when flow is low, and that the spreading is affected and redirected by flow at higher flows, the nature of the communication has not yet been established. Species such as adenosince diphosphate (ADP) released from the adhered platelet could be responsible, but preliminary studies in this laboratory indicate that such release may be very rapid and possibly inconsistent with observed time courses of reaction. It has not yet been proved that actual spreading of platelets may not occur with diffusion velocity and be affected by flow much as solute propagation is. In other studies with human blood, with use of the same apparatus and protocol, on similar polyurethane surfaces, the type of adhesion cited above did not occur. (After 20–25 minutes of spinning, some platelet aggregates believed to have been formed in the bulk did adhere.) Consistent with all of these observations but as yet unproved is the hypothesis that a low molecular weight agent released from platelets affects other platelets, with a perhaps complex dose effect, imparting to them a transient stickiness followed by a period of refractoriness to sticking. Work in progress is aimed at measuring the kinetics of ADP release from platelets consequent to the action of divalent-cation-activated ATP-ase that is responsible for the formation of actomyosin in adsorbed platelets.

Application of Pattern-Recognition Techniques to Analysis of the Adsorption of Radiolabeled Plasma Proteins from Aqueous Solutions to Surfaces Exposed as Discs: Blotching

Protein uptake by biomaterials is considered [1] an important indicator of how subsequent blood-surface interactions will take place. Whether the uptake is studied from solutions of one or more proteins the adsorption is assayed either by (1) counting of an isotopic label previously affixed to one or more of the dissolved proteins, (2) by spectrophotometric approaches, or (3) by a variety of gravimetric techniques (surface titration, disappearance of substances from solution, adsorption of traceable antibodies). All of these methods yield an average over substantial areas and most interpretations from them assume that the distributions are uniform. Systematic, quantitative scanning of protein layers to yield other than average densities on biomaterial surfaces appears not to have been undertaken. In a companion paper [2] is reported a technique for generating autoradiographic images of disk-shaped surfaces exposed, some by simple immersion some by spinning, to radiolabeled proteins. The films were scanned with a Zeiss TLC scanning spectrophotometer using a "window" of approximate size 50 × 50 μm each, the center of each sample being separated from its nearest neighbors by an interval of about 400 μm in one direction and 200 μm in the other. Although closer intervals and more points are possible and perhaps desirable, the present need to punch manually the value of each absorbance onto cards has imposed a temporary, practical limit on resolving power.

Two typical images (both of one autoradiograph of labeled gamma globulin on APTES heparinized silicone rubber, obtained from Carnegie Mellon University) are presented in FIGURE 6 by a pattern of digits representing assignment of the absorbance data into eleven levels designated 0, 1, 2, 3, 4, 5, 6, 7, 8, 9, *, lowest absorbance and thus lowest amount of radioactive protein on the original disc represented as zero, highest absorbance, and highest amount of protein as *. Both patterns were derived from the same image in the same orientation. In the top pattern the lower level (0–1) was set at an absorbance of .150 (cf. .075 in the lower pattern) and the higher level (9–*) was set at an absorbance of .337 (cf. .372 in the lower pattern). The patterns are qualitatively similar, indicating only moderate sensitivity to the levels chosen. Inspection indicates dense blotches ranging in size from 1 to 5 mm in the upper right-hand quadrant and in the center, with considerable additional detail on a millimeter scale. Such patterns are typical of other surfaces scanned, and on the basis of the limited analyses conducted so far cannot be said to be characteristic of the particular material.

The standard deviation of the points representing the picture is a crude measure of the nonuniformity of coverage. It is useful in quantitative comparison of the nonuniformity of different discs. For the circular area of the disc shown in FIGURE 6, the mean is .248 with a standard deviation of 0.076. In order to report the scale and rapidity of variation of these fluctuations quantitatively, however, more detailed information such as is obtained from two-dimensional autocorrelation functions must be obtained. These are closely related to the two-dimensional Fourier Transform discussed below.

Further analysis of these patterns by Fourier analysis [3] is under way; it is encumbered by the fact that the truncation of the analysis imposed by the finite size of the discs is significant because the blotches are so large a fraction of the size of the disc. (Fourier analysis based on spatial distributions measured at one light wavelength as here is different from Fourier analysis based on a wide spectral range of light reflected, transmitted, or absorbed by a specimen; such a procedure has become popular in recent years to gain other types of information.) Spatial Fourier analysis is expected to yield frequency (tantamount to wavelength or size) distributions in two dimensions of variations in protein adsorption over the test surface. These frequency distributions give objective measures of the number of blotches of different sizes, their anisotropic properties, and the sharpness of their edges.

Fourier techniques are also useful in the template matching problem cited above; an example of this problem is considered below for its relevance to the assessment of the blood-foreign material interaction.

Application of Pattern-Recognition Techniques to the Analysis of Relationship between Spatial Patterns on Spun Discs of Proteins Adsorbed From Solution and Platelets Adhered From Canine Blood

As a particular expectation of the belief that protein uptake indicates how subsequent reactions of blood with biomaterials will take place, the adhesion of

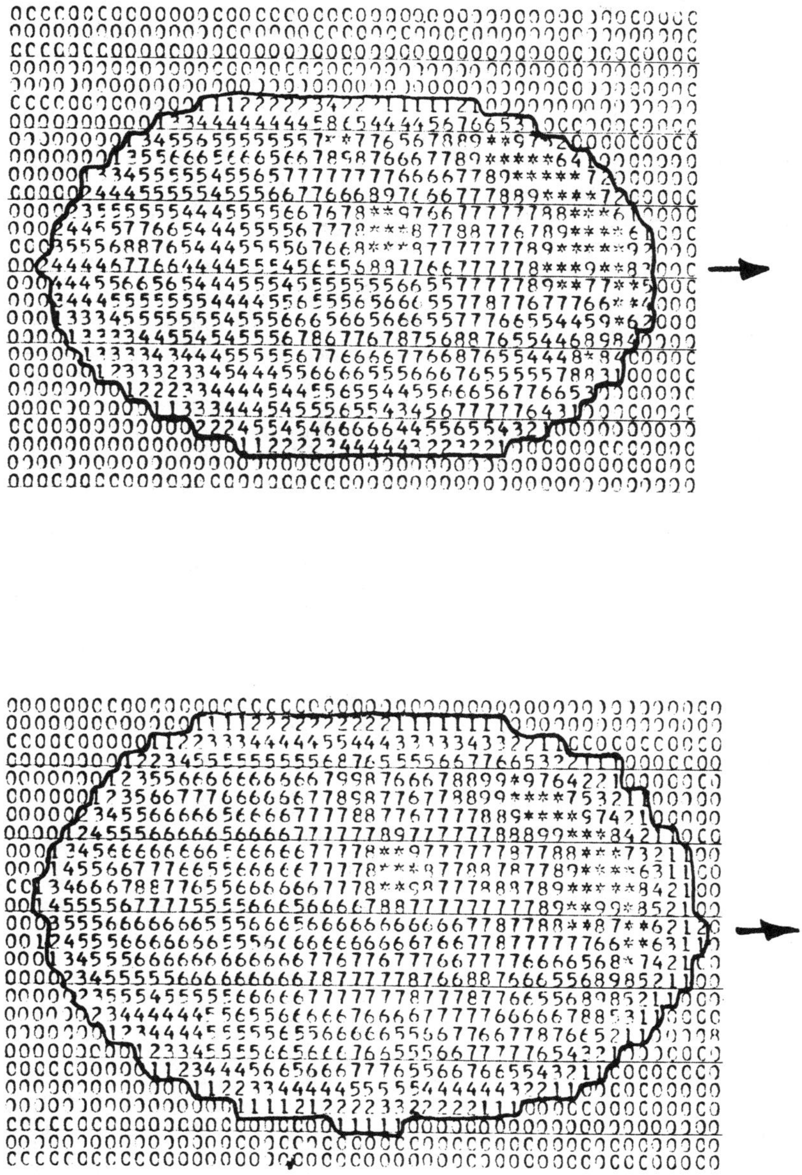

FIGURE 6. Patterns of gamma globulin adsorption on APTES heparinized siliconized rubber (Carnegie Mellon University). The digital pictures are of the same disc similarly oriented but with the absorbances corresponding to transitions from one number to another differently chosen (see text). The patterns are qualitatively very similar.

platelets is judged to be a consequence of what proteins have adhered to a surface and how they have done so. A close corollary of this judgment is that patterns of protein and platelet adhesion should be similar. From an analytical viewpoint such a correlation can be sought either *statistically,* perhaps best by comparing the spatial Fourier transforms of two different but similar surfaces (one on which platelet adhesion is visualized and one on which protein adsorption is observed), or *explicitly,* via a template-matching technique using protein and platelet patterns from exactly the same surface. The latter technique yields a more direct and more powerful test and is discussed here.

The actual experiment was a prototype of that actually desired. Because canine fibrinogen was not available, the test disc of type A polyether urethane from the Stanford Research Institute was first exposed statically to a solution of ^{125}I-labeled human fibrinogen (1 mg/ml in normal saline) for 15 minutes. The test disc was then washed with saline and introduced into a sample of fresh canine blood from a shunted, systemically heparinized canine, and spun for two minutes at 756 rpm. The test disc was then treated with Coomassie blue stain and scanned for platelets with the Zeiss instrument described above. It was then exposed to x-ray film and the autoradiograph scanned. Digitized scans sorted into eleven levels as described above are shown in FIGURES 7A and 7B (platelets and fibrinogen respectively). Inspection suggests that the patterns are correlated.

More quantitative approaches are possible. When good register (positional matching) of the two images can be obtained, a mathematical criterion of correspondence can be specified by summing. If at each point ($x = i$, $y = j$) one picture has an absorbance q_1 and the other an absorbance q_2, a discrepancy q_1-q_2 exists. An overall picture of correspondence can be obtained by some kind of summing of point discrepancies. This summation should not be such that positive deviations in one part of the picture are canceled by negative deviations elsewhere, since both contribute to noncorrespondence. Hence it is common to measure overall noncorrespondence in terms of the mean square deviation

$$\frac{1}{N}\sum_i \sum_j [q_1(i,j) - q_2(i,j)]^2.$$

The procedure requires one further refinement: since the level and range of the absorbances are arbitrary, the absorbance function for each picture must be normalized. We define:

$$\mu_1 = \frac{1}{N}\sum_{ij} q_1(i,j); \quad \mu_2 = \frac{1}{N}\sum_{ij} q_2(i,j).$$

$$\sigma_1 = \left[\frac{1}{N}\sum_{ij}(q_1(i,j) - \mu_1)^2\right]^{1/2}$$

$$\sigma_2 = \left[\frac{1}{N}\sum_{ij}(q_2(i,j) - \mu_2)^2\right]^{1/2}$$

$$\hat{q}_1(i,j) = \frac{q_1 - \mu_1}{\sigma_1}, \quad \hat{q}_2(i,j) = \frac{q_2 - \mu_2}{\sigma_2}$$

and in actual practice use $\hat{q}$'s in place of q's in the mean square expression. This procedure prevents a finding of noncorrespondence simply because one picture is darker than another or because the range of shading in one is larger

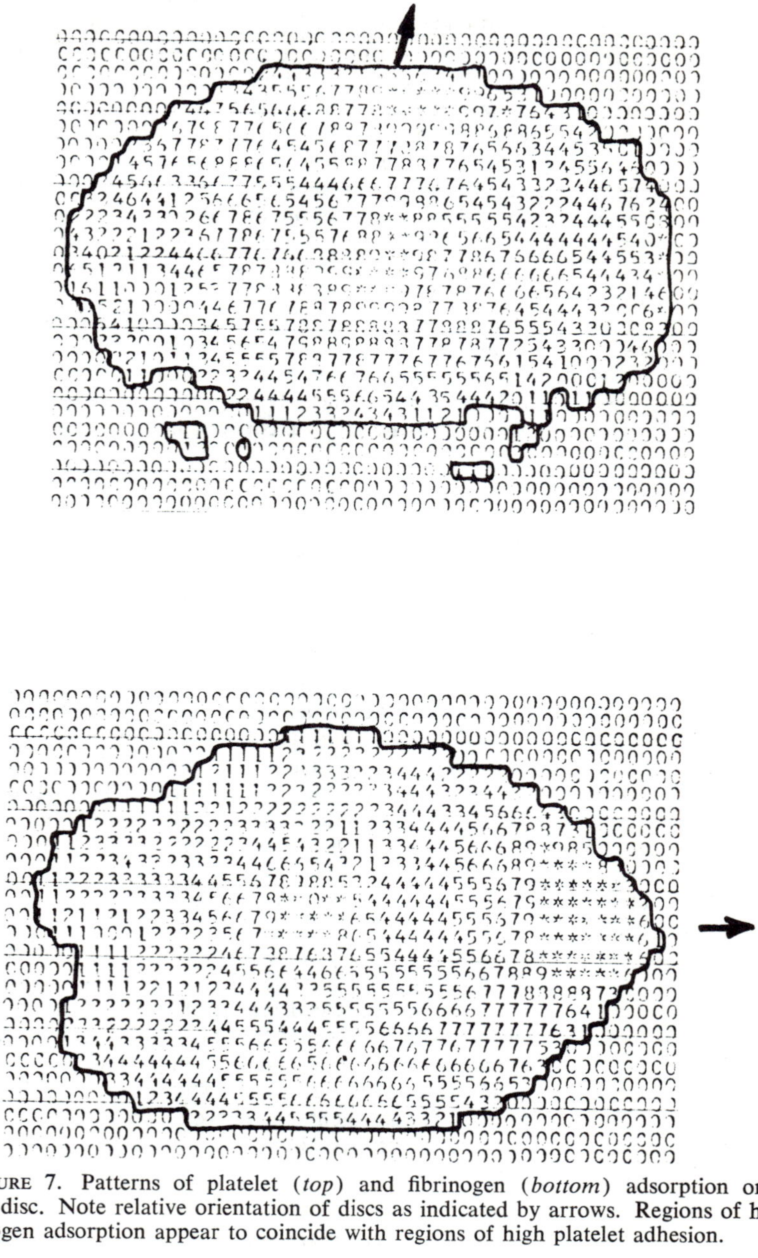

FIGURE 7. Patterns of platelet (*top*) and fibrinogen (*bottom*) adsorption on a single disc. Note relative orientation of discs as indicated by arrows. Regions of high fibrinogen adsorption appear to coincide with regions of high platelet adhesion.

than in the other, as might be caused only by technical differences between autoradiography and staining as methods of preparing surfaces to be scanned.

The assumption of good register cannot generally be guaranteed in practice. The confusing effect of poor register depends on the value of the misalignment relative to the scale (wavelength) of the variations on the surface: with only large-scale variations a small discrepancy in register will have only a small effect. When the register error equals or exceeds the scale of variation, essentially no information can be obtained. Both picture plane and Fourier methods can be used to reduce register error. For the picture plane analysis outlined above, a search process may be used. True noncorrespondence is taken to be the smallest value of the mean square within a population of values computed for small translations, rotations, and magnifications of one picture relative to the other. Computer methods exist for searching within such a population to obtain a minimum value.

It is well recognized that template matching according to correlation techniques like those outlined above is closely related to Fourier transformation.[10] In addition to the digital techniques for correlation analysis that have been stressed here, optical (analog) methods have been employed;[11] their possible application to problems in the present area of concern has not been explored.

Summary

The surface patterns, both deterministic and stochastic, that are an aspect of observable interactions between blood and biomaterials have been remarked upon for many years. Owing to lack of quantification they have, however, offered relatively little insight into either underlying processes or empirical differences among situations and materials. Many other phenomena give rise to surface patterns. Empirical and theoretical methods for extracting information from these patterns have been developed by others. Excerpts from this literature have been discussed here. Yield from these approaches has been obtained in three situations: In studies of platelet clustering, the patterns have served a major role in identifying the kinetic pathway of platelet-surface interactions. New understanding has been obtained of the complex distributions that give rise to the observed, space-average levels of protein adsorption. Greater insight into the relationship between protein adsorption and platelet adhesion seems to be at hand, although only the results of a prototype experiment are presently available.

With expected improvements in the blood compatibility of biomaterials, the role of stochastic processes that generate improbable but important subpatterns should receive more, not less, attention. Occurrences of such lesions should be accompanied both by analysis of the specific pattern and evolution of stochastic models that aid in understanding their cause. New developments beyond those applied in this paper, but not necessarily beyond the state of the art in pattern recognition will be required. Given technical success with these methods, though, it is possible that important new kinds of understanding of blood-biomaterial interactions may evolve.

Acknowledgments

The authors wish to acknowledge the assistance of Robert Estren, Estelle Makuku, and Mark Lauren.

REFERENCES

1. GRABOWSKI, E. F., L. I. FRIEDMAN & E. F. LEONARD. 1972. Effects of shear rate on platelet diffusion and adhesion to a foreign surface. I. & E. C. Fundamentals Vol. 11. May.
2. FELLER, W. 1968. An Introduction to Probability Theory and its Applications. 3d edit. John Wiley & Sons. New York, N.Y.
3. TOU, J. T. & R. C. GONZALEZ. 1974. Pattern Recognition Principles. Addison-Wesley. Reading, Mass.
4. DUDA, R. O. & P. E. HART. 1973. Pattern Classification and Scene Analysis : 263. Wiley-Interscience Pub. New York, N.Y.
5. DUDA, R. O. & P. E. HART. 1973. Pattern Classification and Scene Analysis : 298. Wiley-Interscience Pub. New York, N.Y.
6. BUTRUILLE, Y. A. 1974. Stochastic Interpretation of Platelet Adhesion on Artificial Materials : 134. Doctoral thesis. Columbia University. New York, N.Y.
7. VROMAN, L., A. L. ADAMS, M. KLINGS & G. FISCHER. 1975. Fibrinogen, globulins, albumin, and plasma at interfaces. Adv. Chem. Ser. (145): 255.
8. KOCHWA, S., R. S. LITWAK, R. E. ROSENFIELD & E. F. LEONARD. Blood Elements at Foreign Surfaces. I. A Biochemical Approach to the Study of the Adsorption of Plasma Proteins. This volume.
9. KOCHWA, S., R. S. LITWAK, R. E. ROSENFIELD & E. F. LEONARD. Blood Elements at Foreign Surfaces. II. *In Vitro* Evaluation of Biomaterials in a Spinning Disc Apparatus. This volume.
10. DUDA, R. O. & P. E. HART. 1973. Pattern Classification and Scene Analysis : 305. Wiley-Interscience Pub. New York, N.Y.
11. GOODMAN, J. W. 1968. Introduction to Fourier Optics. McGraw-Hill. New York, N.Y.
12. BAIER, R. E. & R. C. DUTTON. 1969. Initial Events in Interactions of Blood with a Foreign Surface. J. Biomed. Mater. Res. **3:** 191.
13. DUTTON, R. C., R. E. BAIER, R. L. DEDRICK & R. L. BOWMAN. 1968. Initial thrombus formation on foreign surfaces. Trans. Am. Soc. Artif. Intern. Organs **XIV**.
14. PETSCHEK, H., D. ADAMIS & A. R. KANTROWITZ. 1968. Stagnation flow thrombus formation. Trans. Am. Soc. Artif. Intern. Organs **XIV**.

FLUID DYNAMIC FACTORS AFFECTING PARTICLE CAPTURE AND RETENTION *

Perry L. Blackshear, Jr., Kenneth W. Bartelt,† and Richard J. Forstrom ‡

University of Minnesota
Minneapolis, Minnesota 55455

INTRODUCTION

Goldsmith[1] has shown that isolated RBCs § flowing near a wall are repelled from it at a velocity (v_R) that depends upon (among other factors) the proximity of the cell to the wall. Forstrom *et al.*[2] have employed studies of RBCs depositing on filtering walls to infer the nature of the near-wall velocity. The way this wall repulsion velocity depends upon cell size, R, velocity gradient, S, and kinematic viscosity of the suspending phase, ν, led to the selection of the wall repulsion velocity model of Saffman[3,4] as the one providing the best correlation of the data.

Briefly, if the dimensionless distance, y, is given by $y = \frac{h}{R}$, (h = distance of particle center from wall; R = particle radius), then:

$$v_R = 0.343y(1 - f)R^2S^{3/2}/\nu^{1/2}$$

where $y(1 - f)$ is a function of y alone and is given in TABLE 1.[2]

RBC data from a wide range of values of S, R, and ν giving a wide range of v_R/v_f (where v_f is filtration velocity) show that when $v_f < v_R$ ($y = 1.07$) no RBC collect on the surface, whereas for $v_f \geq v_R$, they do.

If these results (i.e., wall contact occurs when $v_f = v_R$ at $y = 1.07$) are applied to platelets ($R = 1\ \mu$, kinematic viscosity $= .01\ cm^2/s$) in normal aortas (v_f of order 10^{-6} to 10^{-5} cm/s), then no platelet deposition would be expected for $S > 50\ s^{-1}$ but would be expected at all sites where $S < 50\ s^{-1}$.

Preliminary results using $R = 1\ \mu$ latex particle suspensions by Bartelt[5] suggested that the extrapolation would be warranted, and a systematic mapping of latex particles in saline, platelets in PRP, and platelets in RBC suspensions was instituted. After a period of data collection the data displayed a strong influence of diffusion that had not been anticipated. In short, the data was not collected in a way to delineate the effects that were discovered important *a posteriore*. They represent concentration polarization data in a transient developing concentration boundary layer in which wall repulsion effects are submerged in the more dominant effects of time and position.

* This work was supported in part by a contract from the Artificial Kidney Program, NIAMDD-NIH.

† Present mailing address: Medtronic, Inc., 3055 Old Highway 8, Minneapolis, Minn. 55418.

‡ Present mailing address: Pharmaseal, 1015 Grandview Avenue, Glendale, Calif. 91201.

§ RBC=red blood cell; PRP=platelet-rich plasma; BSA=bovine serum albumin.

TABLE 1

WALL REPULSION PARAMETER y(1−f)

y	y(1−f)
1	1.000
1.005	0.524
1.05	0.362
1.13	0.263
1.54	0.121
2.35	0.052
3.76	0.021

An effort has been made to account for the factors that hide the influence of wall repulsion.[5] When this is done, the data suggest that concentration polarization theory that neglects the influence of wall repulsion (1) gives an upper bound of the wall particle concentration for latex particle suspensions and PRP, and (2) underestimates platelet wall concentration when RBCs are present.

The present paper presents the data accumulated by Bartelt[5] and introduces a method of estimating the relative importance of platelet diffusion, wall repulsion, ultrafiltration, and RBC distribution on platelet concentration in flowing blood near a filtering wall.

EXPERIMENT

Particle suspensions (alternately 1-micron radius particles, latex particles, or platelets and RBC) flow through a flow cell (see FIGURE 1), one wall of which consists, in part, of a cuprophane membrane suspended on a slotted matrix. The flow channel is 10 cm long and 2 cm wide, with a thickness of alternately 0.10 and 0.025 cm. FIGURE 2 shows the pattern of the matrix and the resulting deposits when ultrafiltration occurs.

Latex particles were suspended in a buffered saline preparation containing BSA designed to minimize particle aggregation but to permit the subsequent glutaraldehyde wash to act as an adhesive. The platelet and RBC suspensions employed native proteins for this purpose.

A typical run would consist of:

1. A preliminary particle-free wash to coat the chamber walls;
2. a ten-minute flow of particle suspension at fixed shear rate and ultrafiltration velocity;

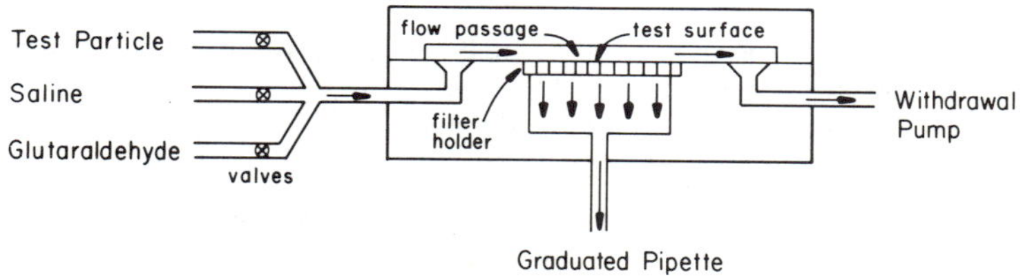

FIGURE 1. Schematic of experimental flow system.

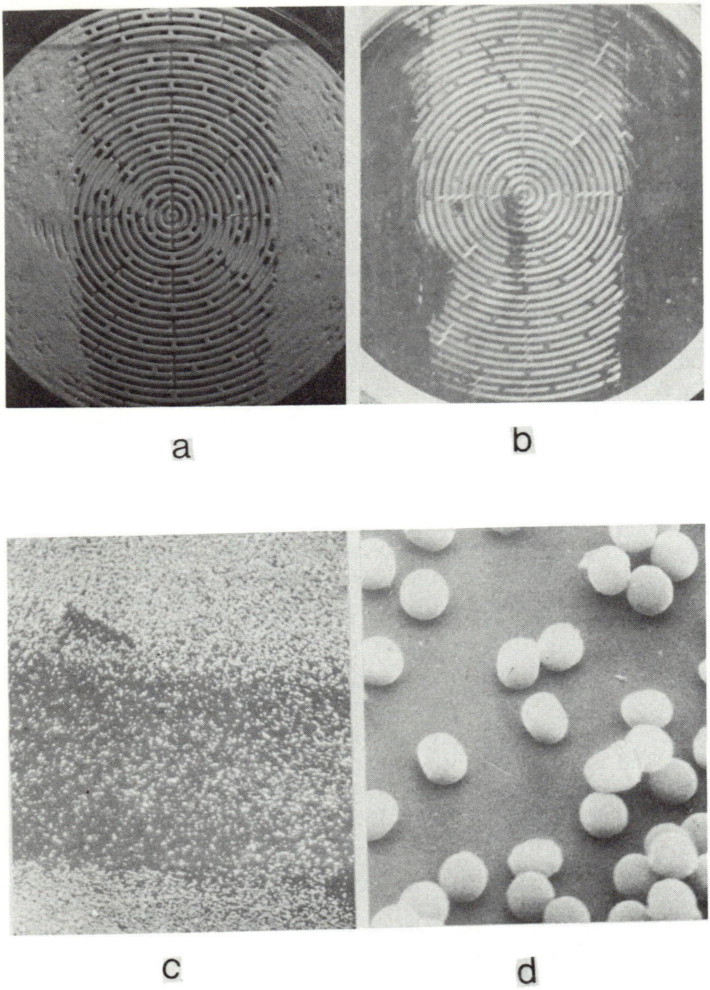

FIGURE 2. Membrane support and patterns of deposition for latex particles. a: membrane support screen; b: membrane (light areas are latex particles); c: magnified view of b (central area is over a support); d: magnification 3900.

3. a three-minute wash with a particle-free fluid while maintaining shear and ultrafiltration constant; and
4. a wash containing glutaraldehyde again maintaining flow and ultrafiltration constant.

Details of the preparation of the cell and of the suspensions are given in Reference 5.

RESULTS

Sample results are shown in FIGURE 3. Here the number of particles per unit area that should have accumulated if the particles had behaved as RBC is given as the pure convection curve. This is contrasted with the experimental results. In the two cases the repulsion velocity is $3.8 \cdot 10^{-7}$ and 10^{-6} for $S = 9.7$, and $19.3\ s^{-1}$, respectively.

It is seen that the concentration measured departs from the purely convective behavior exhibited by the larger RBCs.[2]

Bartelt[6] suggested that diffusion was a factor, that a nonsticky boundary condition should apply (particles on the wall can exchange freely with particles in the stream), and that filtration concentration polarization theory would be of utility in interpreting the data.

Accordingly, Bartelt[5] prepared a computer program that permitted a variety of transient concentration polarization solutions (that neglect wall repulsion) to be generated. From these he prepared a correction factor that permits the comparison of the data (which is for the most part in the time-varying part of the concentration buildup) with steady state solutions of Dresner.[7] These solutions give the ratio of concentration at the wall (c_w) with that in the mainstream (c_o) as functions of a dimensionless parameter.

$$\xi = \frac{v_f^3 x}{SD^2}$$

Dresner's solutions are:

$$\frac{c_w}{c_o} = 1 + 1.536\ \xi^{1/3}, \qquad \xi \leq 0.02$$

$$\frac{c_w}{c_o} = 1 + \xi + 5(1 - e^{-\sqrt{\xi/3}}) \qquad \xi \geq 0.02$$

Because these solutions do not take into account wall repulsion, they are expected to represent an upper bound on c_w, c_o.

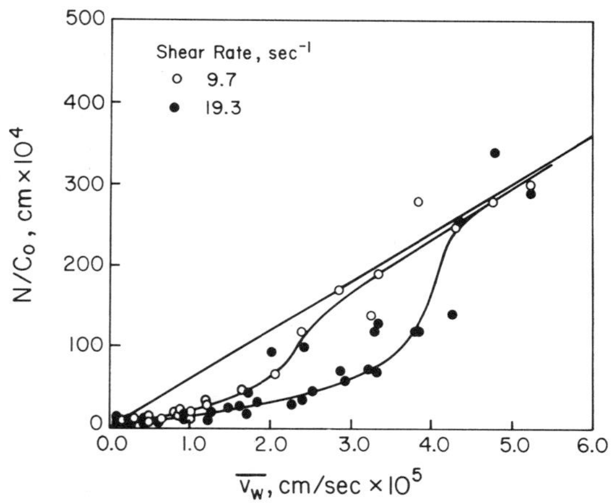

FIGURE 3. Surface concentration of latex particles versus ultrafiltration velocity.

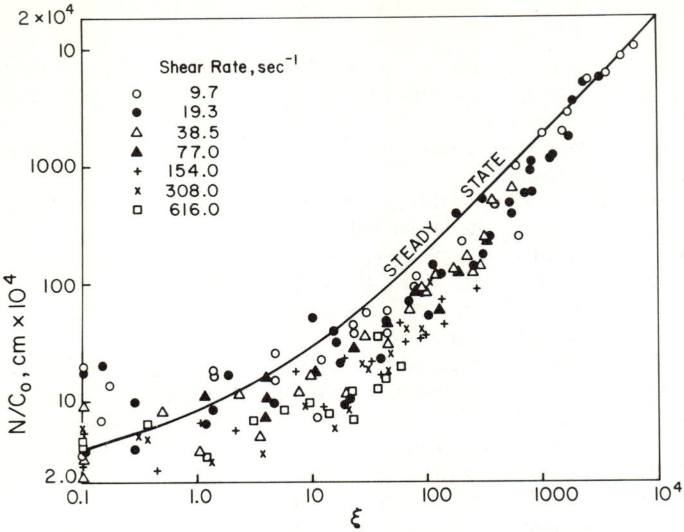

FIGURE 4. Surface concentration of latex particles numerically adjusted for comparison with the steady state.

The data as corrected by Bartelt[5] is given for latex spheres, platelets, and platelets mixed with RBC (in the latter case, only platelets collect on the wall) in FIGURES 4, 5, and 6. Herein the x in ξ is 1/2 the total length of the filtering wall.

The correlation with filtration theory appears persuasive. There seems to

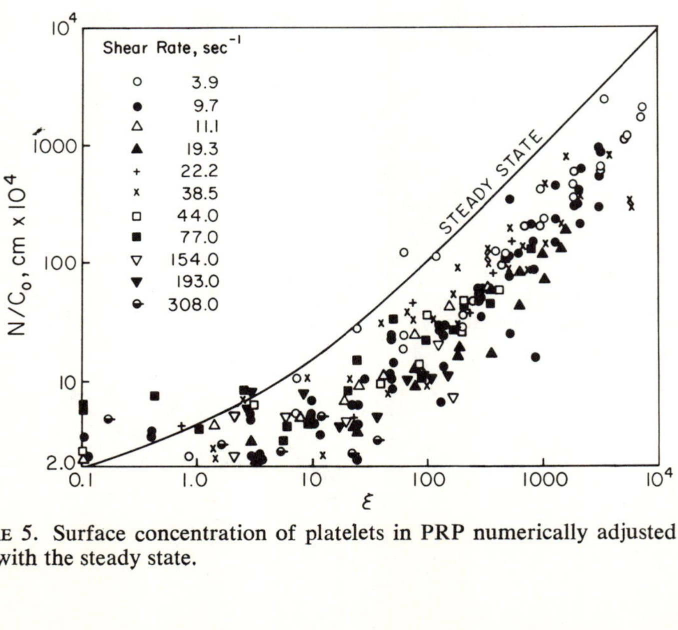

FIGURE 5. Surface concentration of platelets in PRP numerically adjusted for comparison with the steady state.

be a tendency for the higher S wall concentration to be lower than the low S concentrations, suggesting a wall repulsion effect not accounted for in the correlation.

The data when RBCs are present (FIGURE 6) suggest that platelets are in higher concentration near the wall when RBCs are present than would be expected were they uniformly distributed across the flow chamber.

This effect was first reported by Fårhaeus in 1928 [8] and has been quantitated in plane channels by Palmer.[9] The way this phenomenon may be related to hematocrit and flow is discussed below.

The following discussion is designed to provide a framework for interpreting the relevance of these results to flow in the arterial tree as well as in ultrafiltering dialysis equipment.

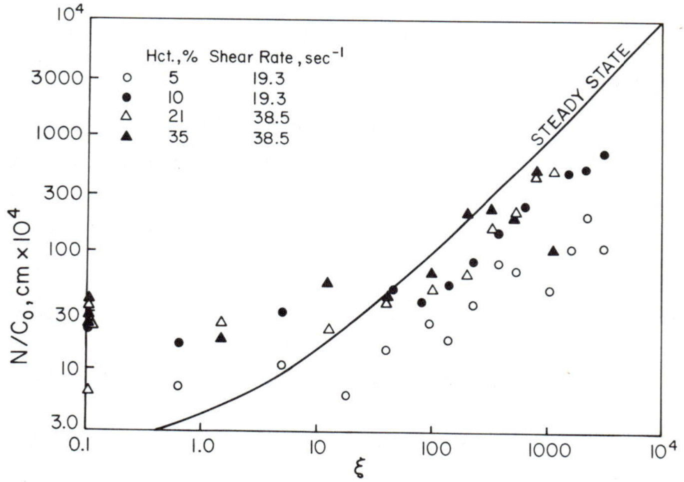

FIGURE 6. Surface concentration of platelets in whole blood numerically adjusted for comparison with steady state.

Discussion

Influence of Wall Repulsive Force and Filtration Velocity on Concentration Distribution Near a Wall

If we consider only the force of repulsion as derived by Saffman,[3,4] we find that any particle at a distance y ($y = h/R$ is dimensionless distance from wall) moves away from the wall with a velocity $v_R = 0.343y(1 - f)R^2S^{3/2}/\nu^{1/2}$ where $y(1 - f)$ is a tabulated function of y (see TABLE 1), R is particle radius, S is shear rate, ν is kinematic viscosity of the suspending fluid. Then in a filtering situation the net particle velocity in positive y direction is:

$$v = v_R - v_f \text{ where } v_f \text{ is filtration velocity.}$$

The flux of particle by convection and diffusion in the positive y direction is:

$vc - (D/R)(dc/dy)$ where c is particle concentration.

It we assume axial convection is negligible and steady state conditions prevail:

$$vc - (D/R)(dc/dy) = 0. \tag{1}$$

To facilitate obtaining an approximate solution to (1) for c(y), we seek an approximate equation for $(1-f)$. Forstrom[2] shows that except for $1 < y < 1.005$, where $y(1-f)$ drops from a value of 1 to 0.4, $y(1-f)$ is closely approximated by $0.4y^{-2}$. This underestimates the v_R at the wall (i.e., at $y < 1.005$), but near the wall (i.e., $y > 1.005$) it is an excellent approximation. Thus:

$$v_R \simeq (0.137/y^2)(R^2S^{3/2}/\nu^{1/2}) = a/y^2. \tag{2}$$

$$\text{Then } v = a/y^2 - v_f \tag{3}$$

and **(1)** becomes:

$$dc/c = (a/y^2 - v_f)(R/D)dy. \tag{4}$$

Note that at the wall $c = c_w$, $y = 1$, $v = a - v_f$. Solving **(4)** we obtain:

$$c/c_w = {}_e(aR/D)\left\{\left(1 - \frac{1}{y}\right) + \frac{v_f}{a}(1-y)\right\} \tag{5}$$

For Nonfiltering Wall

When $v_f/a \simeq 0$, $c_o/c_w = e^{aR/D}$, c_o is concentration where $y \to \infty$ and

$$\frac{c/c_w}{c_o/c_w} = \frac{c}{c_o} = e^{-aR/yD}.$$

Note that for $aR/D \ll 1$ $c_w \simeq c_o$ and no concentration polarization occurs. For $\frac{aR}{D}$ of order magnitude unity or greater, $c_o/c_w > 1$.

In order to examine the influence of particle size we employed Einstein's value of $D = 2.25 \cdot 10^{-13}/R$, where R is in cm and D in cm²/s. Recall $a = 0.237R^2S^{3/2}/\nu^{1/2}$.

For arterial flow $S = 400\ s^{-1}$, $\nu = .01$ cm²/s so that $a \simeq 0.137R^2 \dfrac{400^{3/2}}{(.01)^{1/2}}$ $1.1 \cdot 10^4R^2$. Thus $aR/D = R^4 \cdot 4.87 \cdot 10^{+16}$, R in cm. If platelets behave like spheres of $R = 10^{-4}$ cm, $aR/D = 4.87$ and $c_o/c_w = 130$; i.e., platelet wall concentration would be low.

For low shear regions, e.g. $S = 10$, $aR/D = R^4 \cdot 1.93 \cdot 10^{14}$; for $R = 10^{-4}cm^4$, $aR/D = 1.93 \cdot 10^{-2}$ and platelet $c_o/c_w = 1.019$; i.e., platelet wall concentration will be approximately equal to stream concentration.

On the other hand, the RBC with an effective radius of, say, $4 \cdot 10^{-4}$cm will have a $c_o/c_w > 100$ for the lower shear rate above ($S = 10s^{-1}$) and in excess of 10^{100} for the higher ($S = 400s^{-1}$). Conversely at particles smaller than a platelet, say $R = 0.25 \cdot 10^{-4}$cm, $aR/d \ll 1$ for all physiological shear rates, and no polarization would occur. (Note: At high Hct, other effects influence RBC c_w).

Thus, the platelet occupies a unique size position in respect to the values of aR/D that occur in the human vasculature. Particles an order of magnitude smaller or larger than platelets behave in a uniform manner with respect to the shear rate extremes found in the vasculature, whereas the platelet concentration ranges from $c_o/c_w = 1$ to $c_o/c_w > 100$ for the extremes found in the aorta.

The Effects of RBC Distribution, $v_f/a \ll 1$

As seen above over the entire shear rate range, $c_o/c_w \gg 1$ for the RBC. We may expect (and indeed there is good corroborative evidence) low concentrations of RBC in the near wall region. Thus, in whole blood in tube flow the near wall region should consist of platelets and chylomicra in plasma, because very few RBC will be present.

A value of c_o for platelets for this near wall region can be estimated from the following considerations.

Around each dispersed RBC there is a plasma volume $A_{RBC}R_{platelet}$ that cannot be occupied by platelet centers. The values of $A_{RBC}R_{platelet}/V_{RBC} \simeq 1.5$. When RBC are rouleauxed or packed, only the surface bordering the platelet-rich plasma (PRP) excludes platelets. We designate the concentration of platelets in the PRP over packed RBC as c_{pc}. Let the concentration of platelets, in the plasma volume available to them when red cells are fully dispersed (RBC surfaces are spaced $2R_p$ or greater), be designated by c_o. Then it can be shown that $c_o/c_{pc} = (1 - \text{Hct})/(1 - 2.5\ \text{Hct})$, which goes to ∞ as Hct goes to 0.40. Shear tends to disperse RBC aggregates [10, 11] and thus concentrate the platelets into the plasma volume available to them. The observations concerning RBC-free regions near the tube wall suggest that flowing (and therefore dispersed) RBC tend to force the platelets into the plasma space near the tube walls.[8, 9]

Two results of the experiments reported here suggest such a concentrating effect does occur:

1. At shear rates and ultrafiltration velocities at which RBCs suspended in saline were found to collect on the membrane, only platelets collected when RBC's were suspended in PRP.
2. Platelet wall concentration at low values of ξ were five times as high when RBC were present (at Hct > 10) than when they were not.

In this volume a paper by Turrito *et al.*[12] shows that platelet-deposition rates from whole blood increase with shear. Here we have two competing effects that affect platelet concentrations differently over the different flow regimes.

1. For $aR/D \ll 1$, $c_o/c_w \simeq 1$ ($S < 32\ s^{-1}$); c_o, the platelet concentration in the near-wall regime, would increase with increased S because of the RBC-exclusion effect. Therefore, c_w would tend to increase. In normal cells full RBC dispersion [10] is reached at $S \geq 100$.
2. For $0.11 < aR/D < 0.61$ ($32 < S < 100\ s^{-1}$) c_w/c_o decreases gradually with increasing S (according to $c_w/c_o = e^{-6.09 \cdot 10^{-4} S^{3/2}}$), but this decrease is mitigated by the fact that, at the same time, c_o is increasing with increased

shear (due again to red cells' becoming more dispersed). The net result in this regime is probably an increase in c_w with increased S.

3. $aR/D > .061$ ($S > 100\ s^{-1}$), in this regime $-d(c_w/c_o)/dS$ becomes very large.

In addition, healthy, normal red cells will have reached complete disaggregation at $S \geq 100$ (Reference 9).

Thus, as S increases beyond $S = 100\ s^{-1}$, the platelet concentrations at the wall should decrease.

The concentration of platelets in the near-wall regime should influence the deposition rate of platelets onto sticky walls. In the experiments reported by Turrito,[12] the deposition rate of platelets monotonically increased with increasing S. Next to a filtering nonsticky wall, platelet concentration should increase, then decrease as S increases.

One goal of bioengineering is to determine how the great body of literature on transport phenomena might be most fruitfully employed in solving problems involving the interaction of flowing blood components with stationary surfaces.

In most of the situations in which this body of literature has been accumulated, however, diffusion coefficients in laminar flow are independent of the state of motion; position-dependent forces that impart velocities to solutes are rarely encountered, and rarely are there substantial variations of solubility across a flow chamber. These effects, however, do seem relevant to the use of transport theory in quantitating the flux of platelets toward reacting surfaces in flowing blood.

1. There does appear to be an augmentation of diffusion due to RBC motion.[1, 12, 13, §]

§ Additional background: particles in a flowing suspension are known to diffuse in a shear field at a rate that exceeds the Stokes Einstein estimate, the apparent diffusion coefficient increasing with an increasing shear rate (Thomas, 1955; Pollak, 1956; Pollack, 1957).

THOMAS, H. W. 1955. The diffusion battery method for aerosol particle size determination. J. Colloid Sci. **10:** 247.

POLLAK, L. W., T. C. O'CONNOR & A. L. METNIEKS. 1956. On the determination of the diffusion coefficient of condensation nuclei using the static and dynamic methods. Geofisica Pura e Applicata **34:** 177.

POLLAK, L. W. 1957. O'CONNOR, T. C. & A. L. METNIEKS. 1957. Report on the determination of the diffusion coefficient using the static and dynamic methods. Geofisica Pura e Applicata **36:** 70.

Evidence that this phenomena has an influence on the diffusion of the erythrocyte in flowing blood has been cited by Thomas.

THOMAS, H. W., A. C. G. FRENCH & S. ROWLANDS. 1965. The flow of red cell suspensions through narrow tubes: the extracoporeal determination of the difference in mean velocities of red cells and their suspending phase. Proc. 4th Int. Congr. Rheology. A. L. Copley, Ed.: 381. John Wiley & Sons. New York, N.Y.

Grossly, blood behaves like a Newtonian fluid at shear rates greater than 10 sec^{-1}, and laminar-like flow seems to occur in tubes at Reynolds numbers less than 2000. A closer inspection, however, reveals a pattern of individual red cell spin and migration (Bloch, 1962; Bugliarello, 1962; Merrilll, 1965) that, though certainly not turbulent, is not a pattern one would expect in laminar flow.

BLOCH, E. H. 1962. A quantitative study of the hemodynamics in the living molecular system. Amer. J. Anat. **110:** 125.

BUGLIARELLO, G. & J. W. HAYDEN. 1962. High speed microcinematographic studies of blood in vitro. Science **138:** 1981.

MERRILL, E.W. 1965. Rheology of human blood and some speculation on its role in vascular homeostasis. *In* Biophysical Mechanisms in Vascular Homeostasis and

2. Fårhaeus,[8] Palmer,[9] and the present work suggest that the RBC mass in effect reduces the solubility of platelets, and that this reduction is influenced by hematocrit, state of aggregation (hence, state of motion), and perhaps RBC deformability.

3. Palmer [9] and the present paper suggest that forces of repulsion in flowing particle suspensions impart a velocity normal to the wall that permits a flowing platelet suspension to maintain a concentration gradient near a wall.

The present paper shows these latter effects to be substantial (platelet concentration at the wall is 5–100 times higher (or lower) than that in the bulk blood) in the case where the platelets do not react with (or stick on) the wall. The processes that give rise to these effects must play a role when platelets react and stick to the wall.

Much more work is needed to clarify the role of flow, RBC concentrations and distributions, and motion on platelet interactions with surfaces exposed to flowing blood.

References

1. Goldsmith, H. L. 1971. Red cell motions and wall interactions in tube flow. Fed. Proc. **30:** (5). Sept.-Oct.
2. Forstrom, R. J., G. O. Voss & P. L. Blackshear. 1974. Fluid dynamics of particle (platelet) deposition for filtering walls: relationship to atherosclerosis. J. Fluids Eng. Trans. ASME. June : 168–72.
3. Saffman, P. G. 1956. On the motion of small spheroidal particles in a viscous liquid. J. Fluid Mechanics **1:** 540–553.
4. Saffman, P. G. 1965. The lift on a small sphere in a slow shear flow. J. Fluid Mechanics **22:** 383–400.
5. Bartelt, K. W. 1976. Blood Platelet Deposition onto Filtering Surfaces. Ph.D. thesis submitted to the Graduate School, Univ. Minnesota. Minneapolis, Minn.
6. Bartelt, K. W. 1974. Personal communication.
7. Dresner, L. 1964. Boundary Layer Buildup in the Demineralization of Salt Water by Reverse Osmosis. Oak Ridge National Lab. Rpt. no. 3621. May.
8. Fåhraeus, R. 1928. Die Stromungsverhältnisse and die Verteilung der Blutzellen im Gefässystem. Klinische Wochenschrift **7**(3). Jan. 15.
9. Palmer, A. A. 1966. Platelet and Leucocyte Skimming. Fourth European Conf. on Microcirculation. Cambridge, England. Bibl. anat. **9:** 300–303.
10. Chien, S. 1975. Biophysical behavior of red cells in suspensions. *In* The Red Blood Cell. Vol. **2:** Chapter 26, 1021–1133. Academic Press. New York, N.Y.
11. Schmid-Schoenbein, H. , R. Wells & R. Schildrkraut. 1969. Microscopy and viscometry of blood flowing under uniform shear rate (rheoscopy). J. Appl. Physiol. **26**(5): 676–678.
12. Turrito, V. T. This volume.
13. Blackshear, P. L., F. D. Dorman, J. H. Steinbach, E. J. Maybach, A. Singh & R. E. Collingham. 1966. Shear Wall Interaction and Hemolysis. Trans. Am. Soc. Artif. Intern. Organs. **12:** 113–120.

Intravascular Thrombosis. P. N. Sawyer, Ed. : Appleton Century Crofts. New York, N.Y. 121.

This motion is held responsible for the increased diffusion rate observed. Early studies to quantitate this effect have been conducted by Collingham (1968) and Singh (1968).

Collingham, R. E. 1968. Mass transfer in flowing suspensions. Ph.D. dissertation. Univ. Minnesota. Minneapolis, Minn.

Singh, A. 1968. The thermal conductivity of stationary and flowing suspensions. Ph.D. dissertation. Univ. Minnesota. Minneapolis, Minn.

DISCUSSION

Dr. Salzman: Dr. Leonard, is it possible that the first platelets adherent to a surface have simply become sticky, and that the second layer of platelets has stuck to those platelets so that the preferential concentration of platelet B in the neighborhood of platelet A is a result of interaction directly with platelet A, and not with something diffusable? Can you distinguish between those in your method?

Dr. Leonard: You understood what I was trying to say. I cannot answer that, because our pictures are so bad. The area of preferred interaction of the platelet with the surface is something in the neighborhood of from the edge of the platelet to fourteen microns. That's an area in which platelet pseudopods can be stuck out. We don't see pseudopods in our light micrograms, so I think the answer to your question is yes, it is possible, and we do not have evidence to separate one from the other.

Canine platelet bodies do not stick on top of each other. So one would have to say that it was the pseudopods that were sticky, but not the main membrane body of the platelet. Some people have said that we wouldn't see it because one would be under the other, but I think that we have the depth of field and the ability to tell. They do form monolayers.

Dr. Keller: You wouldn't exclude the possibility that they were potentiated by that contact and then subsequently interacted with the surface.

Dr. Leonard: I think I could not exclude that, right.

Dr. Salzman: In a living microcirculatory preparation, white cells will roll along the wall of the vessel. Dr. Goldsmith has shown us the same thing *in vitro*. I wondered if rheological considerations alone could account for this exclusion of the white cells from the center, or does one also have to postulate that the white cells are sticky?

Dr. Goldsmith: I don't think our research is far enough advanced to answer that. Red cells in the actual stream of a tube exclude white cells into the periphery. But that there should be a tendency to roll along the wall, I don't think you can explain. Besides, most of the phenomena I think you are referring to occur in vessels of the dimensions of an arteriole, and this was a 100-micron vessel, which is just a little bit larger, isn't it?

Dr. E. Ruckenstein (*Univ. of Delaware, Newark, Del.*): A small group in Buffalo, New York, has tried to do some theoretical and experimental research to answer the questions: Why are proteins able to adhere to the surface very quickly, why do platelets follow, and why are the red blood cells never able to arrive at the surface? Because besides the hydrodynamic forces and besides the repulsion forces which we have spoken of, very near to the wall there are attractive forces. Besides this force we have repulsive forces, which are due to double layer forces. The competition between these two types of forces can generate a very strong potential barrier. It is possible to show that this potential barrier is proportional to the diameter of the particle. Assuming a simple geometry, the protein molecules can adhere very quickly to the surface, and the platelets cannot. We have taken particles of two different diameters, and were able to separate them because the smaller particles remained in the center as a result of the velocity distribution. The surface charge that affects this type of interaction potential can be computed taking into account the chemistry of the surface.

DR. LEONARD: In this type of consideration, as you said, Professor Ruckenstein, a major factor is the radius of curvature of the particles that are involved. It is not the principal radius of curvature of the particle, and the surface may have local very small radii of curvature or, for example, bristles of protein fibers sticking up into the solution in such a way that what one would think of initially as an infinite radius of curvature may be replaced by a small finite radius of curvature. There is a concentration of electrostatic and Vander Waals forces affecting the adhesion of materials that one is concerned with.

DR. HOCHMUTH: With respect to Dr. Leonard's rotating disk: although the boundary layer is constant, the shear rate increases linearly with distance from the center, and there is this tremendous augmentation of platelet diffusion, so that you have really a high nonlinear phenomenon there. I wondered if that concerned you.

DR. LEONARD: Yes, the rate of shear does vary across the disk, and this affects the diffusion coefficient so that the disk is not uniformly accessible to shear-sensitive diffusion species, but the diffusivity, we believe, becomes pretty constant with respect to shear rate above a certain value. The one set of curves I showed, and from which most of our analyses were taken, was obtained when we had saturated this phenomenon.

DR. ZUCKER: When physiologists look at blood flow in living blood vessels, one of the criteria they use for not having damaged the blood vessel in any way is the absence of margination of the leukocytes, and this fits with what Dr. Stewart said. I think that white cells along the edge of the blood vessel indicate it has been slightly damaged, and flow is not the only cause of white cell location.

DR. BAIER: Dr. Leonard, with respect to the geometry you assumed for the particle being square, I would have expected that your diffusion would have come out a little bit preferentially from the points of the square, and you wouldn't have had circles around it. Some of the pictures show the pseudopodial platelets giving much irregularity of the boundaries. Should we expect spikes that will influence this randomness or nonrandomness that you're calculating?

DR. LEONARD: We did not have such fineness of grid for calculating the diffusion. If we had little tiny squares, a thousand of them, in which we calculated diffusion on each point, and those thousand little tiny squares added up to the big square that was our pseudoplatelet, we would indeed have seen little funny concentrations in the corner that would have been nonphysiologic and artifactual. But as I said, I believed at the time it was essentially a semiquantitative analysis to deal with what we regard as semiquantitative data.

DR. SAWYER: Cells look at the blood vessel interface at half a million volts per cm potential; closer then 8 angstrom to the blood vessel wall you are at a million volts per cm, and if you get to half of that, you are in 10 million volts per cm. This is what makes it possible to have vascularity in the first place; the blood never sees the blood vessel wall at all. We are statistically unclottable. With actomyosin, pseudopods are thrust out when injury occurs so that the platelet or a tiny portion of it can actually penetrate through this very very dense electric field and actually stick to a point. Otherwise, we would all have died the first time we cut ourselves. Gene Bernstein has done beautiful work with his spinning disk, and I would be much more appreciative if he calculated how much more G's he has to apply to overcome the overvoltage that occurs when the red cells get close to the disk, so we can destroy them and get the answers he has to get.

PART VII. BLOOD AND THE BLOOD VESSEL WALL

INTRODUCTION

Alfred L. Copley

Laboratory of Biorheology
Polytechnic Institute of New York
Brooklyn, New York 11201

I should like to make a few remarks which, I believe, have a direct bearing on the topic of this conference and which are of particular interest to this session. They pertain to our own studies on the endoendothelial fibrin lining as well as to mutual studies with other investigators in other laboratories. I noticed with some gratification that some findings have been reported at this conference that are in support of the concept of the endoendothelial fibrin layer, lining the inner aspects of vessel walls, although no reference has been made at this conference to this concept, which I first proposed in 1953.[1] At present, immunochemical, electron microscopical, surface rheological and surface chemical studies are being made in the above-mentioned mutual studies to provide direct evidence for the occurrence of the endoendothelial fibrin lining.

It appears important to emphasize, what apparently is not sufficiently known, that fibrin surface has antithrombotic action as we found in dogs, employing rubber tubing as prosthesis between the ends of the severed jugular vein.[2] We also found that fibrin surface has strong anticoagulant action *extra vivum*.[3, 4] These findings and the concept of the endoendothelial fibrin lining on the inner aspects of the living vessel wall may explain the long known but poorly understood physiologic antithrombotic action of the endothelium.

The other part of our studies concerns a new concept, which I first proposed in 1971, regarding a hitherto unrecognized form of clotting.[2, 3]

As you all know, for about the past one hundred years two major concepts of clotting have been known, namely, (1) blood cellular clotting, which can be either the reversible aggregation or the irreversible agglutination of platelets, white blood cells or red blood cells; (2) plasma coagulation, which is fibrin formation in all its different phases; and (3) both blood cellular and plasmatic processes mixed.

There is another form of clotting, which I would consider the polymerization and subsequent gelation of fibrinogen without thrombin participation. I conceive this form of clotting, for instance, *in vivo,* as a process occurring on the vessel wall, which begins with the adsorption of fibrinogen to the endoendothelial fibrin lining and then with successive adsorption of fibrinogen as a growth process of layer upon layer, forming a kind of polymerization with subsequent gelation of fibrinogen. This particular form of clotting occurs rapidly, and I consider it to be responsible for the initiation of thrombus formation both in thrombosis and in hemostasis. All other processes of clotting, e.g. platelet clumping and fibrin coagulation, are secondary occurrences.[2]

In our studies, we have been employing the Weissenberg Rheogoniometer, for which Mr. King and I developed modifications for measurements of the viscoelasticity of surface layers of fibrinogen systems without or with the admixture of other plasma proteins, as well as of platelets or red blood cells.[3]

I should like to mention some of our most recent findings concerning this new form of clotting.

In measuring the rigidity of surface layers we obtained high viscous resistance or torque values. These layers, at varying concentrations of fibrinogen from 0.4% down to 0.0004%, were extremely rigid, even at the lowest concentration. In control studies we used oil instead of the air interface, in making certain that the fibrinogen was entirely excluded from air contact, with the result that we obtained identical findings both at the air and oil interfaces.

I should like to refer to the distribution of wall shear rates in different blood vessels. In a compilation of data from three groups of investigators that we presented in a composite figure, which Dr. Turitto will present here, you will note the very high wall shear rates in all blood vessels. On the basis of these findings we applied to fibrinogen solutions steady shear at 1000 sec^{-1} for three minutes. A marked increase in the torque values resulted from testing the surface layers of fibrinogen from six different species—human, rabbit, dog, cat, sheep, and bovine.[3]

In a study on the elastic modulus of surface layers to 0.4% solutions of fibrinogen from sheep, bovine, and human origins, we found high values on dynamic testing. From oscillatory tests of 0.4% fibrinogen of the same origins, we found the surface viscosity, plotted against frequency ranging from 10^{-4} to 10^{0} Hertz, to be extremely high, i.e., values up to more than 10^{8} dynes sec/cm^{2}. These remarkable findings were entirely unexpected. Such values may be similar to those one may expect with materials like layers of steel or of cement of similar thickness.

We found that the fibrinogen surface layers exhibit unusually high elastic rigidity, which, as I proposed earlier, may be an important contributory factor to maintain the patency of blood vessels.[4]

On the basis of our findings of the rigidity of surface layers of fibrinogen, Dr. Birger Blombäck and I developed a hypothesis in which we tried to explain the particular clotting of strong layers of fibrinogen at the vessel wall at high shear rates up to 10,000 sec^{-1}, particularly in the arterioles and capillaries, to produce a conformational change of the fibrinogen. This process of clotting without the activation of the enzyme thrombin may open up polymerization sites, a hypothesis which is now under investigation in Dr. Blombäck's and my laboratory.

References

1. Copley, A. L. On the endoendothelial fibrin layer, fibrin(ogen) polymerization, and thrombosis. *In* Blood Vessels. S. Effert, Ed. Springer-Verlag. New York, N.Y. In press.
2. Copley, A. L. 1964. On the anticoagulant action of fibrin in the prevention of thrombosis. Proc. IX. Congr. Internat. Soc. Hematol. Universidad Nacional Autonoma de Mexico, Mexico City. Vol. **II:** 367.
3. Copley, A. L., P. Steichele, M. Spradau & R. S. Thorley. 1959. The anticoagulant action of fibrin surfaces on mammalian blood. Nature (London) **183:** 1683.
4. Copley, A. L. & B. Becher. 1961. Human, cow and rabbit native fibrin powders as anticoagulants. Nature (London) **192**: 568.
5. Copley, A. L. 1971. Non-Newtonian behavior of surface layers of human plasma protein systems and a new concept of the initiation of thrombosis. Biorheology **8:** 79.
6. Copley, A. L. & R. G. King. 1976. Polymolecular layers of fibrinogen systems and the genesis of thrombosis. *In* Hemorheology and Thrombosis. A. L. Copley and S. Okamoto, Eds. Pergamon Press. New York, N.Y. Thrombosis Research Suppl. **II:** 393.
7. Copley, A. L. 1974. Hemorheological aspects of the endothelium-plasma interface. Microvascular Res. **8:** 192.

PHYSICAL FACTORS INFLUENCING PLATELET DEPOSITION ON SUBENDOTHELIUM: IMPORTANCE OF BLOOD SHEAR RATE *

Vincent T. Turitto

Department of Medicine
Division of Hematology
Roosevelt Hospital
New York, New York 10019

Reto Muggli and Hans R. Baumgartner

Pharmaceutical Research Department
F. Hoffmann-La Roche & Co. Ltd.
Basel, Switzerland

Introduction

Platelets circulate in the blood without attaching to each other or to the intimal lining. Removal of endothelial cells results in platelet deposition on the exposed subendothelial surface, the release of certain platelet constituents, and the formation of platelet aggregates. These platelet events play a basic role in both thrombogenesis and hemostasis. A knowledge of the factors controlling deposition is fundamental to the further understanding of these conditions.

An annular perfusion chamber has been developed for the *in vitro* exposure of subendothelium under controlled blood flow conditions.[1] A range of physical and chemical variables has been studied with this chamber.[2-6] The experimentally obtained values for platelet deposition compared satisfactorily with values predicted by available mass-transport theory. Theoretical analysis has indicated that the platelet attachment rate at the subendothelial surface is controlled predominantly by the transport of platelets through the blood[7] and that this transport is substantially increased by the physical presence of red cells.

The theoretical analysis will be reviewed and the implications of a diffusion-controlled transport situation will be discussed with respect to measurement of platelet kinetics. Preliminary data using a perfusion chamber particularly designed to operate under nondiffusion-controlled conditions will be reported.

Theoretical Considerations

A theory for describing platelet deposition on subendothelium has been previously presented.[7] The flux of platelets to the surface, j_x, can be expressed as a function of physical and chemical parameters:

* This work was supported in part by grant no. HL 14595 from the United States Public Health Service.

$$j_x = \frac{C_\infty}{\frac{1}{K} + \frac{1.48}{\left(\frac{V_o f(k) D_w{}^2}{d_e x}\right)^{1/3}}} \tag{1}$$

(kinetic) (transport)

where C_∞ = bulk platelet concentration, K = reaction (adsorption) rate coefficient, V_o = average blood velocity, D_w = platelet diffusion coefficient near the subendothelial surface, d_e = annular gap spacing, x = axial distance along the vessel segment, and $f(k)$ = a numerical coefficient dependent only on chamber dimensions. As written, the equation is analogous to the electrical analog of current flow through two resistors in a series. The platelet flux (current) which is obtained for a concentration driving force (voltage drop) depends on the sum of kinetic resistance and the transport resistance ($R_1 + R_2$). The kinetic resistance, $1/K$, is dependent on chemical factors and generally exhibits a strong dependence on temperature, whereas the diffusional resistance is classically dependent on fluid dynamical and physical factors and is only a weak function of temperature.

When either the physical or kinetic resistance predominates, two limiting cases occur:

(1). *Reaction-Controlled Transport.* The kinetic resistance is much greater than the diffusional resistance and Equation 1 reduces to

$$j_x = KC_\infty. \tag{2}$$

The platelet flux is dependent only on kinetic rate of adsorption and independent of fluid dynamical and physical parameters.

(2). *Diffusion-Controlled Transport.* The kinetic resistance is now small compared to diffusional resistance, and Equation 1 becomes

$$j_x = 0.67\ C_\infty \left[\frac{V_o f(k) D_w{}^2}{d_e x}\right]^{1/3}. \tag{3}$$

In this case, the platelet flux depends maximally on fluid dynamic factors and is unaffected by moderate changes in the kinetic rate of adsorption.

Equation 1 is referred to as intermediate transport kinetics and is typified by dependence on both kinetic and diffusional resistance. It should be noted that the ratio of kinetic to diffusional resistance can be increased by increasing either the physical or flow parameters or by decreasing the kinetic rate of adsorption.

The effect of the physical and flow parameters may be combined by considering the wall shear rate, γ_w. This term can be thought of as simply the slope of the blood velocity profile at the blood-subendothelium interface and is given by the expression

$$\gamma_w = \frac{2V_o f(k)}{d_e}. \tag{4}$$

Thus, substituting into Equation 3 leads to an expression for the platelet flux in diffusion-controlled transport which depends only on the wall shear rate, platelet diffusivity, axial position, and platelet concentration. Thus, results for chambers of different dimensions may be theoretically combined by determining the wall shear rate.

$$j_x = 0.67\ C_\infty \left[\frac{\gamma_w D_w{}^2}{2x} \right]^{1/3} \qquad (5)$$

A final modification must be considered, since there is strong evidence that platelet diffusivity is dependent on red cell rotation and translational motion in flowing blood.[8-10] This red cell motion is dependent on shear rate, and thus platelet diffusivity has been traditionally expressed as a power-law function of shear rate.

$$D_w = A^{1/2} (\gamma_w)^m \qquad (6)$$

where m is the power-law coefficient and A is a constant. Upon substitution, Equation 5 becomes

$$j_x = 0.67\ C_\infty \left[\frac{A\gamma_w}{2x} \right]^{\frac{2m+1}{3}} \qquad (7)$$

The coefficient m may be determined from a logarithmic plot of platelet flux versus wall shear rate, which gives as indicated by Equation 7, a straight line of slope, $(2m + 1)/3$.

Materials and Methods

Burgunder rabbits from different commercial sources, of either sex, and weighing 2.5–4.0 kg were used as blood donors. They were anesthetized by an intravenous injection of Numal-Roche (70 mg/kg), supplemented with ether as necessary.

Blood Collection. Nine volumes of blood were allowed to flow through a silastic cannula from a carotid artery into polycarbonate centrifuge tubes containing one volume of 90 mM sodium citrate. The tubes were inverted four times against parafilm.

Perfusion Experiments. A description of the basic annular chamber, as well as the general procedure for preparing the subendothelium of everted arterial segments the endothelium of which had been totally removed with a balloon catheter, and exposing them to flowing blood, has been reported previously.[1] A description of the minichamber especially designed for high shear rate studies has been reported.[3] Vessel segments were either 0.7 or 2.0 cm in length. The shorter segments were mounted and exposed in series on the annular core, and a mean value of platelet attachment was determined; the 2.0 cm segments were exposed individually and the mean was determined from deposition at several axial positions.

Briefly, whole blood (25–30 ml) was kept in a plastic reservoir and circulated into the chamber prefilled with phosphate-buffered saline solution (pH 7.4), through the annular space formed by the outer cylinder and vessel segment, and out of the chamber back into the reservoir by a roller pump (Holter). Chamber, reservoir, and buffer were all immersed in a water bath maintained at 37° C ± 1° C by an electronic controller. Platelet count was determined before and after perfusion with a Coulter Counter Model F; hematocrits were determined by centrifugation.

Fixation and Processing of Specimens. After exposure to the whole blood, the vessel segments were rinsed in phosphate-buffered saline solution and fixed in 2.5% (v/v) glutaraldehyde in 0.1M cacodylate buffer while still on the rod. The details of the postfixation, embedding of the exposed segments, and staining of the sections have been described by Baumgartner.[1, 6]

Morphometric Evaluation. Evaluation consisted in determining the percentage of the surface covered with platelets in a section 0.8–0.9 μm in thickness. Three types of platelet interaction with the subendothelial surface have been distinguished: 1) surface devoid of platelets; 2) platelets present at surface but not spread out (contact); and 3) platelets tightly adherent to surface (spread). Platelet adhesion is currently defined as surface coverage with platelets, including contact platelets, and is equivalent to the term "platelet deposition." In addition, platelet-platelet accumulation exceeding 5 μm was arbitrarily defined as mural platelet thrombi.

TABLE 1

SUMMARY OF LOW SHEAR RATE PERFUSION EXPERIMENTS

Chamber	Effective Diameter d_e (mm)	Average Flow Rate Q (ml/min)	Reynolds Number Re	Wall Shear Rate γ_w (sec^{-1})
Small	0.7	2.6	1.8	270.0
Original	2.4	10.0	6.1	52.0
		40.0	24.5	208.0
		160.0	97.5	832.0
Large	15.3	150.0	39.3	11.9*

* This value has been corrected over that previously reported.[7]

RESULTS

Low Shear Rate, $\gamma_w < 1000$ Sec^{-1}

Previous experimental investigations[1, 3, 4] have involved exposure of subendothelial surfaces to flowing blood in annular chambers of various dimensions. As indicated in TABLE 1, wall shear rates, as calculated from the slope of the Newtonian velocity profile, varied from 10 to 850 sec^{-1}, values encountered over a wide range of physiological flow situations. Under these conditions, the blood flow was laminar and fully developed. The following interactions were observed.

Platelet Contact (C). Platelet attachment to the subendothelial surface in a discoid, nonspread manner was significant only at short exposure times. The percentage of platelets in contact decreased rapidly with exposure until after 10 minutes platelets were less than 5% of the surface coverage.[1, 3, 6]

Platelet Deposition (S + C). By contrast, spread platelets (S) increased rapidly with exposure time, so that platelet deposition increased linearly with length of exposure for values less than 60% surface coverage and asymptotically to 100% coverage. Initial rates of platelet deposition were calculated by deter-

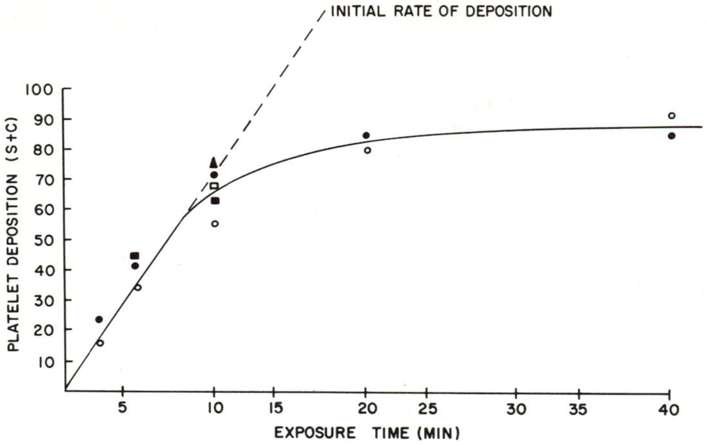

FIGURE 1. Platelet deposition on subendothelium exposed in the standard chamber for various lengths of time to blood flowing at 40 ml/min (wall shear rate of 200 sec^{-1}.) The initial rate of platelet deposition with standard error is determined from linear regression analysis. (Slope$=$7.1$\pm$0.8)

mining the slope of the linear portion of the deposition-exposure time curve by regression analysis (FIGURE 1).

Initial rates of deposition were determined for the three chambers and plotted on logarithmic coordinates versus the wall shear rate, as shown in FIGURE 2. The relationship appears linear, as predicted by Equation 7 for diffusion-controlled transport. The slope of the straight line determined by nonlinear regression analysis is 0.54. This results in a value for *m*, the power law coeffi-

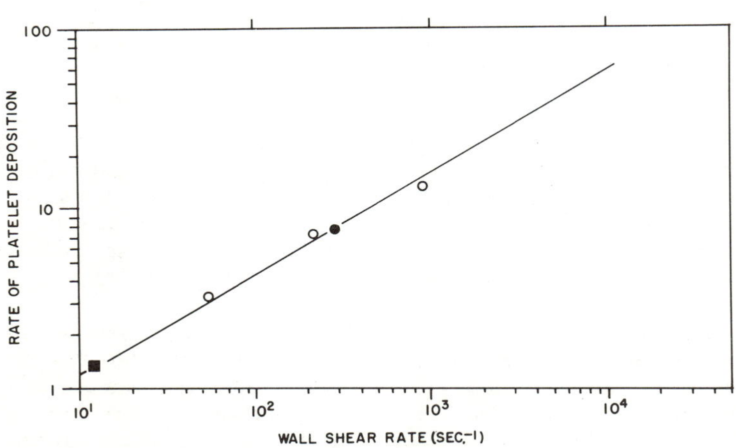

FIGURE 2. Initial rates of platelet deposition on subendothelium determined from large (■), standard (○), and small (●) chambers for various blood flow conditions are plotted versus the wall shear rate. The best straight line, with its 95% confidence limits, is determined by nonlinear regression analysis. (Slope$=$0.54+0.07)

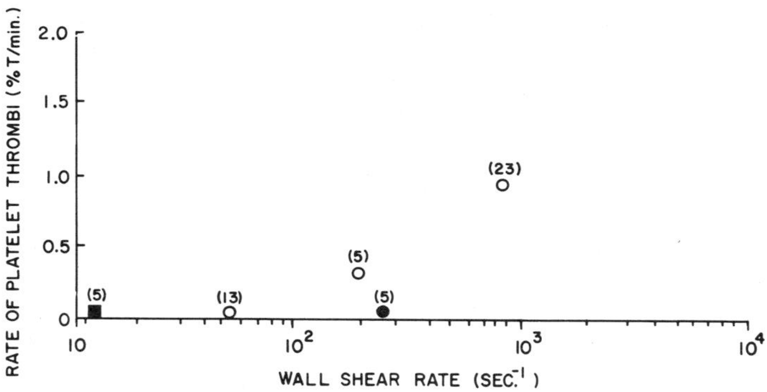

FIGURE 3. Average rates of formation of platelet thrombi on subendothelium exposed in large (■), standard (○), and small (●) chambers to various blood-flow conditions are plotted versus the wall shear rate. Number of experiments is indicated in brackets.

cient indicating dependence of platelet diffusivity on shear rate, $m = 0.31$. In addition, it is important to note that experimental values of platelet deposition obtained under quite different experimental conditions and in perfusion chambers of varying dimensions can be predicted and correlated by means of the shear rate value.

Mural Platelet Thrombi (*T*). Mural thrombi extending more than 5 μm from the subendothelium have several characteristics: (1) they are transient, attaining a maximum number and then disappearing completely within 40 minutes; and (2) they occur in significant numbers only at the higher shear rates (FIGURE 3). Below shear rates of 300 sec^{-1}, platelet thrombi are at most several percent of the platelet-subendothelial interactions. However, at 830 sec^{-1}, the rate of formation of platelet thrombi increases significantly, and 10% of the surface is covered with thrombi after 10 minutes' exposure. These data suggest a plausible explanation for the predominant occurrence of platelet-related thrombi in arterial flow *in vivo* where shear rates are sufficiently high.

High Shear Rate, $\gamma_w > 1000$ Sec^{-1}

Experiments have been conducted in the small chamber under the flow conditions indicated in TABLE 2 for exposure times of less than five minutes.

TABLE 2

SMALL PERFUSION CHAMBER

Flow Rate (ml/min)	Average Velocity (cm/sec)	Wall Shear Rate (sec^{-1})	Reynolds Number (Re)	Entrance Length (cm)
10	3.7	1030	7.5	0.01
20	7.5	2050	15.0	0.02
40	15.0	4100	30.0	0.04
160	60.0	16500	120.0	0.16

This chamber allows high shear rates to be obtained at blood flow rates comparable to those used in the original chamber while still maintaining laminar, fully established flow conditions. Under these shear conditions, the diffusive transport resistance is decreased in order to obtain a more sensitive measurement of kinetic resistance. Several observations have been made in preliminary perfusion experiments; the data in detail will be published elsewhere.

Platelet Contact. This is qualitatively similar to that observed at lower shear rates; in the first minute, platelet contact is approximately 60% of the total interactions, and this decreases to approximately 15% within five minutes.

Platelet Deposition. Spread platelets increase with exposure time in such a way that total platelet deposition increases at first linearly and then asymptotically to complete surface coverage. Rates of deposition, calculated from the linear portion of the deposition-exposure time curve, initially increase with increasing shear rate; the values for 2000 and 4000 sec^{-1} appear to be significantly below those predicted by extrapolation of the straight line indicated in FIGURE 2. Such a finding would be expected in the transition from diffusion-controlled transport to intermediate transport kinetics, where kinetic factors play a greater and shear factors a lesser role. However, at the highest shear rate (16,000 sec^{-1}) the initial rate of deposition decreases so that it is now comparable to the value at shear rate of 1000 sec^{-1}. Apparently, the deposition rate passes through a maximum at wall shear between 4000 and 1600 sec^{-1}. At values greater than the critical wall shear rate, the deposition rate decreases with increasing shear. Several possible mechanisms for this will be discussed later.

Mural Platelet Thrombi. These are formed in significant amounts under these high shear-rate conditions; the rate of surface covered with thrombi increases with shear rate except at the highest shear rate, where the coverage by thrombi (15% after three-minute exposure) is comparable to that at 4000 sec^{-1}. Platelet aggregation, defined as the percentage of spread platelets covered with thrombi ($T/S \times 100$), increases continuously with shear rate, thus indicating that the events that inhibit the rate of platelet attachment at the highest shear rate do not affect platelet thrombi to the same extent.

DISCUSSION

The attachment of platelets to subendothelium has been investigated for a wide range of physical and chemical factors.[2-6] In this present work, available mass-transport theory was used to describe the influence of the physical parameters, and a perfusion system was devised for a more sensitive measurement of platelet kinetics. The theory has indicated that the critical flow parameter for determining platelet transport to the vicinity of the subendothelium is wall shear rate.

For values less than 1000 sec^{-1}, the platelet deposition was adequately described by diffusion-controlled transport, for which the rate of platelet arrival at the surface was determined predominantly by the shear rate and was independent of platelet adhesion kinetics. Thus, under these shear conditions, a reduction in the adsorption coefficient for platelet-subendothelium attachment does not influence platelet deposition (and thus is not sensitive to measurement) until the coefficient is reduced by a factor large enough to substantially increase the reaction rate resistance, its magnitude becoming comparable to that of the diffusive transport resistance (see THEORETICAL CONSIDERATIONS). Indeed, such behavior is suggested in studies of the effect of sodium citrate on platelet deposition.[2, 11] Deposition is unaltered in blood with increasing citrate concentration from that observed for native blood until a high enough citrate level is reached (above 27 mM in plasma), after which deposition decreases rapidly with citrate concentration. The measurement of platelet adsorption kinetics is important in further characterizing the platelet abnormalities in certain bleeding disorders. A defect in platelet adhesion to subendothelium has previously been reported in the perfusion chamber for shear rates of 830 sec^{-1} in von Willebrand's [12] and storage-pool disease [13] and in Bernard-Soulier Syndrome; [14] however, in certain patients with bleeding disorders the defect is slight, and a more sensitive measurement of its magnitude is required. In fact, it has been indicated that the defect in von Willebrand's disease may be masked by shear rate conditions as low as 200 sec^{-1}.[11] Studies are currently in progress at shear rates greater than 1000 sec^{-1}. Baumgartner [15] has indicated that a defect in platelet adhesion caused by an antibody to factor VIII is observed only at shear rates greater than 1000 sec^{-1}.

For shear rates of 2000–4000 sec^{-1}, preliminary experiments suggest that platelet deposition is being influenced by platelet-attachment kinetics in that the deposition rate is decreased below what would be expected at such shear rates for diffusion-controlled transport. At 16,000 sec^{-1} the deposition rate decreases to a value comparable to that obtained at 1000 sec^{-1}. The decrease in the rate of platelet deposition with increasing shear rate is not expected from classical transport considerations which predict a continuous, asymptotic approach to reaction-controlled transport (determined solely by platelet kinetics and independent of fluid dynamical and physical factors). Apparently, an alternate mechanism has become important. There are several possibilities: the shear forces may be altering platelet reactivity in the blood prior to attachment (shear damage); shear may be physically removing platelets from the surface either by tearing off previously adherent platelets whose surface bonds cannot withstand the continued force (fatigue), or by preventing adequate residence time in the vicinity of the subendothelial surface for newly arrived platelets to bond (residence time). The increased percentage of platelets onto adherent platelets (platelet aggregation) at this shear rate suggests that the overall platelet transport has not been significantly diminished; however, transport to the wall may be diminished by the physical presence of the aggregates. Experiments are currently in progress to determine the nature of this shear rate effect and how it might influence the measurement of platelet surface kinetics.

REFERENCES

1. BAUMGARTNER, H. R. 1973. The role of blood flow in platelet adhesion, fibrin deposition and formation of mural thrombi. Microvasc. Res. **5:** 167.
2. BAUMGARTNER, H. R. 1974. The subendothelial surface and thrombosis. Thromb. Diath. Haemorrh. (Suppl.) **59:** 91.
3. TURITTO, V. T. & H. R. BAUMGARTNER. 1974. Effect of physical factors on platelet adherence to subendothelium. Thromb. Diath. Haemorrh. (Suppl.) **60:** 17.
4. TURITTO, V. T. & H. R. BAUMGARTNER. 1975. Platelet interaction with subendothelium in a perfusion system: physical role of red blood cells. Microvasc. Res. **9:** 335.

5. Turitto, V. T. & H. R. Baumgartner. 1975. Effect of temperature on platelet interaction with subendothelium exposed to flowing blood. Haemostasis **3:** 224.
6. Baumgartner, H. R., R. Muggli, T. B. Tschopp & V. T. Turitto. 1976. Platelet adhesion and adhesion induced aggregation: effects of surface properties and blood factors. Thromb. Haem. **35:** 124.
7. Turitto, V. T. & H. G. Baumgartner. 1975. Platelet deposition on subendothelium exposed to flowing blood: mathematical analysis of physical parameters. Trans. Amer. Soc. Artif. Int. Organs **21:** 593.
8. Turitto, V. T., A. M. Benis & E. F. Leonard. 1972. Platelet diffusion in flowing blood. Indust. Engr. Chem. Fund. **11:** 216.
9. Goldsmith, H. L. 1971. Red cell motions and wall interactions in tube flow. Fed. Proc. **30:** 1641.
10. Goldsmith, H. L. 1972. The flow of model particles and blood cells and its relation to thrombogenesis. *In* Progress in Hemostasis and Thrombosis. T. H. Spaet, Ed. : 97. Grune & Stratton, Inc, New York, N.Y.
11. Weiss, H. J., T. Tschopp, V. T. Turitto & H. R. Baumgartner. This volume.
12. Tschopp, T., H. J. Weiss & H. R. Baumgartner. 1974. Decreased adhesion of platelets to subendothelium in von Willebrand's disease. J. Lab. Clin. Med. **83:** 296–300.
13. Weiss, H. J., T. B. Tschopp & H. R. Baumgartner. 1975. Impaired interaction (adhesion-aggregation) of platelets with the subendothelium in storage pool disease and after aspirin ingestion—a comparison with von Willebrand's disease. N. Engl. J. Med. **293:** 619–623.
14. Weiss, H. J., T. B. Tschopp, H. R. Baumgartner, I. I. Sussman, M. M. Johnson & J. J. Egan. 1974. Decreased adhesion of giant (Bernard-Soulier) platelets to subendothelium—further implications on the role of the von Willebrand factor in hemostasis. Am. J. Med. **57:** 920–925.
15. Baumgartner, H. R., T. B. Tschopp & D. Meyer. In press.

INTERACTION OF PLATELETS WITH SUBENDOTHELIUM: A NEW METHOD FOR IDENTIFYING AND CLASSIFYING ABNORMALITIES OF PLATELET FUNCTION *

Harvey J. Weiss,† Hans R. Baumgartner,‡ Thomas B. Tschopp,‡
and Vincent T. Turitto †

† Department of Medicine
The Roosevelt Hospital and
Columbia University College of Physicians and Surgeons
New York, New York 10019
‡ Department of Experimental Medicine
F. Hoffmann-La Roche & Co. Ltd.
Basel, Switzerland

Introduction

Platelets are thought to contribute to hemostasis by adhering to elements of the vessel wall and by forming aggregates that result in the arrest of bleeding. Because of the difficulty of quantifying platelet reactivity *in vivo,* a variety of *in vitro* tests have been developed for the study of platelet function. Among these are measurements of platelet retention in glass bead filters, the aggregation of platelets by various agents in an instrument known as an aggregometer, clot retraction, and the development of platelet procoagulant (platelet factor 3 activity). With these tests, a variety of defects in platelet function have been identified in patients with bleeding disorders (Figure 1).[1] It is tempting to assume that some abnormality of platelet function during the primary arrest of bleeding accounts for the hemostatic defects in these patients. Direct evidence, however, concerning the interaction of platelets with vascular surfaces in these subjects has been lacking. Baumgartner has recently developed a technique for directly assessing the adhesion and aggregation of platelets in citrated whole blood with the subendothelium of rabbit aortic segments under flow conditions similar to those in arteries.[2, 3] We have used this technique to study platelet-subendothelium interaction in a variety of hemostatic disorders and have found abnormalities in adhesion or aggregation that may account for the hemostatic defects in these patients.[4–8] In this paper, we shall review the results of these previously published studies [4–8] and present some more recent observations on the interaction of platelets with the subendothelium.

Materials and Methods

The interaction of platelets in flowing, citrated blood with the subendothelium of rabbit aortic segments was studied by the previously described method of Baumgartner.[2–8] Briefly, venous blood is mixed with 1/10 volume of

* Supported in part by grant HL 15495 from the United States Public Health Service.

108 mM sodium citrate and, after determination of the hematocrit, the plasma citrate concentration is adjusted to 19.7 mM with 108 mM sodium citrate. Forty ml of blood is perfused by means of a roller pump for ten minutes at the rate of 160 ml/minute through a chamber containing everted segments of rabbit aorta previously denuded of endothelium by means of a balloon catheter. Previous studies have shown that this subendothelial surface consists primarily of an amorphous substance that is similar to the basement membrane of small blood vessels, but that does not form a continuous lamina.[9, 10] We also studied the interaction of platelets with subendothelial segments that had been previously incubated with α-chymotrypsin (Worthington, 0.4 mg/ml) for 24 hours at 37° C.[11] α-Chymotrypsin digestion removes both amorphous material and microfibrils and leaves a surface consisting primarily of elastin and islands of fibrillar collagen.[11, 12] Since platelets adhere poorly to elastin and do not spread

Disorder	Feature	Platelet Retention	Platelet Aggregation Collagen	ADP(1°)	Ristocetin
von Willebrand's Disease	▼ Factor VIII	●	○	○	●
Bernard-Soulier Syndrome	Giant Platelets	●	○	○	●
Thrombasthenia	▼ Clot Retraction	●	●	●	○
Storage Pool Disease	▼ Dense Granule Contents	●	●	○	○
Aspirin Ingestion	▼ Cyclo-oxygenase	○	●	○	○

○ = Normal ● = Abnormal (▼)

FIGURE 1. Defects in the primary arrest of bleeding. ADP (1°) signifies primary aggregation by ADP in citrated platelet-rich plasma.

upon this type of surface, platelet interaction with the α-chymotrypsin-digested surface is owing primarily to their interaction with collagen fibrils.[11, 12] Each perfusion rod used in the study contained three undigested vessel segments and two segments that had been digested with α-chymotrypsin. The order of the segments is indicated in FIGURE 2. Following perfusion, the chamber was rinsed with buffered saline and the blood vessel segments were fixed in gluteraldehyde and osmium tetroxide, dehydrated in ethanol, and embedded in Epon.[4] Interaction of platelets with the subendothelium was evaluated by a morphometric method in sections the thickness of which was 0.8 μm and which were stained with toluidine blue and basic fuchsin.[2-8] Four types of interaction are recorded (FIGURE 3) as follows. (a) Naked: no platelet interaction with the subendothelium was observed; (b) contact: platelets contact the subendothelium but are not spread out upon it; (c) spread: platelet is spread out on the subendothelium; and (d) thrombus: a spread platelet has superimposed

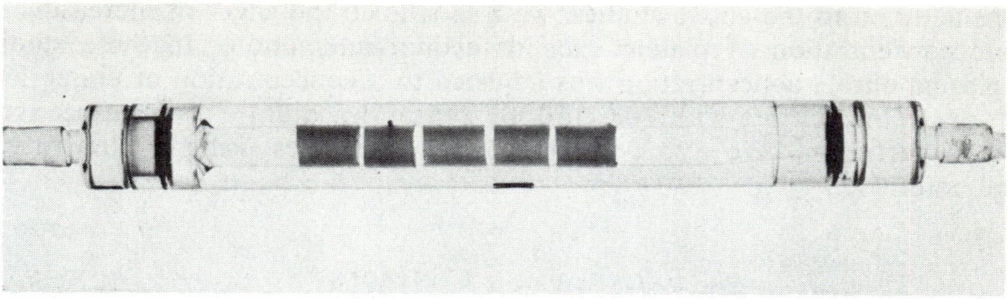

FIGURE 2. Perfusion chamber containing everted segments of deendothelialized rabbit aorta. Anticoagulated blood is perfused through the chamber at a flow rate of 160 ml/mm, exposing the platelets to subendothelium (segments 1, 3, and 5, left to right) or α-chymotrypsin digested subendothelium (segments 2 and 4). Segments are 7 μm long, and for demonstration purposes are shown separated from each other. (In the actual experiments, the segments were mounted without gaps between them.)

upon it a platelet thrombus 5 μm or more in height. Approximately 1000 intersection points were counted for each segment and the percentage of the surface covered by contact platelets, adherent platelets, or thrombi was recorded. In previous studies,[4-7] adhesion was defined as the percentage of coverage with spread platelets, ignoring the small (less than 3%) percent of coverage with contact platelets. In the present study, adhesion is defined as the total deposition, e.g. C + S. All of the segments used in previous studies on undigested subendothelium have been reevaluated in this manner and compared with the results on the α-chymotrypsin-digested segments, as reported elsewhere.[8] The results of these previously reported evaluations [8] are incorporated into the present paper. Aggregation is defined, as in previous studies, as $\frac{100T}{S}$.

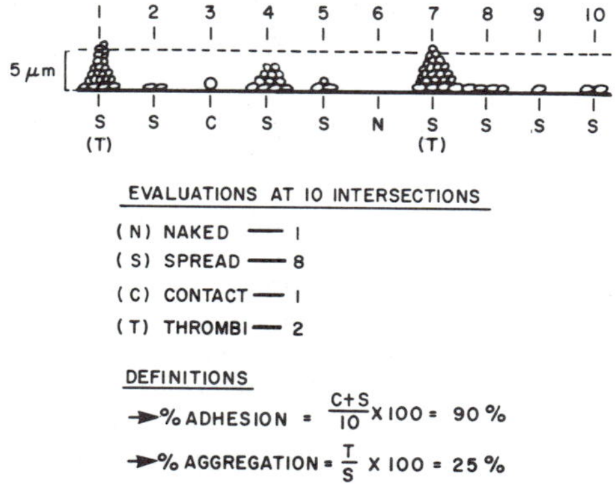

FIGURE 3. Morphometric evaluation of platelet-subendothelium interaction. Figure depicts, schematically, the evaluation of platelet interaction with the subendothelium at 10 intersection points 10 μm apart. (In practice, about 1000 intersections are evaluated per segment.) Platelet adhesion is defined as the percentage of surface coverage. In the example shown, platelets are present (C+S) at 9 of the 10 intersections. Aggregation is defined as the percentage of spread platelets (S) that are covered with thrombi (5 μm or more in height). Values are typical of those obtained on (undigested) subendothelium.

In addition to the above studies, we also studied the effect of increasing the citrate concentration of platelet-subendothelium interaction. In these studies, the plasma citrate concentration was adjusted to a concentration of either 19.7, 27.5, or 45 mM citrate with 108, 150, or 245 mM sodium citrate, respectively, prior to perfusion. We also performed selected studies using a flow rate of 40 ml/minute.

Patients and Controls

We studied nine patients with von Willebrand's disease,[4, 7, 8] two with the Bernard-Soulier syndrome,[6, 8] three Glanzmann's thrombasthenia,[5, 8] six with storage pool disease,[7, 8] and seven normal subjects who ingested aspirin.[7, 8] A general review of these disorders has been recently published.[1] The controls were 18 normal subjects used in previously reported studies.[4, 7] All subjects were asked not to take any drugs for at least one week prior to being studied.

Results

Normal Subjects

In normal subjects 84.0 ± 1.6 (SE)% of the undigested subendothelium was covered with adherent platelets (81.5% spread + 2.5% contact). Platelet aggregation, defined as $\frac{100T}{S}$, was 14.7 ± 1.9 (SE)%. Figure 4A shows a representative section demonstrating the deposition of normal platelets on the subendothelium.

On the fibrillar collagen of the α-chymotrypsin-digested surface, adhesion was 28.2 ± 2.1 (SE)% and aggregation was 80.1 ± 1.5%. The interaction of platelets with this type of surface has been described in detail previously.[8, 11]

Disorders of Platelet Adhesion

von Willebrand's Disease

We studied nine patients with this disorder.[4, 7, 8] As shown in Table 1, all subjects showed the characteristic findings of a prolonged bleeding time, decrease in the factor VIII complex, decreased retention of platelets in glass bead filters, and impaired ristocetin-induced platelet aggregation.[13, 14] The interaction of platelets with the subendothelium in this disorder is shown in Figure 5. Compared with controls, adhesion (C + S) was decreased on both the undigested and the α-chymotrypsin-digested surfaces, ($p < 0.001$), whereas aggregation $\left(\frac{100T}{S}\right)$ was normal.

Analysis of the physical and chemical factors that determine the deposition of platelets on the subendothelium have been recently published.[3, 12, 15, 16] We have begun to study how these factors may influence the magnitude of the adhesion defect in von Willebrand's disease.

1. Surface factors. The magnitude of the adhesion defect (if expressed as

a percentage of control values) is greater on the α-chymotrypsin-digested surface than on the undigested surface (FIGURE 5). This was further demonstrated in one patient (C.M.) who showed consistently low values for adhesion to undigested subendothelium in the initial studies, but in whom we have recently obtained some values that are within the range of normal values. However, we continue to obtain decreased values for the adhesion of his platelets to α-chymotrypsin digested subendothelium. This is demonstrated in FIGURE 6(A), which shows that at the standard flow rate of 160 ml per min, adhesion of this

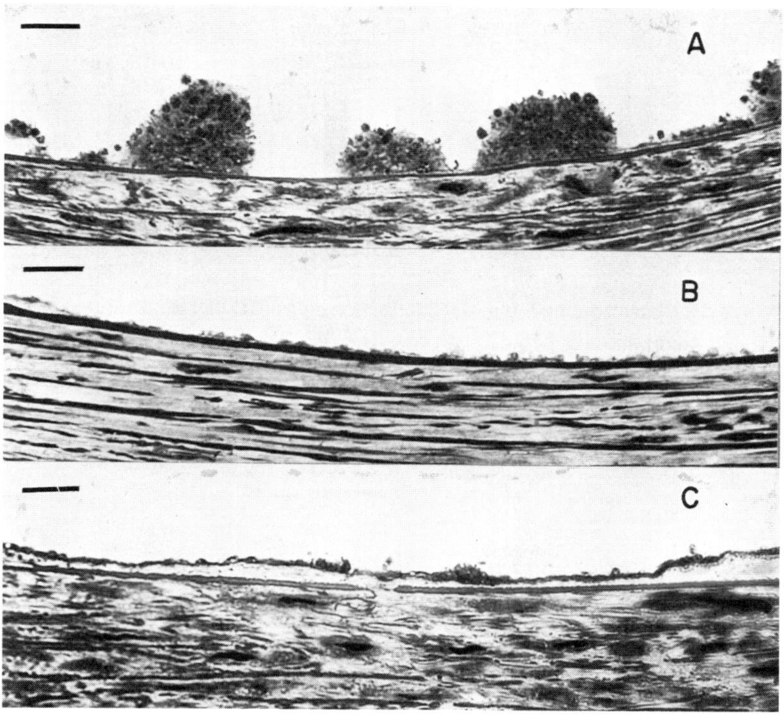

FIGURE 4. Interaction of platelets with the subendothelium. Light micrographs of arterial subendothelium that had been exposed to anticoagulated blood for 10 minutes in the perfusion chamber. A=normal subject; B=thrombasthenia; C=normal subject 2.5 hours after ingesting 0.9 g of aspirin. Bar indicates 10 μm.

patient's platelets to (undigested) subendothelium was the same as for control platelets, whereas adhesion to α-chymotrypsin-digested subendothelium surface was decreased.

2. Flow factors. The demonstration of an adhesion defect in the above patient (C.M.) was also flow rate dependent. Thus, (FIGURE 6(A)), although defective adhesion was demonstrable on the α-chymotrypsin-digested surface at a flow rate of 160 ml/min (shear rate 830 sec^{-1}), it was no longer demonstrable (FIGURE 6(B)) when the flow rate was reduced to 40 ml/min (shear rate 200 sec^{-1}).

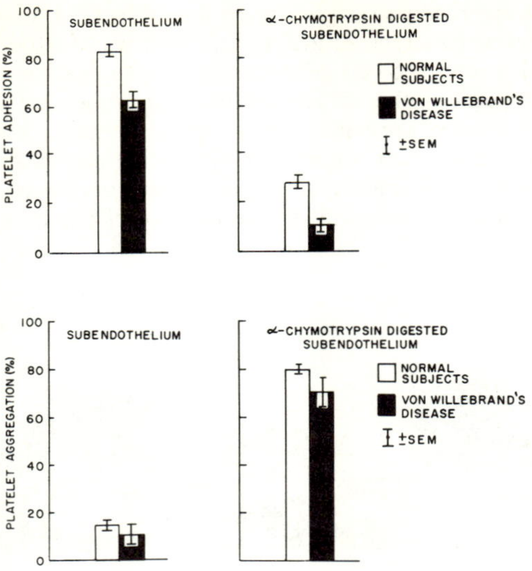

FIGURE 5. Platelet-subendothelium interaction in von Willebrand's disease. Results depict the adhesion (C+S) or aggregation $\left(\frac{100T}{S}\right)$ of platelets on subendothelium or α-chymotrypsin digested subendothelium. Patients studied were those shown in TABLE 1. (Data from References 4, 7, and 8.)

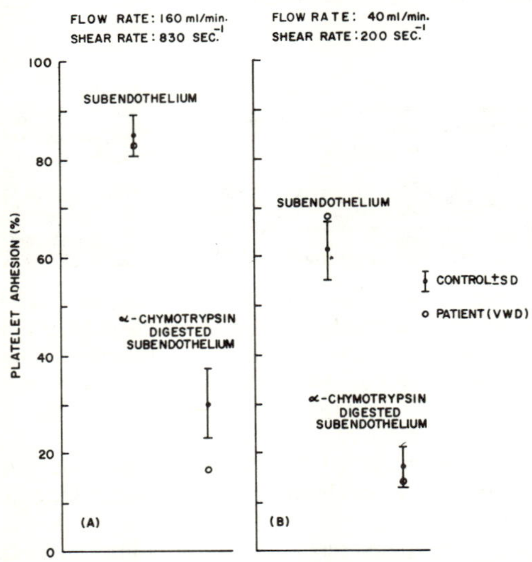

FIGURE 6. Effect of surface and flow rate on platelet adhesion. (A): blood from patient C.M. with von Willebrand's disease (VWD), or control subjects, was perfused at a rate of 160 ml/min (shear rate 830 sec^{-1}) through a chamber containing vessel segments (as in FIGURE 2), thereby exposing platelets to subendothelium and α-chymotrypsin digested subendothelium. (B): same as A, but with a flow rate of 40 ml/min and shear rate of 200 sec^{-1}.

3. Kinetic factors. Increasing the plasma citrate concentration from 19.7 to 45 mM completely eliminated thrombus formation (similar to previous findings using rabbit blood[10, 12]) and decreased the adhesion of normal platelets to the undigested subendothelium from 87 to 66% (FIGURE 7). In patient C.M., the effects of increasing the citrate concentration were more dramatic. Average adhesion values obtained with use of the standard 19.7 mM concentration were 80%, whereas they were 11% when the citrate concentration was 45 mM (FIGURE 7). We then studied platelet adhesion at the two citrate concentrations (19.7 and 45 mM) in six other patients with von Willebrand's disease. As seen in FIGURE 8, the magnitude of the adhesion defect in von Willebrand's disease is greater with the higher citrate concentration.

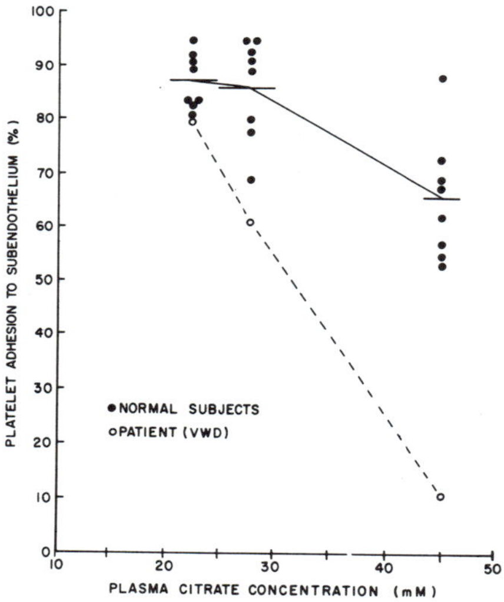

FIGURE 7. Effect of citrate concentration on platelet adhesion to subendothelium. Results on patient C.M. with von Willebrand's disease (VWD) are the average of two separate perfusions.

The results of these preliminary studies demonstrate that both kinetic factors and flow conditions determine the magnitude of the platelet adhesion defect in von Willebrand's disease. This is discussed further below (see DISCUSSION).

Finally, although there is considerable evidence that an abnormality of platelet function accounts for the prolonged bleeding time in von Willebrand's disease, other evidence suggests that the platelets are not inherently abnormal in this disorder. Rather, these patients may be deficient in a plasma factor, associated with factor VIII, that is necessary for normal platelet function.[1] For example, transfusions of plasma or cryoprecipitate often result in a shortening of the bleeding time and a correction of the platelet defects.[17, 18] We have studied the effect of administering cryoprecipitate to a patient (V.M.) with von Willebrand's disease on the adhesion of platelets to subendothelium and α-chymotrypsin-digested subendothelium. As seen in FIGURE 9, adhesion values increased two hours after transfusion, but returned to pretreatment values after 48 hours.

Bernard-Soulier (giant platelet) Syndrome

As in von Willebrand's disease, both ristocetin-induced platelet aggregation and platelet retention are impaired in patients with the Bernard-Soulier Syndrome.[1] Unlike von Willebrand's disease, platelet dysfunction in this disorder is owing to an intrinsic platelet defect (see FIGURE 10), possibly the deficiency of a specific membrane glycoprotein (Type I).[19, 20]

We have studied the interaction of platelets with the subendothelium in two patients with the Bernard-Soulier Syndrome.[6, 8] The findings in this disorder were similar to those in von Willebrand's disease, but of somewhat greater severity.[6, 8] Adhesion is markedly decreased, but aggregation is normal (FIGURE 10). These findings have been confirmed.[19]

TABLE 1

PATIENTS WITH VON WILLEBRAND'S DISEASE *

Subjects	Bleeding Time	Factor VIII †			Platelet Aggregation by Ristocetin (1.2 mg/ml)	Platelet Retention
		AHF	VWF	AGN		
Patients	(min)	(units/100 ml)			(%)	(%)
C.M.	>60	4	4	0.3	0	27
J.H.	>60	4	3	0.4	0	20
D.R.	>60	4	2	0.3	0	6
V.M.	>60	2	0	0.2	0	1
A.S.	28	23	8	7	8	2
J.L.	40	30	6	19	0	10
P.H.	20	9	9	4	13	25
J.W.	15	13	12	11	0	25
M.L.	10	49	40	60	9	8
Normal Values	2–6	50–200	55–135	50–180	51–93	31–81

* Data from References 13 and 14.

† AHF=antihemophilic factor; VWF=von Willebrand factor (ristocetin aggregation assay); AGN=factor VIII antigen.

Disorders of Platelet Aggregation

Some physiologic agents such as adenosine diphosphate (ADP) and epinephrine can aggregate platelets directly. In addition, aggregation by these agents is often followed by a second wave of aggregation, owing to the synthesis of prostaglandin-related substances and the release of endogenous platelet ADP[1] (FIGURE 11A). The latter also accounts for platelet aggregation by collagen (FIGURE 11A).

Studies using the aggregometer have identified a variety of defects in platelet aggregation in patients with bleeding disorders,[1] as depicted in FIGURE 11. Platelet aggregation is impaired most in thrombasthenia; in this disorder, the

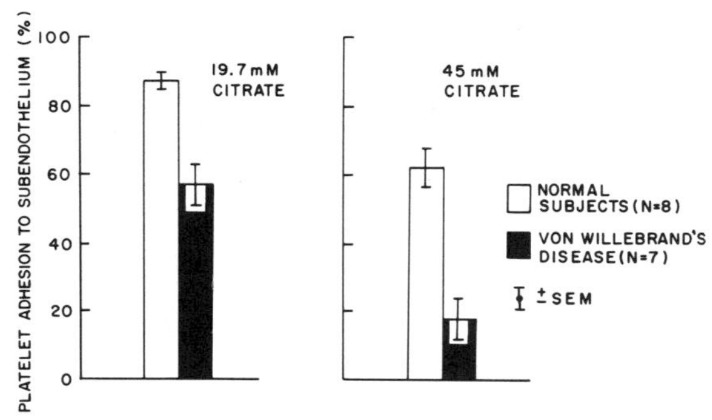

FIGURE 8. Adhesion of platelets to subendothelium at two citrate concentrations. Seven patients with von Willebrand's disease and 8 normal subjects were studied. With each concentration, adhesion is decreased in patients compared with controls ($p < .001$), but the relative magnitude of the defect is greater at the higher citrate concentration.

platelets are not aggregated by ADP, epinephrine, or collagen (FIGURE 11B). In another group of disorders, the platelets can aggregate in response to both ADP and epinephrine, but do not release normal amounts of endogenous ADP.[1] This may be owing to either an absolute deficiency of platelet ADP (e.g., in storage pool disease) or to an impairment of the release mechanism (e.g., normal subjects who ingest aspirin).[1] In both cases, "second-phase" aggregation responses and collagen-induced aggregation are impaired (FIGURE 11C).

We have studied the interaction of platelets with the subendothelium in patients with the above type of defects.

Thrombasthenia

In patients with this disorder, adhesion to the subendothelium was normal, but aggregation was absent[5, 8] (FIGURE 12). In contrast to the findings described below in patients with release defects (in whom small platelet thrombi,

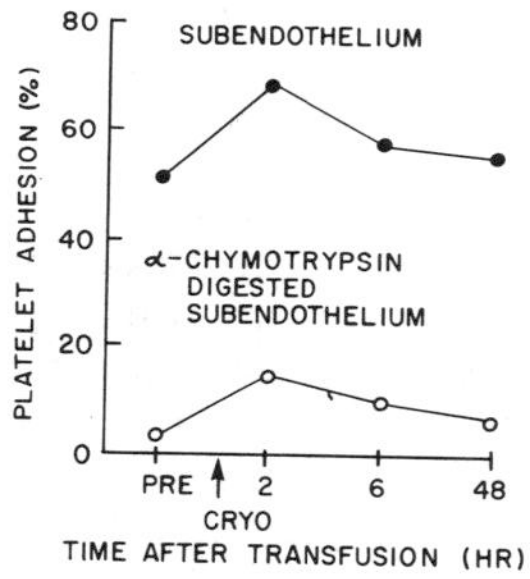

FIGURE 9. Effect of transfusing cryoprecipitate on platelet adhesion in a patient with von Willebrand's disease. Patient V.M. (TABLE 1) was studied before and after transfusion of 9 units of cryoprecipitate.

less than 5 μm in height, were sometimes seen), thrombus formation was completely absent in thrombasthenia.[5, 8] In all three patients, a monolayer of spread platelets adherent to the subendothelium was observed (FIGURE 4B), and, by electron microscopy, platelet-to-platelet interaction was absent.[5]

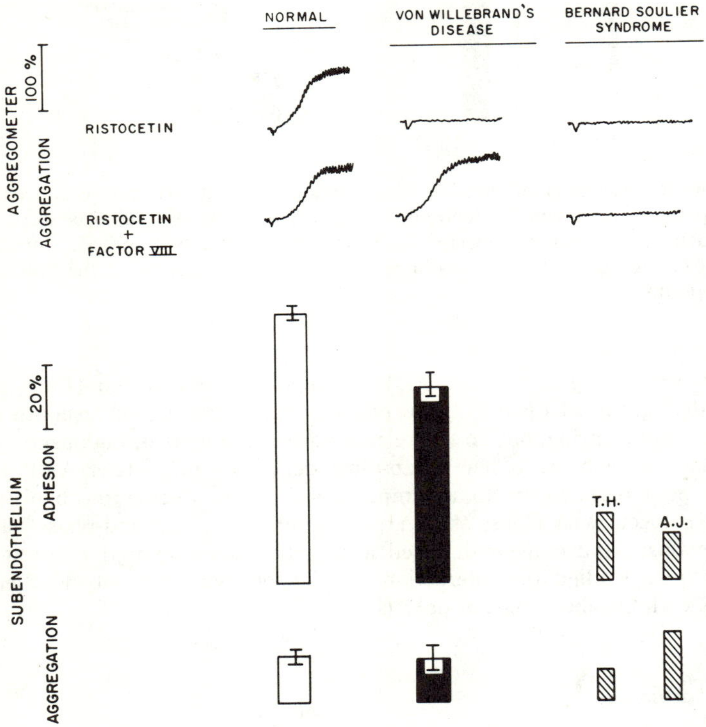

FIGURE 10. Platelet function in the Bernard-Soulier Syndrome (BSS). Findings in two patients (T.H. and A.J.) with the BSS are compared with those in normal subjects and in von Willebrand's disease. *Top:* Ristocetin-induced aggregation, studied in the aggregometer. *Bottom:* Platelet adhesion and aggregation on subendothelium. Bars depict SEM. (Data from References 6 and 8.)

Aspirin Ingestion

Seven normal subjects were studied before and 2.5 hours after ingesting 0.9 grams of aspirin.[7, 8] FIGURE 4C shows a representative light micrograph demonstrating the interaction of platelets with the subendothelium after aspirin ingestion; the complete results of the study are shown in FIGURE 13. Aspirin ingestion did not reduce platelet adhesion to either the subendothelium or the α-chymotrypsin-digested subendothelium. By contrast, aggregates 5 μm or more in height were virtually eliminated (0.1%) on the subendothelium, although platelet-to-

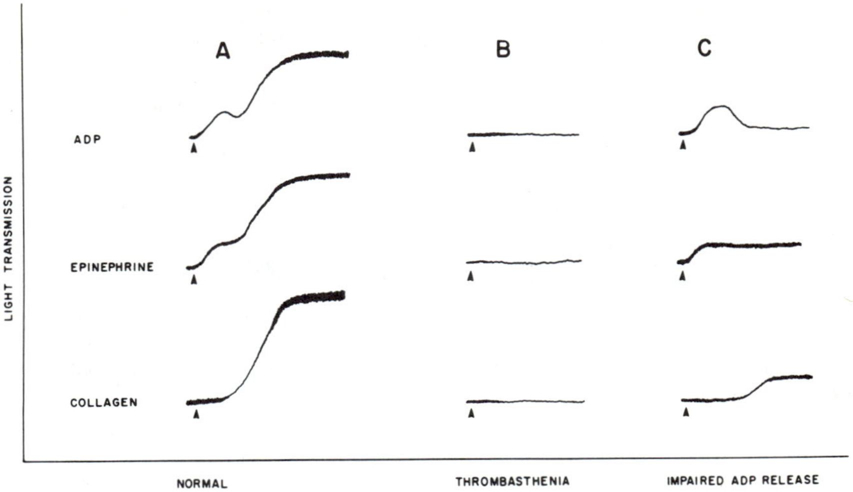

FIGURE 11. Aggregometer patterns in normal subjects and patients with impaired platelet aggregation. A: Normal patterns. B: Glanzmann's thrombasthenia. C: Release defects; these can be due to either impairment of the release mechanism (e.g. aspirin ingestion) or deficiency of endogenous platelet ADP (e.g. storage pool disease). (See Reference 1.)

platelet interaction was not completely eliminated; small platelet thrombi, 2–5 μm in height, were present at an average of 9% of the surface.[7] On the α-chymotrypsin-digested surface, platelet aggregation was reduced from 82.9 ± 2.3 (SE)% to 9.5 ± 3.6% ($p < .001$).[8] As seen by electron microscopy, platelets that had adhered to the surface were depleted of their granules.[7]

Storage Pool Disease

Interaction of platelets with the subendothelium in six patients with this disorder were somewhat more complex[7,8] (FIGURE 14). Aggregation values were similar to those in normal subjects who had ingested aspirin; aggregation

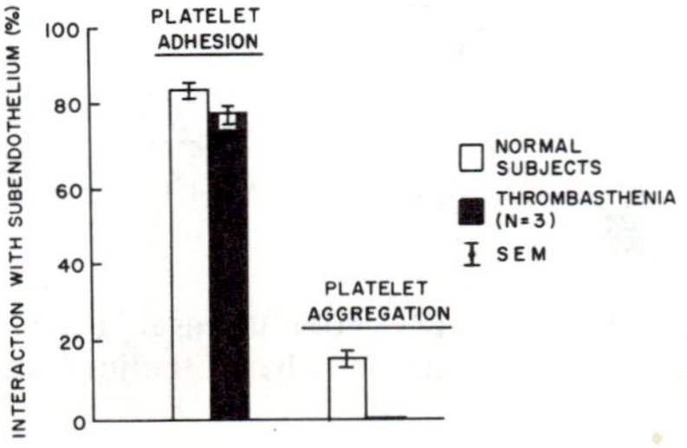

FIGURE 12. Platelet-subendothelium interaction in thrombasthenia. (Data from References 5 and 8.) Platelet aggregation in the patients was 0.0%.

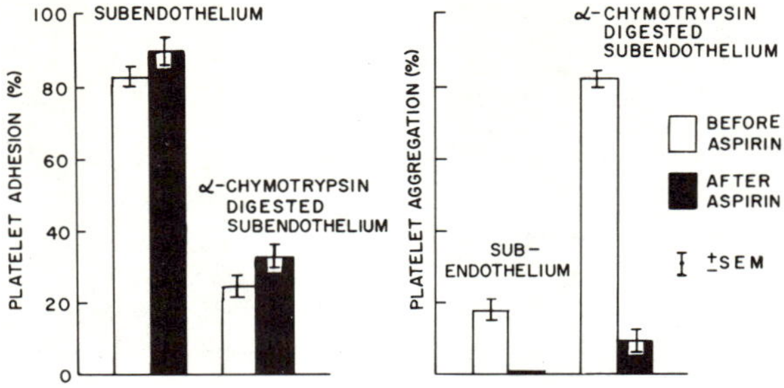

FIGURE 13. Effect of aspirin ingestion on platelet-subendothelium interaction. Seven normal subjects were studied before and 2.5 hours after ingestion of 0.9 grams of aspirin. Aggregation on subendothelium after aspirin ingestion was 0.1%. (Data from References 7 and 8.)

was virtually absent (0.1%) on the subendothelium and was markedly reduced to 9.9 ± 1.7 (SE)% on the α-chymotrypsin-digested subendothelium (normal values 80.1 ± 1.5%). In contrast to the findings after aspirin ingestion, adhesion was decreased in some subjects on both surfaces[7, 8] and the decreased adhesion in the six patients, considered as a group, was significant ($p < .001$).

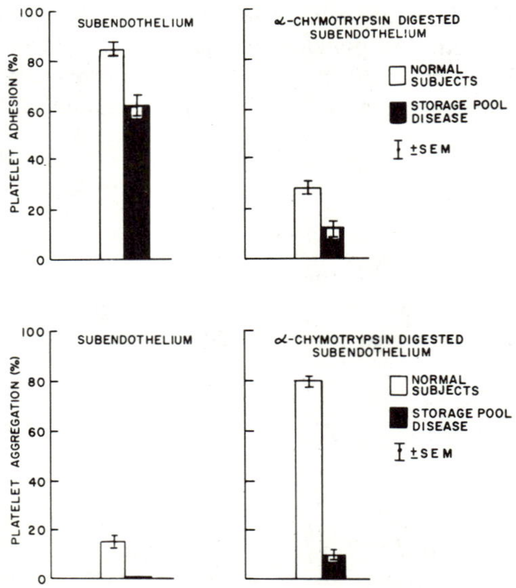

FIGURE 14. Platelet-subendothelium interaction in storage pool disease. Studies were done in 6 patients with this disorder. Aggregation value on subendothelium was 0.1%. (Data from References 7 and 8.)

Discussion

Previous studies using the aggregometer and glass bead retention tests have disclosed abnormalities of platelet function in patients with bleeding disorders and in normal subjects who have ingested aspirin (Figure 1).[1] In some disorders, such as von Willebrand's disease and the Bernard-Soulier syndrome, a physiologic basis for the hemostatic defect has not been apparent. The technique introduced by Baumgartner for studying the interaction of platelets with the subendothelium under flow conditions similar to those in arteries has provided new information about the pathogenesis of these disorders. The findings also suggest a basis for their classification.

Disorders of Adhesion

In von Willebrand's disease[4, 7, 8] and the Bernard-Soulier syndrome[6, 8] the adhesion (C + S) of platelets to the subendothelium was impaired, but thrombus formation $\left(\frac{100T}{S}\right)$ on the (fewer) adherent platelets was normal.[7, 8] Thus, the primary defect is one of platelet adhesion, and a similar impairment in platelet-vessel interaction may account for the hemostatic defect in these disorders. In addition, preliminary studies suggest that von Willebrand's disease in pigs may confer some protection against the development of atherosclerosis.[21] This could be related to an impairment of platelet adhesion to subendothelium and hence lessened availability of the platelet factor that stimulates the proliferation of arterial smooth-muscle cells.[22] Possibly, a drug that inhibited the von Willebrand factor might be useful in the prophylaxis of thromboatherogenesis.

The cause of the impairment in platelet adhesion in von Willebrand's disease and the factors that influence the magnitude of the defect remain to be determined. The magnitude of the defect is greater on the α-chymotrypsin-digested subendothelium than on the untreated subendothelium. Increasing the citrate concentration in the blood also enhances the defect (Figures 7, 8), whereas decreasing the flow rate has the opposite effect (Figure 6). A detailed study of the chemical and physical factors that determine the magnitude of the platelet adhesion defect in von Willebrand's disease is currently in progress. The data obtained thus far suggest the preliminary interpretations discussed below.

Analysis of platelet interaction with subendothelium in rabbits by means of available mass transfer theory has previously indicated that platelet adhesion is adequately described by diffusion-controlled transport kinetics under the standard test conditions.[16, 23] Such a mechanism implies that the transport rate of platelets through blood to the vicinity of the subendothelium, which is controlled by physical factors such as flow rate and chamber dimensions, is significantly less than the potential adsorption rate of platelets at the surface. Thus, physical factors strongly influence platelet adhesion, whereas chemical factors are less effective. The results shown in Figure 7 are consistent with such an analysis: platelet adhesion in the control group is not significantly affected by an increase in citrate concentration to 27.5 mM (although platelet aggregation is significantly reduced). At a citrate concentration of 45 mM, platelet adhesion decreases, presumably because the platelet adsorption rate (reaction kinetics) has been reduced to a level that is comparable to the diffusive transport rate and thus influences the overall adhesion rate (intermediate-transport kinetics). Conversely, the patient with von Willebrand's disease shows a continuous decrease in adhesion with an increase in citrate concentration, which is consistent with expectations for intermediate transport kinetics. Apparently, the defect in platelet exhibited by this patient is not sufficient to be measured under the standard experimental conditions (diffusion-controlled transport); however, when the reaction kinetics are decreased by use of a higher citrate concentration (45 mM), the rate of platelet transport relative to the adsorption reaction rate is increased and the defect in adhesion becomes evident. Alternatively, such a defect could presumably be measured at normal citrate levels by increasing the transport rate physically (by increasing the shear rate) until it was comparable in magnitude to the kinetic rate of adsorption (see Ref. 16 for further discussion). Findings in this and other studies suggest that, for any given surface, the demonstration of a platelet adhesion defect in von Willebrand's disease is strongly shear-dependent; e.g. it may be demonstrable only at a critically high shear rate. Thus, on the α-chymotrypsin-digested subendothelium, an adhesion defect demonstrable at a shear rate of 830 sec^{-1} (our standard flow conditions) was no longer evident when the shear rate was reduced to 200 sec^{-1} (FIGURE 6). Recently, Baumgartner *et al.* have also shown that the defect in platelet adhesion to subendothelium produced in human blood by an antibody to the factor VIII complex (e.g. experimental von Willebrand's disease) is also strongly shear rate-dependent.[24] Since the shear rates in the microvasculature are considerably higher than those we have routinely used, the shear rate-dependence of the adhesion defect in von Willebrand's disease assumes some importance. Studies currently in progress using a high shear rate chamber may help to clarify the question further.

Disorders of Platelet Aggregation

The defects in aggregation $\left(\frac{100T}{S}\right)$ obtained in patients with thrombasthenia[5,8] and storage pool disease,[7,8] and in normal subjects who had ingested aspirin[7,8] confirm previous findings with use of the aggregometer.[1] These findings of impaired platelet aggregation on the subendothelium suggest that a similar abnormality in platelet-vessel interaction after injury may account for the hemostatic defect in these patients. The most striking impairment of aggregation was observed in thrombasthenia. Platelet adhesion, however, was normal in this disorder,[5,8] indicating that adhesion and aggregation on a physiologic surface involve different mechanisms. The reason for the total absence of platelet-to-platelet interaction in thrombasthenia, despite normal platelet degranulation,[5] remains to be determined, but could be related to the recently described absence of a specific-membrane glycoprotein (Type II) in this disorder.[25]

Platelet aggregation was impaired in normal subjects who had ingested aspirin,[7,8] as also reported in aspirin-treated rabbits.[26] These findings are similar to those obtained with the aggregometer[27] and further support the possible use of aspirin as an antithrombotic agent.[28] Contrary to the findings in other studies (in which different techniques were used to study adhesion),[27,29] platelet adhesion was not decreased after aspirin ingestion and platelets that were spread on the subendothelium had lost most of their α-granules.[7] Thus, aspirin does not appear to inhibit either the initial attachment and spreading of a platelet on the subendothelium or the release reaction (e.g. degranulation) of the surface-bound platelet; it inhibits only subsequent steps involved in the formation of a platelet thrombus.

Platelet aggregation was also impaired in storage pool disease, but adhesion may also be impaired in some patients with this disorder.[7, 8] Impaired platelet adhesion has also been described in fawn-hooded rats with storage pool deficiency.[30] Further studies will be necessary to determine whether impaired adhesion is a general feature of the storage-pool deficient platelet disorders [7] and to elucidate the nature of the defect. In this volume, Leonard *et al.* have suggested that platelets adherent to a surface may release a substance that promotes the adherence of nearby platelets.[31] Possibly, storage pool-deficient platelets are deficient in this postulated adhesion-promoting substance.

Summary

The abnormalities of platelet adhesion and aggregation on the subendothelium that we have found in patients with impaired hemostasis suggests a new way to classify these disorders.[7] Further studies on platelet-subendothelium interaction in subjects with well identified biochemical defects may help to determine how platelets interact with the vessel wall in the primary arrest of bleeding. These studies may have important implications for an understanding of thrombosis as well.

Acknowledgment

We wish to acknowledge the technical assistance of Mr. David Cohen, Miss Christine Michael, Miss Käthi Schietinger, and Miss Irene Steck.

References

1. Weiss, H. J. 1975. Platelet physiology and abnormalities of platelet function. New Eng. J. Med. **293:** 531–541, 580–588.
2. Baumgartner, H. R. & C. Haudenschild. 1972. Adhesion of platelets to subendothelium. Ann. N.Y. Acad. Sci. **201:** 22–36
3. Baumgartner, H. R. 1973. The role of blood flow in platelet adhesion, fibrin deposition, and formation of mural thrombi. Microvasc. Res. **5:** 167–179.
4. Tschopp, T. B., H. J. Weiss & H. R. Baumgartner. 1974. Decreased adhesion of platelets to subendothelium in von Willebrand's disease. J. Lab. Clin. Med. **83:** 296–300.
5. Tschopp, T. B., H. J. Weiss & H. R. Baumgartner. 1975. Interaction of platelets with subendothelium in thrombasthenia: normal adhesion, impaired aggregation. Experientia **31:** 113–116.
6. Weiss, H. J., T. B. Tschopp, H. R. Baumgartner, I. I. Sussman, M. M. Johnson & J. J. Egan. 1974. Decreased adhesion of giant (Bernard-Soulier) platelets to subendothelium: further implications on the role of the von Willebrand factor in hemostasis. Am. J. Med. **57:** 920–925.
7. Weiss, H. J., T. B. Tschopp & H. R. Baumgartner. 1975. Impaired interaction (adhesion-aggregation) of platelets with the subendothelium in storage-pool disease and after aspirin ingestion—a comparison with von Willebrand's disease. New Eng. J. Med. **293:** 619–623.
8. Baumgartner, H. R., T. B. Tschopp & H. J. Weiss. 1976. Platelet interaction

with collagen fibrils in flowing blood. II. Impaired adhesion-aggregation in bleeding disorders. A comparison with subendothelium. Thromb. Haemostas. In press.
9. STEMERMAN, M. B. 1974. Vascular intimal components: precursors of thrombosis. Prog. Hemostas. Thromb. **2:** 1–47.
10. BAUMGARTNER, H. R. 1974. The subendothelial surface and thrombosis. Thromb. Diath. Haemorrh. (Suppl.) **59:** 91–105.
11. BAUMGARTNER, H. R. 1976. Platelet interaction with collagen fibrils in flowing blood. I. Reaction of human platelets with α-chymotrypsin-digested subendothelium. Thrombos. Haemostas. In press.
12. BAUMGARTNER, H. R., R. MUGGLI, T. B. TSCHOPP & V. T. TURITTO. 1976. Platelet adhesion—release and aggregation in flowing blood. Effects of surface properties and platelet function. Thrombos. Haemostas. **35:** 124–138.
13. WEISS, H. J., L. W. HOYER, F. R. RICKLES, A. VARMA & J. ROGERS. 1973. Quantitative assay of a plasma factor deficient in von Willebrand's disease that is necessary for platelet aggregation. Relationship to factor VIII procoagulant activity and antigen content. J. Clin. Invest. **52:** 2708–2716.
14. WEISS, H. J. 1975. Factor VIII and platelet function in the pathogenesis of von Willebrand's disease. *In* Haemophilia (Proc. 9th Congr. World Federation of Hemophilia), Excerpta Medica (Amsterdam) : 114–123.
15. TURITTO, V. T. & H. R. BAUMGARTNER. 1974. Effect of physical factors on platelet adherence to subendothelium. Thromb. Diath. Haemorrh. (Suppl.) **60:** 17–24.
16. TURITTO, V. T., R. MUGGLI & H. R. BAUMGARTNER. This volume.
17. WEISS, H. J. & J. ROGERS. 1972. Correction of the platelet abnormality in von Willebrand's disease by cryoprecipitate. Am. J. Med. **53:** 734–738.
18. BOWIE, E. J. W. & C. A. OWEN, JR. 1972. Platelet abnormalities in von Willebrand's disease. Ann. N.Y. Acad. Sci. **201:** 400–420.
19. CAEN, J. P., A. T. NURDEN, C. JEANNEAU, H. MICHEL, G. TOBELEM, S. LEVY-TOLEDANO, Y. SULTAN, F. VALENSI & J. BERNARD. 1976. Bernard-Soulier Syndrome: a new platelet glycoprotein abnormality—its relationship with platelet adhesion to subendothelium and with the factor VIII von Willebrand protein. J. Lab. Clin. Med. **87:** 586–596.
20. JENKINS, C. S. P., D. R. PHILLIPS, K. J. CLEMETSON, D. MEYER, M-J. LARRIEU & E. F. LÜSCHER. 1976. Platelet membrane glycoproteins implicated in ristocetin-induced aggregation. Studies of the protein on platelets from patients with Bernard-Soulier Syndrome and von Willebrand's disease. J. Clin. Invest. **57:** 112–124.
21. BOWIE, E. J. W., V. FUSTER, C. A. OWEN, JR. & A. L. BROWN. 1975. Resistance to the development of spontaneous atherosclerosis in pigs with von Willebrand's disease. (Abstr.) 5th Congr. Int. Soc. Thromb. Haemostas. : 322. Paris, France.
22. ROSS, R., J. GLOMSET, B. KARIYA & L. HARKER. 1974. Platelet-dependent serum factor that stimulates the proliferation of arterial smooth muscle cells in vitro. Proc. Nat. Acad. Sci. USA **71:** 1207–1210.
23. TURITTO, V. T. & H. R. BAUMGARTNER. 1975. Platelet deposition on subendothelium exposed to flowing blood: mathematical analysis of physical parameters. Trans. Am. Soc. Artif. Int. Organs. **21:** 593–600.
24. BAUMGARTNER, H. R., T. B. TSCHOPP & D. MEYER. In preparation.
25. NURDEN, A. T. & J. P. CAEN. 1974. An abnormal platelet glycoprotein pattern in three cases of Glanzmann's thrombasthenia. Br. J. Haematol. **28:** 253–260.
26. BAUMGARTNER, H. R. & R. MUGGLI. 1974. Effects of acetylsalicylic acid on platelet adhesion to subendothelium and on mural thrombus formation in vivo and in vitro. Thromb. Diath. Haemorrh. (Suppl.) **60:** 345–354.
27. WEISS, H. J., L. M. ALEDORT & S. KOCHWA. 1968. The effect of salicylates on the hemostatic properties of platelets in man. J. Clin. Invest. **47:** 2169–2180.

28. WEISS, H. J. 1976. Anti-platelet drugs: a new pharmacologic approach to the prevention of thrombosis. Am. Heart J. **92:** 86:102.
29. CAZENAVE, J.-P., M. A. PACKHAM, M. A. GUCCIONE & J. F. MUSTARD. 1974. Inhibition of platelet adherence to a collagen-coated surface by nonsteroidal anti-inflammatory drugs, pyrimido-pyrimidine and tricyclic compounds, and lidocaine. J. Lab. Clin. Med. **83:** 797–806.
30. TSCHOPP, T. B. & H. R. BAUMGARTNER. 1975. Delayed adhesion to subendothelium and defective aggregation of platelets from rats with storage pool disease (SPD). Thromb. Diath. Haemorrh. **34:** 600.
31. LEONARD, E. F. *et al.* This volume.

FACTORS GOVERNING THE HEALING RESPONSE OF INJURED ARTERIES *

Michael B. Stemerman

Division of Hematology, Department of Medicine
Montefiore Hospital and Medical Center
and The Albert Einstein College of Medicine
The Bronx, New York 10467

Introduction

Arteries, being a conduit for blood, are uniquely situated to have contact with a disparate variety of substances in high concentration at their lumenal surface. It is not surprising that, with these constant chemical as well as mechanical environmental changes, the arterial wall must be an organ with adaptive latitude. The manner in which the arterial wall does alter and reshape itself may ultimately lead from a "naturally" occurring aging process of remodeling to the eventual significant diminution of the caliber of the lumen. Such lumenal narrowing is considered part of the arteriosclerotic process. It is generally accepted that lipid-rich lesions, characteristic of the more complicated, atherosclerotic process further contribute to lumenal narrowing, and complications stemming from this process are the major cause of death in the Western World. Factors that influence this process have recently come under close scrutiny *in vitro* and *in vivo* studies, and form the basis for this report. It is therefore important to describe first the components of the vessel wall and then the arterial response to injury.

The Blood Vessel

The large arterial blood vessel is divided into three components.[1] The outer portion, or adventitia, is composed of connective tissue, fibroblasts, and veil cells (probably a phagocytic cell),[2] as well as small lymphatic vessels and blood vessels.[1,2] The middle layer, or media, is bounded on its intimal surface by the innermost elastic layer, the internal elastica, and on its outer surface by the outermost elastic layer, or external elastica. The media differs in the large elastic arteries from the smaller muscular arteries by the presence of large lamellar units of concentric layers of elastic tissue. This component of the vasculature is nourished in part by vaso vasoram, which are seen only in the outermost layers of the media when the musculoelastic units exceed 29 layers.[3] In the mammal, the smooth muscle cell (SMC) is the only cellular type found in the media; for this reason, it can be used as a source for pure tissue cultures of vascular SMC.[4] The SMC are aligned in a spiral pattern around the long axis of the vessel with interspersed extracellular connective tissue components of elastin, collagen, and glycosaminoglycans.[1] The intima, in its very early forma-

* This study was supported by USPHS grant no. HL 16387 from the National Heart and Lung Institute.

tive state, is a layer of endothelium that lines the vessel lumen. Beneath this monolayer of endothelium lies the subendothelial connective tissue and the internal elastic lamina.[1] Occasionally, pericytes or SMC are seen on the ablumenal side of the endothelium.[1] The connective tissue components of the subendothelium are complex and are involved in the hemostatic mechanism.[1] The manner in which these portions of the wall change with age and stress has been outlined elsewhere.[5] Note that the basic component of arterial growth and modeling is the SMC, which is the cell that participates in arterial change following vascular injury.

TABLE 1

VASCULAR INJURY *

Chemical Agents	Mechanical Means
Homocystinemia	Hemodynamics
Hypoxia	Platelet Emboli
CO	Leukocyte Migration
Changes in Osmolity	Air [7]
Changes in pH	Heat
Immune Injury	Catheter Injury and others [6]
Endotoxemia	Hypertension
Carcinoniatosis	
EDTA	
Enzymes (Collagenase, Trypsin)	
Diabetes	
Cigarette Smoking	
Uric Acid	
Graft Rejection	
Hemodialysis	

* This table is arranged in an arbitrary manner and does not claim to be complete. Underlying the uncertainty of categorizing effects of vascular injury is a lack of understanding of the cellular mechanisms of the processes leading to injury.

ARTERIAL INJURY

Numerous risk factors for atherosclerosis have been identified clinically that include: cigarette smoking, high blood presure, hypercholesterolemia, and diabetes (TABLE 1). In attempting to establish a basis for experimental study of the artery and its response to injury, it has been noted that vessels are especially susceptible to manipulation of any type; [1] this has made isolation of arteries for the study of normal vascular physiology under controlled conditions extremely difficult. Therefore, heading a list of experimental factors that produce vascular damage is mechanical injury. The types and varieties of injurious stimuli is indeed long (TABLE 1). By contrast, the response to vascular injury seems to be similar and will be detailed.

A variety of agents and circumstances have been identified as injurious to the vessel wall and its components. In this manner, the remodeling process already mentioned is either initiated, or accelerated. The common components of most of those agents appear to be either endothelial detachment or dysfunction.

ENDOTHELIUM AND SMOOTH MUSCLE CELLS

Endothelial cells function as a permeability barrier and in terms of atherosclerosis may be of critical importance for the entrance of lipid into the arterial wall. Once endothelial cells are removed or rendered dysfunctional even for a short time, the vessel wall is bathed by concentrations of plasma components that normally are screened out by "properly" functioning endothelium. As previously mentioned, experimental vascular injury usually produces a similar series of events. We have concentrated on using the balloon catheter deendothelialization model,[8, 9] since it is convenient, highly reproducable, seems to damage or remove only the endothelial layer, and produces the same pattern of repair in rabbits,[9] monkeys [10] and rats.[6] Although we do not consider it a physiologic injury, close examination of the process following passage of the balloon catheter allows a step-by-step analysis and thus may enhance our understanding of the pathobiology of arteriosclerosis.

The first observable event following endothelial detachment is the adherence of platelets at places where subendothelial connective tissues are exposed to blood.[1, 9] There appears to be little role for the formation of fibrin in this process unless the vessel has been previously injured or remodeled.[9] In this case, fibrin forms at the denuded surface and may even enter the vessel wall.[9] There follows a period of three to four days after endothelial detachment in which leukocytes are attracted to the injured site.[1, 11] Following this stage, SMC migration occurs, and occasionally platelets can be seen early in this SMC cover (FIGURE 1). The intima is thickened by proliferation of SMC and by the accumulation of extracellular connective tssue components.[9, 10] The thickening is of such extent that by a month, in the rabbit, the intimal hyperplasia is as thick as the media, or about twenty cell layers deep. It appears from tissue culture experiments that the great bulk of the extracellular material is generated by SMC,[4] although evidence is accumulating that endothelial cells do form some types of connective tissue.[12]

A number of techniques have been developed to identify and follow the fibromusculoelastic plaque formation and endothelial regrowth. An antibody marker specific for endothelial cells has been developed that has allowed us to follow the course of reendothelialization.[13] This marker, absorbed antitissue factor, has also been used in tissue culture and has been successful in several instances in the identification of endothelial cells. We have recently combined this technique with the infusion of Evans' blue dye one half hour prior to sacrifice of the animal. The Evans' blue complexes with albumen and apparently is not allowed to permeate the vessel at places in which endothelium is present. In this manner, we have been able to follow reendothelialization and to examine those areas of the healed vessel that are not recovered by endothelium. With the use of these techniques, examination of *en face* preparations of arteries denuded of their endothelium and allowed to heal for various periods of time, a highly reproducable picture of vascular healing has emerged.

The outgrowth of endothelium from the stripped artery commences from branch sites and proceeds to spread out, with endothelial recovery complete by approximately 9–14 months after denudation. A wide degree of biologic

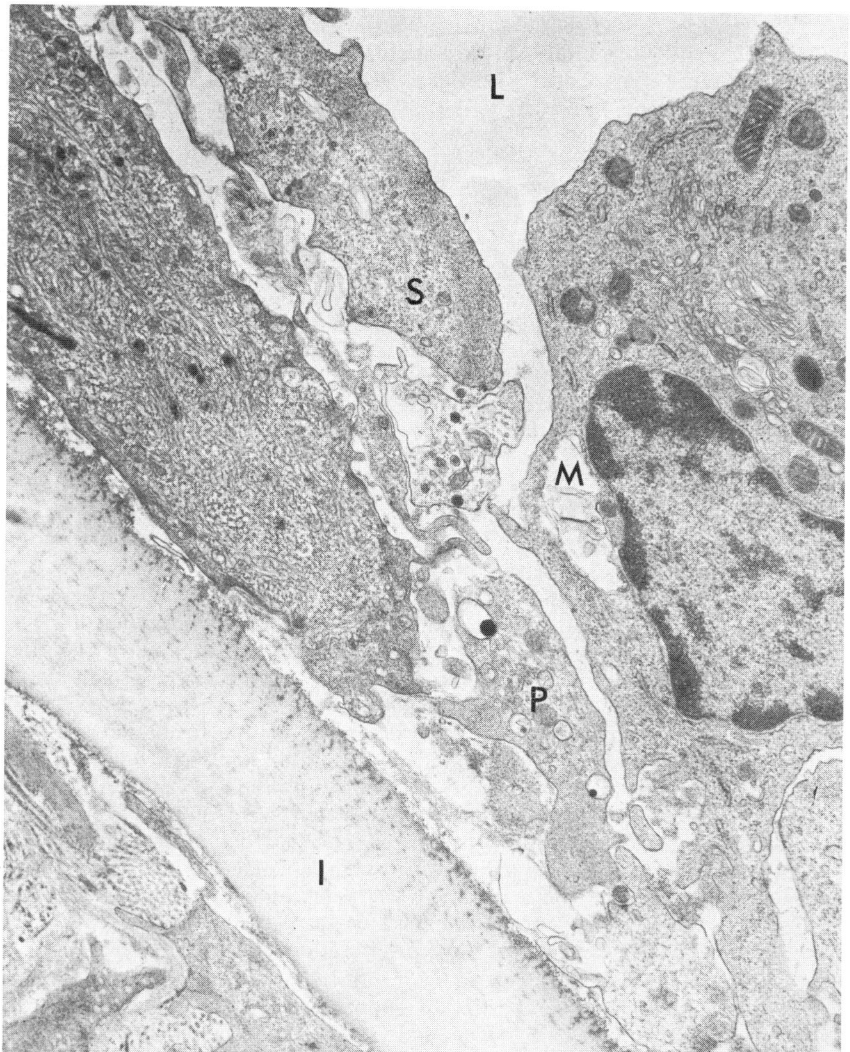

FIGURE 1. Electron micrograph of a rabbit aorta deendothelialized by an intraarterial balloon catheter, allowed to heal for five days, and fixed by perfusion. The internal elastic lamina (I) is seen separating the media below from the early intimal proliferation. Components of the lesion at this stage include modified smooth-muscle cells (S), platelets (P), and mononuclear cells (M). No fibrin can be distinguished morphologically in either the lument (L) or the intima, and the media appears undamaged. ×16,000.

variability is seen which as yet is unexplained. Examination of areas blued by the dye show that smooth-muscle cells remain as lumenal cells for long periods of time.[14] These cells, when examined by electron microscopy, are typical of modified smooth-muscle cells and display a lumenal, moderately electron-dense, amorphous material reminiscent of vascular basement membrane.[1, 14] This material, in turn, is associated with the presence of platelets at the surface, and by scanning electron microscopy the platelets appear spread out upon this smooth-muscle cell surface. The presumed mechanism of platelet attachment is their adherence to this basement membranelike material. Neither this material nor platelets are found in reendothelialized regions. Morphometric measurements of the thickened intima comparing blued and nonblued regions show that the blued areas are thicker than the areas covered by endothelium. This would imply that regression of the fibromusculoelastic plaque is related to reendothelialization and the presence of platelets at the surface; however, studies done at times of greater than four months following injury show spontaneous abatement and gradual regression even in the blued areas not covered by endothelium. Therefore, it seems that although platelets are influencial in plaque formation, as will be described in more detail below, there appear to be other factors that are also important in the process.

Factors Influencing Intimal Proliferation

Experiments in tissue culture have recently described the presence of a platelet component that influences proliferation of SMC.[15] This musculoproliferative factor may be related to a fibroblast proliferative factor that has been identified in the bovine pituitary gland.[16, 17] Whether these factors are the same, and the platelet is a carrier of this low molecular weight cationic protein, is not certain. Friedman *et al.* have shown that thrombocytopenia caused by a sheep anti-rabbit platelet serum inhibited arteriosclerotic plaque formation following balloon injury[18] and atherosclerotic plaque formation following repeated intimal injury caused by an indwelling aortic polyethelene catheter.[19] These *in vivo* findings support the contention that platelets are musculoproliferative. In addition, Tiell, using hypophysectomized rats, has demonstrated that SMC do not proliferate even in the presence of normal platelet counts.[20] This study indicates that there may be a link between the pituitary gland, platelets, and SMC. In all these experiments, it remains unclear if platelets are necessary for the migration or the sustenance of SMC proliferation, or both.

Other agents have been shown to be of influence in this proliferative process. Rhee has demonstrated that estradiol suppresses the intimal thickening of resutured arteries *in vivo*,[21] and Ross and Glomset have demonstrated in tissue culture that SMC proliferation is enhanced by the LDL fraction of serum.[22]

Musculoproliferation appears to be under the influence of other factors which have yet to be identified, as mentioned above. Using [^{3}H]-thymidine following deendothelialization, Burns has demonstrated that SMC proliferation is greatly diminished after 14 days following balloon injury, although platelets have been identified adhering to lumenal SMC.[23] This autoradiographic study confirms the observations we have made, that although intimal proliferation appears to be enhanced by the recovery of endothelial cells over the injured surface, regression begins after a time even in the absence of an endothelial cover and in the presence of platelet adhesion.[14] The factor or factors that govern this process are unknown. At present it is not clear whether this effect is local or systemic. Whether hyperlipidemia and blood pressure interact in this process also remains unclear.

In contrast to SMC, endothelial cells seem to be able to proliferate even in the absence of pituitary or platelet factors.[18, 20] Although a large number of factors do cause endothelial injury, proliferation of these cells seems to depend only on the presence of a high concentration of serum *in vitro*. This leads to the conclusion that endothelioproliferation proceeds by mechanisms markedly different from musculoproliferation.

Conclusion

Although evidence has accumulated that regression of the atherosclerotic lesion may be possible by dietary means,[24–26] it requires prudence not palatable to Western Man's appetite. Under these circumstances, it remains of great importance to continue to explore the pathobiology of vascular healing so that the disease process may be successfully influenced in spite of ourselves.

Acknowledgment

The author wishes to thank Dr. R. J. Friedman, M. Tiell, J. Cintron, and Maria Underwood for their help in the preparation of this manuscript.

References

1. Stemerman, M. B. 1974. Vascular intimal components: Precursors of thrombogenesis. *In* Progress in Hemostasis and Thrombosis. T. H. Spaet, Ed. Vol. **II:** 1–35. Grune & Stratton. New York, N.Y.
2. Jorres, I. & G. Majno. 1974. Cellular breakdown within the arterial wall: An ultrastructural study of the coronary artery in young and aging rats. Virchows Arch. A Path. Anat. Histol. **364:** 111–127.
3. Wolinsky, H. & S. Glagov. 1967. A lamellar unit of aortic medial structure and function in mammals. Circulation Res. **20:** 99–111.
4. Ross, R. & S. J. Klebanoff. 1971. The smooth muscle cell. I. In vivo synthesis of connective tissue proteins. J. Cell Biol. **50:** 159–173.
5. Frist, S. & M. B. Stemerman. Arterial growth and development. *In* Vascular Neuroeffector Systems. J. A. Bevan & S. J. Karger, Eds. In press.
6. Schwartz, S. M., M. B. Stemerman & E. P. Benditt. 1975. The aortic intima. II. Repair of the aortic lining after mechanical denudation. Am. J. Pathol. **81:** 15–48.
7. Fishman, J. A., G. B. Ryan & M. J. Karnovsky. 1975. Endothelial regeneration in the rat carotid artery and the significance of endothelial denudation in the pathogenesis of myointimal thickening. Lab. Invest. **32:** 339–351.
8. Baumgartner, H. R. 1963. Eine neue Methode zur Erzeugung von Thromben durch gezielte Uberdehnung der Gefasswand. Z. Gesamte Exp. Med. **137:** 227–236.
9. Stemerman, M. B. 1973. Thrombogenesis of the rabbit arterial plaque: An electron microscopic study. Am. J. Pathol. **73:** 7–18.
10. Stemerman, M. B. & R. Ross. 1972. Experimental arteriosclerosis. I. Fibrous plaque formation in primates, an electron microscopic study. J. Exp. Med. **136:** 769–793.

11. Spaet, T. H., M. B. Stemerman, F. J. Veith & I. Lejnieks. 1975. Intimal injury and regrowth in the rabbit aorta: Medial smooth muscle cells as a source of neo-intima. Circ. Res. **36:** 58–70.
12. Jaffe, E. A., B. Adelman, R. Minick, C. G. Becker & R. Nachman. 1975. Synthesis of basement membrane by cultured human endothelial cells. Circulation **52:** 235.
13. Stemerman, M. B., F. A. Pitlick & H. B. Dembitzer. 1976. Electron microscopic immunohistochemical identification of endothelial cells in the rabbit. Circ. Res. **38:** 146–156.
14. Stemerman, M. B., T. H. Spaet, F. A. Pitlick, J. R. Cintron & I. Lejnieks. 1975. Reappearance of endothelial cells after extensive arterial de-endothelialization. Fed. Proc. **34:** 411.
15. Ross, R., J. Glomset, B. Kariya & L. Harker. 1974. A platelet-dependent serum factor that stimulates the proliferation of arterial smooth muscle cells in vitro. Proc. Nat. Acad. Sci. USA **71:** 1207–1211.
16. Gospodorowicz, D. 1974. Localization of a fibroblast growth factor and its effect alone and with hydrocortisone on 3T3 cell growth. Nature **249:** 123–127.
17. Gospodorowicz, D. & J. S. Moran. 1975. Mitogenic effect of fibroblast growth factor on early passage culture of human and murine fibroblasts. J. Cell. Biol. **66:** 451–457.
18. Friedman, R. J., M. B. Stemerman, T. H. Spaet, S. Moore & J. Gauldie. 1976. The effect of thrombocytopenia on arteriosclerotic plaque formation. Fed. Proc. **35:** 207.
19. Moore, S., R. J. Friedman, D. P. Singal, J. Gauldie, M. Blajchman & R. Roberts. Inhibition of injury induced thromboatherosclerotic lesions by antiplatelet serum in rabbits. Thromb. et Diath. Haemorrh. In press.
20. Tiell, M. Personal communication.
21. Rhee, C. Personal communication.
22. Ross, R. & J. A. Glomset. 1973. Atherosclerosis: a problem in the biology of the arterial smooth muscle cell. Science **180:** 1332–1335.
23. Burns, E. Personal communication.
24. National Heart and Lung Institute Task Force on Arteriosclerosis Report. 1972. Arteriosclerosis. DHEW Publication no. 72–219, 13.
25. Eggen, D. A., J. P. Strong, W. P. Newman, M. S. Catsulis, G. I. Malcolm & M. G. Kokatnur. 1974. Regression of diet-induced fatty streaks in rhesus monkeys. Lab. Invest. **31:** 294–301.
26. Armstrong, M. L. 1975. Regression of atherosclerosis. *In* Current Research in Atherosclerosis. A. Gotto & R. Paoletti, Ed. Raven Press. New York, N.Y.

PLATELET KINETIC EVALUATION OF PROSTHETIC MATERIAL *IN VIVO* *

Laurence A. Harker, Stephen R. Hanson, and Allan S. Hoffman

Departments of Medicine and Chemical Engineering and the Regional Primate Research Center University of Washington Seattle, Washington 98195

Thrombosis and thromboembolism constitute the major deterrent to the use of cardiovascular prostheses.[1-5] The process of platelet thrombogenesis predominates in the development of thrombotic complications when grafts are positioned in the arterial system as shown by: 1) direct visualization of prosthetic luminal surfaces after exposure to circulating blood;[6-10] 2) renal microinfarction produced by platelet microemboli following prosthetic aortic grafts;[11, 12] 3) selective platelet consumption regularly observed in patients with cardiovascular devices;[13-15] and 4) interruption of platelet consumption and thromboembolism by antiplatelet drugs.[13-19]

Traditionally the thrombogenicity of vascular grafts *in vivo* has been assessed by measuring the amount of thrombus present at some point in time after surgical placement. The uncontrolled variables that seriously compromise the quantitative usefulness of this measurement include: 1) loss of thrombus by embolization; 2) loss of thrombus by fibrinolysis; 3) differences in effects of surgery; 4) timing of observations; and 5) hemodynamic characteristics of the test system.[5, 12, 13, 23, 24] In order to quantify the overall rate of graft-induced thrombus formation *in vivo* in a manner that includes thromboembolization and thrombolysis and that is free of surgical and nonsteady state effects, the rate of platelet consumption by prosthetic material is being measured.

In this paper we discuss the development of the platelet kinetic approach in baboons to the *in vivo* evaluation of prosthetic materials, antiplatelet drugs, and graft endothelialization.

In Vivo *Evaluation of Prosthetic Materials*

Platelet Survival and Turnover Measurements

Male disease-free baboons weighing 10–14 kg with normal hematocrits and leukocyte counts are used after placement of a femoral arteriovenous (A-V)

* Supported by research grants (HL-11775 and RR-00166) from the U.S. Public Health Service and contract E-(45-1)-2225 no. 22 from the U.S. Energy Research and Development Administration. A portion of this work was conducted through the Clinical Research Center's facility of the University of Washington with the support of grants (FR-37 and FR-133) from the National Institutes of Health. Reprint requests and correspondence should be addressed to: Dr. L. A. Harker, Division of Hematology, Harborview Medical Center, 325-9th Ave., Seattle, Washington 98104.

Silastic® cannula (FIGURE 1) with 0.2 cm internal diameter and Dacron® sewing cuffs at skin exit sites.[25, 26] To protect these A-V shunts and to facilitate frequently repeated blood sampling, the animals are maintained in restraining chairs during the period of study.

Platelet survival is determined by measurement of the disappearance of radioactivity from blood sampled 10–15 times after injection of autologous ^{51}Cr-labeled platelets. In this procedure 100 ml of autologous whole blood is collected directly into plastic bags (TA-6, Fenwal, Morton Grove) containing 20 ml ACD anticoagulant. The blood is centrifuged at $200 \times g$ at room temperature for 10 minutes. The supernatant platelet-rich plasma is transferred to a second transfer bag by a plasma extractor and the pH is adjusted to 6.5 with 0.15 M citric acid (0.1 ml/10 ml plasma). Platelets are then formed into a

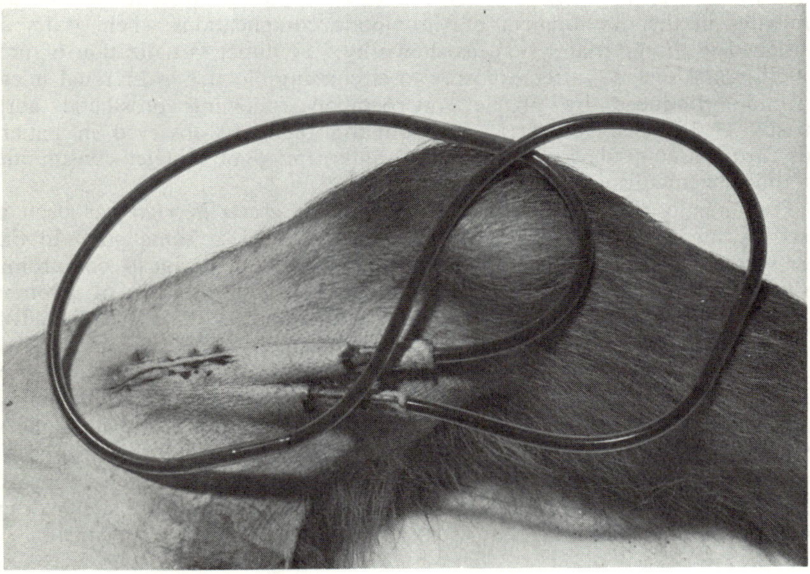

FIGURE 1. Femoral arteriovenous cannula in baboons.

pellet by centrifugation at 3,000 *g* for 15 minutes. The supernatant plasma is removed except for 2 ml residual plasma into which the platelets were carefully resuspended. This platelet suspension is then incubated with 50 μCi of radiochromium (New England Nuclear, Boston, Mass.) for 30 minutes. Most of the nonradioactive platelet-poor plasma and an equivalent volume of sterile air are then added, and the pellet is reformed by centrifuging at 3,000 *g* for 15 minutes. The residual radioactive platelet-poor plasma is completely decanted without disturbing the pellet. Ten ml of nonradioactive platelet-poor plasma is carefully layered over the platelet pellet and then discarded by decantation. This maneuver washes the bag of more than 99% of the residual nonplatelet bound ^{51}Cr. The presence of air in the bag facilitates this process by maintaining the overall configuration of the bag during decantation. The labeled platelet pellet is gently suspended in 2 ml of nonradioactive platelet-poor plasma. Contaminating red cells are largely removed by a final slow centrifugation of 100 × *g* for five minutes. A known amount of ^{51}Cr-platelet suspension is administered by intravenous injection after the preparation of a standard. Three-ml samples of whole blood, collected in EDTA twice daily for three days and daily for three additional days, are lysed with 0.1 ml of SDS and counted for radioactivity in a gamma spectrometer (Nuclear Chicago, Chicago, Ill.).

Platelet survival time is analyzed by computer fitting to a gamma function as described by Murphy[27–29] and is 5.5 ± 0.2 days in 24 normal male baboons. The proportion of labeled platelets remaining within the systemic circulation after infusion (i.e., "recovery") is calculated from the platelet activity per milliliter, extrapolated to zero time, multiplied by the estimated blood volume, and divided by the platelet ^{51}Cr activity injected. Platelet consumption, measured as platelet turnover per μl of blood per day, is calculated from the peripheral platelet count divided by the platelet survival time in days and corrected for recovery. Platelet recovery averages 85 ± 5% and platelet turnover is 59,000 plat/μl/day ± 7,000 in 24 normal male baboons.

Testing Prosthetic Materials

For *in vivo* testing in baboons, various prosthetic materials are obtained in tubular form, or are prepared by coating the luminal surface of Silastic tubing of varying diameters and lengths that can be inserted as extension segments in the arteriovenous cannula. Studies have shown that proximal and distal Silastic connections with the artery and vein do not add significantly to platelet consumption.

Mathematical Analysis

Platelet consumption in baboons supporting thrombogenic cannulae is dependent on both the rate of platelet consumption by the arteriovenous shunt material and the rate of platelet removal through senescent mechanisms. Since the relative contribution of each process of platelet elimination may depend significantly on the test situation, the following mathematical model was developed to separate these effects and allow estimation of the rate of platelet destruction by test materials only.

The Mills-Dornhorst[30, 31] approach to the interpretation of platelet survival curves states that if $\phi(t)$ is the probability that a platelet will reach or exceed age t, then the average platelet survival time, τ, is:

$$\tau = \int_0^\infty \phi(t)\,dt \qquad (1)$$

and the survival curve for the population of the labeled platelets is:

$$\frac{c(t)}{c(c)} = \frac{\int_t^\infty \phi(t)\,dt}{\int_0^\infty \phi(t)\,dt} \qquad (2)$$

where c(t) is the concentration of labeled platelets at time t. It then follows that when t = o

$$\frac{d}{dt}\left(\frac{c(t)}{c(o)}\right) = \frac{-1}{\tau} \quad (3)$$

i.e., the initial slope of the platelet survival curve intersects the time axis at τ, the average platelet survival time.

The utility of this model results from the fact that Equation 3 is valid regardless of the mechanism of platelet destruction, assuming steady state rates of platelet production, and that labeled and unlabeled platelets behave identically. To further model the baboon-arteriovenous shunt system, mechanisms must be postulated for platelet destruction by the shunt and by senescent removal.

Assuming that all platelets become senescent and die at exactly 5.50 days, senescence is described by

$$\underset{\text{senescence}}{\phi(t)} = \begin{cases} 1, & t \leq 5.50 \text{ days} \\ 0, & t > 5.50 \text{ days.} \end{cases} \quad (4)$$

Integrating this function via Equation 2 results in the observed linear survival curve intersecting the t axis at 5.50 days.

For animals supporting arteriovenous cannula, we assume that the reactivity of individual platelets toward the shunt is independent of their age, and that platelet destruction by the shunt is kinetically limited and the reaction is first order. Thus:

$$V\frac{dc}{dt} = -K'Ac \quad (5)$$

where V = blood volume of baboon (ml),
A = shunt surface area (cm^2),
c = concentration of labeled platelets (platelets/ml), and
K′ = rate constant (cm/day),

which states that the number of labeled platelets consumed per unit time by the cannula is proportional to the product of shunt surface area and the concentration of labeled platelets. If consumption is kinetically limited, the same number of platelets must be consumed per unit time for a given shunt, regardless of variations in platelet count or shunt hemodynamic parameters between animals.

The rate of consumption of all platelets (labeled plus unlabeled) is K′A(PC) where (PC) is the platelet count. Since this rate is independent of (PC), we define:

$$K' = \frac{K}{(PC)}. \quad (6)$$

The rate of platelet consumption by a shunt is now KA, and K is independent of shunt flow rate, geometry, and platelet count. Substituting Equation 6 into Equation 5 and integrating:

$$\frac{c(t)}{c(o)} = e^{\frac{-KAt}{V(PC)}}. \quad (7)$$

Equation 7 is the platelet survival curve, assuming an operative A-V cannula without other destructive mechanisms. It follows from Equations 1–3 that:

$$\underset{\text{shunt}}{\phi(t)} = e^{\frac{-KAt}{V(PC)}}. \quad \textbf{(8)}$$

In the case where both physiological and cannula mechanisms of platelet elimination operate simultaneously:

$$\phi(t) = \underset{\text{senescence}}{\phi(t)} \times \underset{\text{shunt}}{\phi(t)} .$$

Substituting from Equations 4 and 8 and integrating according to Equation 1, yields:

$$\tau = \frac{1 - e^{\frac{-5.5\,KA}{V(PC)}}}{\frac{KA}{V(PC)}} \quad \textbf{(9)}$$

and the overall rate of platelet consumption is:

$$\frac{V(PC)}{\tau} = \frac{KA}{1 - e^{\frac{-5.5\,KA}{V(PC)}}} \quad \textbf{(10)}$$

It follows from Equations 9 and 10 that with no shunt ($A = O$) or non-consumptive shunts ($K = O$), platelet survival is 5.5 days. Conversely, when the rate of platelet consumption by the shunt alone, (KA), is very large compared to the total number of platelets, (V(PC)), the overall rate of platelet consumption approaches KA; i.e., relatively few platelets are removed by senescence.

To test this approach, thrombogenic shunt material (0.104 in. i.d. × 0.192 in. o.d.) was studied at lengths of 20, 50, and 100 cm resulting in exposed surface areas of 16.6 cm^2, 41.5 cm^2, and 83 cm^2. Larger diameter shunts (0.125 in. i.d. × 0.250 in. o.d.) of the same material were also studied at 100-cm lengths and exposed areas of 100 cm^2.

The survival curves were computed by nonlinear regression analysis computer programs to obtain unbiased values of the platelet survival time, τ, that were independent of any assumptions in the foregoing model.[27–29] Platelet counts were done frequently, and blood volume was estimated as 7% of body weight. Given independent determinations of τ, V, PC, and A, Equation 9 was used to calculate values of K. Overall platelet consumption was calculated as $\frac{V(PC)}{\tau}$ and shunt consumption was calculated as KA.

Results are shown in TABLE 1. FIGURE 2 shows that overall average platelet survival time decreases in a nonlinear relationship with increasing shunt area. FIGURE 3 shows that platelet consumption by the prosthetic material alone is directly proportional to surface area exposed to circulating blood.

The model also predicts that the rate of platelet consumption by materials is independent of platelet count, and hence for shunts of a given surface area, survival time will be approximately proportional to platelet count. FIGURE 4 shows this relationship for the 41.5-cm^2 shunts. Similar correlations were found for other cannula luminal surface areas.

Flow rate ranging from 50 to 220 ml/minute had no effect on survival, which supports the assumption that consumption is kinetically limited.

TABLE 1

ANALYSIS OF PLATELET KINETIC MEASUREMENTS

			Cannula Platelet Consumption		
Cannula Surface Area (cm^2)	Platelet Survival Time (days)	Overall Platelet Turnover (platelets/ day x 10^{-10})	KA (platelets/ day x 10^{-10})	$\frac{KA\ \tau}{V(PC)}$ (fraction of overall turnover)	K (platelets/ cm^2 per day x 10^{-8})
0	5.50±0.12	4.96±0.31	0	0	0
16.6	4.13±0.61	6.75±0.57	2.8±1.3	0.41	16.8±7.6
41.5	2.80±0.23	9.48±0.63	7.3±0.8	0.73	17.6±1.9
83.0	1.81±0.31	13.67±1.76	12.8±1.9	0.94	15.4±2.3
100.0	2.23±0.42	16.19±1.99	14.3±2.7	0.88	14.3±2.7

In the survival studies with 100-cm shunts, consumption is predominately by the shunt. Fitting the survival curves to the general reaction equation $dc/dt = Kc^n$ yields $n = 0.981 \pm 0.163$ (±SEM). This justifies the first order assumption, and it can be shown that within the observed range of reaction orders, assumption of an order other than 1.0 affects the calculated value of K to only a small degree.

^{51}Cr-platelets obtained from animals with shortened autologous platelet survivals due to vascular prostheses give normal survivals in normal recipients

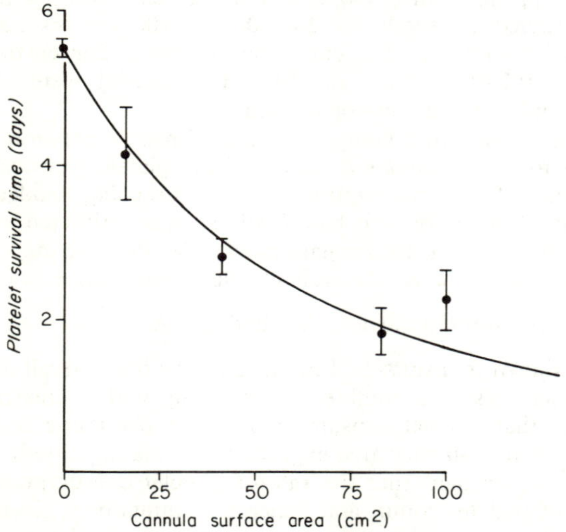

FIGURE 2. Effect of cannula surface area on platelet survival. Platelet survival is predictably shortened by increasing the arteriovenous cannula surface area that is exposed to circulating blood. However, the relationship is not linear. Each point is the mean of at least 4 studies (±1 SEM).

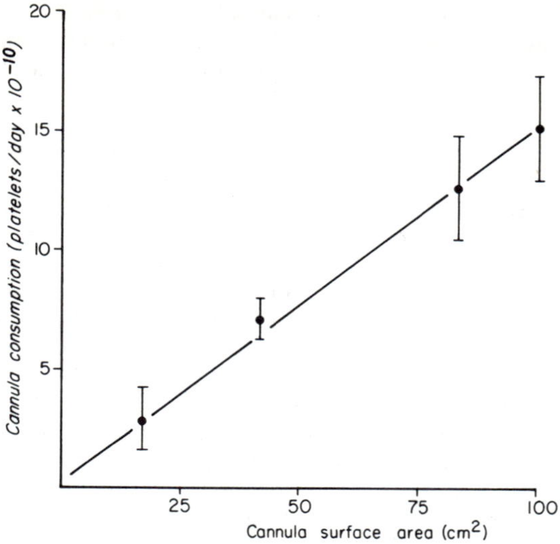

FIGURE 3. Direct relationship between cannula consumption and cannula surface area. When platelet consumption by the cannula is separated from physiologic senescence, a linear relationship is found between luminal cannual surface area and cannula platelet consumption.

and vice versa, indicating that the platelet survival is reduced by all-or-none consumption rather than by cumulative intrinsic changes in circulating platelets. Heparin (35 U per kg/hr, 3,000 U loading dose) increases the clotting time to over 20 minutes but does not affect platelet consumption. The steady state assumption is justified by the fact that platelet counts vary by less than 10% during the course of an experiment, and since serial weekly survivals are equivalent.

This approach to the evaluation of biomaterials offers an objective, *in vivo,* steady state comparison of material thrombogenicity that is not affected by surgical variables or limited to the initial deposition of thrombotic material.

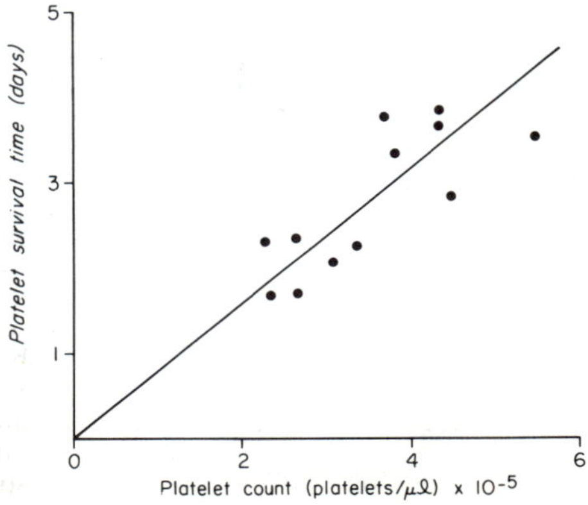

FIGURE 4. Effect of platelet concentration on platelet survival. Since the reaction between platelets on prosthetic surface appears to be saturated in this system, a reduction in circulating platelets results in a shortening in platelet survival when the canual length is held constant.

The use of a given thrombogenic cannula also provides a means to study the effects of oral antiplatelet drugs on reducing thrombus formation on prosthetic surfaces.[32] This approach has obvious direct application to man.[13, 15, 33]

Endothelialization of Arterial Prosthesis

The thrombogenic mechanism of arterial prostheses and its interruption is usefully characterized by determining the relative involvement of platelets, coagulation, and fibrinolysis in human arterial prostheses, and by direct examination of arterial grafts in a baboon model. Serial survival and turnover measurements of ^{51}Cr-platelets, ^{131}I-fibrinogen and ^{125}I-plasminogen in ten patients with aortofemoral knitted Dacron prostheses demonstrate selective platelet consumption after graft placement (platelet survival 4.2 days $\pm$ 0.5 and turnover 68,000 plat/μl/day $\pm$ 10,000 compared with 8.2 days $\pm$ 0.3 and 35,000 plat/μl/day $\pm$ 5,000, respectively, for control subjects, $p < 0.01$) without significantly increased consumption of fibrinogen or plasminogen. *In vitro* platelet function test results are normal. Platelet consumption is interrupted by dipyridamole inhibition of platelet function, and normalized spontaneously over nine months postoperatively (Figure 5).

Placement of impervious filamentous velour Dacron aortic prostheses into baboons predictably shortens platelet survival from 5.5 days $\pm$ 0.2 to 2.3 days $\pm$ 0.3 ($p < 0.001$) when studied one week following surgery; platelet turnover is reciprocally increased 2½-fold over baseline values, i.e. 153,000 plat/μl/day $\pm$ 21,000 vs. 59,000 plat/μl/day $\pm$ 7,000. Sham-operated control animals show normal platelet survival times when studied one week following surgery. Fibrinogen survival and turnover are not significantly altered; baseline values of 2.6 days $\pm$ 0.2 and 1.0 mg/ml $\pm$ 0.1 compare with 2.4 days $\pm$ 0.4 and 1.2 mg/ml/day $\pm$ 0.3 one week postoperatively. Both platelet survival and turnover progressively normalize over the subsequent five weeks.

When the underlying mechanism responsible for this spontaneous normalization of platelet survival is studied in baboons by serial direct microscopic examination of impervious aortic prostheses after grafting, following *in vivo* pressure-perfusion fixation with 0.3% $AgNO_3$, patchy islands of endothelial-like

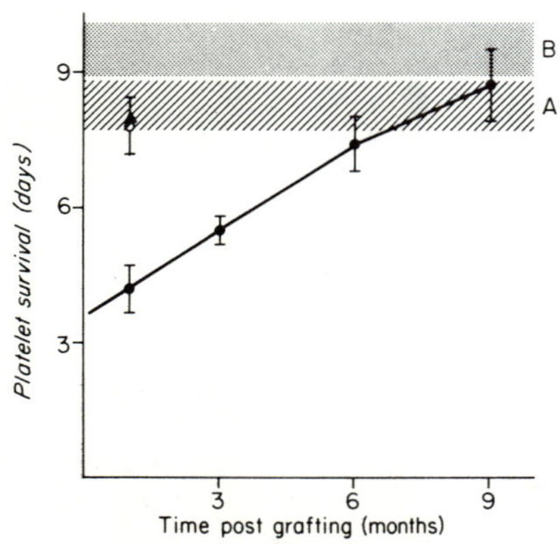

Figure 5. Platelet survival measurements in patients with arterial grafts. Platelet survival was consistently reduced one month after surgery and spontaneously normalized during the following nine months, as shown by the solid circles ($\pm$1 SD). Platelet consumption was interrupted by dipyridamole (open circle) or a combination of dipyridamole and ASA (closed triangle). Baseline platelet survival times in control patients with severe but stable peripheral vascular disease ($\pm$1 SD) is shown by the hatched area (A) and the results with young normal subjects is indicated by the stippled area (B).

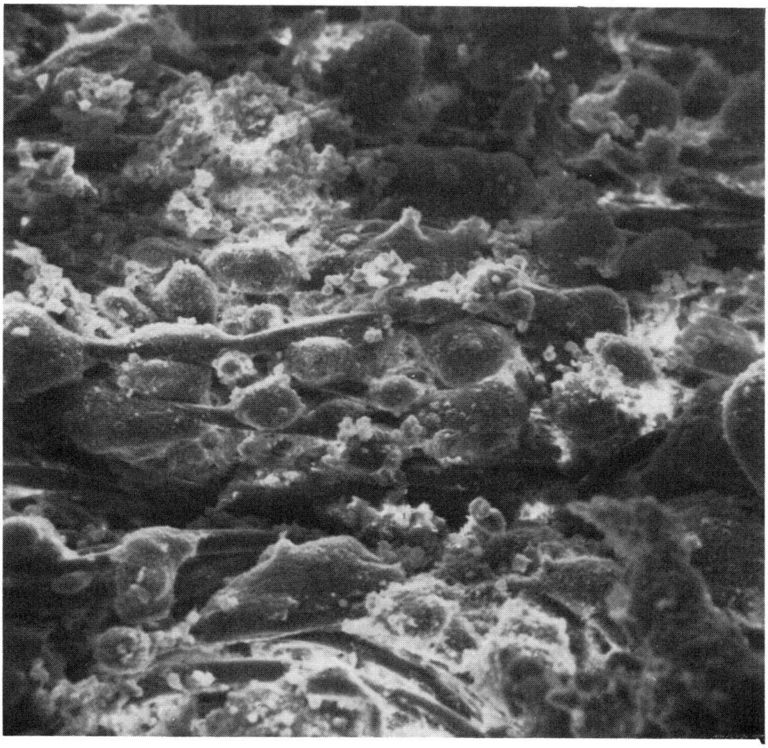

FIGURE 6. Scanning electron micrograph of luminal graft surface. Endothelial cell coverage of the luminal prosthetic surface after 3 weeks *in vivo* is partial with adjacent areas showing platelet thrombus.

cells are distributed randomly over the luminal prosthetic surface within a week of grafting. These lining cells appear to be endothelial cells morphologically, as indicated by the presence of tight intercellular junctions and the cell-specific organelle, Weibel-Palade bodies (FIGURE 6).

The three-week partially healed prosthetic surface demonstrated areas showing endothelial cell coverage and adjacent as yet exposed and persistently thrombogenic areas (FIGURE 7). Endothelialization of the graft surface resulted from coalescence of proliferating islands of endothelial cells with one another and with endothelial ingrowth across the anastomoses from the host aorta.[34, 35] Normalization of platelet survival correlates directly with the coverage of the luminal surface of the graft by endothelial cells (FIGURE 8), and appears to reflect the substitution of the thrombogenic prosthetic surfaces by nonthrombogenic endothelial cells. The shortening in platelet survival appears to be due to the formation of platelet thrombus and microembolization *in vivo,* as evidenced by direct examination of the prosthetic surface and the formation of microinfarcts distal to the site of arterial grafting.[11–12] From these data we conclude that a reduction in platelet survival may be a useful *in vivo* indicator of exposed nonendothelialized thrombogenic surface.

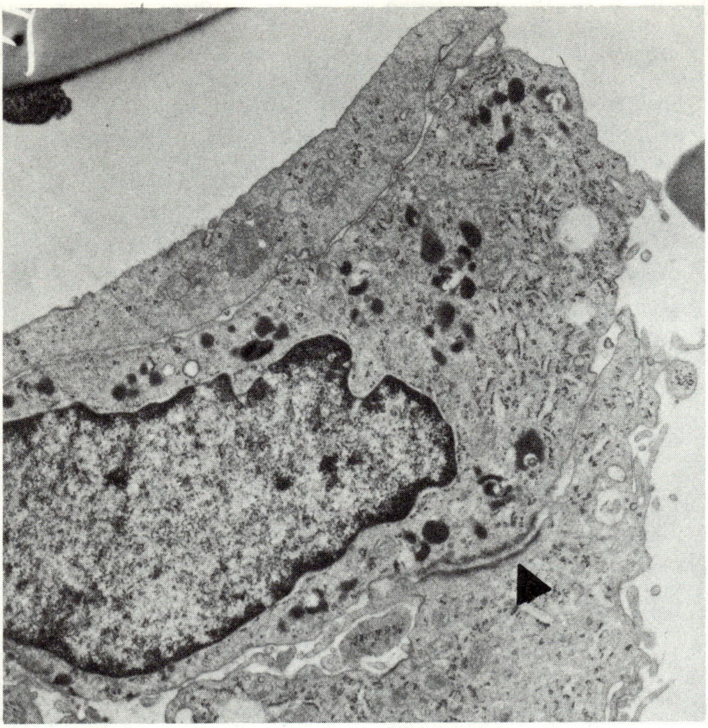

FIGURE 7. Photomicrograph of luminal graft cells. Tight intercellular junctions (arrow) and the presence of membrane bound lamellar organelles (Weibel-Palade bodies) identify the luminal cells as vascular endothelium.

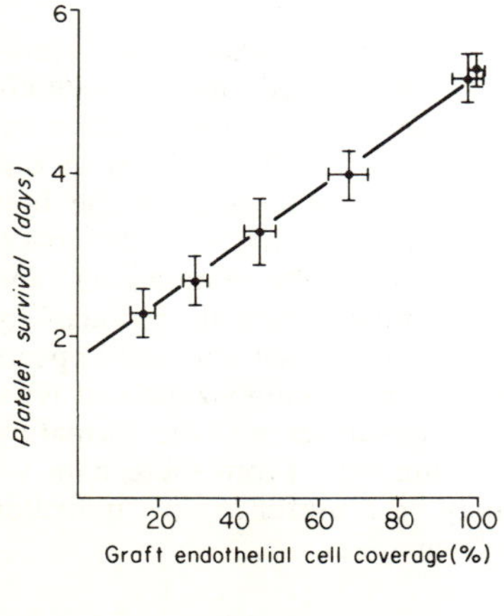

FIGURE 8. Direct relationship between platelet survival and graft endothelialization. Normalization of platelet survival correlated directly with the coverage of the prosthetic surface by endothelial cells (solid circles ±1 SD).

These data in nonhuman primates suggest that the progressive normalization of platelet survival in patients with prosthetic arterial grafts reflects endothelialization of the prosthetic luminal surface within nine months of surgery. Although this interpretation is supported by the appearance of partial endothelial coverage in some patients with arterial grafts,[36, 37] other studies have failed to demonstrate endothelial cells on arterial prosthetic flow surfaces after long healing intervals in man.[38-40] It should be recognized, however, that many of these studies involved older style prosthetic materials and designs. Furthermore, the absence of endothelial coverage might also have been related to the delays in obtaining autopsy material or the lack of pressure perfusion fixation *in vivo,* since endothelium lying directly on a noncellular base may be particularly susceptible to injury-induced desquamation.

In summary, platelet survival and turnover studies are useful objective *in vivo* measurements of: 1) the rate of arterial graft thrombogenesis; 2) antithrombotic efficacy of antiplatelet drugs in association with cardiovascular prostheses; and 3) the rate of endothelialization of luminal graft surfaces. These studies further suggest that the most promising practical approach to solving the problems of prosthesis-induced thrombus formation involves the combination of: 1) selection of the least thrombogenic material; 2) pharmacologic inhibition of platelet function using oral agents during the period of greatest thrombogenicity; and 3) the use of grafts that promote luminal endothelialization.

References

1. Wesolowski, S. A., C. C. Fries, G. Hennigar *et al.* 1964. Factors contributing to long-term failures in human vascular prosthetic grafts. Presented at Symposium on the Late Results of Reconstructive Arterial Surgery, Rome, Italy, 1963. J. Cardiovas. Surg. **5:** 544–567.
2. De Bakey, M. E., G. L. Jordan, J. P. Abbott *et al.* 1964. The fate of Dacron vascular grafts. Arch. Surg. **89:** 757–782.
3. Scarborough, D. E. 1971. The pathogenesis of thrombosis in artificial organs and vessels. Curr. Top Pathol. **54:** 95.
4. Mason, R. G. 1972. The interaction of blood hemostatic elements with artificial surfaces. *In* Progress in Hemostasis and Thrombosis. T. H. Spaet. Ed. Vol. **1:** 141. Grune & Stratton. New York, N.Y.
5. Berger, S. & E. W. Salzman. 1974. Thromboembolic complications of prosthetic devices. *In* Progress in Hemostasis and Thrombosis. T. H. Spaet, Ed. Vol. **2:** 273–309. Grune & Straton. New York, N.Y.
6. Mason, R. G., D. E. Scarborough, S. R. Saba, K. M. Brinkhouse, L. Ikenberry, J. J. Kearney & H. G. Clark. 1969. Thrombogenicity of some biomedical materials: platelet-interface reactions. J. Biomed. Mater. Res. **3:** 615.
7. Friedman, L. I. & E. F. Leonard. 1971. Platelet adhesion to artificial surfaces: consequences of flow, exposure time, blood condition and surface nature. Fed. Proc. **30:** 1641.
8. Jacobsson, B., S. E. Bergentz & U. Ljungqvist. 1969. Platelet adhesion and thrombus formation on vascular catheters in dogs. Acta Radiol. (Stockh.) **8:** 221–227.
9. Lessin, L. S., W. N. Jensen, G. A. Kelser, T. Motomiya & G. H. Nachnani. 1972. Scanning electron microscopy of thrombogenesis on vascular catheter surfaces. N. Engl. J. Med. **286:** 139.
10. Takebayashi, J., M. Kamatani, S. Namba *et al.* 1974. Early reparative process of implanted arterial prosthesis: a morphological and hematological study. J. Surg. Res. **17:** 102–110.

11. KUSSEROW, B. K., R. LARROW & J. NICHOLS. 1970. Observations concerning prosthesis-induced thromboembolic phenomena made with an *in vivo* embolus test system. Trans. Am. Soc. Artif. Int. Organs **16:** 58.
12. KUSSEROW, B. K. 1972. The use of pathologic techniques in the evaluation of emboli from prosthetic devices. Bull. N.Y. Acad. Med. **48:** 468.
13. HARKER, L. A. & S. J. SLICHTER. 1970. Studies of platelet and fibrinogen kinetics in patients with prosthetic heart valves. N. Engl. J. Med. **283:** 1302–1305.
14. WEILY, H. S. & E. GENTON. 1970. Altered platelet function in patients with prosthetic mitral valves. Effects of sulfinpyrazone therapy. Circulation **42:** 967.
15. HARKER, L. A. & S. J. SLICHTER. 1972. Platelet and fibrinogen consumption in man. N. Engl. J. Med. **287:** 999–1005.
16. SULLIVAN, J. M., D. E. HARKEN & R. GORLIN. 1968. Pharmacologic control of thromboembolic complications of cardiac-valve replacement. A preliminary report. N. Engl. J. Med. **279:** 576–580.
17. ARRANTS, J. E., P. HAIRSTON & W. H. LEE, JR. 1970. Use of dipyridamole (Persantine) in preventing thromboembolism following valve replacement. Chest **58:** 275.
18. SULLIVAN, J. M., D. E. HARKEN & R. GORLIN. 1971. Pharmacologic control of thromboembolic complications of cardiac-valve replacement. New Engl. J. Med. **284:** 1391–1394.
19. KAEGI, A., G. F. PINEO, A. SHIMIZU, H. TRIVEDI, J. HIRSH & M. GENT. 1974. Arteriovenous-shunt thrombosis: prevention by sulfinpyrazone. N. Engl. J. Med. **290:** 304–306.
20. SEVITT, S., N. G. GALLAGHER. 1959. Prevention of venous thrombosis and pulmonary embolism in injured patients. A trial of anticoagulant prophylaxis with phenindione in middle-aged and elderly patients with fractured necks of femur. Lancet **2:** 981–989.
21. SHERRY, S., K. M. BRINKHOUS, E. GENTON & J. M. STENGLE, Eds. 1969. Thrombosis. National Academy of Science. Washintgon, D.C.
22. HARKER, L. A. & S. J. SLICHTER. 1974. Arterial and Venous thromboembolism: kinetic characterization and evaluation of therapy. Thromb. Diath. Haemorrh. **31:** 188–203.
23. GOTT, V. L. & A. FURUSE. 1972. Standardized methods for the *in vivo* evaluation of artificial surfaces. Bul. N.Y. Acad. Med. **48:** 482–490.
24. MASON, R. G., R. H. WOLF, W. H. ZUCKER, B. A. SHINODA & S. F. MOHAMMAD. 1976. Effects of antithrombotic agents evaluated in a nonhuman primate vascular shunt model. Am. J. Pathol. **83:** 557–568.
25. HARKER, L. A., S. J. SLICHTER, C. R. SCOTT & R. ROSS. 1974. Homocystinemia: Vascular injury and arterial thrombosis. N. Engl. J. Med. **291:** 537–543.
26. HARKER, L. A., R. ROSS, S. J. SLICHTER & C. R. SCOTT. 1976. Homocystine-induced atherosclerosis: the role of endothelial cell injury and platelet response in its genesis. J. Clin. Invest. **58:** 731–741.
27. MURPHY, E. A. & M. E. FRANCIS. 1971. The estimation of blood platelet survival. II. The multiple hit model. Throm. Diath. Haemorr. **25:** 53–80.
28. MURPHY, E. A. 1971. The estimation of blood platelet survival. III. The robustness of the basic models. Throm. Diath. Haemorr. **26:** 431–454.
29. MURPHY, E. A., M. E. FRANCIS & J. F. MUSTARD. 1972. The estimation of blood platelet survival. IV. Characteristics of the residual errors from regression. Throm. Diath. Haemorrh. **28:** 447–456.
30. MILLS, J. N. 1946. The life-span of the erythrocyte. J. Physiol. **105:** 16P.
31. DORNHORST, A. C. 1951. The interpretation of red cell survival curves. Blood **6:** 1284–1292.
32. HARKER, L. A. & S. J. SLICHTER. 1973. Arterial thromboembolism—quantitation and prevention. Int. Soc. Hem. Thromb. Vienna, Austria.
33. HARKER, L. A. 1974. *In vivo* evaluation of antithrombotic therapy in man. Thromb. Diath. Haemorr. (Suppl.) **60:** 481–495.

34. Florey, H. W., S. J. Greer, J. Kiser *et al.* 1962. The development of the pseudointima lining fabric grafts of the aorta. Brit. J. Exp. Pathol. **43:** 655–660.
35. Sun, C. N. & J. J. Ghidoni. 1973. Fibrinous pseudo-intimas within impermeable silastic-nylon velour. II. Development of "Neointima." Exp. Pathol. Bd. SS 323–330.
36. Sauvage, L. R., K. Berger, L. B. Beilin *et al.* 1975. Presence of endothelium in an axillary-femoral graft of knitted Dacron with an external velour surface. Ann. Surg. **182**(6): 749–753.
37. DeBakey, M. E., J. P. Abbott, R. M. O'Neal *et al.* 1964. Endothelial lining of a human vascular prosthesis. Cardiovascular Res. Center Bull. **3:** 7–12.
38. Sauvage, L. R., K. Berger, Y. Nakagawa *et al.* 1971. An external velour surface for porous arterial prostheses. Surgery **70:** 940–953.
39. Berger, K., L. R. Sauvage, A. M. Rao *et al.* 1972. Healing of arterial prostheses in man: its incompleteness. Ann. Surg. **175:** 118–127.
40. Sun, C. N. & J. J. Ghidoni. 1973. Fibrinous pseudointimas within impermeable silastic-nylon velour. I. Ultrastructure of cell components at intimal stages and cell population changes in the earlier pseudointima. Exp. Path. Bd. SS 266–275.

DISCUSSION

Dr. Baier: Dr. Turitto, in the early part of your experiment you showed that you had used both platelet-rich plasma and whole blood, and you said that the rate of events was very much retarded in the platelet-rich plasma. But then most of the discussion was involving whole blood, and you showed that the rate of events was a little bit beyond the theory. I'm wondering if you did enough experiments to say whether theory was in fact met when you didn't have the larger cells to augment the diffusion of the platelets.

Dr. Turitto: No, we didn't do any experiments with platelet-rich plasma other than the ones we showed. We compared the rate of deposition from platelet-rich plasma and from whole blood under the same single experimental condition. As far as the augmentation caused by red cells in flow is concerned, yes, we could expect some enhancement of diffusion coefficient of, say, plasma proteins, but we have to remember that the diffusion coefficients of the proteins are already quite large compared to the value that the platelet is enhanced to: the platelet diffusion coefficient of 10^{-7} without the enhancement would be some two orders of magnitude smaller than it is with the enhancement, whereas the plasma proteins are already in the range of 10^{-7}, and we might see an enhancement of maybe fifty to seventy-five percent. But we haven't done any measurements about the augmentation of plasma proteins.

Unidentified Speaker: Dr. Stemerman, does the enzyme system play a part in endothelial proliferation? And would Dr. Harker say something about utilization of antiplatelet drugs before surgery and continuing these drugs during the surgical procedure and postoperatively for about ten days?

Dr. Stemerman: *In vivo,* so far everything that we've tried does not influence endothelial proliferation. *In vitro,* endothelial cell rate of growth appears in some way influenced by throwing platelets on these cells after a certain number of passages. The only other material that I am aware causes endothelial proliferation in tissue culture is a substance mentioned in a recent Science article; it is an extract of a neurogenic tumor. This is a substance different from tumor angiogenesis factor, which causes capillary proliferation and is an RNA-like material derived from tumors.

Dr. Harker: Our experience would indicate that anticoagulants represent the appropriate preventive for venous thromboembolism, whereas antiplatelet drugs would only have a potential in the prevention of arterial thrombotic disease. Heparin given in doses of 5,000 units subcutaneously every eight hours, starting before surgery, probably provides satisfactory prevention of pulmonary emboli for most operative procedures in those patients who have particular propensity for that complication.

Unidentified Speaker: Dr. Harker, I have a question about the hydraulics of the bypass tube. I believe there is a difference in the rate of *in vivo* endothelial cell turnover in the rabbit aorta, depending on the region of the aorta, and that it is greatest where the hydraulic stress is greatest: in the ascending aorta, and least in the terminal aorta. Is there any evidence in the work that you have done thus far to suggest that the rate of endotheliazation of your bypass grafts is influenced by hydraulic factors as well? If there is a little more of a curve in the tube, for example, do you see different rates of endothelialization?

Dr. Harker: The endotheliazation of those grafts proceeds from scattered islands of what we are regarding as endothelial cells; these proliferate randomly, rather than growing from both ends. There is a high incorporation of tritiated thymidine in those cells, but we are unable to demonstrate any hemodynamic correlations so far.

Dr. Schultz: We have been doing experiments similar to Dr. Turitto's, using an *ex vivo* shunt system in measuring the rate of platelet and fibrinogen deposition without the use of anticoagulants, and with a very similar analysis we found a rate of approach of platelets to the surface about a factor of ten greater than Dr. Turitto's, which makes us wonder if there may be some factors other than simple diffusion involved which accelerates the rate of platelet transfer to a growing thrombus in a more or less *in vivo* situation.

Dr. Turitto: You are measuring total platelet deposition: not only platelets that interact with your surface, but platelets that have attached to the platelets that have already interacted. Past a certain height of thrombus, I think other fluid dynamic forces come into play and make the analysis much more complex. Other forces besides simple diffusion could enhance the rate of deposition; direct contact of the particles by flow, and trapping between thrombi would enhance deposition rate.

Dr. Stemerman: Dr. Harker noticed blood-derived colonies of endothelial cells, but the other intriguing possibility, which I think Dr. Harker has thought about, is that endothelial cells can be pulled off and can circulate, as has been demonstrated by the late Dr. E. Gaynor; they can certainly alight upon anything. In other words, "blood-borne" does not mean "bone marrow-derived." We have not noticed endothelial cells in any kind of fancy random distribution with scanning microscopy of the injured surface.

CURRENT ACTIVITIES AND FUTURE DIRECTIONS IN BIOMATERIALS RESEARCH *

Stephen D. Bruck

National Heart, Lung, and Blood Institute
National Institutes of Health
Bethesda, Maryland 20014

INTRODUCTION

Polymeric biomaterials include both naturally and synthetically derived products that may be useful for a variety of prosthetic applications and can serve as models for the study of the complex interactions with blood. The components of the vascular wall are mostly biopolymers, which, together with the endothelium, perform vitally important functions in maintaining normal blood flow patterns and the prevention of thrombosis. Thus, the proper understanding of blood compatibility and the development of prosthetic materials require the investigations of both natural and synthetic materials. The study of biomaterials is also important for the better understanding (and the eventual prevention) of arteriosclerosis and aging. Extensive *in vitro, ex vivo,* and *in vivo* testing in suitable animals and considerations of the important species-related differences between the properties of blood components of animals and humans are essential in order to insure the maximum safety of medical devices.

The close interrelationship between biomaterials research and development, test, and evaluation, and short- and long-term applications are schematically illustrated in FIGURE 1. The major components of current activities involving biomaterials research and development for cardiovascular applications are illustrated in FIGURE 2. Although each area represents an important aspect of the entire program, there is a close interdependence and interrelationship between them, as shown by the solid and dotted connecting lines. A detailed discussion of each area will be presented in a later section of this paper.

DISCUSSION

Interactions of Blood Components with Synthetic and Natural Materials

Coagulation and Thrombosis

Among the initial events that occur when materials come in contact with whole blood is the very rapid adsorption of plasma proteins. This process seems to be completed in less than three seconds and effectively influences the subsequent interactions of the formed blood elements, especially the platelets, with the

* The views expressed in this paper are those of the author and do not necessarily represent those of the NHLBI, NIH, or the Department of Health, Education, and Welfare.

proteinated surfaces.[1] In particular, this rapid adsorption of proteins probably influences the activation of factor XII and other coagulation factors, and affects the adhesion and activation of the platelets. The adsorption of proteins from plasma is influenced by the type of surface, the properties of blood components, species-related differences, hemorheological parameters, and the large number of small ionic species present in plasma which are expected to arrive at a given surface prior to proteins. Hence, the adsorption of proteins may be mitigated by a number of parameters, including other plasma components. The adsorbed proteins do not become permanently immobilized on the surface on a material in the physiological environment, but may be enzymatically degraded, replaced by other proteins, or may undergo various conformational and configurational changes, and denaturation.[2] All these play a dominant role in the activation of

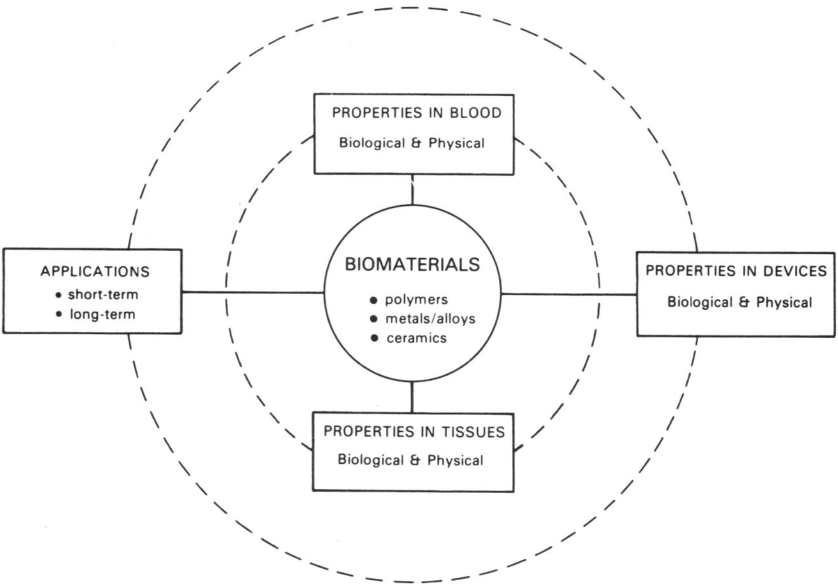

FIGURE 1. Relationship between biomaterials R&D and applications.

plasma coagulation factors, and affect the formed blood elements, especially the platelets. When platelets adhere to proteinated surfaces, they may become activated depending on the molecular stimuli and hemorheological factors, extrude their granules, and liberate adenosine nucleotides, serotonin, and other coagulation activators.[3] As a consequence, irreversible platelet aggregation results, leading to thrombosis. As indicated schematically in FIGURE 3, coagulation and thrombosis involve at least three major steps when flowing blood contacts synthetic surfaces: (1) adsorption of and subsequent changes in plasma proteins, (2) clotting of the plasma proteins via a complex series of reactions involving the various clotting factors, and (3) activation of the platelets and their aggregation in conjunction with the other formed blood elements. Low shear conditions lead to the formation of "red" thrombus, which is chiefly an

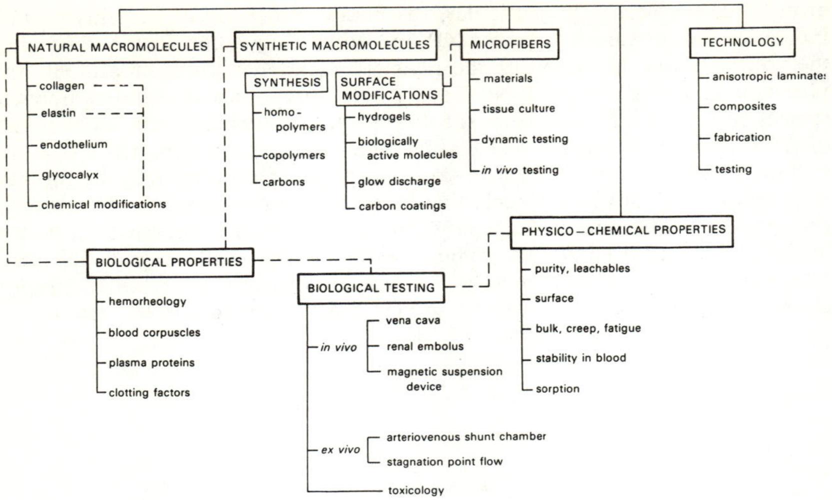

FIGURE 2. Blood-compatible materials R&D.

interwoven mesh of red cells in fibrin, whereas high shear conditions give rise to "white" thrombus, which is mainly an interwoven mesh of white cells in fibrin.

In the case of natural surfaces, it is well known that when the endothelial cells are damaged, platelets adhere to the sites of injured blood vessels as the result of exposure of the subendothelial tissue and native collagen.[3] The endothelial cells have a surface coating, the glycocalyx. It has been shown that even slight trauma to this surface coating, without gross injury to the endothelial cells, can activate the coagulation mechanism and fibrinolysis with or without platelet aggregation.[4] Using cultured endothelial and smooth-muscle cells, and

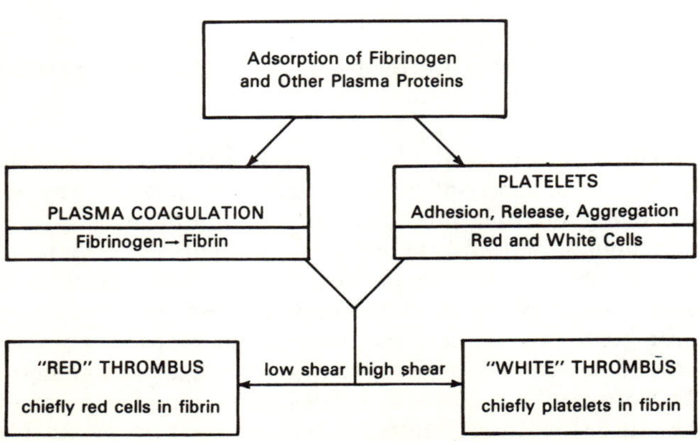

FIGURE 3. Coagulation and thrombosis when flowing blood contacts synthetic surfaces.

fibroblasts, Pitlick [5] found that endothelial cells have about 5% as much tissue factor activity as smooth-muscle cells.

As a result of the interaction with subendothelial tissue, following injury to the endothelium, the platelets release ADP, which causes their aggregation. During the aggregation process, platelets also release phospholipids which are essential for the coagulation process. The property of collagen to activate and aggregate the platelets appears to be related to its native, highly ordered structure because denatured collagen neither promotes the aggregation of platelets nor initiates the clotting process. The ability of native, fibrillar collagen to aggregate the platelets may be related also to the particular architecture of the collagen molecule because monodisperse tropocollagen with its triple helix is apparently insufficient for platelet aggregation.[6] This does not rule out the possibility that the more complex triple helical structure of multimeric tropocollagen or collagen fibrils is not involved in platelet aggregation.

Although platelet aggregation depends on the fibrillar structure of collagen, Silberberg and Miller [7] recently found that tropocollagen adsorbed onto glass support can bind platelets without aggregating them. On the other hand, Gordon and Dingle [8] concluded that tropocollagen *in solution* does not bind platelets. However, subsequent work by Silberberg and Miller,[7] who used competitive binding experiments with protein solutions, indicates that tropocollagen in solution can in fact bind platelets. Furthermore, experiments by Silberberg and Miller [7] and by Michaeli [9] and Katzman *et al.*[10] suggest that platelets can interact with α-chains derived from collagen.

Collagen and Its Structural Aspects

The fundamental structural unit of collagen appears to be the tropocollagen molecule, having a diameter of 15 Å, length of 2800 Å, and a molecular weight of about 300,000. The tropocollagen molecules are organized into fibrils, approximately 5000 Å long, in such a way that they overlap by a quarter of their length. The tropocollagen molecule forms a triple helix, the structure of which was established by Rich and Crick,[11] and by Ramachandran.[12] The individual chains are nearly extended so that only intermolecular hydrogen bonding is possible between them. One third of collagen is glycine, and one quarter is composed of proline and hydroxyproline. Collagen contains one intermolecular hydrogen bond via the N-H . . . O=C group, plus one intermolecular hydrogen bond via a water molecule per three residues. This is in contrast to other proteins, the architecture of which permits a greater amount of hydrogen bonding to occur. Chang and Chien [13] have shown that a variety of electrolytes can affect the stabilization and destabilization of the rodlike superstructure of reconstituted collagen.

The triple-stranded helical structure of collagen is formed by intracellular processes involving the three α-polypeptide chains which constitute the collagen subunits. The precursor procollagen consists of polypeptide chains with molecular weight in the range of 120,000–125,000. The cysteine residues in the procollagen give rise to disulfide crosslinks between the α-polypeptide chains. These crosslinks seem to have a stabilizing effect on the formation of the triple-stranded helix, which has a molecular weight of ~360,000.[14] Work by Schofield *et al.*[15] and by Uitto and Prockop [16] suggests that the α-polypeptide chains of procollagen are linked by disulfide crosslinks prior to the formation of the triple helix. In other words, it appears that without such crosslinks, the production of a triple-helical structure would not be possible. The triple-helical conformation of procollagen polypeptides is apparently stabilized by the presence of hydroxyproline in the molecule and contributes to the thermal stability of the collagen.[17]

Electrical Conduction and Semiconduction in Collagen and Other Biopolymers

Before discussing this phenomenon of electrical conduction in collagen, some fundamental considerations are in order. In general, electrical conductivity may be either electronic or ionic. *Electronic* conduction is characteristic of metals in which electrons are the current carriers. On the other hand, *ionic* conduction is characterized by the presence of charged atoms or groups of atoms, which are the current carriers. Semiconductors are characterized by two energy bands, one that is filled with electrons (valence band), and the other that is empty (conduction band). These two bands are separated by a forbidden energy gap. If an electron acquires sufficient energy, it can jump into the upper conduction band. Electronic conduction may occur that is accompanied by the removal of electrons from the valence bands, leaving empty levels and creating the appearance of a flow of positively charged electrons (holes). In a perfect *intrinsic* semiconductor, the number of electrons in the conduction band is equal to the number of holes. In such a case, electrical conduction will depend on the inherent atomic and crystal structure of the material. On the other hand, in an *extrinsic* semiconductor, electrical conduction by electrons and holes is caused by impurity atoms present in the crystal lattice. Depending on whether or not the impurity atom (or atoms) donates or accepts an electron (or electrons) from the valence band, the semiconducting material will be *n*-type (because of the negative charge of the carriers) or *p*-type (because of the positive charge of the holes).

Electrical conductivity, σ, may be expressed as:

$$\begin{aligned}\sigma &= |e|\, n(\mu_h + \mu_e)\\ &= |e|\, n(1 + c)\\ &= \sigma_o \exp\,(E/2kT)\end{aligned}$$

where, $|e|$ = electronic charge, n = concentration of current carriers, μ_h and μ_e = mobilities of holes and electrons, respectively, $c = \mu_e/\mu_h$, σ_o = pre-exponential factor, E = activation energy to form charge carriers, k = Boltzmann constant, T = absolute temperature, e = base of natural logarithm.

It is apparent that electrical conduction and semiconduction in proteins are involved in a number of biochemical reactions, and has been reported for many biopolymers, including collagen.[18-21] It seems that the electrical properties of these macromolecules are strongly influenced by their water "structure," which in turn depends on the particular molecular architecture of the biopolymers. A number of proteins and synthetic polymers in the dry state exhibit electrical semiconduction. For example, in the case of β-proteins, Evans and Gergely[22] calculated that the energy gap (ΔE) between the top of the filled bands and the bottom of the unfilled bands leads to a value of 3.05 eV. Beta-proteins are characterized by hydrogen bond structures that presumably enable the movement of electrons and holes through the system. Cardew and Eley[19] have suggested that α-proteins may have similar electrical properties due to their helical structure.

TABLE 1

ACTIVATION ENERGIES FOR SEMICONDUCTION OF SELECTED DRY PROTEINS

Protein	Δ E, e. V.	Ref.
Hemoglobin (methanol denatured)	2.89	Eley & Spivey [21]
Hemoglobin (natural)	2.66	Eley & Spivey [21]
Hemoglobin (crystalline)	2.3–2.4	Rosenberg [20]
Globin (mixture of native and denatured)	2.97	Cardew & Eley [19]
Thrombin	2.59	Eley & Spivey [21]
Fibrinogen	2.69	Eley & Spivey [21]
Elastin	2.91	Eley & Spivey [21]
Collagen	2.73	Eley & Spivey [21]
Bovine plasma albumin	2.78	Eley & Spivey [21]

TABLE 1 represents a summary of the activation energies for semiconduction of several dry proteins and shows that the values fall within the range of ~2.3 to 3.0 eV. The corresponding mobility of charge carriers as calculated by Eley and Spivey [21] are between 10^3 and 10^5 cm^2V^{-1} sec^{-1} at 400°K. These values are much larger than those of many synthetic aromatic compounds and compare favorably with those of inorganic semiconductors. The specific electroconductivities of selected proteins observed by Eley and Spivey [21] and some synthetic polymers reported by Topchiev,[23] Marvel and Rassweiler,[24] and Bruck [25] are shown in TABLE 2. Apparently, the observed electroconductivities are caused by the π-electrons in the hydrogen-bonded C=O . . . H-N systems.

The fact that water has great influence on the electrical conduction properties of proteins is shown by the lowering of the activation energy of conduction.[20, 26] In the case of collagen, Dehl [27] found that about 0.54 g of water/g of collagen does not freeze and retains high mobility to −50° C, which represents about 2.6 molecules of unfreezable water per residue of the collagen

TABLE 2

SPECIFIC ELECTROCONDUCTIVITIES OF SOME PROTEINS AND SELECTED SYNTHETIC POLYMERS

Material	Sp. Electroconductivity ohm^{-1} cm^{-1}	Temp. ° C	Ref.
Thrombin	3.8×10^{-12}	27	Eley & Spivey [21]
Fibrinogen	1.6×10^{-12}	27	Eley & Spivey [21]
Bovine plasma albumin	1.3×10^{-12}	27	Eley & Spivey [21]
Hemoglobin (natural)	1.8×10^{-12}	27	Eley & Spivey [21]
Collagen	3.4×10^{-14}	27	Eley & Spivey [21]
Poly [N,N′-(p,p′-oxydiphenylene) pyromellitimide] (pyrolytic product)	0.2×10^2	25	Brucks [25]
Polyphenyleneaminoquinone	7×10^{-7} to 9×10^{-7}	25	Topchiev [23]
Polymeric copper phthalocyanine	2.5×10^{-2}	25	Marvel & Rassweiler [24]

molecule. Further work by Dehl [28] with $MgCl_2$ and $MgSO_4$ in conjunction with nuclear magnetic resonance (nmr) spectroscopy and the use of D_2O suggested that neither the so-called two-state nor the structured water concept can satisfactorily explain the D_2O nmr doublet spectrum or the effects of salts on it. According to the two-state concept of water in collagen, there would be a rapid exchange between bound and free water in collagen, and furthermore, the nmr doublet splitting factor, $\Delta\nu$, should vary linearly with water content. Fung and Siegel,[29] however, have recently shown that this is not the case. In view of these results, it is unlikely that the amount of adsorbed (anisotropic) water in collagen is sufficient to be in equilibrium with an isotropic liquid phase, and that there is a significant quantity of "structured" water present in collagen.[28] In the case of collagen, the observed electrical conduction at low water content is probably electronic. However, at a water content between about 20% and 45%, Bardelmeyer [30] has recently proposed that the current carriers are probably protons rather than electrons. At higher water content (above approximately 65%), the conduction may be due to small inorganic ions.[30] The evidence that at low water content (below approximately 20%) the conduction is caused by electrons is supported by the observation that good linearity exists between current and voltage without polarization effects.[30] Between 45% and 65% water content, there is a sharp discontinuity in the plot of the activation energy vs. water content, indicating that the main charge carriers are probably protons.[30] Such protonic conduction may occur along the chains of collagen mediated by both the water molecules adsorbed on polar groups and the C=O . . . H-N hydrogen bond system.

Since collagen exhibits electrical conduction both in the dry and hydrated states, it is interesting to offer some speculative thoughts about this property and a hypothesis of its consequences. As has been shown, water held by the collagen molecule has a decisive effect on the conduction. Any disturbance to the native structure of this protein (such as increased ionic concentration and dehydration) would be expected to affect the particular condensed fibrillar structure of the molecule, and ultimately even its triple-helical structure by disrupting at least some of the hydrogen bonds. It is possible that the electrical conduction is enhanced by the dense, fibrous structure of the molecule by creating the type of close "overlap" that is necessary for efficient electron mobility. If this is the case, then a severe enough disturbance may cause a disruption of this organization. This in turn should be reflected in increased ion-binding propensity and in changes in the electrical conduction in the molecule. It is possible that a sufficient alteration in the water structure may be brought about by changes in the immediate milieu of the collagen fibers or by injury to the endothelium of blood vessels. In such circumstances, the altered collagen fibers (and other macromolecular subendothelial components) would be expected to become modified by the inorganic ions and organic polyelectrolytes of blood. The adsorption of these could subsequently affect the platelets which normally carry a net negative charge density and affect the coagulation factors. In other words, fundamental changes may occur in the native collagen molecule when it changes from the milieu that prevails underneath the normal endothelium to the one that becomes operative when collagen is exposed to blood constituents as the result of injuries to the endothelial lining of the blood vessel. These changes may by themselves be insufficient to cause gross denaturation of collagen, but sufficient to initiate the complex biochemical events that lead to platelet activation, aggregation, thrombosis, and blood compatibility.

A possible relationship between intrinsic electroconduction and blood compatibility was observed by this author.[31, 32] By thermally converting a specially purified aromatic polyimide, poly [N,N′-(p,p′-oxydiphenylene) pyromellitimide], into semiconducting and conducting condensation products at temperatures well below graphitization conditions,[31-34] showed that these materials exhibit quite different biological properties *in vitro* than their unconverted precursor insulators. The *in vitro* results are summarized in TABLE 3. These preliminary tests consisted of the Lee-White blood coagulation times, partial thromboplastin times (PTT), and platelet activation and aggregation with human platelet-rich plasma. The Lee-White blood coagulation times and PTT were compared with those of siliconized glass. The data indicate that the conducting and semiconducting pyrolytic polymers have clotting times two to three times longer than

TABLE 3

PHYSICAL AND *in Vitro* BIOLOGICAL PROPERTIES OF INSULATING SEMICONDUCTING AND ELECTROCONDUCTING POLYPYROMELLITIMIDES (PPMI)*

Sample	Specific Electro-conductivity $(\text{ohm cm})^{-1}$, 25°C	No. of Spins g^{-1}	Lee-White Coagulation Index †	PTT Index *	Platelet Aggregation and Activation
Unmodified PPMI	$<10^{-12}$	—	0.3	0.5	heavy and activated
Pyrolitic PPMI	0.1	$>10^{19}$	2.1	1.3	very light to none, not activated
Pyrolitic PPMI	11.1	$>10^{19}$	2.6	1.3	very light to none, not activated
Pyrolitic PPMI	20.0	$>10^{19}$	2.5	1.4	very light to none, not activated

* Compiled from Bruck.[31, 33]

† Expressed as ratio of clotting times for test specimens and those of siliconized glass (average of three).

those of siliconized glass, whereas the nonconducting (control) sample had a clotting time of approximately one third that of siliconized glass. Similarly, the semiconducting and electroconducting pyropolymers show very low or no platelet aggregation in contrast to the control sample. This behavior may be the result of the electrical properties of the pyropolymers that affect the initial adsorption and conformation of plasma proteins, which in turn should affect the interactions with platelets. Although the above observations are preliminary and should not be generalized, they may be important not only to the interactions of blood components with natural and synthetic surfaces, but possibly also to the better understanding of the molecular properties of the vascular endothelium and to the pathogenesis of arteriosclerosis.

In addition to the role of *intrinsic* conductors, above, there is evidence in the literature that *extrinsic* conductors also have biological relevance. It is recalled that extrinsic conduction, as opposed to intrinsic conduction, is not a molecular property, but depends on the presence of dispersed conducting particles, such as carbon black or metals, within the polymer matrix. Following the initial report by this author [31] with *intrinsically* conducting pyropolymers, Kolobow *et al.*[35] observed that conducting carbon particles dispersed in a matrix of silicone rubber exhibit greatly improved blood compatibility in comparison to unmodified silicone rubber. Previously, Sharp and colleagues [36] reported that "Electrolour" (Goodyear), a polyurethane containing dispersed conducting carbon particles, exhibits improved biological properties.

Electroconduction appears to be involved also in other biomedical areas. For example, McGinness *et al.*[37] have recently shown that melanins exhibit threshold switching, which until now has been restricted to intrinsic amorphous inorganic semiconductors. Melanins are polymeric pigments present in skin, hair, retina of the eye, midbrain, and inner ear. They have condensed, unsaturated ring structures, and are formed by the polymerization of oxidation products of tyrosine and dopa(3,4-dihydroxyphenylalanine). At the critical threshold voltage, switching occurs that is manifested by "on" and "off" states in the current vs. voltage plots. This property of melanin may be related to diseases such as Parkinsonism and schizophrenia.[37] Similar electrical switching was also observed with equine cytochrome c. The electroconductivity of melanins is in the order of 10^{-5} ohm^{-1} cm^{-1} that increases greatly in the "on" state. Water absorbed by these pigments is necessary for electrical switching to occur, since dried samples lose this property, apparently as the result of alteration in the dielectric constant of the system.

Synthetic and Chemically Modified Natural Biomaterials

Derivatives of Collagen

Collagen, when chemically crosslinked and modified, can be made both blood compatible and mechanically useful for prosthetic applications. Yannas [38] has prepared a series of crosslinked collagen/mucopolysaccharide (glycosaminoglycan) composite materials aimed at achieving reasonable mechanical properties with good blood compatibility. The rationale behind these studies is the fact that collagen fibers of the vascular wall are imbedded in a polysaccharide matrix that normally prevents contact between blood components and collagen; however, as a result of injury to the vascular wall, the polysaccharide matrix may be disturbed, thus enabling direct contact between collagen and blood components, including the platelets.

Among the mucopolysaccharides used by Yannas [38] was chondroitin-6 sulfate having the following chemical structure:

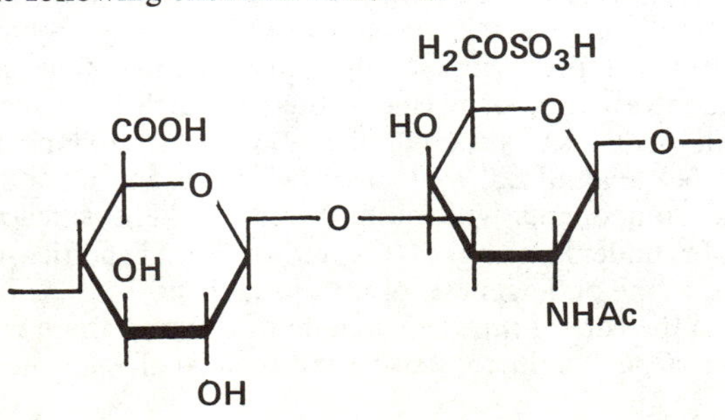

The collagen/chondroitin-6 sulfate composite was crosslinked either by glutaraldehyde or thermally in a vacuum. As seen in TABLE 4, the molecular weight between crosslinks ranges from 1,200 to 6,800, Young's moduli from 253 to 700 psi elongation at break from 11% to 21%, and ultimate tensile strength from 92 to 631 psi.

Biological evaluation *in vitro* indicates that the collagen/chondroitin-6 sulfate composite material strongly suppresses the usual coagulant and platelet-aggregating activity of unmodified collagen without leaching.[38] *In vivo* and *ex vivo* tests are in progress. The combined biological and mechanical properties of the collagen/chondroitin-6 sulfate and similar composite materials may make them suitable in the fabrication of tubular and other prostheses.

TABLE 4

PHYSICAL PROPERTIES OF COLLAGEN/CHRONDROITIN-6 SULFATE COMPOSITE MATERIALS *

Chrondroitin-6 Sulfate	$\overline{M}_c$	1% Modulus psi	Elong. at Break %	Ultimate Tensile Strength psi
3.5 †	2,500	253± 92	11±3	133±30
3.9 †	6,800	343±120	21±1	130±10
9.6 ‡	1,200	700± 65	20±1	631±28

* Data of I. V. Yannas.[38]
† Glutaraldehyde-crosslinked.
‡ Thermally-crosslinked in vacuum.

Synthetic Polymers

There is considerable interest in extracorporeal circulatory assistance devices, such as blood oxygenators, for which polymeric membranes are needed having both good blood compatibility and high gas transmission rates toward oxygen and carbon dioxide. Among such polymers is ethyl cellulose perfluorobutyrate, the structure of which is shown below:

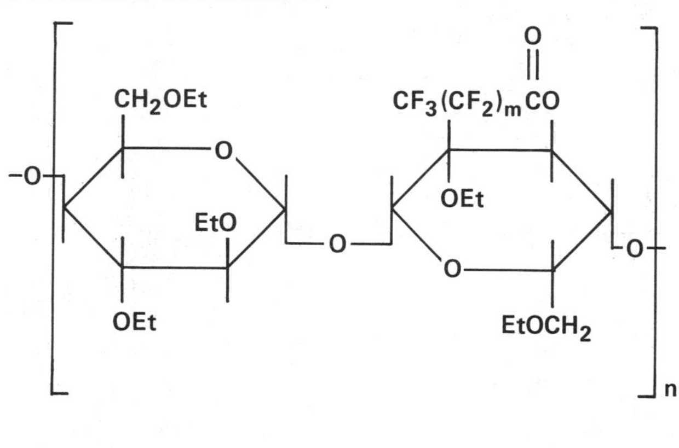

This is an amorphous polymer that exhibits neither a glass transition nor a melting temperature, has good tensile properties, and dissolves readily in a number of organic solvents. Typically, the number-average molecular weight ($\overline{M}_n$) is 73,000 and the weight-average molecular weight is 250,000, yielding a value for $\overline{M}_w/\overline{M}_n = 3.44$. The hydrolytic stability of the fluorinated ethyl cellulose is excellent, as indicated by tests carried out up to two weeks, and longer tests are in progress. The vena cava and renal embolus tests (to be discussed in more detail below), showed very promising thromboresistance in dogs, and the polymer also exhibited low shear-induced hemolysis *in vitro* with human blood. These properties compare favorably to low temperature isotropic (LTI) carbons (developed at General Atomic Corporation) that are widely used in artificial heart-valve prostheses with excellent success.

Although the gas-to-gas *permeabilities* toward oxygen and carbon dioxide are low in comparison to polydimethylsiloxane, ultrathin membranes in the range of 1–3 μm can be prepared and laminated to porous materials, for example, porous polypropylene ("Celgard," Celanese Corp.), to give the membrane adequate physical support. Other porous polymers may also be suitable. Such ultrathin membranes exhibit approximately a fourfold increase in the gas-to-gas *transmission rates* toward oxygen and carbon dioxide in comparison to polydimethylsiloxane. The gas-to-blood permeabilities and gas-to-blood transfer rates toward oxygen are at least as high as those exhibited by polydimethylsiloxane under typical clinical flow conditions. The combination of the promising biological properties and high gas transfer rates toward oxygen and carbon dioxide make the ethyl cellulose perfluorobutyrate membranes potentially useful candidates for blood oxygenators and for blood-compatible surface coatings. Experiments performed by Zapol (Massachusetts General Hospital) with 0.8 m^2 spiral coil oxygenators in an awake lamb showed an oxygen transfer rate of 60 ml/m^2-min and a carbon dioxide transfer rate of 67.5 ml/m^2-min. Lifetime studies performed with ^{51}Cr-labeled platelets showed that in three out of five experiments, 63%–69% of the platelets prior to bypass were still in circulation after 24 hours of perfusion. This compares with 67% ± 6% platelet survival in the case of silica-free silicone membrane devices, and significantly surpasses those made from commercial silicone rubber, which typically showed a platelet survival of 47% ± 5%. This development could eliminate the need to use heparinized materials in oxygenator applications to prevent thrombosis. While polydimethylsiloxane has many desirable attributes (such as flexibility, relative inertness to body fluids, nontoxicity, and sterilizability by steam autoclaving), its overall blood compatibility is relatively poor.

Other polymers with possible applications for membrane oxygenators and surface coatings are the polyalkylsulfones.[40] Polymers and copolymers of polyalkylsulfones can be prepared from the C_{16} and C_{18} straight chain α-olefins and sulfur dioxide yielding and general structure illustrated below:

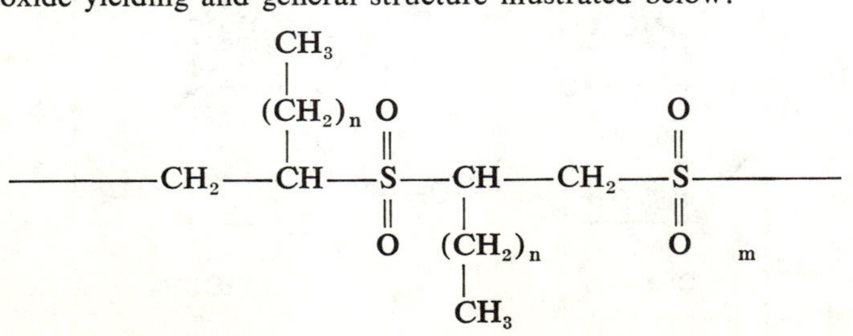

Although gas-to-gas permeabilities toward oxygen and carbon dioxide are about one-tenth of those of polydimethylsiloxane, ultrathin (2.5 μm) membranes can be made and coated onto a microporous polypropylene. This composite membrane exhibits gas-to-gas *transfer rates* toward oxygen that are approximately double of those of polydimethylsiloxane. The gas-to-blood transfer rates (measured with a large spiral channel membrane cell) are approximately 20% higher with oxygen and approximately three times higher with carbon dioxide in comparison with polydimethylsiloxane. Experiments performed by Zapol (Massachusetts General Hospital) with 0.54 m^2 spiral coil oxygenators in an awake lamb showed an oxygen transfer rate of 75 ml/m^2-min and a carbon dioxide transfer rate of 192.6 ml/m^2-min at a blood flow rate of 900 ml/min. At a blood flow rate of 1000 ml/min, the oxygen transfer rate was 95.24 ml/m^2-min and the carbon dioxide transfer rate was 251.9 ml/m^2-min.

Polyalkylsulfones have molecular weights above one million and $\overline{M}_w/\overline{M}_n$ ratios between 5 and 7. Thermal decomposition begins at approximately 200° C and the polymer starts to soften between 75° and 90° C. Because of these properties, steam autoclaving cannot be used. However, ethylene oxide gas gives a staisfactory means for sterilization, provided that a careful outgassing procedure is followed and the temperature is kept to a minimum. The biological properties of the polyalkylsulfones based on the vena cava test in dogs appear fairly promising, and additional evaluations are in progress involving other tests.

Surface Modifications of Polymers

One approach to the preparation of blood-compatible surfaces involves hydrogels. These are coherent three-dimensional polymeric networks that can imbibe large quantities of water without dissolution of the polymeric network. Wichterle and Lim [41] in 1960 were the first to call attention to the potential biological use of hydrogels based on 2-hydroxymethylmethacrylate (HEMA). Until recently, a major problem with hydrogels was their lack of good mechanical strength. In 1971, a microwave discharge grafting technique was developed by Scott *et al.*[42] Also in 1971, Halpern *et al.*,[43] using chemical means, successfully grafted polyacrylamide hydrogels onto polyurethanes and other polymers. On this author's recommendation, the grafting technique was applied to cardiovascular prosthetic devices that extended the usefulness of the otherwise weak hydrogels by combining mechanical strength with good blood compatibility. Following these developments, other investigators, using high energy irradiation, have grafted hydrogels onto polymeric substrates.[44]

I have recently dealt [45] with the physical and biological aspects of polymeric materials, including hydrogels for biomedical applications. The evidence strongly suggests that the presence of negatively charged ionic groups on certain synthetic hydrogels is not essential for blood compatibility. The biological performance of hydrogels apparently depends on a critical level of water uptake, chemical composition, purity, crosslinking density, porosity, the possible existence of a quasiorganized water "structure," and on the thermodynamic interaction parameters between the components of the biological environment and the gel. The possible existence of a quasiorganized water "structure" in certain hydrogels was subsequently also proposed by others; [46] however, solid experimental evidence is lacking to support this.

Small amounts of impurities can influence the blood compatibility of hydrogels. In the case of grafted polyacrylamide hydrogel, optimum blood compatibility was achieved only with highly purified monomers and small quantities of crosslinking agent and will be discussed below. It should be stressed that not all hydrogels perform well biologically and therefore, each of these materials must be treated individually. This is especially important since it is likely that blood components (especially proteins) interact differently with the various types of hydrogel surfaces.

Recent evidence suggests that there is practically no penetration by plasma proteins into the covalently grafted hydrogels based on polyacrylamide. Smaller molecules, ions, and oxygen and carbon dioxide can penetrate into the network. These properties of covalently grafted hydrogels permit their use in oxygenators where high gas-transfer rates and good blood compatibility are essential. Also under development are hydrogels of poly(vinyl acetate-*co*-2% crotonic acid) 60% sodium ionomer grafted onto polymeric surfaces by high energy irradiation from a ^{60}Co source.[47] These hydrogels are anionic, and their biological performance will be discussed in a later section of this paper.

In addition to the covalent grafting of hydrogels, glow discharge techniques can also be used to treat polymer surfaces with or without the deposition of polymer coatings.[48] The technique permits the preparation of very low as well as very high surface-energy polymeric surfaces. Some of these exhibit interesting biological performance in preliminary tests and will be presented below.

Still another approach to the surface modification of polymers involves the ionic bonding of heparin.[49, 50] Ionically bonded heparin surfaces have been used successfully clinically, especially in short-term applications. Although heparin has been covalently bonded to hydrogels and other polymers, the biological activity of these is diminished in comparison to ionically bonded heparin surfaces.

Investigations are also being conducted to deposit carbons onto appropriate polymeric and nonpolymeric substrates by vacuum-vapor and ion-plating techniques,[51] and by ion-beam processes.[52] Both the vacuum-vapor and the ion-plating techniques yield carbon surfaces on polymeric substrates which are nearly impermeable to gases at a thickness of 0.1 μm. The coatings adhere well to a number of polymers, including poly*i*mides, cellulose acetate, and segmented polyether-urethanes. The biological properties of these composite carbon structures are under investigation.

Biological Performance of Selected Biomaterials

The biological performance of candidate biomaterials cannot be assessed reliably from a single experimental procedure. Materials that seemingly perform well in one type of test may fail in others. Therefore, the proper assessment of the biological performance of biomaterials must rely on the analysis of data based on a variety of test procedures. Although simplified toxicological screening tests are valuable, these cannot be equated to blood compatibility.

Heparinized Polymers. TDMAC/heparin complex † was tested on various substrate polymers. In the vena cava test,[53] very good results were obtained

† Tridodecylmethylammonium chloride (Battelle Memorial Institute).

with both 2.0% and 3.6% TDMAC/heparin complex, with somewhat better performance shown by the former (TABLE 5). All in all, only two of 37 specimens were thrombosed completely in two hours. Without heparin, all of the substrate polymers thrombosed. However, the same TDMAC/heparin complexed polymers performed poorly in the renal embolus test system [54] (TABLE 5). Of the seven rings implanted, all showed various levels of thrombotic deposits on the rings. These were generally distributed throughout the ring lumen rather than toward the rim, as is often the case. Although the aorta below the ring remained usually clean, there was severe infarction affecting both kidneys. There was no particular difference between the performance of the 2.0% and the 3.6% TDMAC/heparin complex.

These results underline the difference between the vena cava and the renal embolus tests. Even more importantly, the data show that just because there

TABLE 5

In Vivo BIOLOGICAL PROPERTIES OF HEPARINIZED POLYMERS

	TDMAC/Heparin *		
	2%	3.6%	APTES/HEPARIN †
Vena Cava			
2 Hours	flow normal, not sacrificed	flow normal, not sacrificed	flow normal in most, not sacrificed
2 Weeks ‡	excellent	moderate	excellent
Renal embolus			
Ring thrombus	thin coating or thick deposit	thin coating or thick deposit	thin coating
Aorta below ring	mostly clean	clean	mostly clean
Renal infarcts	numerous, large	numerous, large	numerous, small and large

* TDMAC=tridodecylmethylammonium chloride (Battelle).
† APTES=γ-aminopropyltriethoxysilane (Carnegie-Mellon).
‡ Code for 2-week vena cava test: excellent=75–100% of rings essentially clot-free; good=50–75% of rings essentially clot-free; moderate=25–50% of rings essentially clot-free; poor=less than 25% of rings clean.

may be no evidence of thrombotic deposit on the rings, a material may not necessarily be blood compatible. Often, the thrombotic deposit is merely washed downward with no evidence of thrombus on the rings themselves, but causing severe infarction at distant sites, with serious organ damage. The implications of this phenomenon to device performance cannot be underrated.

Rotating disk experiments [55] carried out *in vitro* with TDMAC/heparin complex on polyvinyl chloride substrate showed an initial delay in platelet adhesion up to approximately six minutes, followed by a rapid increase in platelet adhesion. The TDMAC/heparin complex on silicone rubber substrate showed a similar trend, but platelet adhesion started after approximately two minutes. Photomicrographs show blotchy patterns of platelet uptake, in contrast to certain other materials studied. This may be due to the uneven distribution of the TDMAC/heparin complex on the polymer surface.

TABLE 6

In Vivo BIOLOGICAL PROPERTIES OF ETHYL CELLULOSE PERFLUOROBUTYRATE

	Results
Vena Cava	
2 Hours	flow normal, not sacrificed
2 Weeks *	excellent
Renal Embolus	
Ring thrombus	none or thin coating
Aorta below ring	clean
Renal infarcts	few to moderate

* Code for 2-week vena cava test: excellent=75–100% of rings essentially clean; good=50–75% of rings essentialy clean; moderate=25–50% of rings essentially clean; poor=less than 25% of rings clean.

The APTES-heparinized ‡ polymers showed also good performance in the vena cava test (TABLE 5). Of the 15 rings evaluated, 13 exhibited normal flow behavior after two hours (without sacrificing the animals), and only two rings were occluded. In the two-week vena cava test, nine rings were essentially clot-free, three were partially occluded, and one was totally occluded. In the renal embolus test (TABLE 5), of the three rings tested, the extent of renal infarction was about the same as in the case of the TDMAC/heparinized polymers.

Fluoroesters of Ethyl Cellulose. Ethyl cellulose perfluorobutyrate coated onto "Delrin" vena cava rings was evaluated in dogs. None of the eight rings tested thrombosed after two hours, six showed no thrombus deposit after two weeks, and two exhibited only moderate occlusion, with blood flow remaining essentially unimpaired (TABLE 6).

In the renal embolus test system (TABLE 6), all six rings tested exhibited a noteworthy absence of mural thrombotic deposit on the rings, and two of the rings were entirely free of any thrombotic deposit. The extent of renal infarction was slight in the case of four rings, but more extensive with the two other rings that were prepared at a later date. These results compare favorably with the performance with LTI carbons that are among the best available biomaterials. It should be mentioned, however, that two other homologs, ethyl cellulose perfluoropropionate and ethyl cellulose perfluorooctanoate, showed much more extensive renal embolism than the ethyl cellulose perfluorobutyrate. Preliminary *in vitro* shear-induced hemolysis experiments with human blood showed a low level of hemolysis for the polymer in comparison with control specimens.[57]

Hydrogels. Major efforts involved the biological evaluation of three types of hydrogels: neutral polyacrylamide, polyvinyl acetate-*co*-2% crotonic acid) 60% sodium ionomer polyelectrolyte hydrogel, and "Ioplex 101" polyelectrolyte. Prior to the development of grafted hydrogels, biological evaluation was conducted on neutral polyacrylamide and "Ioplex 101" polyelectrolyte hydrogels involving not only the vena cava and renal embolus tests but also a number

‡ γ-Aminopropyltriethoxysilane (Carnegie-Mellon University).

of *in vitro* test procedures that since have been superseded by others. A summary of these earlier biological test results is shown in TABLE 7. It should be noted that the original vena cava test procedure developed by Gott *et al.*[56] involved the sacrifice of the dogs after two hours and after two weeks, respectively, regardless of whether or not the test rings were occluded. This enabled the physical examination of the rings after each period of testing, as shown in TABLE 7. Recent developments by Daniels and Mortensen[53] include the monitoring of the blood flow with the dogs allowed to live until 14 days, unless the experiment must be terminated earlier because of thrombotic occlusions. The reliance on blood flow measurements as an indication of clot-formation on the rings after shorter periods does not permit physical visualization but eliminates the sacrifice of the animals. It should be kept in mind, however, that blood flow measurements without autopsy data lead only to approximations without providing detailed information about the presence or absence of small clots on the rings. The data in TABLE 7 indicate that the neutral polyacrylamide hydrogel shows a somewhat better performance than the 0.5 meq anionic "Ioplex 101" polyelectrolyte hydrogel. This suggests that anionic groups on certain hydrogels may not be essential for blood compatibility.

The best biological results to date were obtained with chemically grafted

TABLE 7

BIOLOGICAL PROPERTIES OF SOME HYDROGELS

	Polyacrylamide * (neutral)	"Ioplex" 101 † (0.5 meq. excess anionic)
In Vivo		
Vena Cava		
2 Hours	excellent	excellent ‡
2 Weeks	very good	very good ‡
Renal Embolus	—	—
In Vitro		
Effect on Plasma Proteins (17) §	none	none (except fibrinogen)
Effect on Plasma Enzymes (8) §	none	some (alkaline phosphatase)
Calcium Replacement Clotting Times §	not prolonged	not prolonged
Adherence of ¶		
Erythrocytes (WB)	~70,000/cm^2	~510,000/cm^2
Leucocytes (WB)	0	0
Platelets (PRP)	~256,000/cm^2	~320,000/cm^2
Platelet Aggregation and activation	none	—
Cell Growth (amnion)	slightly less than control	—
Zeta Potential (Krebs)	—	negative
Critical Surface Tension	—	—

* Polysciences, Inc.

‡ Amicon, Inc.

‡ Sterilized by EtO; shipped in glycerin and equilibrated in isotonic saline for 2 hours.

§ 20% acrylamide.

¶ 15% acrylamide.

TABLE 8

PLATELET ADHESION FROM HEPARINIZED WHOLE CANINE BLOOD TO POLYACRYLAMIDE HYDROGEL COVALENTLY GRAFTED ONTO POLYURETHANE IN ROTATING DISC EXPERIMENTS AT 400 RPM AFTER 3 MINUTES *

	Platelet Density/900μ^2 (approximate)
Nongrafted polyurethane †	28
Chemically grafted polyacrylamide with no crosslinker	negligible

* Data from Leonard *et al.*[55]
† Block polyether-urethane, type 3-1000/425(70–30)–1–X (SRI).

polyacrylamide hydrogels.[43] As seen in TABLES 8 and 9, recent results indicate that polyacrylamide, chemically grafted onto specially prepared polyether-urethanes, elicits no platelet adhesion in rotating-disk experiments and absorbs the least plasma proteins, especially fibrinogen, gamma globulin, and albumin.[55] Shear-induced hemolysis under low shear stresses was least in the case of chemically grafted polyacrylamide hydrogels in comparison to unmodified segmented polyether-urethane, polyethylene, silicone rubber, and polyvinyl chloride.[57]

Similar shear-induced hemolysis experiments conducted with the grafted poly(vinyl acetate-*co*-2% crotonic acid) 60% sodium ionomer onto polypropylene substrate showed that this ionic hydrogel is inferior to the grafted neutral polyacrylamide hydrogel.[57] Renal embolus tests carried out with grafted poly(vinyl acetate-*co*-2% crotonic acid) 60% sodium ionomer hydrogel were not impressive (TABLE 10). Eleven rings implanted showed only moderate

TABLE 9

UPTAKE OF SINGLE ^{125}I-LABELED PROTEINS BY HYDROGELS COVALENTLY GRAFTED ONTO POLYURETHANES IN STATIC EXPERIMENTS *

	Proteins, μg/cm^2		
	Albumin	Fibrinogen	γ-Globulin
Nongrafted Polyurethane †	0.58	0.92	0.93
Polyurethane Chemically Grafted with Polyacrylamide with Crosslinker ‡	0.19	0.18	0.29
Polyurethane § Chemically Grafted with Polyacrylamide without Crosslinker	0.97	0.11	0.09
Polyurethane Microwave-Discharge Grafted with HEMA with Crosslinker ¶	0.38	0.33	0.58

* Data from Leonard *et al.*[55]
† Block polyether-urethane, type 3–1000/425(70/30)–1–X (SRI).
‡ 2% N, N′-methylene-bis-acrylamide.
§ Block polyether-urethane, type 3–2000–1–E (SRI).
¶ 2% ethylene glycol dimethacrylate crosslinker.

thromboresistance, with a thin thrombotic deposit forming on approximately 50% or more of the ring lumen and the renal infarction was rather extensive, with both kidneys affected. These results seem to be general for all samples, even though the preparative radiation dose varied between 0.1 and 0.17 Mrad. Vena cava tests with 43 rings showed that 11 were either totally clot-free or showed some clot formation at the ring edges after two weeks, 17 were partially occluded after two weeks, four were occluded after two weeks, and the remaining 11 rings were essentially occluded after two hours (TABLE 10). Optimum results were shown by those rings that were grafted at a dose rate of 0.1 Mrad.

Glow-Discharge Polymers. Glow-discharge deposition of polymers onto various substrates can be achieved by the introduction of vapors of organic monomers into ionized gases (plasma), such as argon or helium.[48] Alternately, the organic vapor may be ionized to form a plasma that requires no extraneous

TABLE 10

In Vivo BIOLOGICAL PROPERTIES OF POLY(VINYL ACETATE-CO-2%-CROTONIC ACID) 60% SODIUM IONOMER GRAFTED ONTO POLYPROPYLENE BY ^{60}Co IRRADIATION

	Dose, Mrad		
	0.7	0.1	0.17
Vena Cava			
2 hours	majority occluded	flow normal, not sacrificed	flow normal in most, not sacrificed
2 weeks *	moderate	moderate	poor
Renal Embolus			
Ring Thrombus	not tested	thin coating	thin coating
Aorta Below Ring	not tested	clean	clean
Renal Infarcts	not tested	substantial	substantial

* Code for 2-week vena cava test: excellent=75–100% of rings essentially clean; good=50–75% of rings essentially clean; moderate=25–50% of rings essentially clean; poor=less than 25% of rings clean.

addition of ionized gases. Among the various systems investigated were the glow-discharge polymers of hexa- and tetramethyldisiloxane and polymers of acetylene/N_2/H_2O.

The vena cava tests (TABLE 11) of glow-discharge polymer of hexamethyldisiloxane deposited onto Pyrex® glass showed that of the seven rings, three remainder clot-free after two weeks, one was partially occluded after two weeks with blood flow normal, one was essentially occluded after two weeks, and the remaining two rings were essentially occluded between two hours and two weeks. The 11 rings of glow-discharge polymer of tetramethyldisiloxane (TABLE 11) deposited onto polypropylene showed that four were entirely clot-free after two weeks, four were partially occluded after two weeks with blood flow essentially normal, and three were essentially occluded. In the case of the eight rings of the glow-discharge polymer of acetylene/N_2/H_2O system, three remained clot-free after two weeks and the rest clotted after two hours. The above data indicate that the glow-discharge polymer of tetramethyldisiloxane performed best in the vena cava rings. It should be mentioned also that the glow-discharge polymer of tetrafluoroethylene deposited onto Pyrex glass rings performed poorly, with seven out of eight rings essentially occluded (not shown in TABLE 11). This is in line with the known thrombogenic property of polytetrafluoroethylene.

In the renal embolus test (TABLE 11), of the six rings of glow-discharge polymer of tetramethyldisiloxane deposited onto Delrin-rings coated with a segmented polyether-urethane (3–1000/425 (70/30)–1–X, SRI), almost all were either free of thrombus or showed only minimal thrombus after three days. The kidneys showed only slight to moderate infarcts (4 rings) with two rings causing severe damage. In contrast, the six rings of glow-discharge polymer of acetylene/N_2/H_2O showed more extensive thrombus formation and substantial renal infarctions.

TABLE 11

In Vivo BIOLOGICAL PROPERTIES OF POLYSILOXANE GLOW-DISCHARGE POLYMERS

	HMDSiO *	TMDSiO †
Vena Cava		
2 Hours	flow normal in most, not sacrificed	flow normal in most, not sacrificed
2 Weeks ‡	good	good to moderate
Renal Embolus		
Ring Thrombus	thin coating	thin coating
Aorta Below Ring	mostly clean	mostly clean
Renal Infarcts	moderate to numerous	moderate

* Hexamethyldisiloxane.

† Tetramethyldisiloxane.

‡ Code for 2-week vena cava test: excellent=75–100% of rings essentially clean; good=50–75% of rings essentially clean; moderate=25–50% of rings essentially clean; poor=less than 25% of rings clean.

Preliminary shear-induced hemolysis experiments with human blood conducted with the glow-discharge polymers of hexamethyldisiloxane and tetramethyldisiloxane indicate somewhat better performance with the latter material, although the results may reflect surface effect.[57] Further work is in progress to clarify the situation.

Microfiber-Tissue Culture Approach

Although woven fabrics, velours, and flocked surfaces have been used in clinical practice (especially in large blood-vessel replacements), the blood compatibility of these materials depends on the formation of a fibrin layer and subsequent vascularization. In prosthetic devices that undergo repeated flexing and stretching, such an approach is not entirely satisfactory.

In the case of porous woven or knitted materials, Sauvage *et al.*[58] showed that the extent of pannus ingrowth (tissue extending across the anastomosis into the area of blood flow) is extremely slow in man compared to various animals. Additionally, man has the slowest ability to grow tissue through the pores of woven or knitted materials by the process called transinterstices ingrowth. When these highly thrombogenic surfaces first come in contact with blood, a thrombus-fabric complex forms on the inside, and the pores of the fabric become clogged by thrombus. In contrast to many animals, especially calves and baboons, the healing process in man is extremely slow and incomplete, even over a period of many years.

Another approach involves the use of impervious (nonporous) materials, the inside blood-contacting surfaces of which consist of millions of tiny polyester fibrils, constituting what is termed a "flocked" surface.[59] Since the material is nonporous, no transinterstices ingrowth is possible. However, when blood first contacts the highly thrombogenic fibril surface, a compacted layer of fibrin-red cell mesh is deposited onto it. This compacted fibrin-red cell layer works fairly well in high blood-flow velocity regions, but it is not suitable even for short periods of time in slow blood-flow areas because of the so-called thrombotic threshold velocity. There are, however, other potential problems associated with nonintegral flocked surfaces. For example, the tiny fibrils may separate from the surface and the fibrin clot may break up, especially during repeated flexing, leading to embolization and thrombosis at distant sites. Furthermore, the significant hematological differences between the calf (favorite test animal with some medical devices) and man, as observed by Marzec and coworkers,[60] suggest the need to evaluate the performance of biomaterials also with blood obtained from primates and humans.

An important alternate approach is the use of microfibers as scaffold structures for the anchoring of viable cells and for the production of a vascular intima.[61, 62] Such cellular linings must be capable of surviving the shearing forces of blood and the systolic and diastolic pressure differentials. To date, the best results were obtained by Kahn *et al.*[62] with diploid WI-38 cells from embryonic human lung tissue and epidermal cells which were uniformly seeded onto nonwoven microfibers, including those made from specially prepared poly-(tetramethylene terephthalate) and microwave-discharge tested parylene-C-coated polypropylene. The microwave-discharge treatment converts the hydrophobic parylene-C to a hydrophilic surface that is essential for proper cellular adhesion and growth. In order to use the microfiber-scaffold cellular linings for prosthetic applications *in vivo,* autologously derived cells must be seeded onto appropriate surfaces. Work is currently under way to accomplish this objective.[62]

Anisotropic Systems

The components of the cardiovascular system, including arteries, veins, and heart valves, are composite materials, the stress-strain properties of which vary in the transverse and longitudinal directions. This stiffness *anisotropy* is important in the performance of physiological functions, since it prevents buckling of the blood vessels and provides for the accommodation of the vessels to systolic and diastolic blood pressure changes. This anisotropy also plays an important role in the operation of natural heart valves.

To imitate some of the mechanical properties of the components of the cardiovascular system, investigations are under way with specially prepared, pure, noncommercial, segmented polyether-urethanes.[63] It should be stressed that the aim is to provide the required mechanical properties, rather than blood compatibility. Although polyether-urethanes have shown fairly good blood compatibility, especially in short range applications, their overall biological performance for longer use can be enhanced further by various surface modifications. To impart anisotropy, segmented polyether-urethanes are cast in films (plies) with the careful removal of the residual solvent. The individual plies are then stretch-oriented to produce the desired stiffness anisotropy. After quenching, the stretched plies are stacked at 0°, 90°, 90°, and 0° and compression-molded at a moderate temperature to form composite laminates. Exposure of the plies to whole blood for several months showed no significant change in the anisotropy and only slight relaxation occurred. Cyclic biaxial straining experiments indicated some irreversible creep for the earlier segmented polyether-urethane, but this has been greatly reduced by the careful purification of the polymer prior to fabrication. Furthermore, an improved family of segmented polyether-urethane was developed that shows practically no creep.

Summary

It is proposed that *intrinsic* electroconduction and semiconduction may be involved in the compatibility of some materials with blood and its components, as evidenced by the biological behavior of intrinsically electroconducting conversion products of an aromatic polypyromellitimide. This molecular property may relate not only to blood compatibility but also to arteriosclerosis and other diseases. Although some conducting carbon black-containing polymers exhibit improved biological properties, these are *extrinsic* and not intrinsic conductors. Pure, noncommercial, segmented polyether-urethanes enabled the fabrication of anisotropic laminates with mechanical stiffness ratios similar to tissues with applications in leaflet heart valves and arterial prostheses. Excellent blood compatibility is exhibited by a chemically modified collagen, chemically grafted polyacrylamide hydrogels, ethylcellulose perfluorobutyrate, and glow-discharge polymers of pure, silica-free tetramethyldisiloxane. Tissue culture techniques with nonwoven microfibers should enable the creation of a living blood compatible surface for long-term applications.

Ackowledgment

The author thanks his wife, Mrs. A. Katherine Bruck, for typing the manuscript.

References

1. Vroman, L. & A. L. Adams. 1969. J. Biomed. Mater. Res. **3:** 43.
2. Vroman, L., A. L. Adams & M. Klings. 1971. Fed. Proc. Fed. Am. Soc. Exp. Biol. **30:** 1494.
3. Nemerson, Y. & F. A. Pitlick. 1972. *In* Progress in Hemostasis and Thrombosis. E. H. Spaet, Ed. Vol. **1:** 1. Grune and Stratton. New York, N.Y.
4. Ashford, R. P. & D. G. Freeman. 1968. Amer. J. Pathol. **53:** 599–603.
5. Pitlick, F. A. Activation of Coagulation by the Cell Surface Coat (Glyco-

calyx). Ann. Rep. July 1975. Contract NIH–NO1–HB–4–2968, PB 244279. (Public document available from the National Technical Information Service, 5285 Port Royal Road, Springfield, Va. 22161.)
6. MUGGLI, R. & H. R. BAUMGARTNER. 1973. Thrombosis Res. **3:** 715.
7. SILBERBERG, A. & I. R. MILLER. Interactions of Natural and Chemically Modified Biopolymers with Blood. Ann. Rep. Dec. 1975. Contract NIH–NO1–HB–5–2907. (Public document available. See Ref. 5.)
8. GORDON, J. L. & J. T. DINGLE. 1974. J. Cell Sci. **16:** 157.
9. MICHAELI, D. Studies on the Molecular Basis of Collagen-Platelet Interaction and Synthesis of Peptides That Will Inhibit This Interaction. Ann. Rep. July 1975. Contract NIH–NO1–HB–4–2984, PB 244843. (Public document available. See Ref. 5.)
10. KATZMAN, R. L., A. H. KANG & E. H. BEACHEY. 1973. Science **181:** 670.
11. RICH, A. & F. H. C. CRICK. 1961. J. Mol. Biol. **3:** 483.
12. RAMACHANDRAN, G. N. 1967. *In* Treatise on Collagen. G. N. Ramachandran, Ed. Vol. **1**, Ch. 3. Academic Press. New York, N.Y.
13. CHANG, E. P. & J. C. W. CHIEN. 1973. Biopolymers **12:** 1063.
14. MONSON, J. M. & P. BORNSTEIN. 1973. Proc. Nat. Acad. Sci. USA **70:** 3521.
15. SCHOFIELD, J. D., J. UITTO & D. J. PROCKOP. 1974. Biochemistry **13:** 1801.
16. UITTO, J. & D. J. PROCKOP. 1973. Biochem. Biophys. Res. Commun. **55:** 904.
17. JIMENEZ, S., M. HARSCH & J. ROSENBLOOM. 1973. Biochem. Biophys. Res. Commun. **52:** 106.
18. SZENT-GYÖRGYI, A. 1946. Nature **157:** 875.
19. CARDEW, M. H. & D. D. ELEY. 1959. Faraday Soc. Discussions **27:** 115.
20. ROSENBERG, B. 1962. J. Chem. Phys. **36:** 816.
21. ELEY, D. D. & D. I. SPIVEY. 1960. Trans. Faraday Soc. **56:** 1432.
22. EVANS, M. G. & J. GERGELY. 1949. Biochim. Biophys. Acta **3:** 188.
23. TOPCHIEV, A. V. 1963. J. Polym. Sci. **A1:** 591.
24. MARVEL, C. S. & J. H. RASSWEILER. 1958. J. Amer. Chem. Soc. **80:** 1197.
25. BRUCK, S. D. 1965. Polymer **6:** 319.
26. ELEY, D. D. & R. B. LESLIE. 1964. *In* Electronic Aspects of Biochemistry. B. Pullman, Ed. Academic Press. New York, N.Y.
27. DEHL, R. E. 1970. Science **170:** 738.
28. DEHL, R. E. 1973. Biopolymers **12:** 2329.
29. FUNG, B. B. & M. M. SIEGL. 1972. Biochim. Biophys. Acta **278:** 185.
30. BARDELMEYER, G. H. 1973. Biopolymers **12:** 2289.
31. BRUCK, S. D. 1973. Nature **243:** 416.
32. BRUCK, S. D. 1975. Polymer **16:** 25.
33. BRUCK, S. D. 1965. Polymer **6:** 319.
34. BRUCK, S. D. 1967. J. Polym. Sci. (C) **17:** 169.
35. KOLOBOW, T., T. TOMLINSON, J. PIERCE & L. GATTINONI. 1975. (Abstr.) Vol. 4, 21st Ann. Mtg. Amer. Soc. Artif. Int. Organs. April 17–19. San Francisco, Calif.
36. SHARP, W. V., C. TAYLOR & J. W. WRIGHT. 1970. Trans. Amer. Soc. Artif. Int. Organs **16:** 435.
37. MCGINNESS, J., P. CORRY & P. PROCTOR. 1974. Science **183:** 853.
38. YANNAS, I. V. Crosslinked Collagen—Glycosaminoglycan Composite Materials: Biological and Mechanical Properties. Ann. Rep. July 1975. Contract NIH–NO1–HB–4–2969, PB 243772. (Public document available. See Ref. 5.)
39. PETERSEN, R. J. & L. T. ROZELLE. 1975. Trans. Amer. Soc. Artif. Int. Organs **21:** 242.
40. KETTERINGHAM, J., W. ZAPOL, J. BIRKETT, L. NELSEN, A. MASSUCCO & C. RAITH. 1975. Trans. Amer. Soc. Artif. Int. Organs **21:** 224.
41. WICHTERLE, O. & D. LÍM. 1960. Nature **185:** 117.
42. SCOTT, H., P. L. KRONICK & E. E. HILLMAN. Active-Vapor Grafting of Hydrogels in Medical Prostheses. Ann. Rep. August 1971. Contract NIH–NO1–

HB–1–2017, PB 206499; also Ann. Rep. February 1973. PB 221846; and Ann. Rep. Jan. 1974. PB 230308. (Public documents available. See Ref. 5.)

43. HALPERN, B. D., M. K. AKKAPEDDI & S. L. LEDIS. Polymer Studies Related to Prosthetic Cardiac Materials Which Are Non-Clotting at a Blood Interface. Ann. Rep. Jan. 1971. Contract NIH–NO1–HB–6–1124, PB 200987; see also Ann. Rep. Feb. 1974, PB 230310. (Public documents available. See Ref. 5.)
44. HOFFMAN, A. S., G. SCHMER, C. HARRIS & W. G. KRAFT. 1972. Trans. Amer. Soc. Artif. Int. Organs **18:** 10.
45. BRUCK, S. D. 1974. Blood Compatible Synthetic Polymers—An Introduction. Charles C Thomas. Springfield, Ill.
46. ANDRADE, J. D., H. B. LEE, M. S. JHON, S. W. KIM & J. B. HIBBS, JR. 1973. Trans. Amer. Soc. Artif. Int. Organs **19:** 1.
47. KWIATKOWSKI, G. T. Blood Compatible Polyelectrolytes. Ann. Rep. Nov. 1974. Contract NIH–NO1–HB–3–2950, PB 238814. (Public document available. See Ref. 5.)
48. YASUDA, H. A Study of Electrodeless Glow Discharge as a Means of Modifying the Surface of Polymers. Ann. Rep. Jan. 1975. Contract NIH–NO1–HB–3–2918, PB 042041. (Public document available. See Ref. 5.)
49. LEININGER, R. I. Development of Blood Compatible Materials: Heparinized Surfaces and Platelet Protective Agents. Ann. Rep. Dec. 1974. Contract NIH–NO1–HB–3–2918, PB 238763. (Public document available. See Ref. 5.)
50. MERKER, R. L., L. J. ELYASH, S. H. MAYHEW & J. Y. C. WANG. 1969. The heparinization of silicone rubber using aminoorganosilane coupling agent. *In* Proceedings of the Artificial Heart Program Conference. R. J. Hegyeli, Ed. National Institutes of Health. June 9–13. U.S. Government Printing Office. Washington, D.C.
51. MEYER, C. H., JR. Development of Carbon Fiber Composites for Use in Prosthetic Devices. Ann. Rep. Dec. 1974. Contract NIH–NO1–HB–3–2954, PB 238753. (Public document available. See Ref. 5.)
52. AISENBERG, S. Ion Beam Deposited Carbon Coatings for Biocompatible Materials. Ann. Rep. Nov. 1974. Contract NIH–NO1–HB–3–2919, PB 238761. (Public document available. See Ref. 5.)
53. DANIELS, A. U. & J. D. MORTENSEN. Vena Cava Ring Tests of Biomaterials in Dogs. Ann. Rep. Nov. 1975. Contract NIH–NO1–HB–4–2979, PB 248222. (Public document available. See Ref. 5.)
54. KUSSEROW, B. T. Analysis and Measurement of the Effects of Materials on Blood Leucocytes, Erythrocytes and Platelets. Ann. Rep. Jan. 1976. Contract NIH–NO1–HB–5–2939. See also Annual Reports, March 1975, PB 244250, and Jan. 1974, PB 233685. (Public document available. See Ref. 5.)
55. LEONARD, E. F., S. KOCHWA, R. S. LITWAK & R. E. ROSENFELD. Coordinated Studies of Platelet and Protein Reactions on Artificial Materials. Ann. Rep. Jan. 1975. Contract NIH–NO1–HB–3–2910, PB 241333. (Public document available. See Ref. 5.)
56. GOTT, V. L., M. D. RAMOS, F. B. NAJJAR, J. L. ALLEN & K. E. BECKER. 1969. The in vivo screening of potential thromboresistant materials. *In* Proc. Artif. Heart Program Conf. R. J. Hegyeli, Ed. National Institutes of Health. June 9–13. U.S. Government Printing Office. Washington, D.C.
57. WILLIAMS, M. C. Shear-Induced Hemolysis: Materials and Blood Composition. Ann. Rep. Dec. 1975. Contract NIH–NO1–HB–3–2952. (Public document available. See Ref. 5.)
58. SAUVAGE, L. R., K. E. BERGER, S. J. WOOD, S. G. YATES, II., J. C. SMITH & P. B. MANSFIELD. 1974. Arch. Surg. **109:** 698.
59. KEISER, J. T. Development and Testing of Flocking Materials. Ann. Rep. April 1974. Contract NIH–NO1–HV–3–2915, PB 233915. (Public document available. See Ref. 5.)

60. Marzec, U., G. G. Johnston & E. F. Bernstein. 1975. Trans. Amer. Soc. Artif. Int. Organs **21:** 581.
61. Mansfield, P. B., A. R. Wechezak & L. R. Sauvage. 1975. Trans. Amer. Soc. Artif. Int. Organs **21:** 264.
62. Kahn, R. H., W. E. Burkel & J. C. Stanley. Development and Testing of Pseudointimal-Lined Vascular Devices. Ann. Rep. Jan. 1976. Contract NIH–NO1–HB–1–2054. (Public document available. See Ref. 5.)
63. Kardos, J. L., C. Thies, R. E. Clark & S. F. Apostolou. Development and Mechanical Characterization of Anisotropic Polymeric Biomaterials. Ann. Rep. Jan. 1975. Contract NIH–NO1–HB–3–2909, PB 240765. (Public document available. See Ref. 5.)

HYDROPHOBIC POLYMER SURFACES AND THEIR INTERACTIONS WITH BLOOD *

J. L. Brash

Departments of Chemical Engineering and Pathology
McMaster University
Hamilton, Ontario, Canada L8S 4L7

Introduction

For the purposes of this review the designation "hydrophobic" is taken to mean solid surfaces on which water and aqueous fluids will not spontaneously spread but will form separated drops having a nonzero contact angle. In a word, they are "nonwettable." This definition serves to set such surfaces apart from their antithetic category the hydrophilic surfaces, the latter being distinguished by the fact that water will spread on and be absorbed into the bulk of the material. Such materials are the subject of other presentations and will not be discussed further, except for comparative purposes, in this paper. Hydrophobic surfaces are to be taken also as essentially smooth, or at least as having a topography that is not of any specific form. This stipulation again separates them from another major category of materials that have been used in blood-contact situations. These latter are surfaces that have been purposely designed with a roughened topography to promote development of a thin fibrin layer or other pseudoendothelium when placed in flowing blood. The material of such surfaces is frequently hydrophobic in nature, e.g. Dacron® and Teflon®,[1] and although they may have microscopic behavior identical to that to be discussed in this paper, they again behave grossly in a different fashion and are dealt with in detail elsewhere in this volume. The purpose of this paper is to review the current status of hydrophobic surfaces as blood-interfacing materials and to discuss the nature of their interactions with various key components of blood.

Early recognition of the potential benefit of hydrophobicity in minimizing blood response was provided by the observation of Lister in 1863[2] that blood coagulation was slower in a rubber container than in glass. Similarly, it was reported by Bordet and Gengou[3] that paraffin-coated surfaces retarded plasma coagulation relative to glass. In more recent times, hydrophobicity has been exploited in the practice of siliconizing glassware in the coagulation laboratory. These observations serve to emphasize that it was blood coagulation that was seen by early workers as the effect to be avoided, and hydrophobic surfaces seem principally to have been proposed in this context. When the search for a blood-compatible surface was intensified in the early 1960s it was widely believed that if coagulation could be avoided, nonthrombogenic surfaces would be achieved.

Such thinking may account in part for the use of nonwettable or hydrophobic materials in blood-contact devices. For example, silicones are used in the construction of prosthetic heart valves and the arteriovenous shunts used by

* Supported by the Medical Research Council of Canada and the Ontario Heart Foundation.

hemodialysis patients, Teflon is used as a tip material for the shunts; polyethylene is a material frequently chosen for tubing to carry blood and for intravascular catheters; polyurethanes are used for the construction of intraaortic balloons following favorable reports of their blood compatibility.[4–6]

Of more importance than their blood compatibility are perhaps their physical and formability properties. Hydrophobic polymers exhibit a very broad range of mechanical behavior, from rigid to flexible with good strength and flex-fatigue properties, in many instances. TABLE 1 shows some relevant data for a number of typical hydrophobic polymers, most of which have been proposed or used for blood-contact applications. As can be seen, these materials range from high-strength, brittle types like polystyrene, to low-strength, compliant materials like silicones. It should be noted with respect to polyvinyl chloride that, while this is generally thought of as a compliant material, it is

TABLE 1

PHYSICAL PROPERTIES OF SOME UNMODIFIED HYDROPHOBIC POLYMERS

	Tensile Strength (dyne cm^{-2}) $\times 10^{-8}$	Elongation at Break %	Tensile Modulus (dyne cm^{-2}) $\times 10^{-9}$
Polyethylene (High Density)*	2.1–3.8	20–1300	4.1–12.4
Polypropylene *	3.0–3.8	200–700	11.0–15.1
Polystyrene	3.4–8.3	1.0–2.5	27.6–34
Polyvinylchloride	5.5	30	25
Polytetrafluoroethylene *	1.4–3.4	200–400	4.0
Polymethylmethacrylate	7.0	3	40
Polycarbonate (bisphenol A)	5.3	80	23.5
Nylon 66® *	8.3	60–300	1.5
Polyether-urethane †	4.1	700	6.9
Polydimethylsiloxane ‡	0.7	350	—

* Data from Modern Plastics Encyclopedia. 1975. Vol. 52. McGraw Hill. New York, N.Y.
† Based on polyoxypropylene.[6]
‡ Silastic® 372 Medical Grade Silicone.[7]

somewhat rigid in the unmodified state and requires the addition of plasticizer to become flexible. In general the strength of these polymeric materials is about an order of magnitude less than that of metals, but of course, their flexibility is much greater. With respect to use in contact with blood, it is also very important that hydrophobic polymers do not absorb water to any appreciable extent (typically less than 0.1%) and thus retain their physical strength and compliance when immersed in aqueous media. Whether physical properties can be maintained over periods of months or years in various implant locations where conditions may be acid or alkaline is essentially unknown, although there is some data suggesting that silicones[7] and segmented polyether urethanes[5] are resistant to alteration in tissue-implant situations.

Hydrophobic polymers also have an important advantage in their ready formability. Complex shapes can be formed by molding techniques for thermoplastic materials and casting techniques for thermosets. Machining, milling, and solution methods can also be used where appropriate.

Surface Physical Properties: Surface Free Energy, Critical Surface Tension, and their Correlation with Blood Clotting

In terms of a blood-contact application one can think of hydrophobic surfaces as being essentially "inert"; since they are water-repellent, they should interact only minimally with any contacting aqueous medium. The concept of inertness finds a somewhat more precise expression in terms of surface free energy or interfacial tension. Hydrophobic solids are in general possessed of relatively low surface free energies and one can think of inertness as being a reflection of this fact. Surface free energy can be defined as the work required to increase a surface by unit area at constant temperature, pressure, and composition of the contacting phases. For liquids the surface tension can be defined similarly to the surface free energy, although conceptually it is thought of as the force existing in the surface per unit length of an imaginary line; it therefore has units in the c.g.s. system of dyne cm^{-1}, whereas surface free energy has units of erg cm^{-2}. These units are, of course, equivalent. As thermodynamic quantities, surface free energy and surface tension imply conditions of thermodynamic equilibrium and reversibility, and these are difficult conditions to satisfy for solids. The free energies and tensions of solid surfaces are thus difficult to determine and recourse to approximations or simplifications is generally made. Typical of this approach is the concept of critical surface tension (CST) developed by Fox and Zisman [8] for low-energy solids. CST may be defined simply as the value of liquid surface tension below which liquids will spread on a given solid. Zisman found that if a series of liquids such as the *n*-alkanes were used, the cosine of the contact angle decreased linearly as surface tension increased. Extrapolation to zero contact angle—i.e., the critical spreading condition—gave the value of CST. It can readily be appreciated that the CST gives an indication of a surface energy term and can be used as a relative ranking device in a series of solids where the concept is applicable. Typical values are shown in Table 2 for both low-energy surfaces, typified by hydrophobic polymers, and high-energy surfaces such as glass.

Among the earliest guiding principles in the search for surfaces that would delay clotting was the correlation proposed by Lampert [9] which claimed to show that the clotting time of blood was inversely proportional to the "wettability" of the surface. Wettability by water could crudely be taken as an indication of surface energy, but would also be influenced by other factors, e.g. hydrogen bonding. The validity of this correlation was repeatedly challenged, for example by Rose and Broida [10] and Ross *et al.*,[11] who found numerous examples that did not fit the correlation. In view of what is now known about protein adsorption to surfaces, it is, of course, not surprising that the correlation should fail. Nonetheless, the idea persisted that wettability, surface tension, or some other energy-related surface parameter would be important in ranking surfaces with respect to their blood coagulation response. Thus Lyman and coworkers [12] adapted the critical surface-tension concept for correlative purposes and found that for simple hydrophobic surfaces (whose intermolecular forces are predominantly of the London dispersion type and do not have hydrogen bonding or ionic bonding capabilities) the clotting time for human or dog blood decreased linearly with the logarithm of CST. A few exceptions were noted: Teflon, for example, had a relatively short clotting time and did not fit the correlation. This deviation was attributed to high-energy impurity sites on the Teflon surface. Such a correlation suggests that minimization of surface energy is a valid approach to nonclotting surfaces. It should, however, be noted that parameters based on contact angles are representative of a large area of surface and can be meaningful at the molecular level only if the surface is molecularly uniform over the area of measurement. If blood response is also at the molecular level, then correlations between parameters based on contact angle and blood interactions would be expected only if the surface is molecularly uniform.

In practice, the lowest value of CST exhibited is about 5 dyne cm^{-1} for a monolayer of perfluorolauric acid [13] with a surface composed effectively of $—CF_3$ groups and this has not been tested with respect to coagulation of blood. The lowest CST polymeric material tested is in fact Teflon, which, as indicated,

TABLE 2

CRITICAL SURFACE TENSION (CST) OF VARIOUS HYDROPHOBIC POLYMERS *

Polymer	CST (dynes cm^{-1})
Poly (hexafluoropropylene)	17.0
Poly (tetrafluoroethylene)	18.0
Siliconized Glass	24.0
Paraffin hydrocarbons	22–26
Polyethylene	31–33
Poly (trifluorochloroethylene)	31
Poly (methylmethacrylate)	39.0
Poly (vinylchloride)	39.0
Polystyrene	33–43.3
Nylon 66	42.0–46.0
Pyrex® Glass	170

* Data taken from Reference 12.

has a clotting time short enough to be of no particular practical interest. Extrapolation of the Lyman *et al.*[12] CST correlation would lead to the expectation that the clotting time is infinite at zero CST. Zero CST is, of course, a hypothetical abstraction implying that the interface vanishes. That real surfaces must indeed have finite positive CST or energy associated with them is obvious, so that ultimately this concept must break down.

Thus "inertness" or "low surface energy" provides whatever rationale exists for the use of hydrophobic polymers in blood-contact situations. Just how inert such materials are in contact with blood will be explored in some detail in the remaining sections of this paper.

BLOOD SURFACE INTERACTIONS

As has already been implied, an important reaction of blood with hydrophobic surfaces is coagulation. A gross measure of surface-induced coagulation is the time taken to form a clot. Numerous measurements of clotting time have been made, and some of these have already been mentioned.[9–12] The precise mechanism of initiation of coagulation is essentially unknown, but the early stages are very likely involved, particularly the activation of factors XII and XI. No studies have been performed on the activation of these factors by hydrophobic polymers. Perhaps the most relevant and detailed recent research in this area has been carried out by Cochrane *et al.*,[14] who studied the activation of factor XII by kaolin surfaces and found that no molecular weight change was associated with activation. They concluded from indirect evidence that the activation did involve a change in conformation of the molecule. Falb *et al.*[15] studied the adsorption of Hageman factor to several surfaces, including a polystyrene-like surface, a positively charged polypropylene surface, and a heparinized surface. They found that the smallest amount was adsorbed to the polystyrene and most to the positively charged surface. These studies were performed with labeled proteins that had been prepared by attaching di-isopropylfluorophosphate to the protein, and the effects of this on biological activity were not determined.

Difficulties in the purification of the clotting factors involved in the early stages make such studies very difficult to interpret. Therefore, more detailed work has been carried out with clotting factors like fibrinogen and thrombin, which are available in pure form and in useful quantities. This work will be reviewed under *Protein Interactions*.

Protein Interactions

The area of protein adsorption in general is covered in other papers. It is perhaps relevant, however, to discuss protein effects with respect to hydrophobic polymers in particular. Adsorption of protein is a pervasive phenomenon for any surface in contact with blood. However, little is known of the composition of the layers adsorbed, of the dependence of the composition on surface properties, of the biological status of the adsorbed proteins, or of the time-dependence of adsorption phenomena, e.g. the rates of adsorption from blood and the change in composition with time over relatively long periods.

Early work by Brash and Lyman [16] suggested that on hydrophobic polymers, molar surface concentration of the common plasma proteins would be identical and would not vary from surface to surface. It was also concluded that adsorbed proteins retain globular form, and would be adsorbed from mixtures, e.g. blood, in proportion to their solution concentration. More recent work in several laboratories has upheld some and required abandonment or modification of others of these conclusions.

With respect to the influence of surface composition on adsorption, TABLE 3 shows recent data obtained in our laboratory with radioiodinated albumin, a method that allows greater accuracy and precision in measuring small quantities of protein than does the infrared reflectance spectroscopy method used in the earlier work.[16] TABLE 3 also shows, for comparison, data on a number of surfaces that are not hydrophobic. Among the hydrophobic surfaces there are differences in the plateau surface concentration, with a hydrophobic segmented polyurethane showing higher surface concentration than polyethylene, polystyrene, or siliconed glass. The surfaces showing a value of about 0.2 μg cm^{-2} all possess effectively a hydrocarbon composition (aside from any impurities).

The polyurethane surface undoubtedly contains a high proportion of ether oxygen and urethane functionalities as well as hydrocarbon. Indeed, segmented polyurethanes have been shown to possess morphology of the domain type, in which the segment types (the polyether and polyurethane-urea) form segregated microdomains due to thermodynamic incompatibility.[17] The surface may thus consist of a mosaic of polyether-rich and polyurethane-rich regions, and this may be responsible for high albumin adsorption. The hydrophilic surfaces all show uniformly low surface concentrations, although it should be noted that since desorption on these surfaces also occurs, there is uncertainty associated with any method that involves rinsing prior to surface evaluation, since rinsing can remove adsorbed protein as well as adherent solution. Horbett and Hoffman,[18] also using a technique involving rinsing, found that grafting of hydrophilic hydroxyethylmethacrylate to polydimethylsiloxane decreased fibrinogen adsorption. Also, MacRitchie [19] using an *in situ* method, showed that adsorption of bovine serum albumin on hydrophilic silica is of the order of 0.02 μg cm^{-2} at pH 7.5, and that complete desorption occurs in this system.

TABLE 3

ADSORPTION OF ALBUMIN TO VARIOUS SURFACES

Surface	Steady State Surface Concentration (μg cm$^{-2}\pm$S.D.)*
Polyethylene	0.18±0.005
Polystyrene	0.18±0.04
Siliconed Glass	0.18±0.004
Glass	0.04±0.037
Segmented Polyurethane	0.60±0.17
Hydrophilic Polyurethane	0.02±0.009
Collagen-coated glass	0.09±0.007

* Solution concentration was 100 mg/100 ml in each case.

On a hydrophobic methylated silica, surface concentrations were much higher and there was evidence of coagulation at the surface. Virtually no desorption took place from hydrophobic surfaces. Brash *et al.*[20] have shown that on polyethylene, although the protein does not desorb, there is continuous turnover of protein between the surface and the solution. The rate of turnover is dependent on flow conditions and concentration and increases with shear rate and concentration. These results suggest that in flowing blood the rate of turnover could be considerable. In general it was found that a fraction of surface sites do not undergo exchange, and again this fraction decreases with increasing shear rate and concentration. It is not yet known if protein that has been adsorbed and returned to solution is biologically altered.

With respect to the alteration of adsorbed proteins from the native state, little information is available. Morrissey and Stromberg [21] reported "bound fraction" measurements for adsorption to colloidal silica. Bound fraction refers to the fraction of carbonyl groups in the protein molecule that have undergone a characteristic infrared spectral shift attributable to formation of hydrogen bonds with the silica. For albumin and prothrombin, the bound fraction was low (about 0.1) and did not change with the amount adsorbed, whereas with fibrinogen the bound fraction increased with the amount adsorbed. Recently Morrissey and Fenstermaker[22] found that γ-globulin bound fraction decreased with increasing surface concentration. These results are interpreted as showing a retention of conformation for albumin and prothrombin, a type of coagulation phenomenon for fibrinogen, and a loss of native conformation for γ-globulin at low surface coverage.

Studies by Vroman and coworkers have focused on "conversion" of adsorbed proteins as an indication of biological alteration in the adsorbed state. "Conversion," as used by Vroman and Adams,[23] means destruction of the antigenicity of the adsorbed protein (assumed to occur by interaction with plasma factors) which presumably can be taken as an indication of biological alteration. This effect is observed for fibrinogen adsorption on silicon and tantalum surfaces that are either in the natural state or modified in some way to become hydrophobic or hydrophilic. Fibrinogen adsorbed on hydrophilic silicon was "converted" to a greater extent than when adsorbed on hydrophobic silicon. Conversion of γ-globulin also occurred. This data is consistent with the maintenance of native form in proteins adsorbed at hydrophobic surfaces.

Bearing on the question of the composition of the layer adsorbed from blood, several studies have recently been reported (some on hydrophobic polymers) on the amounts adsorbed from mixtures of proteins. Thus Lee *et al.*[24] studied adsorption from mixtures of albumin, γ-globulin, and fibrinogen on hydrophobic polymers such as Teflon, silicone, and polyurethane. Changes in layer composition with time were studied, and fibrinogen was found to be preferentially adsorbed in relation to its solution concentration. Its predominance was especially noted in the early stages of adsorption prior to establishment of a steady-state layer composition. Horbett and Hoffman[18] studied competitive adsorption between albumin and fibrinogen and between γ-globulin and fibrinogen. They found that at mole ratios (γ-globulin or albumin to fibrinogen) less than about 1.0, the adsorbed layer contained almost 100% fibrinogen. No difference in this regard was observed between hydrophilic and hydrophobic surfaces.

Vroman *et al.*[25] studied the competition adsorption between albumin and fibrinogen on an oxidized silicon surface and also found enrichment of fibrinogen in the adsorbed layer. Similar results were found in the author's laboratory[26] for the albumin-fibrinogen competition on glass or polyethylene. The preference of glass for fibrinogen over albumin was even stronger than that of polyethylene. Thus on a wide variety of surfaces it appears that fibrinogen is a major component in the layer adsorbed from simple mixtures. There is evidence, as discussed below, that fibrinogen is also a major component of the adsorbate from blood on various surfaces, and this fact may strongly influence the development of thrombus, with respect to both its coagulation and platelet components.

Studies of adsorption from plasma or blood itself are comparatively rare. Vroman and Adams[27] have shown that fibrinogen is adsorbed strongly from plasma to either hydrophobic or hydrophilic surfaces and Vroman *et al.*[25] have suggested that contrary to previous speculation,[16] albumin is adsorbed in only minor quantities, if at all. Horbett and Hoffman[18] found that the surface concentration of fibrinogen adsorbed from plasma to a silicone surface was much reduced compared to that adsorbed from fibrinogen solutions or binary mixtures of albumin or γ-globulin with fibrinogen, and attributed the reduction to "unknown plasma factors" and not to a simple competitive effect among the proteins in plasma. Limber *et al.*[28] have studied adsorption from plasma by elution of adsorbed proteins, and identification of proteins in the eluate. This work showed that albumin and IgG are among the proteins that are strongly adsorbed. Overall, the results suggested that adsorption would bear some relation to bulk concentration. However, factor XII and fibrinogen were implicated as playing roles greater proportionately than their concentration, based on the fact that fewer proteins were adsorbed from plasmas deficient in either of these proteins. Conclusions with respect to fibrinogen are somewhat tenuous because of the unknown but possibly deleterious effect of the detergents (SDS and Triton X-100) used to elute the proteins.

In summary, with respect to protein adsorption on hydrophobic polymers the following can reasonably be concluded: Adsorption occurs quickly and is limited in extent to a layer about one molecule thick, even at bulk concentrations similar to those in blood. There is evidence that the surface chemistry of the polymer may influence the surface concentration and composition of the protein layer. Proteins are strongly held on hydrophobic polymers and are not readily desorbed. There is evidence, however, for the occurrence of turnover and possibly exchange, even when the concentration and composition are at steady state. Fibrinogen is probably a major component of the layer on most surfaces and is adsorbed in amounts greater than its proportion of the bulk concentration of protein. The exact composition may vary from surface to surface and is generally unknown. There is little detailed information on the conformational or biological state of adsorbed proteins.

Platelet Interactions

The adhesion of platelets to surfaces is another important effect involved in thrombogenesis. In this regard hydrophobic polymers are not different from other types of foreign surface, except perhaps with respect to quantitative aspects of the phenomenon. Tests of platelet adhesion to glass surfaces have been conducted for many years with the objective of diagnosing platelet abnormalities such as von Willebrand's disease. The work of Wright,[29] Hellem,[30] and Salzman[31] was motivated in this regard. It is only in the past ten years that attention has been paid to platelet adhesion as an indication of a property of the contacting surface as opposed to a property of the platelet. Studies of platelet adhesion are beset by particular experimental difficulties that do not affect studies of protein adsorption. In particular, there are difficulties with respect to the wide variation in possible experimental conditions, particularly regarding composition of the fluid medium. Another problem arises from the fact that under certain conditions, the adhesion process can be transport-limited as opposed to surface reaction-limited. This is to say that the number of platelets seen to adhere under given conditions is limited by the rate of transport of platelets from bulk to surface and not by the rate of reaction of the platelet with the surface. Obviously such conditions should be avoided if one wishes to study the adhesion reaction itself. There are few studies, however, in which this problem has been recognized, and efforts made to characterize the experimental system so that its transport features are well defined.

Among the first reports on adhesion of platelets as a means of investigating surface thrombogenicity were those of Lyman *et al.*[32-34] This work involved exposure of the test surface to flowing whole blood from humans with no anticoagulant. It was found that the number of platelets per unit area adhering in one minute of flow increased with increasing critical surface tension for a group of hydrophobic polymers including silicone, Teflon, polyethylene, acrylics, and polystyrene. Segmented polyurethanes did not conform to the correlation and showed adhesion considerably less than would be expected. It was also observed that adhesion was reduced when the surfaces were preexposed to plasma proteins including albumin, fibrinogen, and γ-globulin. In this test, observations could not be carried beyond about four minutes because of the elaboration of thrombus at longer times. Flow conditions in the test cell have been characterized[35] as mild, with wall shear rates of the order of 3–4 sec^{-1}. Classically, these conditions would tend to lead to transport limitation and indeed would suggest the presence of red cell aggregates. However, since dependence on surface properties was observed, it does not seem likely that transport limitation was operative. Arguments involving red-cell augmented platelet transport and adhesion are also relevant to these experiments and will be elaborated on below.

Work by Friedman *et al.*[36] on a wide variety of surfaces including hydrophobic, hydrophilic, heparinized materials, and others, showed that under their experimental conditions the process of platelet adhesion was transport-limited. Flow conditions were vigorous in these experiments, with wall shear rates of the order of 1000 sec^{-1}, and with use of dog blood, sometimes heparinized, sometimes without anticoagulant. The surface concentration of platelets was very much higher than observed by Lyman *et al.*,[34] and recent work by Grabowski *et al.* has shown that this difference may be explained in terms of a species difference between dog and human platelets.[37] Later work by Turitto *et al.*,[38] in which a spinning disc apparatus at lower shear rates was used, showed that in this system also, with a glass surface, adhesion is transport-limited.

More recently Feuerstein *et al.*[39] and Brash *et al.*[40] have conducted experiments using a rotating probe apparatus that functions in a couette flow mode. This apparatus has been used in conjunction with washed platelet suspensions[41] which have the advantage that they can be manipulated with respect to platelet concentration, protein content, and red cell concentration, and the platelets can be labeled to facilitate evaluation of the surface. Additionally, platelet adhesion can be observed independently of aggregation. This system has been shown not to be transport-limited, even though low shear rates (about 20 sec^{-1}) are used.[39] With polymer surfaces, in the absence of red cells the kinetics of adhesion are not readily accessible, since saturation levels are reached within a minute. These levels are low and indistinguishable from surface to surface. When red cells are present the saturation levels are higher and the polymer surfaces are again indistinguishable, but fibrinogen- and collagen-coated surfaces are of higher reactivity. These results are explained in terms of red cell-augmented transport of platelets and augmentation of adhesion itself via increased collision energy imparted by red cell motion. More recent work with this apparatus has shown very low platelet adhesion to hydrophilic surfaces.[42] It is concluded that early platelet adhesion *per se* is not a strong determinant of ultimate thrombogenicity, which instead may be controlled by synergisms that exist among various factors, including protein adsorption, coagulation, and platelets.

Effects of red cells on platelet transport have been observed by other workers. Thus Keller[43] has shown that red cell rotation caused by fluid shear can augment mass transport of relatively large species in the immediate vicinity of the cells, and his analysis suggests that platelet transport could be enhanced. Turitto *et al.*[44] showed that platelet diffusion coefficient is strongly dependent on hematocrit in flowing blood with a variation between 0.5 and 2.5×10^{-7} cm^2 sec^{-1}. A similar range of values was observed by Feuerstein *et al.*[39] In addition to rotational motion, Goldsmith has demonstrated the motion of red cells perpendicular to flow streamlines.[45] This is a fluctuating random-walklike motion which could give rise to additional augmentation of platelet transport. It has been suggested recently that red cell motions by increasing the collision energy between platelet and surface, could also influence the adhesion reaction itself.[40] If this is true, then the classic picture of high flow leading to reaction limitation and slow flow leading to transport limitation may not always hold. The net result in any situation will depend on the relative magnitude of the flow/red cell effects on transport on the one hand and reaction on the other. If the effect is greater on reaction, then low flow may lead to reaction limitation, but if the effect is greater on transport, then low flow may lead to transport limitation. There is of course no *a priori* way at present to predict these relative magnitudes.

Another approach to the study of platelet adhesion has been reported by George.[46] In this method the platelets are transported to the surface in a high-level centrifugal force field. The platelets are present in very low concentration (about 200-fold dilution relative to plasma), so that they appear well separated on the surface for microscopic evaluation. This is a somewhat artificial situation but has the advantage of allowing the study of adhesion *per se* in a situation uncomplicated by transport effects. After contact has occurred, the centrifugal force field is reversed and platelets that are strongly adherent remain attached, while those that are loosely held are removed. Most of the data reported with this device pertain to a glass surface, but it was observed that siliconization of glass did not affect the adhesion of platelets from serum, plasma, or washed suspensions. On the other hand, a surface of polyethylene oxide, presumably strongly hydrophilic, showed greatly decreased adhesion.

Studies by Lee and Kim[47] have focused attention on the mechanism by which adsorbed plasma proteins influence platelet adhesion. They proposed that platelets adhere via enzyme-substrate complex formation between platelet glycosyl transferases and incomplete heterosaccharide chains of adsorbed glycoproteins, and obtained adhesion data on desialylated and degalactosylated protein coatings to support this contention. This mechanism is closely parallel to that suggested by Jamieson *et al.*[48] for adhesion of platelets to collagen. More recently Lee and Kim[49] have shown that platelet adhesion to silicone rubber is inhibited by incubation of the platelets with cyclic AMP, dibutyryl cyclic AMP, and prostaglandin E_1, thus placing adhesion to hydrophobic surfaces and to plasma protein layers on a similar mechanistic basis to other platelet responses such as ADP-, thrombin-, and collagen-induced aggregation.

Little is known of the detailed events leading from initial platelet adhesion to the elaboration of a thrombotic structure. Various workers have observed the deployment of pseudopods adherent to surfaces, suggesting that the same metabolic and shape changes that presage aggregation are triggered by adhesion also. In general, hydrophobic surfaces seem less likely than other types of surface to cause pseudopod formation at short contact times.[50] Little is known of the tendency to undergo the release reaction by platelets that adhere to foreign surfaces. Packham *et al.*[51] have demonstrated that platelets in contact with γ-globulin-coated glass surfaces undergo considerable release of serotonin, whereas fibrinogen- and albumin-coated glass elicit this response only minimally. Whether release had taken place only from platelets that had adhered or from platelets that had contacted the surface without adhering could not be determined. Siliconization of the glass caused an increase in adhesion whether or not the glass was subsequently coated with protein. Siliconization appeared to have no effect on release.

Recent work in the author's laboratory[42] has attempted to quantitate release of constituents from platelets that have adhered to surfaces. The approach used was to label platelets with ^{51}Cr, which is bound mainly to the cytoplasmic nucleotides,[52] and ^{14}C-serotonin, which is located mainly in intracellular granules. By counting both isotopes on the surface after exposure to the platelets, an indication of adhesion and of release subsequent to adhesion can be obtained. In preliminary work it was found that surfaces that support adhesion tend to induce little release, and considerable release occurs on surfaces that do not support much adhesion. In addition "environmental" factors such as hematocrit and protein content of the platelet medium appear to have opposite effects on adhesion and release. Of particular note is the strong inhibitory effect of fibrinogen on release compared with its enhancing effect on adhesion.

Baumgartner *et al.*[53] have measured disappearance of amine storage granules from platelets adhering to various surfaces and have noted an effect on all surfaces studied. By far the greatest effect was observed with collagen and subendothelial surfaces with an epoxy resin surface showing only minimal degranulation.

Red Cell Interactions

Red cells are important in blood surface interactions in two principal ways. First, as already discussed, they play a role in thrombogenesis by their effects on transport of thrombotic material, by forming a major component of thrombi (particularly in the venous circulation), and by providing a source of ADP, which can accelerate platelet aggregation. Second, they can interact directly with a surface to produce hemolytic damage to the cell. It is the second of these mechanisms that remains to be discussed. Bernstein[54] has given a review of red-cell surface interactions to about 1971 and Blackshear[55] has published a recent comprehensive review on hemolysis originating from prosthetic heart valves.

For many years there was considerable debate as to whether red cell damage in blood-contact devices was occasioned by fluid shear or by "wall effects." Most investigators now agree that shear stress of very high magnitude acting for a short time can produce hemolysis, but the levels of shear stress required to do this are much higher than are normally met in artificial organ systems.[55,56] The most important hemolytic mechanism is now believed to occur via cell-wall contact. Blackshear has postulated that such hemolysis may occur via the forming and breaking away of "tethers."[55] These are filamentous structures that can extend in length to several red cell diameters, and can form an attachment between cell and wall. The ultimate breaking of the tether can lead to hemolytic damage. Tethers, of which the origins are unknown but which may be derived from the membrane, are less likely to be formed in protein-containing media,[55] thus reinforcing the concept of the protective effects of adsorbed protein layers. Hochmuth *et al.*[57] and Mohandas *et al.*,[58] in additional studies of red cell-surface interaction, again demonstrated the existence of tethers and showed that, in protein-free systems, the critical shear stress for detachment of red cells that have settled on a surface increases with increasing CST of the surface.

Additional information about the effect of surface properties on hemolytic damage is provided by the work of Lampert and Williams.[59] For a group of metals and polymers such as polycarbonate, polymethylmethacrylate, and Teflon it was found that hemolysis in a spinning disc apparatus could be correlated with time via an empirical relation involving a surface-sensitive parameter. This parameter in turn could be correlated with the critical surface tension, the hemolytic tendency increasing with decreasing CST. These results were discussed in relation to protein adsorption, which, it was concluded, would be such as to make the properties of the surface itself of secondary importance only, although a few results demonstrated a direct effect of surface properties on red cell adhesion. Weiss and Blumenson [60] showed that adhesion to siliconized glass was much less than to glass itself in protein-free conditions, although the presence of protein in the medium, by reducing adhesion to the glass surface, tended to eliminate any differences.

The role of proteins in red cell-surface interactions has been noted in several reports, including that of George *et al.*,[61] who showed that adhesion of red cells in washed suspensions to a glass surface is greatly diminished when small amounts of serum or plasma are added. In later work [62] George showed that fibrinogen inhibits adhesion in this system, since less adhesion was observed with plasma than with serum. Furthermore, it was demonstrated that the action of fibrinogen was probably via adsorption to the glass, since no adsorption to the cell surface could be detected.

More recently we have examined these phenomena from the opposite point of view, namely, the effect of red cells on protein adsorption.[63] We have shown that adsorption of fibrinogen and albumin is significantly reduced in the presence of red cells and that the preference of polyethylene for fibrinogen over albumin is enhanced in the presence of red cells. We postulated that via surface contact the red cells are able to deposit material on the surface which is inhibitory to protein adsorption. The concept of deposits occurring from red cells is supported by the observation of tethers already referred to, and by the work of Keller and Yum,[64] who showed a decrease of exchange of cholesterol between the cells and a contacting surface with time. This was interpreted in terms of a deposit from the red cell.

Summary

Hydrophobic polymers, defined as having nonzero water-contact angles, have more a historic than a rational basis for their application as materials for interfacing with blood. They were originally regarded as causing a minimal clotting response and as being inert. They possess great advantages in terms of mechanical strength, flexibility, and formability over most other materials. Unmodified hydrophobic polymers that have proved to be reasonably blood-compatible are the segmented polyether polyurethanes, silicones, and some fluorinated polymers. The molecular basis for compatibility in these materials is not understood.

In terms of their interactions with blood, hydrophobic polymers in general initiate coagulation, support protein adsorption and platelet adhesion, and cause lysis of red cells. Much of the detail of these interactions, which might enable the mechanism of thrombogenesis to be understood, is only beginning to emerge. Thus, although it is known that protein adsorption is limited to a single molecular layer it is not known what the composition of the layer is, or how this depends on surface properties within the hydrophobic series. It is also known that although protein binding is strong enough to prevent desorption (in contrast to hydrophilic polymers) there may well be turnover occurring under steady-state conditions of concentration and composition. Definitive data on the state of biological alteration of adsorbed proteins have yet to be obtained.

Experiments on platelet-surface interaction are complicated by the effects of transport from bulk to surface, and these can obscure surface reactivities in certain situations. Such effects may also occur in prosthetic or other blood circulation devices. From limited evidence it seems that adhesion of platelets to hydrophobic polymers occurs more readily than to hydrophilic surfaces, and there is evidence of a direct relationship with critical surface tension. On the other hand, release of granule contents may occur more readily from platelets adhering to hydrophilic surfaces. Plasma proteins play an important mediatory role in platelet adhesion. Fibrinogen, which is a major component of protein layers adsorbed from blood, is known to enhance adhesion but appears to inhibit release of granule contents from adherent platelets. Considerable gaps remain in our knowledge of events leading from adhesion of platelets to the formation of a thrombus.

Interaction of red cells with hydrophobic polymers is also important as a thrombosis-related effect (via augmentation of platelet transport), and because of hemolytic damage caused by surface contact. From limited data it appears that adhesion decreases with decreasing CST while hemolysis increases. Protein layers again serve to reduce red cell surface interactions.

References

1. Wesolowski, S. A., C. C. Fries, A. Martinez & J. D. McMahon. 1968. Arterial prosthetic materials. Ann. N.Y. Acad. Sci. **146**(1): 325–344.
2. Lister, J. 1863. Proc. Roy. Soc. **B12:** 580.
3. Bordet, J. & O. Gengou. 1903. Recherches sur la coagulation du sang. Ann. Inst. Pasteur **17:** 822–833.
4. Boretos, J. W. & W. S. Pierce. 1967. Segmented polyurethane: a new elastomer for biomedical applications. Science **158:** 1481–1482.
5. Boretos, J. W., D. E. Detmer & J. H. Donachy. 1971. Segmented polyurethane II. Two years experience. J. Biomed. Mater. Res. **5:** 373–388.
6. Brash, J. L., B. K. Fritzinger & S. D. Bruck. 1973. Development of block copolyether-urethane intra-aortic balloons and other medical devices. J. Biomed. Mater. Res. **7:** 313–334.
7. Braley, S. 1968. The silicones as subdermal engineering materials. Ann. N.Y. Acad. Sci. **146**(1): 148–157.
8. Fox, H. W. & W. A. Zisman. 1952. The spreading of liquids on low-energy surfaces. II. Modified tetrafluoroethylene polymers. J. Colloid Sci. **7:** 109–121.
9. Lampert, H. 1930. Muench. Med. Wochschr. **77:** 586.
10. Rose, J. C. & H. P. Broida. 1954. Effects of plastic and steel surfaces on clotting time of human blood. Proc. Soc. Exp. Biol. Med. **86:** 384–386.
11. Ross, J., L. J. Greenfield, R. L. Bowman & A. G. Morrow. 1961. The chemical structure and surface properties of certain synthetic polymers and their relationship to thrombosis. *In* Prosthetic Valves for Cardiac Surgery. K. A. Merendino, Ed. : 212–223. Charles C Thomas, Springfield, Ill.

12. Lyman, D. J., W. M. Muir & I. J. Lee. 1965. The effect of chemical structure and surface properties of polymers on the coagulation of blood. I. Surface free energy effects. Trans. Amer. Soc. Artif. Int. Organs **11:** 301–306.
13. Osipow, L. I. 1962. Surface Chemistry. Reinhold Publishing Corp. New York, N.Y.
14. Cochrane, C. G., S. D. Revak & K. D. Wuepper. 1973. Activation of Hageman factor in solid and fluid phases. J. Exp. Med. **138:** 1564–1583.
15. Falb, R. D., M. T. Takahashi, G. A. Grode & R. I. Leininger. 1967. Studies on the stability and protein adsorption characteristics of heparinized polymer surfaces by radioisotope labeling techniques. J. Biomed. Mater. Res. **1:** 239–251.
16. Brash, J. L. & D. J. Lyman. 1969. Adsorption of plasma proteins in solution to uncharged, hydrophobic polymer surfaces. J. Biomed. Mater. Res. **3:** 175–189.
17. Koutsky, J. A., N. V. Hien & S. L. Cooper. 1970. Some results on electron microscope investigations of polyether-urethane and polyester-urethane block copolymers. J. Polymer. Sci. **138:** 353–359.
18. Horbett, T. A. & A. S. Hoffman. 1975. Bovine plasma protein adsorption to radiation grafted hydrogels based on hydroxyethylmethacrylate and N-vinyl pyrrolidone. *In* Applied Chemistry at Protein Interfaces. R. E. Baier, Ed. : 230–254. American Chemical Society. Washington, D.C.
19. MacRitchie, F. 1972. The adsorption of proteins at the solid-liquid interface. J. Colloid Interface Sci. **38:** 484–488.
20. Brash, J. L., S. Uniyal & Q. Samak. 1974. Exchange of albumin adsorbed on polymer surfaces. Trans. Amer. Soc. Artif. Int. Organs **20:** 69–76.
21. Morrissey, B. W. & R. R. Stromberg. 1974. The conformation of adsorbed blood proteins by infrared bound fraction measurements. J. Colloid Interface Sci. **46:** 152–164.
22. Morrissey, B. W. & C. A. Fenstermaker. 1976. Conformation of adsorbed γ-globulin and β-lactoglobulin. Effect of surface concentration. Trans. Amer. Soc. Artif. Int. Organs **22:** 278–283.
23. Vroman, L. & A. L. Adams. 1969. Identification of rapid changes at plasma-solid interfaces. J. Biomed. Mater. Res. **3:** 43–67.
24. Lee, R. G., C. Adamson & S. W. Kim. 1974. Competitive adsorption of plasma proteins onto polymer surfaces. Thromb. Res. **4:** 485–490.
25. Vroman, L., A. L. Adams, M. Klings & G. Fischer. 1975. Fibrinogen, globulins, albumin and plasma at interfaces. *In* Applied Chemistry at Protein Interfaces. R. E. Baier, Ed. : 255–289. American Chemical Society. Washington, D.C.
26. Brash, J. L. & V. J. Davidson. 1976. Adsorption on glass and polyethylene from solutions of fibrinogen and albumin. Thromb. Res. **9:** 249–259.
27. Vroman, L. & A. L. Adams. 1967. Possible involvement of fibrinogen and proteolysis in surface activation. Thromb. Diath. Haemorr. **18:** 510–524.
28. Limber, G. K., C. H. Glenn & R. G. Mason. 1974. Studies of proteins elutable from certain artificial surfaces exposed to human plasma. Thromb. Res. **5:** 735–746.
29. Wright, H. P. 1941. Adhesiveness of blood platelets in normal subjects with varying concentrations of anticoagulants. J. Pathol. Bacteriol. **53:** 255–262.
30. Hellem, A. J. 1960. The adhesiveness of human blood platelets in vitro. Scand. J. Clin. Lab. Invest. **12**(Supp. 51)**:** 1.
31. Salzman, E. W. 1963. Measurement of platelet adhesiveness. J. Lab. Clin. Med. **62:** 724–735.
32. Lyman, D. J., J. L. Brash, S. W. Chaikin & M. Carini. 1968. The effect of chemical structure and surface properties of synthetic polymers on the coagulation of blood. II. Protein and platelet interaction with polymer surfaces. Trans. Amer. Soc. Artif. Int. Organs. **14:** 250–255.
33. Lyman, D. J., K. G. Klein, J. L. Brash & B. K. Fritzinger. 1970. Interaction

of platelets with polymer surfaces. I. Uncharged hydrophobic polymer surfaces. Thromb. Diath. Haemorr. **23:** 120–128.

34. LYMAN, D. J., K. G. KLEIN, J. L. BRASH, B. K. FRITZINGER, J. D. ANDRADE & F. BONOMO. 1971. Platelet interaction with protein-coated surfaces: an approach to thromboresistant surfaces. Thromb. Diath. Haemorr. (Supp.) **42:** 109–114.
35. DAY, R. C., I. A. FEUERSTEIN & J. L. BRASH. 1976. Flow patterns in a platelet adhesion test cell and their effect on adhesion measurements. Thromb. Res. **9:** 133–142.
36. FRIEDMAN, L. I., H. LIEM, E. F. GRABOWSKI, E. F. LEONARD & C. W. MCCORD. 1970. Inconsequentiality of surface properties for initial platelet adhesion. Trans. Amer. Soc. Artif. Int. Organs **16:** 63–73.
37. GRABOWSKI, E. F., K. K. HERTHER & P. DIDISHEIM. 1976. Human versus dog platelet adhesion to cuprophane under controlled conditions of whole blood flow. J. Lab. Clin. Med. To be published.
38. TURITTO, V. T. & E. F. LEONARD. 1972. Platelet adhesion to a spinning disc. Trans. Amer. Soc. Artif. Int. Organs **18:** 348–354.
39. FEUERSTEIN, I. A., J. M. BROPHY & J. L. BRASH. 1975. Platelet transport and adhesion to reconstituted collagen and artificial surfaces. Trans. Amer. Soc. Artif. Int. Organs **21:** 427–434.
40. BRASH, J. L., J. M. BROPHY & I. A. FEUERSTEIN. 1976. Adhesion of platelets to artificial surfaces: effect of red cells. J. Biomed. Mater. Res. **10:** 429–443.
41. MUSTARD, J. F., D. W. PERRY, N. G. ARDLIE & M. A. PACKHAM. 1972. Preparation of suspensions of washed platelets fro mhumans. Brit. J. Haematol. **22:** 193–204.
42. BRASH, J. L. & S. J. WHICHER. 1976. Interaction of platelets with surfaces: a factorial study of adhesion and associated release of serotonin. Proc. Strathclyde Bioengineering Seminar Series. Second Seminar, Aug. 1976. *In* Biomedical Engineering Approaches to the Artificial Lung, Kidney and Liver. To be published.
43. KELLER, K. H. 1971. Effect of fluid shear on mass transport in flowing blood. Fed. Proc. **30:** 1591–1599.
44. TURITTO, V. T., A. M. BENIS & E. F. LEONARD. 1972. Platelet diffusion in flowing blood. Ind. Eng. Chem. Fundam. **11:** 216–232.
45. GOLDSMITH, H. L. 1971. Red cell motions and wall interaction in tube flow. Fed. Proc. **26:** 1578–1588.
46. GEORGE, J. N. 1972. Direct assessment of platelet adhesion to glass: a study of the forces of interaction and the effects of plasma and serum factors, platelet function, and modification of the glass surface. Blood **40:** 862–874.
47. LEE, R. G. & S. W. KIM. 1974. The role of carbohydrate in platelet adhesion to foreign surfaces. J. Biomed. Mater. Res. **8:** 393–398.
48. JAMIESON, G. A., C. L. URBAN & A. J. BARBER. 1971. Enzymatic basis for platelet: collagen adhesion as the primary step in haemostasis. Nature [New Biol.] **234:** 5–7.
49. LEE, R. G. & S. W. KIM. 1976. Cyclic AMP and platelet adhesion to silastic surfaces. Thromb. Res. **8:** 111–114.
50. HUM, O. S., A. W. NEUMANN & W. ZINGG. 1975. Platelet interaction with smooth solid substrates determined by an open static method. Thromb. Res. **7:** 461–470.
51. PACKHAM, M. A., G. EVANS, M. F. GLYNN & J. F. MUSTARD. 1969. The effect of plasma proteins on the interaction of platelets with glass surfaces. J. Lab. Clin. Med. **73:** 686–697.
52. STEINER, M. & M. BALDINI. 1970. Subcellular distribution of ^{51}Cr and characterization of its binding sites in human platelets. Blood **35:** 727–739.
53. BAUMGARTNER, H. R., R. MUGGLI, T. B. TSCHOPP & V. T. TURITTO. 1976. Platelet anhesion, release and aggregation in flowing blood: effects of surface properties and platelet function. Thromb. Diath. Haemorr. **35:** 124–138.

54. Bernstein, E. F. 1971. Certain aspects of blood interfacial phenomena—red blood cells. Fed. Proc. **30:** 1510–1515.
55. Blackshear, P. L. 1972. Hemolysis at Prosthetic Surfaces. *In* The Chemistry of Biosurfaces. Vol. 2. M. L. Hair, Ed. : 523–562. Marcel Dekker Inc. New York, N.Y.
56. Leverett, L. B., J. D. Hellums, E. C. Lynch & C. P. Alfrey. 1972. Red blood cell damage by shear stress. Biophys. J. **12:** 257–273.
57. Hochmuth, R. M., N. Mohandas, E. E. Spaeth, J. R. Williamson, P. L. Blackshear, Jr. & D. W. Johnson. 1972. Surface adhesion deformation and detachment at low shear of red cells and white cells. Trans. Amer. Soc. Artif. Int. Organs **18:** 325–332.
58. Mohandas, N., R. M. Hochmuth & E. E. Spaeth. 1974. Adhesion of red cells to foreign surfaces in the presence of flow. J. Biomed. Mater. Res. **8:** 119–136.
59. Lampert, R. H. & M. C. Williams. 1972. Effect of surface materials on shear-induced hemolysis. J. Biomed. Mater. Res. **6:** 499–532.
60. Weiss, L. & L. E. Blumenson. 1967. Dynamic adhesion and separation of cells in vitro. II. Interactions of cells with hydrophilic and hydrophobic surfaces. J. Cell Physiol. **70:** 23–32.
61. George, J. N., R. I. Weed & C. F. Reed. 1971. Adhesion of human erythrocytes to glass: the nature of the interaction and the effect of serum and plasma. J. Cell Physiol. **77:** 51–60.
62. George, J. N. 1972. Fibrinogen inhibits red cell adhesion to glass. J. Cell Physiol. **79:** 457–462.
63. Brash, J. L. & S. Uniyal. 1976. Adsorption of albumin and fibrinogen to polyethylene in presence of red cells. Trans. Amer. Soc. Artif. Int. Organs **22:** 253–259.
64. Keller, K. H. & S. I. Yum. 1970. Erythrocyte-tube wall interactions in laminar flow of blood suspensions. Trans. Amer. Soc. Artif. Int. Organs **16:** 42–47.

INTERACTIONS OF BLOOD AND BLOOD COMPONENTS AT HYDROGEL INTERFACES *

Allan S. Hoffman, Thomas A. Horbett, and Buddy D. Ratner

Center for Bioengineering and Department of Chemical Engineering University of Washington Seattle, Washington 98195

Introduction

A hydrogel can be defined as a polymeric material which exhibits the ability to swell in water and retain a significant fraction (e.g., >10–20%) of water within its structure, but which will not dissolve in water. Hydrogel materials resemble, in their physical properties, living tissue more than any other class of synthetic biomaterial. In particular, their relatively high water contents and their soft, rubbery consistency give them a resemblance to living soft tissue. Based upon these properties, a number of advantages, some obviously real and others somewhat speculative, can be cited for hydrogel materials.

With respect to the real advantages, two in particular stand out. First, the expanded nature of the hydrogel structure and its permeability to small molecules allows polymerization initiator molecules, initiator decomposition products, polymerization-solvent molecules, and other extraneous materials to be efficiently extracted from the gel network before the hydrogel is placed in contact with a living system. The *in vivo* leaching of additives used during the fabrication of polymeric materials has been cited as a cause of inflammation and eventual rejection of implanted biomaterials.[1] Second, the rather soft and rubbery consistency of most hydrogels can contribute to their biocompatibility by minimizing mechanical (frictional) irritation to surrounding cells and tissue.

The most intriguing of the potential advantages for hydrogels is the low interfacial tension that may be exhibited between a hydrogel surface and an aqueous solution. This low interfacial tension should reduce the tendency of the proteins in body fluids to adsorb and to unfold upon adsorption.[2] Minimal protein interaction may be important for the biological acceptance of foreign materials, since the denaturation of proteins by surfaces may serve as a trigger mechanism for the initiation of thrombosis or for other biological rejection mechanisms.

Clearly, the presence of large amounts of water within a polymeric network is not the sole factor controlling the "biocompatibility" of such materials, although it is considered to be related to the biological interactions of those hydrogels which are "biocompatible" and "reasonably nonthrombogenic" (or nonthromboadherent).[3] The nature or organization of the water within the

* Supported by the Energy Research and Development Administration (contract no. AT-45-1-2225); the National Heart and Lung Institute, NIH (contract NIH-NO1-HB-4-2970); and the National Institute of General Medical Sciences, NIH (grant 16436–5 to 7).

hydrated polymeric network may be one of the key factors that influence the interactions that occur between biological systems and the hydrogel.[4–6]

The ability of small molecules to diffuse through hydrogels may also be advantageous for hydrogel *in vivo* performance. The diffusion of important low molecular weight metabolites and ions through the implant and to the surrounding tissue would occur with hydrogels, but not with relatively hard, less permeable plastics.

A wide variety of compositions is possible for synthetic hydrogels, since they may be synthesized from monomer mixtures or by chemical modifications of existing polymers. Hydrogels can often be prepared in the form of highly porous sponges, less porous gels, optically transparent films, liquids that can be subsequently crosslinked to form gels, and coatings bound by either chemical covalent bonds or physical noncovalent forces to a substrate polymer material. Ratner and Hoffman have recently reviewed the synthesis, properties, and biomedical applications of hydrogels.[7, 8]

There are a number of techniques that can be used to coat substrates with hydrophilic polymers or copolymers, as follows:

1. Dip-coat in prepolymer + solvent
2. Dip in monomer(s) (±solvent, polymer) then polymerize, using catalyst ± heat.
3. Preactivate surface ("active vapor," ionizing radiation in air) then contact with monomer(s) ± heat to polymerize.
4. Irradiate with ionizing radiation while in contact with vapor or liquid solution of monomer(s).

The first technique yields a physically deposited coating; the others probably lead to covalent bonding (grafting) of the hydrogel on and within the substrate polymer surface. By covalently bonding a hydrogel to the surface of another polymer, a new composite material is formed whose mechanical properties more closely resemble those of the base polymer than the thin, grafted hydrogel layer, whereas the interfacial properties are closer to those of the hydrogel.

In summary, it should be emphasized that a particular hydrogel composition suitable for one biomedical application may have to be significantly modified in composition and form for a different application. That is, the hydrogel system must always be matched to each biomedical use.

Interaction of Specific Hydrogels with Blood and Blood Components

Poly(hydroxyalkyl methacrylates)

Included in this class of compounds are poly(2-hydroxyethyl methacrylate) (P-HEMA), poly(2-hydroxyethyl acrylate) (P-HEA), poly(glyceryl methacrylate) (P-GMA), and poly(hydroxypropyl methacrylate (P-HPMA). A review article with particular emphasis upon hydroxyalkyl methacrylate hydrogels has been published.[9]

Poly(2-hydroxyethyl methacrylate) (P-HEMA) hydrogels were first described and synthetized by Wichterle and Lim in the early 1960s.[10] To date, P-HEMA hydrogels have probably been among the most widely studied and used of all the synthetic hydrogel materials. Because of the poor mechanical properties of P-HEMA gels, there have always been experimental difficulties in evaluating the blood compatibility of these materials by accepted *in vivo* testing techniques (e.g., the vena cava ring test or the renal embolus ring test). However, the blood compatibility of P-HEMA was observed in a few studies either *in vitro* or with less conventional *in vivo* techniques.[11-15] It was found, in all cases, to be a "relatively nonthrombogenic" (or at least nonthromboadherent) material, although the *in vivo* tests which were used do not allow a systematic grading of thrombogenicity, and did not compare the performance of P-HEMA to a number of other commonly used materials.

A number of researchers have stressed the importance of initial protein adsorption followed by cellular interactions with the adsorbed proteinaceous layer when blood is exposed to a foreign interface (e.g. Refs. 16–19); it is for this reason that protein adsorption and cell adhesion studies on hydrogel surfaces are relevant to the design of blood-compatible hydrogels.

P-HEMA hydrogels have been radiation-grafted to various polymer sub-

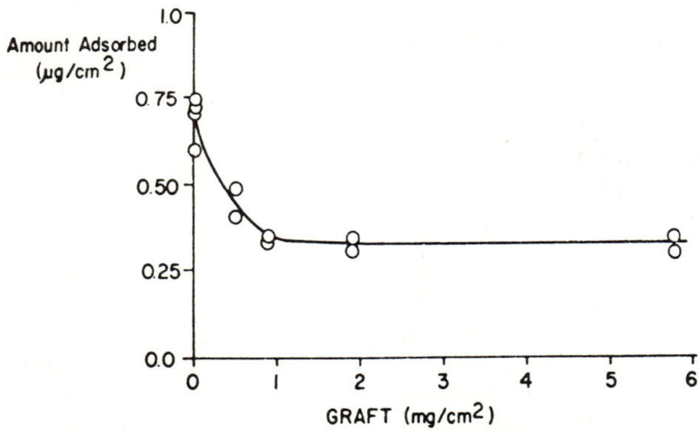

FIGURE 1. Fibrinogen adsorption to radiation-grafted P-HEMA hydrogels on Silastic films as a function of the extent of grafting.[22]

strates, and protein adsorption, cellular adhesion, and vena cava thrombus formation have all been studied for these materials.[20-25] Horbett and Hoffman have noted a reduction in fibrinogen adsorption with increasing levels of graft on Silastic® films (FIGURE 1).[22] The fibrinogen is also desorbed more readily from the grafted surface. When tagged fibrinogen is mixed with plasma there is an apparent reversal in the adsorption levels noted with pure fibrinogen solutions, and a significant decrease in fibrinogen adsorption on the ungrafted Silastic is seen, relative to the almost unchanged adsorption on the P-HEMA grafted Silastic. Although albumin and γ-globulin were found to compete with fibrinogen for adsorption sites when these proteins were in very high molar excess over fibrinogen (in mixed protein solutions), it was concluded that other, unknown plasma constituents may be effectively competing with fibrinogen for adsorption sites on the untreated Silastic surface.[22]

Holly and Refojo have investigated the effects of protein adsorption on the wettability of P-HEMA and P-HEA hydrogels relative to the hydrophobic poly(methyl methacrylate) and polyethylene surfaces.[25] They concluded that

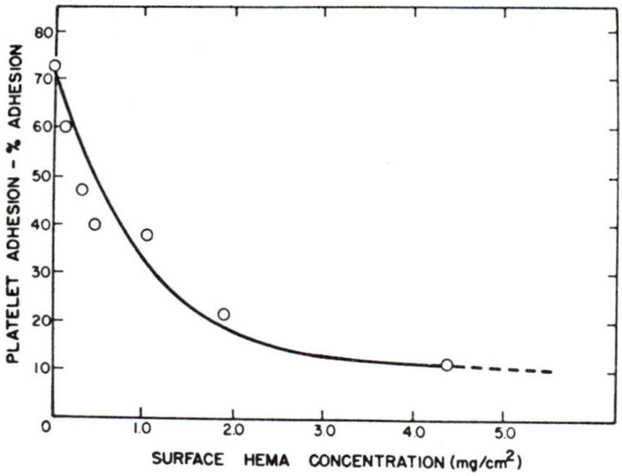

FIGURE 2. Platelet adhesion to radiation-grafted P-HEMA hydrogels on cellulose acetate films.[26]

the effect of protein adsorption on the hydrogel-water interfacial tension is negligible when compared to the extensive adsorption at the hydrophobic solid-water interfaces.

Ratner *et al.*[23] have observed a decrease in chick embryo myoblast adhesiveness to the radiation-grafted P-HEMA/Silastic films, and Muzykewicz *et al.*[26] have noted a gradual decrease in platelet adhesiveness with increasing levels of grafted P-HEMA on cellulose acetate films (FIGURE 2; compare to FIGURE 1). Ratner *et al.*[23] also noted a significant increase in myoblast adhesion on all surfaces, both hydrogel-grafted and ungrafted Silastic, after preadsorption of fibrinogen on these surfaces. Preadsorption of albumin or γ-globulin did not produce significant changes in cell adhesion on any of the hydrogel surfaces studied.[23]

When P-HEMA hydrogels are grafted to Silastic vena cava rings, there is a sharp reduction in the amount of thrombus deposited in comparison to the untreated Silastic rings[24] (FIGURE 3). The above studies all tend to support the concept that such hydrogels have a low thromboadherence. Indeed, in the

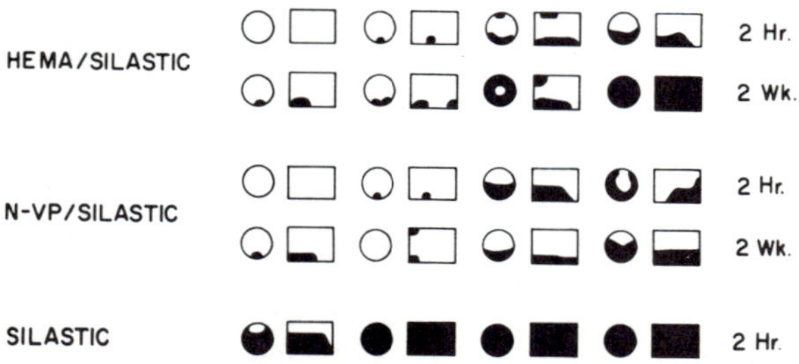

FIGURE 3. Results of vena cava ring tests on untreated Silastic rings and radiation-grafted hydrogels on Silastic rings.[24] (Data of Dr. James D. Whiffen. Department of Surgery, University of Wisconsin Medical School, Madison, Wis.)

renal embolus test, although little thrombus is found within most grafted hydrogel-treated test rings, the kidneys almost always show moderate to extensive embolus damage.[27]

Hoffman *et al.* have immobilized streptokinase, albumin, and heparin on radiation-grafted copolymer hydrogels based upon HEMA and N-vinyl-2-pyrrolidone (NVP).[28] Streptokinase immobilized via an "arm" demonstrated significant fibrinolytic activity. Immobilized heparin, on the other hand, did not seem to retain biological activity when immobilized to these surfaces with use of either BrCN or carbodiimide chemical techniques.

Poly(acrylamide) and Derivatives

Gels of poly(acrylamide) (P-AAm) and of some N-substituted derivatives of P-AAm can be readily prepared by the free radical polymerization of an aqueous solution of acrylamide containing a small fraction of crosslinking agent (often *N,N*-methylenebisacrylamide). The gels formed are optically transparent and mechanically weak, and can have extremely high water contents (>95%). The water content is dependent upon the per-cent crosslinker in the system, unlike the homogeneous P-HEMA gel system. Another technique was recently described for preparing gels composed primarily of polyacrylamide with smaller fractions of poly(acrylonitrile) and poly(acrylic acid).[29] This technique involves polymerizing acrylonitrile in concentrated aqueous zinc chloride and then partially hydrolyzing the resulting gel. The high water contents attainable with acrylamide gels prepared by solution polymerization or by hydrolysis make them attractive for biomedical applications.

The thrombogenicity of a number of P-AAm gels was investigated *in vitro* by the Lee-White coagulation-time test.[15] While the coagulation time of fresh blood samples in glass tubes was approximately 12 minutes, blood in P-AAm tubes prepared with singly recrystallized acrylamide monomer showed a clotting time of ~45 minutes. When gels formed from triply-recrystallized acrylamide monomer were tested, they showed clotting times in excess of 24 hours. The deleterious effects of incomplete removal of initiator by-products on the thrombogenicity of acrylamide materials was also noted in this study. The effect of varying the crosslinking agent concentration in the P-AAm gel was found not to alter significantly the Lee-White clotting times for the system. Interesting effects of other comonomers incorporated into the P-AAm gels on the clotting times were noted. Some of these effects are discussed below. In general, the P-AAm system prepared with triply-recrystallized monomer gave the best results, although systems containing dimethylaminoethyl methacrylate were shown to demonstrate excellent Lee-White clotting times. The thrombogenicity of these particular gels was found to be extremely sensitive to crosslinker concentration and total gel water content. Bruck has recently reviewed three types of biomedical hydrogels.[30] In particular, the pore size and water content of P-AAm is discussed in relation to various measures of its biocompatibility.

Nguyen and Wilkes have described a fibrinolytic surface made by immobilizing brinolase to Enzacryl®, a particulate, crosslinked, modified polyacrylamide.[31] Significant brinolase activity was maintained. The authors suggest a grafted polymer, utilizing acrylic acid and *N*-acryloyl para-phenylene diamine as a more practical material for both immobilizing brinolase and constructing useful devices.

Kearney *et al.* have studied the blood compatibility of radiation-grafted P-AAm surfaces with some indications of improved performance of the hydrogel surfaces.[32]

Leonard *et al.* have studied the adhesion of platelets on ceric ion-grafted acrylamide/polyurethane surfaces (Polysciences), using the *in vitro* spinning disc apparatus with platelet-rich plasma.[33] They observed negligible platelet adhesion on the hydrogel surface after about seven to eight minutes' exposure, for a disc speed of 400 rpm., but the untreated polyurethane (Stanford Research Institute) exhibited greater than 28 platelets/900 μ^2 after two minutes' exposure under similar conditions.

Poly(N-*vinyl-2-pyrrolidone*)

Poly(*N*-vinyl-2-pyrrolidone) (P-NVP) is a somewhat unique polymer in that in its uncrosslinked form it is extremely soluble in water and is also soluble in many other polar and nonpolar solvents. Because of its strong interaction with water it can be used for preparing gels that will exhibit high water contents.

P-NVP gels are also of interest for biomedical applications, since the soluble polymer has had a long history of use in the medical and pharmaceutical fields. One of the most important uses for P-NVP solutions has been as a plasma expander.[34] When infused intravenously, P-NVP is nontoxic and nonthrombogenic and can be used to maintain circulatory fluid volume in cases of severe injury or trauma. Some retention of P-NVP in the liver, spleen, lungs, and kidneys has been noted.[35] In a review of the world literature on P-NVP in 1962, it was concluded that P-NVP could be used orally or intravenously with complete safety.[36] At the present time, however, P-NVP is no longer used as a plasma expander in humans because it is not metabolized and is not retained in circulation as well as other plasma expanders (e.g. Dextrans). P-NVP has also been used in blood volume determinations[37] and in the preservation of blood and blood components.[38]

Hydrogels consisting only of P-NVP have not often been described in the biomedical literature, possibly because high concentrations of crosslinker (5–20%) are needed to produce a material with useful mechanical properties. P-NVP gels crosslinked with methylene bis(4-phenyl isocyanate) were evaluated for use as hemodialysis membranes.[39] Faster metabolic waste transfer was obtained with these membranes than with conventional cellulose films.

In vitro evaluation of the thrombogenicity of P-NVP gels and P-NVP/P-AAm copolymer gels by the Lee-White test showed some extension of clotting times, although problems with residual NVP monomer in the gels was noted.[15] Fibroblast adhesiveness to P-NVP gels has also been measured *in vitro*.[40] It was determined that increasing the concentration of the gel (relative to water) from 40% to 96% renders it more adhesive to the cells.

The difficulties involved in preparing homogeneous P-NVP materials makes NVP an ideal monomer for use in covalent surface grafting systems. Both NVP and NVP/HEMA mixtures have been radiation-grafted to Silastic substrates.[21, 23, 28] Results for myoblast cell adhesion were similar to those noted above for P-HEMA grafts. Radiation-grafted P-NVP on Silastic vena cava rings showed greatly reduced thrombus deposits relative to the untreated ring[24] (FIGURE 3), although renal embolus ring studies showed moderate to extensive embolus damage, similar to the grafted P-HEMA rings.[41]

Poly(vinyl Alcohol)

Poly(vinyl alcohol) (PVA) is a water-soluble polymer formed by the partial hydrolysis of poly(vinyl acetate). A number of uses in the biomedical field have been found for crosslinked gels of PVA.

A crosslinked, highly porous sponge of PVA can be formed by reacting formaldehyde with soluble PVA and blowing air through the solution before the polymerization-crosslinking process is completed. This material was commercially available under the name Ivalon® and had been extensively used in hernia treatment, duct replacement, cardiovascular surgery, plastic surgery, and reconstructive surgery. Healing problems with Ivalon sponges were encountered, and it was concluded that Ivalon did not merit the early enthusiasm expressed for it, and that other synthetics would be more satisfactory in similar situations.[42]

A hydrogel consisting of PVA and the anticoagulant heparin, crosslinked together with glutaraldehyde/formaldehyde mixtures has been synthesized, and demonstrated low thrombogenicity in *in vitro* tests.[43] Experiments with ^{35}S-labeled heparin indicated that heparin does not leach out of the crosslinked gel. A potential problem with this material is that, possibly due to the presence of heparin, it shows a tendency to adsorb blood platelets. PVA-heparin hydrogels have also been evaluated for use as hemodialysis membranes.[44] They may show promise for this application, since the permeability to "middle-molecular weight" molecules such as inulin is much higher for PVA-heparin hydrogels than for Cuprophan® cellophane hemodialysis membranes.

Charged Hydrogels

Anionic and cationic hydrogels may be formed by the copolymerization of small amounts of anionic or cationic monomers with neutral hydrogel monomers. They can also be prepared by modification of polymeric hydrogels, such as the partial hydrolysis of polyacrylonitrile, polyacrylamide, or poly(hydroxyalkyl methacrylates) or, in the case of polyelectrolyte complexes, the addition of an excess of the polyanion or polycation component.

The interest in such hydrogel systems stems from observations on the surface charges on blood cells, blood vessel walls, and other tissue types. Under normal conditions the blood vessel walls and blood cells have a negative charge. It is generally thought that negatively charged surfaces should be less thrombogenic than positively charged ones, and experiments have been performed that support this contention.[46] However, results indicating decreased thrombogenicity for positively charged surfaces have also been presented.[15, 47] The role of charge density (as opposed to total charge) has been suggested as an important factor with respect to the thrombogenicity of surfaces.[48] At the present time, the importance of surface charge in blood-hydrogel interactions is not at all clear.

Polyelectrolyte complexes are polysalts formed by the coreaction of a cationic polymer [such as poly(vinyl benzyltrimethyl-ammonium chloride)] and an anionic polymer [such as sodium poly(styrene sulfonate)]. The complex formed from these two particular polyelectrolytes was developed by the Amicon Corporation and is referred to as Ioplex 101®. It has received biomedical evaluation in a number of situations.[49, 50]

Because of mechanical strength limitations, such polyelectrolyte complexes have been generally used as coatings on fabrics and other supports. In order to be used for coatings, the gel must be solubilized in a complex multicomponent solvent system usually containing water, a polar, water soluble organic solvent, and a strong electrolyte. Ioplex solvent solutions have often been strongly acidic and have been shown to degrade certain plastics such as nylon 6,6, thus making the requirements for a suitable reinforcing substrate for the polyelectrolyte complex more stringent.[51] Hoffman has suggested a way to radiation-graft a polyelectrolyte complex onto a polymer substrate, in a two-step process using monomeric precursors.[52]

Difficulties have been found in the sterilization of Ioplex materials. Autoclave sterilization of these complexes can result in disintegration of the gel structure, and gas sterilization can leave entrapped ethylene oxide in the matrix.[51] The problems encountered in sterilizing these hydrogels have been reviewed.[3, 53]

Despite these problems, however, there remain certain advantages in the use of these materials. For example, a net charge (anionic or cationic) can readily be incorporated in the system. This is done by adding stoichiometrically greater or lesser amounts of one of the two polymeric components during formulation. It was determined with the *in vivo* vena cava ring test that Ioplex 101 containing 0.5 meq excess anionic component showed the greatest thromboresistance.[51] Cationic Ioplexes and gels containing an increased number of anionic sites were more thrombogenic.

Horbett and Hoffman have demonstrated significant effects of increasing hydrogel anionic charge (by adding increasing amounts of methacrylic acid in P-HEMA gels) on plasma protein adsorption, particularly in the absence of added salt.[22] Rosen *et al.* have noted important differences in the density and thickness of the collagenous encapsulation around extravascular implants of neutral, cationic and anionic P-HEMA hydrogels.[54]

The *in vitro* thrombogenicity of hydrogels of AAm copolymerized with a number of anionic and cationic monomers was studied by Halpern and coworkers[15] and Halpern and Blessings,[45] using the Lee-White technique. Only the dimethylaminoethyl methacrylate-acrylamide hydrogel showed a significant extension in clotting times. As mentioned above, polyelectrolyte complexes containing a small excess of the anionic component were found to have the lowest thrombogenicity in *in vivo* studies.[48] These two results seem to be contradictory, since the dimethylaminoethyl methacrylate-acrylamide hydrogel would be positively charged at physiological pH, but the anionic polyelectrolyte complex would have a negative charge.

A radiation-grafted copolymer of 98% vinyl acetate with 2% crotonic acid (of which 60% is subsequently ionized to the Na^+ form) has shown negligible thrombus accumulation in the vena cava ring test after 14 days' implantation.[55] This supports the arguments in favor of a small negative charge on the surface.

"Hydrophilic/Hydrophobic Hydrogels"

It is also possible to synthesize hydrogels with varying water contents by either of two techniques: 1) mixing hydrophilic and hydrophobic monomers in varying ratios and then bulk- or graft-copolymerizing the mixtures, or 2) converting a hydrophobic (or hydrophilic) polymer by, for example, hydrolysis (or esterification, acylation). Very little is known about the effects of such compositional variations on the interaction of blood or blood components.

In one recent study Sasaki *et al.* have prepared radiation-grafted copolymers of ethyl methacrylate (EMA) and HEMA on Silastic surfaces.[56] Weathersby has found that fibrinogen adsorption to these surfaces decreases with increasing HEMA/EMA ratio in the grafting solution (note that the data has been normalized assuming a planar surface) (FIGURE 4).[57] He has also studied the molecular weights of the proteins adsorbing from plasma on P-EMA and P-HEMA surfaces, by radiotagging after adsorption, eluting with sodium dodecyl sulfate, running acrylamide gel electrophoresis on the eluate and then slicing and counting the poly(acrylamide) gel.[58] One major difference noted between the two surfaces is the presence of a small peak at ca. 102,000 molecular weight on P-EMA; this peak was absent on P-HEMA. Another striking feature of his results is that two protein peaks observed on both surfaces were at ca. 26,000 and 12,000 molecular weights. Neither of these peaks is from albumin, γ-globulin or fibrinogen. In fact, these two low molecular weight proteins have not been mentioned in the literature of plasma or blood interactions with foreign surfaces. At the present time these peaks remain unidentified, but the investigation into their composition and significance is continuing.[57]

[**Note Added in Proof:** It is possible that the 12,000 molecular weight peak is hemoglobin; this could have significant implications for nonthrombogenic vs. thrombogenic surfaces.]

Dr. James Whiffen (University of Wisconsin) has implanted vena cava rings of the same compositions as those studied by Sasaki *et al.*[56] and Weathersby[57] (FIGURE 5). The pure EMA grafts (FIGURE 5)[56] or untreated Silastic rings (FIGURE 1)[24] both show extensive thrombus deposits, but as little as 1 HEMA/3 EMA in the grafting solution is sufficient to render the surface thromboresistant (or nonthromboadherent) by this test. Two-week vena cava tests or renal embolus tests have not yet been performed, but these preliminary results suggest that materials with mixed hydrophilic/hydrophobic character ought to be investigated further.

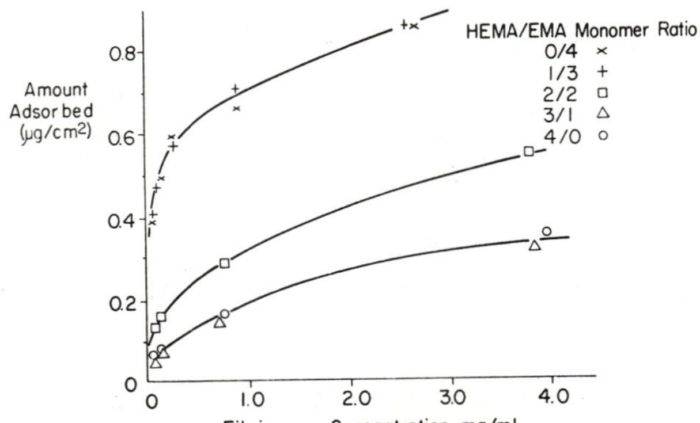

FIGURE 4. Adsorption isotherms for fibrinogen on radiation-grafted HEMA/EMA mixtures on Silastic films.[57]

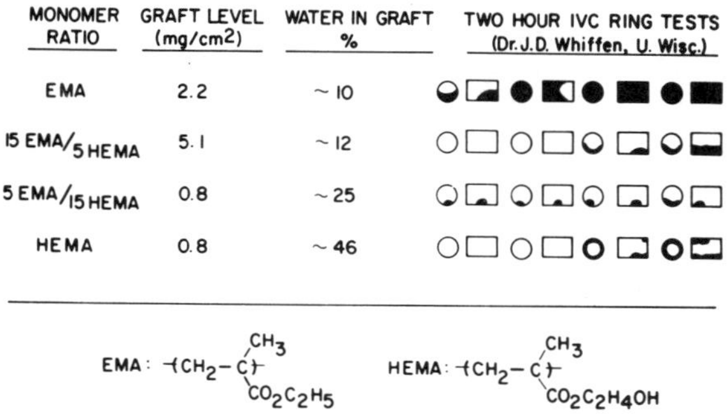

FIGURE 5. Results of vena cava ring tests for radiation-grafted HEMA/EMA mixtures on Silastic rings.[56] (Data of Dr. James D. Whiffen. Department of Surgery, University of Wisconsin Medical School, Madison, Wis.)

ACKNOWLEDGMENTS

The authors would like to thank Dr. James D. Whiffen for his collaboration in the vena cava ring studies (FIGURES 3, 5).

They would also like to express their appreciation to the personnel of the Chemical Engineering Department (Prof. S. Sideman, Head), Technion, Haifa, Israel, and the Laboratoire de Chimie Macromoléculaire sous Rayonnement (C.N.R.S.) (Dr. A. Chapiro, Head) for help in preparing this manuscript.

REFERENCES

1. HOMSY, C. A. 1970. J. Biomed. Mater. Res. **4:** 341.
2. HOFFMAN, A. S. 1974. J. Biomed. Mater. Res. Sympos. no. **5** (Part 1)**:** 77.
3. BRUCK, S. D. 1973. Biomat. Med. Dev. Artif. Organs **7:** 387.
4. LEE, H. B. *et al.* 1974. ACS Polymer Preprints **15**(1)**:** 706.
5. LEE, H. B. *et al.* 1975. J. Colloid Interface Sci. **51:** 225.
6. KHAW, B. *et al.* 1975. ACS Polymer Preprints **16**(2)**:** 446.
7. HOFFMAN, A. S. 1975. Hydrogels, a broad class of biomaterials. *In* Polymers in Medicine and Surgery. R. L. Kronenthal *et al.,* Eds. : 33–34. Plenum Press. New York, N.Y.
8. RATNER, B. D. & A. S. HOFFMAN. 1976. Synthetic hydrogels for biomedical applications. *In* Hydrogels for Medical and Related Applications. J. D. Andrade, Ed. ACS Symposium Series 31. ACS. Washington, D.C.
9. WICHTERLE, O. 1971. *In* Encyclopedia of Polymer Science and Technology. H. F. Mark & N. G. Gaylord, Eds. Vol. **15:** 273. J. Wiley & Sons. New York, N.Y.
10. WICHTERLE, O. & D. LIM. 1960. Nature **185:** 117.
11. LEVOWITZ, B. S. *et al.* 1968. Trans. Amer. Soc. Artif. Int. Org. **14:** 82.
12. WARREN, A. *et al.* 1967. Surgical Forum **18:** 183.
13. SINGH, M. P. 1969. Biomed. Eng. **4:** 68.
14. SINGH, M. P. & D. G. MELROSE. 1971. Biomed. Eng. **6:** 157.
15. HALPERN, B. D. *et al.* 1969. *In* NHLI Artif. Heart Prog. Conf. Proc. R. J. Hegyeli, Ed.: 87. U.S. Government Printing Office. Washington, D.C.
16. VROMAN, L. *et al.* 1971. Fed. Proc. Fed. Amer. Soc. Exp. Biol. **30:** 1494.
17. BAIER, R. E. & R. C. DUTTON. 1969. J. Biomed. Mater. Res. **3:** 191.

18. MADRAS, P. N. *et al.* 1971. Fed. Proc., Fed. Amer. Soc. Exp. Biol. **30:** 1665.
19. FRIEDMAN, L. I. *et al.* 1970. Trans. Amer. Soc. Art. Int. Org. **16:** 63.
20a. HOFFMAN, A. S. & W. G. KRAFT. 1972. ACS Polymer Preprints **13**(2): 723.
20b. HOFFMAN, A. S. & C. HARRIS. 1972. ACS Polymer Preprints **13**(2): 740.
21a. RATNER, B. D. & A. S. HOFFMAN. 1974. J. Appl. Polymer Sci. **18:** 3183.
21b. RATNER, B. D. & A. S. HOFFMAN. 1975. *In* Biomedical Applications of Polymers. H. P. Gregor, Ed. : 159. Plenum Press. New York, N.Y.
22. HORBETT, T. A. & A. S. HOFFMAN. ACS Advances in Chemistry Series. R. E. Baier, Ed. Vol. **145:** 230. ACS. Washington, D.C.
23. RATNER, B. D. *et al.* 1975. J. Biomed. Mater. Res. **9:** 407.
24. RATNER, B. D. *et al.* 1975. Biomat. Med. Dev. Artif. Org. **3:** 115.
25. HOLLY, F. J. & M. F. REFOJO. 1975. ACS Polymer Preprints **16**(2): 426.
26. MUZYKWICZ, K. J. et al. 1975. J. Biomed. Mater. Res. **9:** 487.
27. KUSSEROW, B. K. *et al.* 1972. Annual Report for 1972 to NHLI, NIH. Contract PH 43–68–1427.
28. HOFFMAN, A.S. *et al.* 1972. Trans. Amer. Soc. Artif. Int. Org. **18:** 10.
29. KUDELA, K. *et al.* 1974. Europ. Polymer J. **10:** 905.
30. BRUCK, S. D. 1973. Biomat. Med. Dev. Artif. Org. **1:** 79.
31. NGUYEN, A. & G. L. WILKES. 1974. J. Biomed. Mater. Res. **8:** 261.
32. KEARNEY, J. J. *et al.* 1975. *In* Biomed. Appl. of Polymers. H. P. Gregor, Ed. : 75. Plenum Press. New York, N.Y.
33. LEONARD, E. *et al.* 1975. Annual Report for 1974 to NHLI, NIH. Contract 1–HB–3–2910–1.
34. JENKINS, L. B. *et al.* 1956. A.M.A. Arch. Surg. **72:** 612.
35. MOHN, G. 1960. Acta Histochem. **9:** 76.
36. BURNETTE, L. W. 1962. Proc. Sci. Section T.G.A. **38:** 1.
37. RIVANO, R. *et al.* 1957. Path. (Genoa) **49:** 301
38. RICHARDS, B. & H. PERSIDSKY. 1964. J. Cardiovasc. Surg. **5:** 313.
39. LUTTINGER, M. & C. W. COOPER. 1967. J. Biomed. Mater. Res. **1:** 67.
40. MAROUDAS, N. G. 1975. Nature **254:** 695.
41. KUSSEROW, B. K. 1974. Personal communication. Oct. 31.
42. ALDER, R. H. & C. DARBY. 1960. U.S. Armed Forces Med. J. **11:** 1349.
43. MERRILL, E. W. *et al.* 1970. J. Appl. Physiol. **29:** 723.
44. MERRILL, E. W. *et al.* 1972. ACS Polymer Preprints. **13**(1): 511.
45. HALPERN, B. D. & H. W. BLESSINGS. 1973. Annual Report for 1972 to NHLI, NIH. Contract PH 43–66–1124.
46. SAWYER, P. N. & S. SRINIVASAN. 1969. *In* NHLI Artif. Heart Prog. Conf. Proc. R. J. Hegyeli, Ed. : 243. U.S. Govt. Print. Off. Washington, D.C.
47. WALTER, C. W. *et al.* 1951. Surg. Forum. **2:** 289.
48. LEONARD, F. 1969. Trans. Amer. Soc. Artif. Int. Org. **15:** 15.
49. MARKLEY, L. L. *et al.* 1968. J. Biomed. Mater. Res. **2:** 145.
50. MARSHALL, D. W. *et al.* 1970. J. Biomed. Mater. Res. **4:** 357.
51. BIXLER, H. J. *et al.* 1969. *In* NHLI artif. Heart Prog. Conf. Proc. R. J. Hegyeli, Ed. : U.S. Govt. Print. Office. Washington, D.C.
52. HOFFMAN, A. S. 1970. Isotopes & Rad. Tech. **8**(1): 84.
53. BRUCK, S. D. 1971. J. Biomed. Mater. Res. **5:** 139.
54. ROSEN, J. J. *et al.* 1975. ACS Polymer Preprints **16**(2).
55. KWIATKOWSKI, G. T. *et al.* 1973. Annual Report for 1972–1973 to NHLI, NIH. Contract NO1–HL3–2950 T.
56. SASAKI, T. *et al.* 1975. ACS Polymer Preprints **16**(2): 435.
57. WEATHERSBY, P. 1976. Ph.D. Thesis. Chem. Eng. Dept. Univ. of Washington. Seattle, Wash.
58. WEATHERSBY, P. K., *et al.* 1976. Trans. Amer. Soc. Artif. Int. Organs **22:** 242.

CARBON IN PROSTHETICS

Axel Haubold

Medical Products Division
General Atomic Company
San Diego, California 92121

The passive nature of carbon in tissue has been known since ancient times. Charcoal and lampblack were used for ornamental and official tattoos by many.

Over the past ten years, other forms of carbon have been studied for possible biomedical applications stimulated primarily by Gott's original studies.[1] The various common forms of carbon that have received attention are artificial graphites, vitreous or glassy carbons, carbon fibers, pyrolytic carbons, composites, and vacuum vapor-deposited carbon coatings. Among the pure forms of carbon, the pyrolytic carbons and the glassy carbons have been studied in detail and have been subjected to extensive testing. These materials have found clinical applications in the cardiovascular, orthopedic, and dental areas as well as long-term transcutaneous applications. This is a result not only of the biocompatibility and inertness demonstrated by these materials but also of the fact that the physical properties can be controlled and in many cases tailored to fit the intended application.

The biological properties of pyrolytic carbons have been well-summarized by Bruck[2, 3] and others,[4-13] and Benson[14] surveyed the data on vitreous carbons and other types of carbon. The physical and engineering properties necessary for effective utilization of the various types of carbon have been documented and compared.[15-29] These studies have led to the development and use of prosthetic carbon devices. This paper reviews the current clinical applications of pyrolytic and vitreous carbons, presents applications undergoing preclinical trials, and describes some new forms of carbon under development.

Cardiovascular Applications

It has been almost a quarter of a century since Hufnagel and Harvey[30] implanted the first artificial heart valve. Since that time, open-heart procedures have become not only a technical reality but also commonplace. The use of prosthetic valves has been successful in salvaging otherwise hopeless patients.

The earliest prosthetic valves were simple check valves, polymeric balls in metal cages. In the short term, these valves functioned well. With increasing usage, however, thromboembolic complications, valve malfunctions, and mechanical failures became more common.[31-34] The polymeric balls were found to be susceptible to biochemical degradation. Replacement of the polymeric poppets with hollow metal balls limited the biodegradation but resulted in other difficulties because of the galling tendency of metal-to-metal contacts.[35-40] Other valve designs emerged gradually. These were primarily low-profile valves with tilting, pivoting, or free-floating disk-shaped occluders. These valves have been shown to have superior hemodynamic characteristics but were susceptible to many of the same problems encountered with ball valves. Disk wear and variance were particularly important complications.

The use of carbon in place of polymeric occluders has virtually eliminated the problems associated with wear, distortion, and biodegradation, because of the mechanical durability, inertness, and biocompatibility of carbon. Through February 1976, more than 130,000 pyrolytic carbon components have been produced for clinical use in prosthetic valves. Probably more than 100,000 components have been implanted since the first clinical prosthetic valve utilizing a hollow, pyrolytic carbon ball was implanted by DeBakey in 1969. There have been no failures of the pyrolytic components in normal use.[12]

Some valves currently utilize pyrolytic carbon coatings for all blood-contacting surfaces. Still other valves are being developed to use the properties of

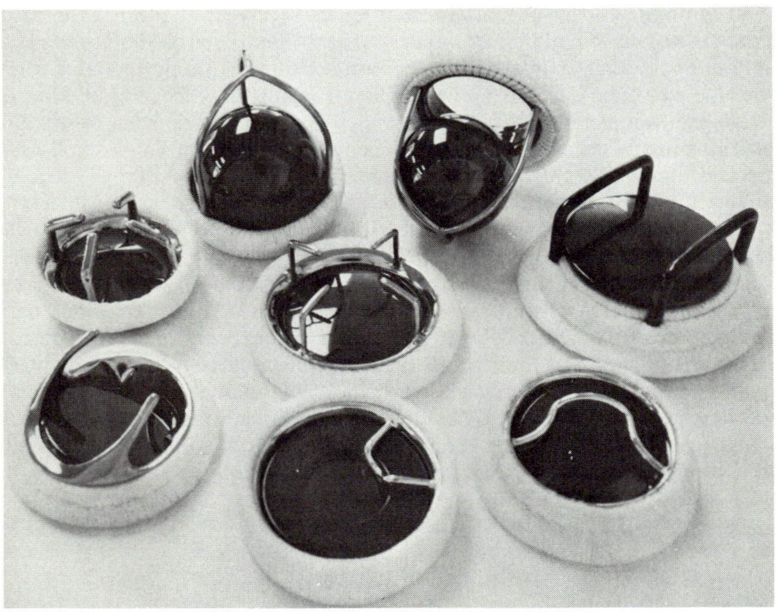

FIGURE 1. Prosthetic heart valves with pyrolytic carbon components.

pyrolytic or glassy carbons to produce an all-carbon valve. An excellent status report on valve replacements through 1975 is available.[41] FIGURE 1 shows a number of clinical prosthetic heart valves that use pyrolytic carbon components.

Since x rays are not absorbed to any great extent by carbon, methods are under development to make the various carbon components visible on an x ray. Some components such as hollow ball or hollow conical occluders have been visible in an x ray because of the presence of a tungsten screen in the hollow cavity. Disk occluders with a thin metal foil embedded in the substrate are currently undergoing tests. The thin metal foils are radiopaque and reveal the disk position as a white ring in an x ray.

The large number of valve designs and types that have appeared over the years indicate, however, that many problems still exist. To complicate the situa-

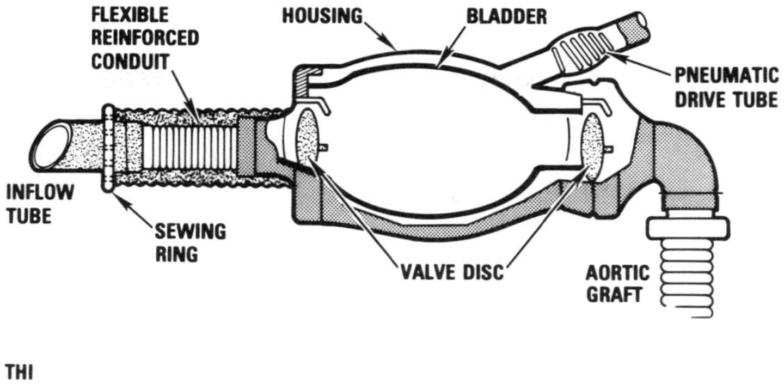

FIGURE 2a. Intracorporeal left ventricular assist device (Texas Heart Institute, Houston, Texas). Schematic.

tion further, long-term implications often show the existence of unanticipated problems. Nevertheless, the eight-year clinical history of pyrolytic carbon in prosthetic heart valves has been encouraging and has proved the value of this material.

Pyrolytic carbon components are being considered for use in left-ventricular assist devices. A schematic of an intracorporeal left-ventricular assist device undergoing clinical trials at the Texas Heart Institute, Houston, Texas, is shown in FIGURE 2a. The inlet tube (see FIGURE 2b) and the valve occluders will, in all likelihood, be pyrolytic carbon.[42]

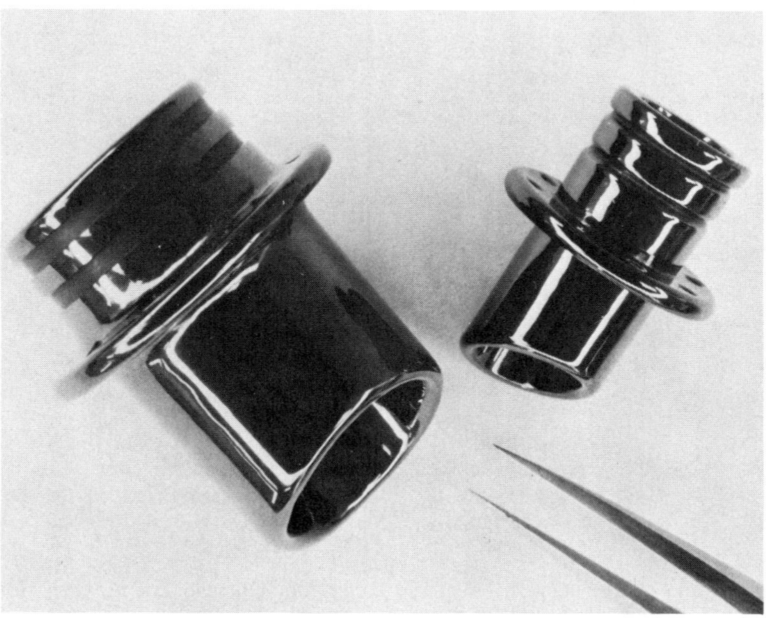

FIGURE 2b. Prototype of pyrolytic carbon inlet tubes. See FIGURE 2a legend.

Through-the-Skin Access

In 1967, it was suggested that carbon might provide the means for gaining chronic access through the skin.[14] Work during the past ten years has shown that both vitreous carbon and pyrolytic carbon conduits can be used successfully for electrical and mechanical access. A number of researchers have used carbon devices for neural stimulation and blockage, muscle stimulation, skeletal attachments, and provision of access ports.

Researchers and clinicians at Rancho Los Amigos Hospital, Downey, Calif., have used carbon and titanium pedestals for a variety of applications.[43-47] Shown in Figure 3a is a typical external electrode/transcutaneous device pair. A magnetic coupling to hold the external wire in physical contact has minimized the stress on the through-the-skin device. This advancement has overcome previous problems encountered with wires inadvertently becoming snagged and putting excessive load on the tissue/device interface, with resultant trauma. Devices of this type have been used for the chronic control of pain as well as the control of contractures. More recently, a number of these electrode assemblies have been used in a biofeedback system for myoelectric control of a prosthesis (see Figure 3b).

The neuroprosthesis program at the University of Utah, Salt Lake City, Utah, is using pyrolytic carbon buttons to house special high-density electrical connectors to allow chronic stimulation of the cochlea for artificial hearing. Deaf volunteers have been implanted for more than a year with typically six to eight electrodes, all contained in a single transcutaneous device. These electrodes

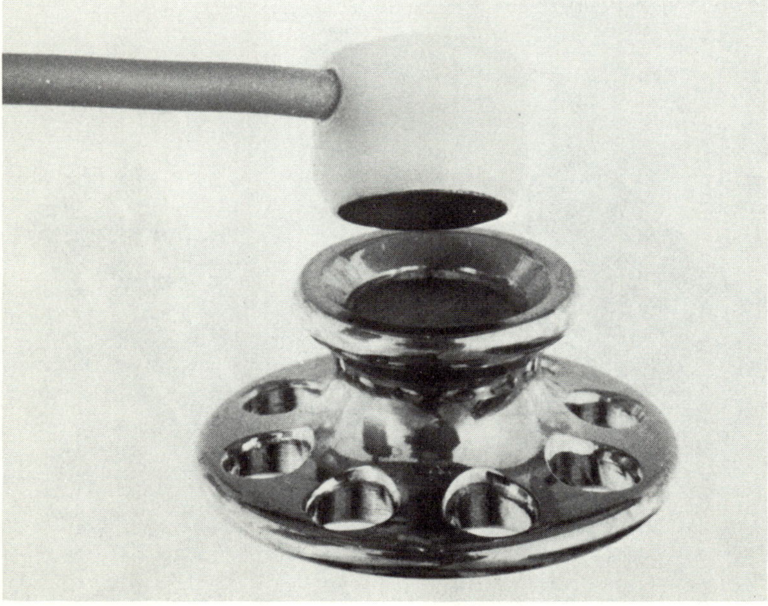

Figure 3a. Transcutaneous electrical connectors (Rancho Los Amigos Hospital, Downey, Calif.), typical external electrode/transcutaneous device pair.

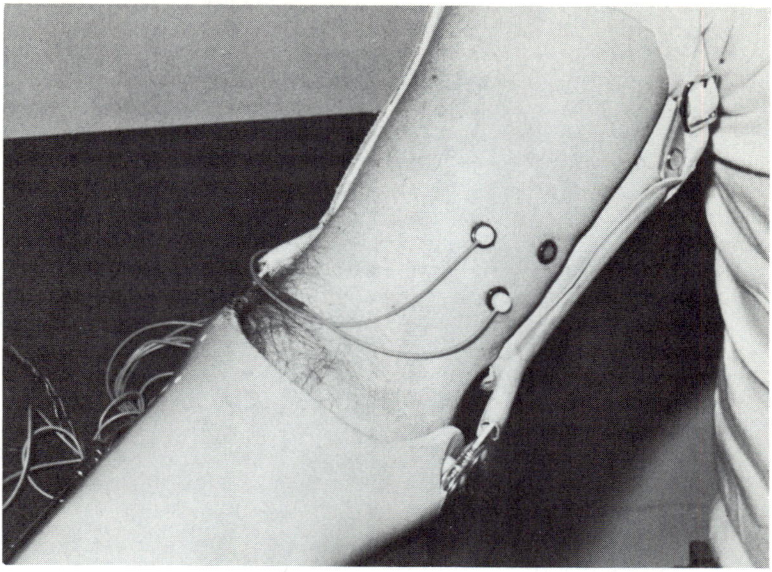

FIGURE 3b. Connectors in use for myoelectric control of a prosthesis (four months after insertion). See FIGURE 3a legend.

are placed at various points in the cochlea to take advantage of the cochlea's tonotopic spatial organization. The initial results are very encouraging and have shown not only that the tonotopic spatial organization can be effectively used for artificial hearing but also that it may be possible to achieve a pitch continuum through the use of both place stimulation and pitch modulation.[48]

Using a similar multiple electrode approach, researchers in the artificial vision program have been able to transmit useful visual information directly to the brain through stimulation of the visual cortex.[49] In this case, 64 electrodes (embedded in a Teflon® matrix) terminate in a special high-density connector housed in a relatively small (15-mm-diameter) pyrolytic carbon through-the-skin device (see FIGURE 4).

Carbon has recently been proposed as a possible urinary conduit.[50] Urinary diversion or bypassing of obstructions, either acquired or congenital, has been moderately successful but is frequently unsatisfactory in the long run because of skin irritation and infection. One of the primary difficulties is the inability to seal the collection device effectively around a stoma, resulting in stomal inflammation and peristomal skin changes.

A carbon conduit that extends well above the skin line may alleviate this problem by allowing the formation of a good mechanical seal with the collection device, thereby eliminating the tissue adhesives currently in use. The rigid conduit should also be relatively easy to clean. This potential application results not only from the compatibility of pyrolytic and vitreous carbons with tissue but also from the fact that, in addition to their compatibility, the materials' mechanical properties allow the formation of complex shapes.

Researchers have long sought a permanent blood-access device. The demon-

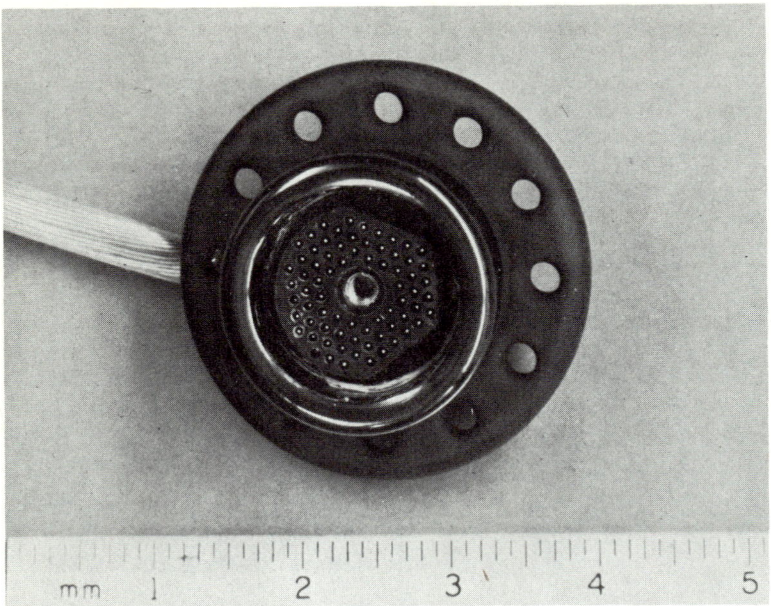

FIGURE 4. Transcutaneous electrical connector (University of Utah, Salt Lake City, Utah).

strated blood compatibility of pyrolytic carbon and its ability to function transcutaneously have resulted in several potential designs suitable for single-needle dialysis. Animal trials have been initiated; but this development is still in its infancy, and designs are changing as more is learned.

Pyrolytitc and vitreous carbons have been studied since 1971 as a possible artificial tooth root,[51] i.e., an implantable support for a single tooth, a bridge, or even a complete denture. This is a considerably different application from those described above but is, nevertheless, an important through-the-skin application.

A number of metals and ceramics in a variety of configurations have been used for this purpose. Porous coatings designed to allow bone ingrowth to secure the implant and to distribute stresses have been tested. The mechanical properties of the implant are crucial to long-term success, since the formation and resorption of bone are influenced by stresses.[52] The elastic properties of many types of carbon have been measured and are in the range reported for bone,[20] whereas most metals are an order of magnitude stiffer. This means that a carbon/bone composite will be a more uniform load-bearing member than a metal/bone composite.

Blade-type implants fabricated from pyrolytic carbon have evolved as a result of exploratory studies. Details of the design evolution, mechanical properties, and animal test results have been reported.[53, 54] The blade design is currently undergoing clinical trials. Vitreous carbon supports have been in use for several years. Schematics of both types of implants are shown in FIGURE 5. The differences in designs are necessitated by the differences in the mechanical properties of the two types of carbon. The vitreous carbon post design has worked reasonably well in healthy bone for single-tooth replacements[55, 56] and for securing bridges, but the thinner, blade-design pyrolytic carbon device can be used where some bone degeneration has already taken place.

The above-mentioned experiences certainly demonstrate that carbon can function well in chronic through-the-skin applications, but more work remains to be done. The transcutaneous devices used by Rancho Los Amigos Hospital researchers and most other researchers are free-floating in tissue secured only by tissue ingrowth into holes in the device specifically provided for this purpose. In this way, the device can move to some extent with the tissue. The risk of excess stress at the tissue/device interface is an ever-present problem but has been minimized by the use of magnetic coupling for the electrical leads. Other researchers, notably those at the University of Utah, fix the device securely to bone with screws. It would at first appear that this technique could increase the probability of high stresses at the tissue/device interface, since the implant is not allowed to move, but this conjecture is not borne out by experience. Volunteers have "worn" the devices for more than a year with no pain, discomfort, or infection.

The optimum surface topography that is required to form the best bacterial seal has not been identified,[57] primarily because no systematic study has been carried out. Nevertheless, the use of carbon devices has been shown to be a feasible technique for chronic through-the-skin access.

Orthopedics

Carbon devices, because of their biological and mechanical properties, were very early considered for orthopedic applications. However, since the metallic implants commonly in use at that time seemed to function well, this area was not pursued. Indeed, total or partial replacement of joints with metallic prostheses had resulted for many patients in relief of pain and had allowed new freedom of movement for others.

Long-term implantations unfortunately have shown that degradation of metal

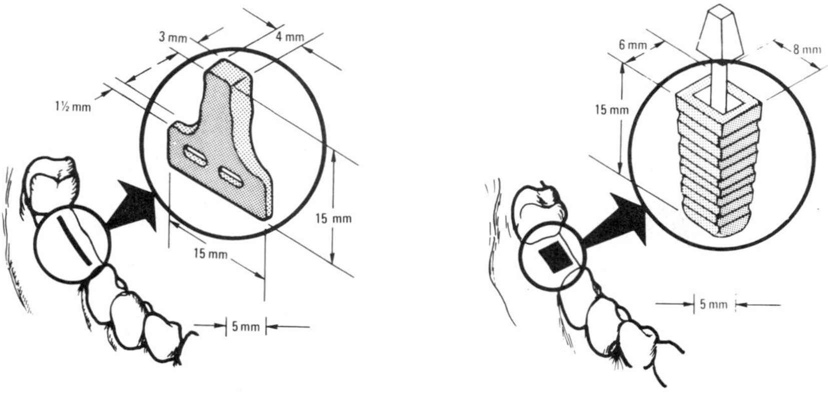

FIGURE 5. Typical carbon dental implants: pyrolytic carbon (on left) and vitreous carbon (on right).

prostheses does occur. Finely divided metal particles are often found in the surrounding soft tissue.[58, 59] These particles may result because of galling of the metal-to-metal contacts or because of wear.[59, 60] Furthermore, it has been found that although the bulk material may be reasonably well-tolerated by the body, finely divided particles of the same material can lead to severe and even carcinogenic complications[61] in test animals. Consequently, prostheses were developed which are composed of a metallic member and a polymeric member (typically high-density polyethylene). This combination has essentially eliminated *in-vivo* galling of the metal, but a suitable nonwearing polymer for high-load-bearing conditions has not yet been found. Another complication with metallic load-bearing prostheses is a result of the mismatch between the elastic properties of metals and bone. This is the same situation which has caused problems with metallic endosseous dental implants.[62]

For some applications, such as finger joints, an all-polymeric prosthesis made of pure silicon rubber was developed.[63, 64] These devices seem to function well in low-load applications but are not useful in active individuals.

Because of the long-term results described above, there has been a renewed interest in carbons for orthopedic applications. The success of pyrolytic carbon dental implants confirms the need for a close match of the elastic properties of the implant and the bone to prevent bone resorption. Shown in FIGURE 6 are two examples of orthopedic devices fabricated from pyrolytic carbon.

The wear properties of pyrolytic carbon indicate that the higher-density pyrolytic carbons should be more durable than high-density polyethylene. The lower-density pyrolytic carbons and vitreous carbons probably are unsuited for orthopedic applications. Wear products, presumably finely divided carbon par-

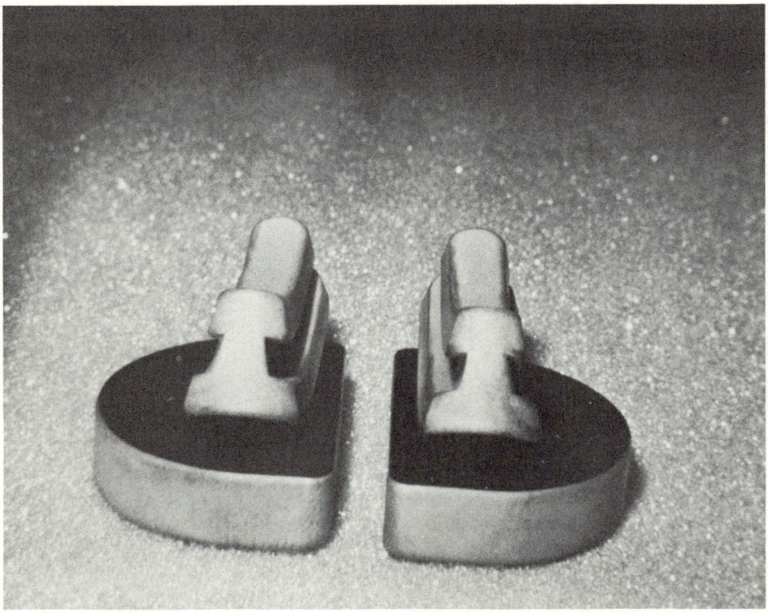

FIGURE 6a. Experimental orthopedic device: kneejoint.

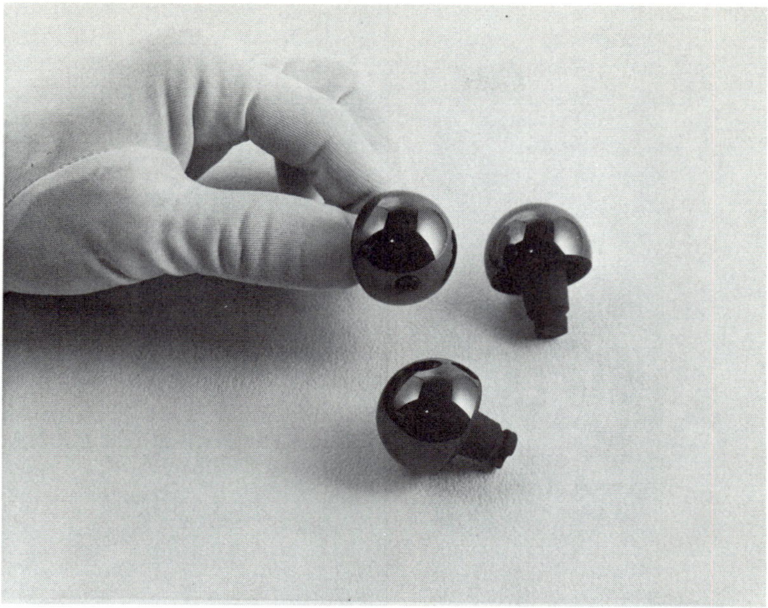

FIGURE 6b. Experimental orthopedic device: femur head.

ticles (which may be unavoidable), should not result in the formation of foreign-body giant cells in the synovial lining of joints, as in the case with polyethylene,[65] or possible cytotoxic effects, as is the case with metals,[66] since even finely divided carbon particles have been shown to be well-tolerated by the body.[14]

VACUUM VAPOR-DEPOSITED CARBONS

The properties of vacuum vapor-deposited carbons are being investigated. This material has the potential of complementing pyrolytic carbon and may result in a new class of biocompatible surfaces. Thin carbon coatings deposited under vacuum conditions can be applied to metals and polymers and on geometries that cannot reasonably be fabricated from pyrolytic carbon, vitreous carbon, or other bulk forms.

Although the mechanisms responsible for the biocompatible properties demonstrated by pyrolytic carbon are not well-understood, the physical and chemical properties of this material are well known. Consequently, as a starting point, the physical and chemical properties of vacuum vapor-deposited films are being tailored by appropriate processing parameters to resemble, as closely as possible, the measured properties of pyrolytic carbon. In this respect, thin carbon films have been produced that are isotropic, have a density of about 1.8 g/cm^3, have a crystallite size on the order of 8 to 15 Å, are impermeable to gases at film thicknesses of $>$1000 Å, have high purity, are not susceptible to fluid friction erosion, and bond well to many substrates.[67]

In-vivo and *in-vitro* tests sponsored by the National Institutes of Health,

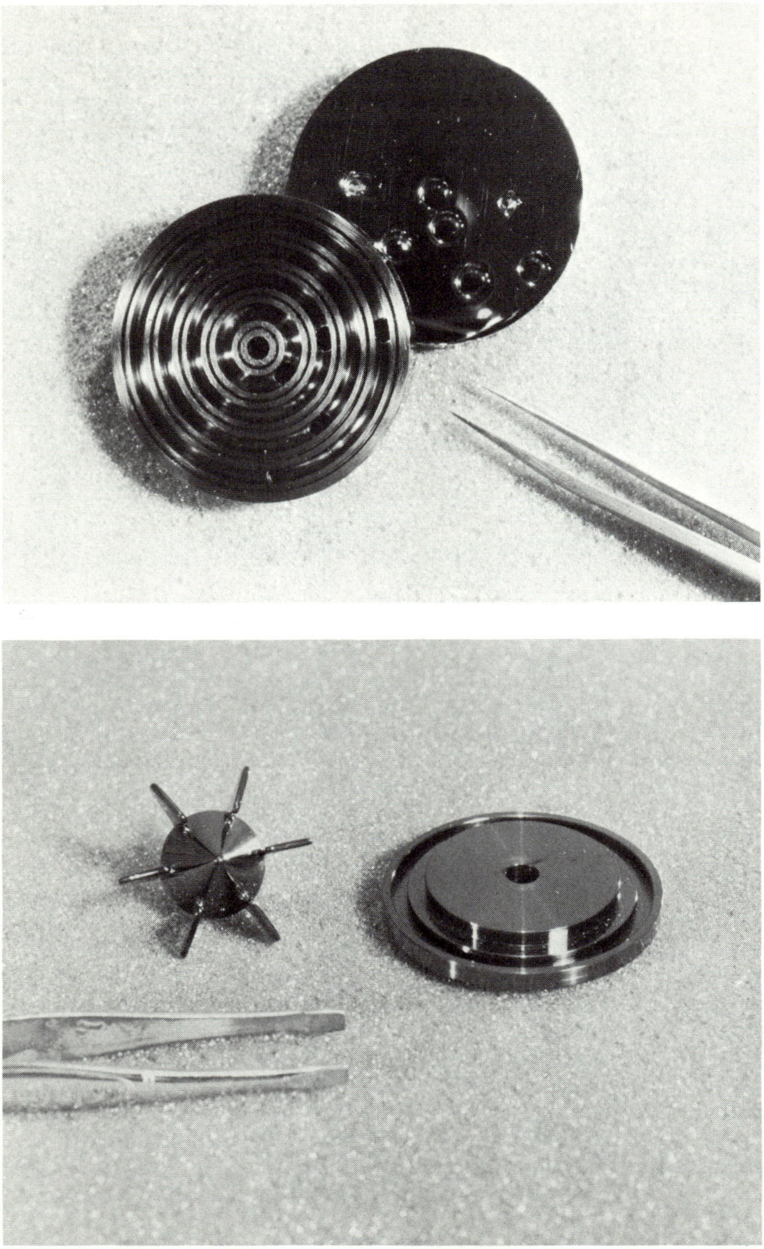

FIGURE 7. *Top* and *bottom:* Experimental metallic blood-handling device components coated with a thin layer of isotropic carbon.

Bethesda, Maryland, are beginning to show that the original assumptions are valid. Vena cava test results are mixed to very good; renal embolus results are very good.[10, 68] Adherence and interaction with blood proteins are being studied. Corrosion experiments currently under way indicate that the thin impermeable carbon coating may well prevent biodegradation and galvanic degradation of metallic implants. Not only are the mechanical properties of an implant retained, but furthermore, the thin carbon coating presents an inert surface to tissue. Metallic components of experimental blood-handling devices coated with a thin layer of isotropic carbon are shown in FIGURE 7, *top* and *bottom*.

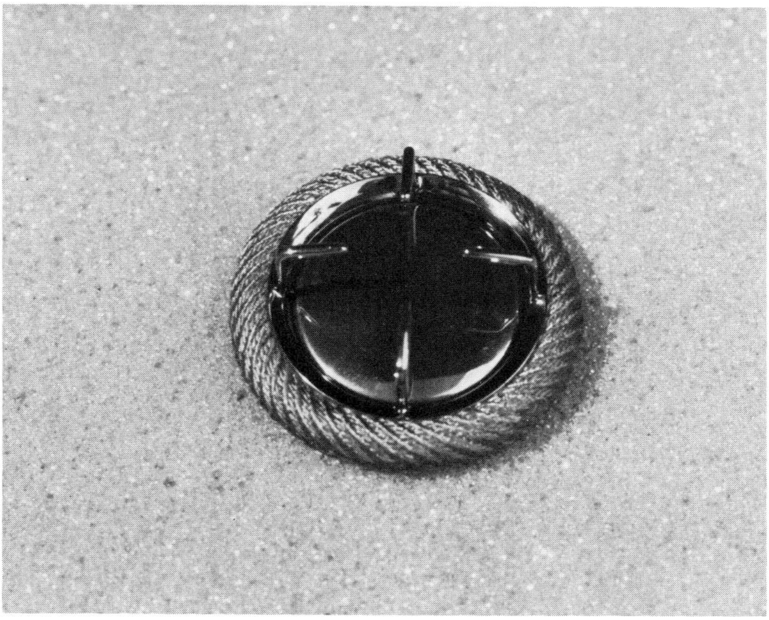

FIGURE 8. Experimental prosthetic heart valve (all components carbon-coated).

In addition to rigid components, devices requiring a certain degree of flexibility can also be coated. Fabrics of Dacron®, polypropylene, and Teflon have been successfully coated with a well-adherent layer of carbon. The biological properties of these coated fabrics are unknown at present but are being studied. Coated, knitted tubes, for example, are being evaluated for use as autogenous reinforced artery grafts. An experimental prosthetic heart valve is shown in FIGURE 8. Both the metallic portion and the sewing ring are carbon-coated; the occluder is pyrolytic carbon. As more is learned about thin carbon films, it is reasonable to conclude that additional uses will be found for carbon, a truly versatile biomaterial.

REFERENCES

1. GOTT, V. L. *et al.* 1961. Surgery **50:** 382.
2. BRUCK, S. D., S. RABIN & R. J. FERGUSON. 1973. Biomater. Med. Dev. Art. Organs **1:** 191.
3. BRUCK, S. D. 1974. Blood Compatible Synthetic Polymers. Charles C Thomas. Springfield, Ill.
4. GOTT, V. L. & A. FURUSE. 1973. Med. Instr. **7:** 121.
5. WHALEN, R. L., D. L. JEFFERY & J. C. NORMAN. 1973. Trans. Am. Soc. Artif. Intern. Organs **19:** 19.
6. HALBERT, S. P., M. ANKEN & A. E. USHAKOFF. 1969. Compatibility of Blood with Materials Useful in the Fabrication of Artificial Organs. National Institutes of Health Annual Rpeort. Contract PH–43–66–980. Cordis Laboratories. Miami, Fla.
7. HEGYELI, R. J., R. GALLAGHER & L. K. PETERSON. 1969. Further studies of the interaction of blood and tissue cells with artificial heart implant candidate materials *in-vitro*. *In* Artificial Heart Program Conference. : 203. National Institutes of Health. Bethesda, Md.
8. SCHOEN, F. J. 1971. Surface studies of carbons for prosthetic applications. *In* Proceedings of 4th Annual Scanning Electron Microscope Symposium. Part **I:** 385. IIT Research Institute. Chicago, Ill.
9. DE PALMA, V. A. *et al.* 1972. J. Biomed. Mater. Res. Symp. **6:** 37.
10. KUSSEROW, B. K., R. W. LARROW & J. E. NICHOLS. 1972. Analysis and Measurement of the Effects of Materials on Blood Leukocytes, Erythrocytes, and Platelets. National Institutes of Health Annual Report. Contract PH–43–68–1427. University of Vermont. Burlington, Vt.
11. BOKROS, J. C., L. D. LAGRANGE & F. J. SCHOEN. 1972. Control of structure of carbon for use in bioengineering. *In* Chemistry and Physics of Carbon. P. L. Walker, Jr. & P. A. Thrower, Eds. Vol. **9:** 103–171. Dekker. New York, N.Y.
12. BOKROS, J. C. *et al.* 1975. Carbon in prosthetic devices. *In* Petroleum Derived Carbons. M. L. Deviney & T. M. O'Grady, Eds. ACS Symposium Series no. **21:** 237–265. American Chemical Society. Washington, D.C.
13. BOKROS, J. C. & R. J. AKINS. 1971. Applications of pyrolytic carbon in artificial heart valves: a status report. *In* Proceedings of 4th Buhl Conference on Materials : 243. Carnegie Press. Pittsburgh, Pa.
14. BENSON, J. 1969. Pre-Survey on Biomedical Applications of Carbon. Report R–7855. North American Rockwell Corp. Canoga Park, Calif.
15. KOTLENSKY, W. V. 1972. Deposition of pyrolytic carbon in porous solids. *In* Chemistry and Physics of Carbon. P. L. Walker, Jr. & P. A. Thrower, Eds. Vol. **9:** 173–261. Dekker. New York, N.Y.
16. KAAE, J. L. 1972. J. Biomed. Mater. Res. **6:** 279.
17. KAAE, J. L. & T. D. GULDEN. 1971. J. Am. Ceram. Soc. **54:** 606.
18. SHIM, H. S. & F. J. SCHOEN. 1974. Biomater. Med. Dev. Art. Org. **2:** 103.
19. SHIM, H. S. 1974. Biomater. Med. Dev. Art. Org. **2:** 55.
20. BOKROS, J. C. 1969. The preparation, structure, and properties of pyrolytic carbon. *In* Chemistry and Physics of Carbon. P. L. Walker, Jr., Ed. Vol. **5:** 1. Dekker. New York, N.Y.
21. GEBHARDT, J. J. & J. M. BERRY. 1965. AIAA J. **3:** 302.
22. COWLARD, F. C. 1970. Design Eng. March : 49.
23. KAAE, J. L. 1971. Carbon **9:** 291.
24. KAAE, J. L. 1975. Carbon **13:** 55.
25. KAAE, J. L. 1975. Carbon **13:** 246.
26. KENNER, G. H. *et al.* 1975. J. Biomed. Mater. Res. **9:** 111.
27. BOKROS, J. C. 1965. Carbon **3:** 201.
28. SCHOEN, F. J. 1973. Carbon **11:** 413.
29. KAAE, J. L. 1971. J. Nucl. Mater. **38:** 42.

30. Hufnagel, C. A. & W. P. Harvey. 1952. Bull. Georgetown Univ. Med. Center **4:** 128.
31. Hylen, J. C. et al. 1970. Ann. Intern. Med. **72:** 1.
32. Roberts, W. C. & A. G. Morrow. 1968. Am. J. Cardiol. **22:** 614.
33. Mellenry, M. M. et al. 1970. J. Thorac. Cardiovasc. Surg. **59:** 113.
34. Hylen, J. C. 1971. Am. Heart J. **81:** 299.
35. Cooley, D. A. *et al.* 1967. Trans. Am. Soc. Artif. Intern. Organs **13:** 93.
36. Starr, A., R. Herr & J. H. Wood. 1969. Accumulated experience with the Starr-Edwards prosthesis 1960–1968. *In* Prosthetic Heart Valve. L. A. Brewer, Ed. Chap. **13:** 468–482. Charles C Thomas. Springfield, Ill.
37. Detmer, D. E. & N. S. Braumwald. 1971. J. Thorac. Cardiovasc. Surg. **61:** 175.
38. Anon. 1968. J. Am. Med. Assoc. **205:** 28.
39. Reis, R. L. *et al.* 1970. J. Thorac. Cardiovasc. Surg. **59:** 84.
40. Schottenfeld, M. *et al.* 1971. Thorax. **26:** 195.
41. Rahimtoola, S. H., Ed. 1975. Am. J. Cardiol. 35 (5 & 6).
42. Norman, J. C. Texas Heart Institute. Houston, Tex. Private communication.
43. Moony, V. *et al.* 1974. Arch. Surg. **108:** 148–153.
44. Kadefors, R. & J. B. Reswick. 1970. Med. Biol. Eng. **8:** 129–135.
45. Mooney, V. & D. B. Hartmann. 1974. Percutaneous passage. *In* Biomedical Electrode Technology. H. A. Miller & D. C. Harrison, Eds. : 329–339. Academic Press. New York, N.Y.
46. Mooney, V. & A. M. Roth. Advances in permanent percutaneous electrode systems. To be published.
47. Reswick, J. B. & V. Mooney. 1975. Amputee Clin. **7:** 5.
48. Mladejovsky, M. G. *et al.* 1975. Trans. Am. Soc. Artif. Intern. Organs **21:** 1–6.
49. Dobelle, W. H. *et al.* 1976. Nature **259:** 111.
50. Longley, J. R. *et al.* Carbon urinary conduits—animal experiments. Unpublished data.
51. Grenoble, D. E. 1973. Ariz. St. Dental J. **19:** 12.
52. Bassett, C. A. 1971. *In* The Biochemistry and Physiology of Bone. 2nd edit. G. H. Bourne, Ed. Vol. **3:** 1. Academic Press. New York, N.Y.
53. Hamner, J. E. & O. M. Reed. 1973. Pyrolite carbon dental implants in baboons: a preliminary report. *In* Medical Primatology. Part **II:** 177. Krager. Basel, Switzerland.
54. Hulbert, S. F. *et al.* 1975. Oral Implant **6:** 79.
55. Grenoble, D. E. & R. L. Kim. 1973. Oral Implant **4:** 216.
56. Reedy, M. T., D. T. Devore & V. P. Thompson. 1974. Oral Implant **5:** 85.
57. Winter, G. D. 1974. J. Biomed. Mater. Res. Symp. **8:** 99.
58. Charosky, C. B., P. G. Bullough & P. D. Wilson. 1973. J. Bone Joint Surg. **55–A:** 49–58.
59. Young, H. H. 1971. J. Bone Joint Surg. **53–A:** 1658.
60. Amstutz, H. C., R. Contini & R. Johnson. 1975. Clin. Orthop. **106:** 131–139.
61. Heath, J. C., M. A. R. Freeman & S. A. V. Swanson. 1971. Lancet. **1:** 564–566.
62. Natiella, J. R. *et al.* 1972. J. Am. Dental Assoc. **84:** 1358.
63. Brody, G. S. & W. L. White. 1963. J. Plastic Recon. Surg. **32:** 45.
64. Swanson, A. 1968. Surg. Clin. N. Am. **48**(5): 1113–1127.
65. Charnley, J. 1969. *In* Reconstruction Surgery and Traumatology. Vol. **2:** 9. Phiebig. New York, N.Y.
66. Winter, G. D. 1974. J. Biomed. Mater. Res. Symp. **8:** 11.
67. Meyer, C. H., Jr. *et al.* 1974. The Compatibility of Carbon with Blood. National Institutes of Health Annual Report. Contract NO1–HB–3–2954. General Atomic Company. San Diego, Calif.
68. Kusserow, B. K., R. W. Larrow & J. E. Nichols. 1974. Analysis and Measurement of the Effects of Materials on Blood Leukocytes, Erythrocytes, and Platelets. National Institutes of Health Annual Report. Contract PH–43–68–1427. University of Vermont. Burlington, Vt.

MATERIALS WITH CHEMICALLY ACTIVE SUBSTITUENTS

Richard D. Falb,* R. I. Leininger,
and James P. Crowley

Battelle, Columbus Laboratories
Columbus, Ohio 43201

It has been observed for many years that the nature of the surface contacting blood profoundly affects the rate at which that blood will coagulate. Two hundred years ago, William Hewson[1] found that blood contained within an isolated venous segment remained fluid for hours but coagulated quickly when placed in a glass container. Later, Lister found that blood clotted more rapidly in a glass tube than in a rubber tube.[2] It was subsequently found that coating a glass tube with paraffin significantly increased the clotting time of blood placed in the tube. A host of studies has been conducted attempting to relate the surface properties of materials to their propensity to induce blood coagulation. The early studies were necessarily empirical, since little was known about mechanisms of blood coagulation. In spite of the greatly expanded knowledge in the field of blood coagulation, the work at the present time remains largely empirical. One cannot now, from first principles, design a surface that will have ideal blood compatibility.

Over the last several years, a number of different surface features has been linked empirically to the process of surface-induced blood coagulation. The longest standing of these is the concept of surface-free energy. Lyman and his associates have postulated that a surface having a very low free energy would have a minimal interaction with components of blood and thus have good blood compatibility. They obtained a rough correlation between the surface-free energy and the coagulation time of contact of blood for a given series of materials.[3] Notable exceptions to this correlation, however, can be found in the work of Baier and Dutton,[4] who showed that extremely low surface-energy materials had adverse interactions with components of blood.

Another surface feature that has been linked with blood compatibility is surface charge. The early work of Sawyer and Pate[5] suggested that normal endothelium owes its nonthrombogenic character to its negative charge. *In vivo* thrombosis resulting from injury was attributed to the formation of a positive charge. Further work by Sawyer and Deutsch[6] indicated that electrodes placed in the cardiovascular system did not induce coagulation if a negative charge was imposed. When an electrode was positively charged, coagulation did occur. Subsequent to this work, a great deal of experimental work was devoted to investigation of the effect of surface charges on blood coagulation. Unfortunately, much confusion has ensued over the years because of the failure to distinguish between an impressed charge in an electric field such as induced by Sawyer, an ionized surface group, a negative surface streaming potential, and a charge polarization. Numerous surfaces containing ionized species have been evaluated, and a few of these do exhibit reasonably good blood compatibility.

* Present address: Research & Development, Ames Co., Division of Miles Laboratories, Elkhart, Ind. 46514.

It is not possible, however, in any way to relate compatibility with the number of negatively charged groups present on a given surface.

At the present time, the picture is not at all clear with respect to the relationship of surface chemistry and configuration to blood compatibility. The literature is rife with contradictory data. Confusion can be attributed to several factors. In the first place, surfaces quite often are not well characterized. It is not possible to deduce from the chemical structure of a given polymer what the surface properties of the processed polymer will be. Additives to the polymer, impurities, or processing aids may be present at the surface and completely obscure the effect of the base polymer. Furthermore, even if the polymer is completely pure, it could conceivably have a number of different surface configurations. For example, a polymer such as polystyrene sulfonic acid could be oriented at the surface so that the ionized sulfonic acid groups were present at the surface or could be oriented in such a way that the hydrophobic backbone was at the surface.

The surface of a polymer may or may not be homogeneous. It may contain areas of high surface energy resulting from its fissures or cracks. These areas could serve as a stimulus for blood coagulation and could obscure the effect of of the remaining portion of the surface.

Another source of confusion can come from the actual test methods used in the evaluation of a given surface. If an air interface is present, a layer of denatured protein can easily deposit on the surface, and this denatured layer can impart surface incompatibility. A good correlation does not exist between *in vitro* and *in vivo* test methods, since a clot formed in a test tube is different from a white thrombus formed *in vivo*. Most surfaces considered to be relatively nonthrombogenic are passive surfaces; that is, they do not themselves initiate blood coagulation. If, however, another stimulus for coagulation such as tissue trauma is present, they cannot prevent the formation of a clot.

In spite of the confusion that abounds on factors contributing to blood compatibility, a number of surfaces have been developed that have considerable compatibility with blood. Heparinized materials belong to this category. The first report of surface-attached heparin was in 1963 by Gott and co-workers,[7] who attached heparin through formation of a complex with a quaternary ammonium salt adsorbed to graphite. Shortly after Gott's work, our group at Battelle's Columbus Laboratories began research to develop methods of attaching heparin to the surfaces of a large number of synthetic and natural polymers. These materials included silicone rubber, poly(vinyl chloride), Teflon®, polyethylene, polypropylene, polyesters, and nylon. In the initial experimental approach, quaternary ammonium groups were covalently attached to the surfaces of these polymers. Heparin was attached by taking advantage of the fact that it forms highly nondissociable complexes with quaternary ammonium salts. Many different routes for the attachment of quaternary ammonium salts and amines to polymer surfaces were developed. After heparin complexation, these polymers were evaluated both *in vivo* and *in vitro* and demonstrated considerably improved blood compatibility as a result of the surface modification.[8] In the *in vitro* coagulation assay, recalcified blood in contact with the heparinized surface did not clot during a several-hour test period. When the blood was subsequently placed in a glass container, clotting occurred normally. The nonthrombogenicity of the surface as judged by this assay could not be related to the amount of heparin attached, except that surfaces containing less than 1 $\mu g/cm^2$ were thrombogenic. In some instances, surfaces with amounts of heparin as high as 5 $\mu g/cm^2$ were thrombogenic, presumably because of nonhomogeneous coverage of the surface. A typical reaction for the attachment of heparin is shown below.

$$\xrightarrow[\text{AlCl}_3]{\text{ClCH}_2\text{OCH}_3} \quad \text{CH}_2\text{Cl} \xrightarrow{\text{R}_3\text{N}} \quad \text{CH}_2\text{–}\overset{\overset{\text{Cl}^-}{+}}{\text{NR}_3}$$

Analysis of the heparinized surfaces indicated that heparin was slowly leached from the surface by dissociation of the complex. Since the resulting surface-bound quaternary ammonium group was incompatible with blood elements, we next set out to develop ways of covalently binding the heparin molecule itself to polymeric surfaces. The heparin molecule has carboxylic acid, hydroxyl, and amine groups available for covalent attachment. In our experimental work, a number of different reagents and heparin derivatives was employed [8] such as the acid hydrazide of heparin, ethylenimine-heparin derivatives, a carbodiimide-heparin derivative, and a heparin-cyanuric chloride adduct. The best results in terms of the amounts of heparin attached were achieved using the cyanuric chloride adduct. In this reaction scheme, heparin was first reacted with cyanuric chloride to form a derivative that had approximately seven residues per heparin molecule and that retained 85% of its anticoagulant activity. This derivative could be covalently attached to any polymeric surface that had bound amine groups. For example, silicone rubber was treated with aminopropyltriethoxysilane to attach surface-bound amine groups. It was then subsequently reacted with the cyanuric chloride-heparin adduct to form covalently attached heparin in amounts ranging from 50 to 100 $\mu g/cm^2$. These amounts were more than adequate to impart nonthrombogenicity to the surface based on previous experience with ionically bound heparin. Surprisingly, the *in vivo* results with covalently bonded heparin were not as good as those obtained with ionically bonded heparin. Possible reasons for this will be discussed later.

Once the *in vivo* tests had established the reduction in thrombogenicity that could be obtained by heparin bonding, we then turned our attention to the development of methods to obtain simple and rapid surface heparinization. All of the early methods required chemical modification of the surface. The processes could often be time-consuming and in some cases could result in damage to the surface such as crazing, roughness, or opacification. Many of the heparinization processes were specific for a given material. Thus, if one wished to heparinize a composite device, a separate process for each different material in the device would be required. In seeking a more generally applicable and simpler method, we investigated adsorption of a quaternary ammonium salt to the surface. Quaternary ammonium salts containing a single long-chain alkyl are easily displaced from the surface and thus would not be acceptable. However, salts with three long alkyl groups are water-insoluble and are not easily displaced from a surface in contact with an aqueous phase. For this reason, tridodecylmethyl ammonium chloride (TDMAC) was investigated as a means of attaching heparin to a large number of polymers. In a very simple technique, a solution of TDMAC in an organic solvent was used to contact the material. After drying, the surface was exposed to a 0.25% solution of heparin in water. This method was generally applicable for a large number of different polymers [9] and resulted in the attachment of large amounts of heparin, as shown in TABLE 1.

TABLE 1

ATTACHMENT OF HEPARIN TO POLYMERS WITH TDMAC

Polymer	Amount of Heparin on Surface, μg/cm² Initial	Percentage After 100 hr in Saline	Percentage After 4 hr in Plasma
Poly (vinyl chloride)	25	100	95
Polycarbonate	4	93	90
Mylar®	18	95	90
Silicone rubber	22	91	—
Polyurethane	186	100	98
Polyethylene	25	100	94
Polypropylene	8.2	92	91
Teflon®	1.1	99	87

As can be seen from the table, the heparin attached to the surface was quite stable, and very little was removed after four hours' contact with blood plasma. This technique had the advantage over previous methods of heparinization in its simplicity and speed, and also because it enables the treatment of composite devices containing several different polymers. Further improvement has been made on the TDMAC process by the development of the one-step treatment.[10] Heparin forms an organic-soluble complex with TDMAC at appropriate ratios of heparin to quaternary ammonium salt. In the one-step process, the material to be heparinized is simply dipped for a short time into a 2% solution of the complex in an appropriate solvent and then air-dried. The length of exposure time varies according to the polymer, but that of most materials is only a few seconds. The resulting surfaces are stable and can be sterilized by either autoclaving or ethylene oxide. Surfaces heparinized with the TDMAC process are stable during short-term exposure to blood; however, after longer implantation times, a considerable portion of the heparin is lost, as shown in TABLE 2.

TABLE 2

SURFACE ELUTION FROM TDMAC/HEPARIN A–V SHUNTS

Experiment No.	Mean Complex Content: Heparin mg/cm²±SD	Mean Complex Content: TDMAC mg/cm²±SD	Percentage Remaining: Heparin	Percentage Remaining: TDMAC
976 (Control)	0.41±0.15	1.20±0.46	—	—
976 (Sheep)	0.09±0.10	0.34±0.32	21.4	28.2
970 (Control)	0.81±0.42	2.39±1.29	—	—
970 (Sheep)	0.21±0.21	0.67±0.64	25.5	27.9
972 (Control)	1.13±0.31	3.31±0.91	—	—
972 (Sheep)	0.38±0.26	1.18±0.81	33.6	35.6
971 (Control)	1.15±0.20	3.44±0.60	—	—
971 (Sheep)	0.25±0.18	0.81±0.60	21.7	23.5

In spite of the fact that heparin is lost, materials of this type retain nonthrombogenicity during implantation periods of several months and even years. The reason for this is not clear but may be due to the fact that a passivated surface consisting of adsorbed proteins renders the material nonthrombogenic even after some of the heparin is gone.

One of the commonly observed results of exposure of heparinized surfaces to blood either *in vivo* or *in vitro* is the accumulation of platelets on the surface. In *in vitro* experiments, fresh platelet-rich plasma was eluted though a column consisting of heparinized silicone rubber particles. In the first fractions recovered from the column, virtually all the platelets were missing.[11] In subsequent fractions, the platelet count returned to normal. These data seem to indicate that platelets were adsorbed to the surface until saturation was reached. Similarly, in *in vivo* experiments, surfaces exposed to the bloodstream when examined microscopically after removal showed a surface coverage with blood platelets. The data indicated that exposure to heparinized surfaces did not stimulate release of platelet intracellular factors such as platelet factor 3.

In order to determine the mechanism for the effectiveness of surface-bound heparin, we then conducted a study of the effect of various surface functional groups on compatibility with blood. The experiments were designed to remove as many artifacts as possible by changing only the variable of surface chemistry. To accomplish this, a number of different functional groups were attached to the surface of cross-linked polystyrene beads of uniform particle size. The functional groups that were attached were hydroxyl, sulfate, sulfate ester, sulfhydryl, carboxylic acid, amino, sulfamino, and nitro. Nitro groups were produced by nitration of the beads in a sulfuric-nitric acid mixture. Amine groups were produced by reduction of the nitro groups with sodium dithionite. Surface hydroxyl groups were produced by reaction in an electrophilic alkylation of polystyrene with chloromethyl methyl ether in the presence of aluminum chloride. To produce aromatic carboxylic acid groups, the hydroxyl groups were oxidized with permanganate. Hydroxyl groups also were reacted with chlorosulfonic acid to make a sulfate ester. Aliphatic carboxylic acid groups were attached to the polystyrene beads by reacting them with succinic anhydride in the presence of aluminum chloride. Sulfhydryl-containing polystyrene beads were produced by reacting chloromethylated polystyrene with a saturated solution of hydrogen sulfide in methanol. A polyglutamic acid surface was attached to the polystyrene by reacting the aminated polystyrene with the *N*-carboxy anhydride derivative of glutamic acid.

The presence of the above-cited groups on the derivatives was ascertained either by titration or by infrared adsorption analysis. To investigate the effect of these surfaces on various blood components, an experimental scheme employing a column was used. The various derivatized polystyrene beads were packed into columns thermostated at 37° C. Sufficient numbers of particles were placed in the column so that the surface area measured approximately 500 cm^2. Platelet-rich and platelet-poor plasma were then eluted through the columns and the effluents collected in 4-ml fractions. These fractions were then analyzed for specific components which were used as an index of interaction of blood components with the derivatized polystyrene surfaces. With the platelet-rich plasma, platelet counts were made as a measure of platelet adsorption. To assess platelet rupture, measurements of platelet factor 3 were estimated by Stypven clotting times. With the platelet-poor plasma, a rough estimation of clotting factor interaction was obtained by measuring prothrombin times and partial thromboplastin times. A summary of these data is shown in TABLE 3.

Discussion

The results show that surfaces containing a nonionizable group appear to have the least effect on blood constituents. Those containing groups that ionize to form a negative charge, such as carboxylic acids and sulfonic acids, had a moderate effect on platelet adsorption and partial thromboplastin times. The most dramatic effect comes from the surface containing amino groups. Large amounts of platelets were adsorbed on this surface, and significant platelet rupture was observed. The amine groups, however, did not appear to activate the coagulation mechanism in the absence of platelets. This is not particularly surprising in view of the earlier results of Nossel and associates, who showed that Hageman factor activation was inhibited by quaternary ammonium salts.[12] The thrombogenicity of quaternary surfaces *in vivo* could be explained on the basis of the adverse interactions that occur with blood platelets.

Table 3

Results of Various Functional Groups on Blood Components

Surface	Platelet Adsorption	Platelet Rupture	Change in Prothrombin Time	Change in Partial Thrombo-plastin Time
Polyglutamic acid	+, 0 *	++	0	++
Aliphatic CO_2H	+	++	0	++
Aromatic CO_2H	+, 0	+	0	++
$-NH-SO_3H$	++	+	0	++++
$-SO_3H$	++	++	+, 0	+, 0
$-NH_2$	++++	++++	0	+, 0
$-OH$	+, 0	+	0	+, 0
$-NO_2$	0	0	0	+, 0
$-SO_3Me$	+	+	0	+, 0
$-SH$	0	0	0	+, 0
Polystyrene	+, 0	+	0	+, 0

* 0=none observed; +=slight effect; ++=moderate effect; +++=large effect; and ++++=very large effect.

The attractiveness of the negatively charged groups such as carboxylate and sulfonate for platelets may, in some way, account for the adhesion of platelets to heparinized surfaces. This effect may be the result of a general reaction with negative groups, and not a specific effect of the heparin molecule itself. The mechanism responsible for the effectiveness of heparinized surfaces is still unknown. The fact that covalently bonded heparin was not as effective as the ionically bound heparin might be explained by two different points of view. It may be essential that a very small amount of heparin be free in solution in the microenvironment of the surface. This heparin could then serve to block any activation of the coagulation mechanism, much as heparin normally does in solution. In fact, certain other workers claimed that the release of heparin from a surface must exceed a certain minimal rate in order for the surface to be effective.[13, 14] From another point of view, covalently bonded heparin may not be effective because its attachment was effected in such a way as to restrict molecular mobility. This, in turn, could inhibit heparin from complexing with heparin cofactor or other molecules that would enable it to be an effective anticoagulant.

The deleterious effect of quaternary ammonium groups on platelets make such groups on a surface highly undesirable. In surfaces bearing ionically bound heparin, the possibility of dissociation of the complex in producing unbound quaternary ammonium salts may account for any deleterious effects that heparinized surfaces have on platelets.

In spite of the fact that many questions remain unanswered, surfaces heparinized by the TDMAC/heparin process have been used to considerable advantage in medical practice.[15-17] The process is now in commercial production in an increasing number of applications. This process may not be useful for every application in which blood must contact a foreign surface. It is likely that a number of different types of surfaces will be essential for various applications in the body. Many questions remain unanswered regarding the reason for the failure or success of various types of surfaces; but in the absence of a definitive theory of blood-surface interaction, one must be content at the present time with empirically derived solutions to a very complex problem.

References

1. Gulliver, G., Ed. 1846. Works of William Hewson. London Sydenham Society. London, England.
2. Lister, J. 1863. On the coagulation of blood. Proc. Roy. Soc. of London **12:** 580.
3. Lyman, D. J., J. L. Brash, S. W. Chakin, K. G. Klein & M. Carini. 1968. Effect of chemical structure and surface properties of synthetic polymers in the coagulation of blood. Trans. ASAIO **XXIV:** 250.
4. Baier, R. E. & R. C. Dutton. 1969. Initial events and interactions of blood with foreign surface. J. Biomed. Mater. Res. **3:** 191.
5. Sawyer, P. N. & J. W. Pate. 1953. Electric potential distance across the normal aorta and aortic grafts of dogs. Am. J. Physiol. **175:** 118.
6. Sawyer, P. N. & B. Deutsch. 1956. Use of electric current to delay intravascular thrombosis in experimental animals. Am. J. Physiol. **187:** 473.
7. Gott, V. L., J. D. Whiffen & R. C. Dutton. 1963. Heparin bonding on colloidal graphite surfaces. Science **142:** 1297.
8. Falb, R. D., G. A. Grode, H. M. Grotta, R. A. Wright, R. H. Poirier, M. T. Takahashi & R. I. Leininger. March 30, 1967. Development of blood-compatible materials. PM 175 668; October, 1967, PB 183 317; October, 1968, PB 188 108; and October, 1969, PB 188 111.
9. Grode, G. A., *et al.* October, 1970. Biocompatible materials for use in the vascular system. PB 195 727; and November, 1971, PB 205 475.
10. Leininger, R. I., R. D. Falb, J. P. Crowley & G. A. Grode. 1972. Three years' experience *in vivo* and *in vitro* with surfaces and devices treated by the heparin complex method. Trans. ASAIO **XVIII:** 312.
11. Grode, G. A., *et al.* December, 1973. Development of blood-compatible polymeric materials. PB 228 789.
12. Nossel, H. L., H. Rabin, M. Grilling & R. Hsieh. 1968. Inhibition of Hageman factor activation. J. Clin. Invest. **46:** 1172.
13. Idezuki, E., *et al.* 1975. Mechanism of antithrombogenicity of a new heparinized hydrophilic polymer: Chronic *in vivo* studies and clinical application. Trans. ASAIO **XXI:** 436.

14. Schmer, G. Personal communication.
15. Krause, A. H., T. B. Ferguson & C. S. Weldon. 1972. Thoracic aneurysmectomy utilizing the TDMAC-heparin shunt. Ann. Thor. Surg. **14:** 123.
16. Brenner, W. I., R. M. Engelman, C. D. Williams, A. D. Boyd & G. E. Reed. May, 1974. Nonthrombogenic aortic and vena caval bypass using heparin-coated tubes. Am. J. Surg. **127:** 555.
17. Mobin-Uddin, K., J. R. Utley, L. R. Bryant, M. Dillon & D. L. Weiss. 1974. Experimental and clinical evaluations of heparin-impregnated cloth-covered cardiac valves used without system anticoagulation. Ann. Thor. Surg. **17:** 351.

HEPARINIZED SURFACES—A COMMENT*

Robert D. Rosenberg

Department of Medicine, Beth Israel Hospital
Boston, Massachusetts 02115
Sidney Farber Cancer Institute, Harvard Medical School
Boston, Massachusetts 02115

Lun H. Lam

Sidney Farber Cancer Institute, Harvard Medical School
Boston, Massachusetts 02115

Introduction

Heparin acts as an anticoagulant by dramatically accelerating the rate at which antithrombin-heparin cofactor neutralizes series proteases of the hemostatic mechanism.[1-5] This is accomplished via binding of heparin to lysyl residues of antithrombin-heparin cofactor, which probably induces a conformational alteration of the inhibitor that renders its reactive site more accessible to the active center of these enzymes.[6] Considerable effort has been expended in defining the linear sequence and three-dimensional configuration of heparin.[7-9] However, the precise relationship between its structure and anticoagulant properties remains elusive. Heparin preparations exhibit considerable polydispersity in molecular size,[10] variations in the ratio of glucuronic acid to iduronic acid,[11] alterations in the amount of ester and *N*-sulfation,[12] and differing extents of *N*-acetylation.[13] Changes in each of these parameters correlate to only a limited degree with anticoagulant potency.

These heparin preparations have been bonded to a variety of materials. They exhibit varying degrees of effectiveness as nonthrombogenic surfaces. In this communication, we provide evidence that only a small fraction of a given heparin preparation can bind to antithrombin-heparin cofactor and is responsible for its distinctive anticoagulant effect.[14] We suggest that the bulk of the mucopolysaccharide, with little anticoagulant activity, could interact with other blood components such as platelets and might endow "heparinized surfaces" with undesirable thrombogenic properties. We therefore believe that the active fraction of heparin must be utilized in constructing artificial surfaces if meaningful data is to emerge.

Materials

Human antithrombin-heparin cofactor and human thrombin were obtained in physically homogeneous form by methods previously reported from this laboratory.[6, 15] Heparin of porcine intestinal origin (Riker Laboratories, Lot

* Supported by grants from The National Institutes of Health (NHLI 19131) and from the Riker Laboratories. The latter grant was provided for developing new techniques for the fractionation of heparin.

no. 56913), utilized for the anticoagulant therapy of human subjects, was employed throughout these studies. This mucopolysaccharide was characterized by its susceptibility to degradation by crude heparinase (sonicated flavobacterium heparinum), and resistance to cleavage with chondroitinase ABC (Miles Laboratory). Incubation conditions and assay techniques have been described previously in detail.[16] Furthermore, chromatography of this heparin product on DEAE-cellulose demonstrated that the mucopolysaccharide eluted at LiCl concentrations above 1.0 M. This behavior is similar to that obtained with other preparations of this mucopolysaccharide.[16] All other chemicals were reagent grade or better.

Methods

Assay of Heparin Concentration. The mucopolysaccharide concentration of a heparin sample was determined colorimetrically by assay of uronic acid via the carbazole method of Bitter and Muir[17] and by a modification of the Azure A method of Jaques.[18] When this latter method was utilized, 50 μl of a sample (0–5 μg) was added to 1 ml of Azure A (0.01 mg/ml in distilled water). The resultant mixture was agitated and absorbance at 500 nm was measured. Sucrose concentrations from 10% to 50% (w/v) and antithrombin-heparin cofactor levels from 20 μg/ml to 290 μg/ml had, essentially, no effect upon this assay. The heparin concentration of all fractionated samples was determined by comparison with the initial starting material. The standard titration curve of this unfractionated sample exhibited a linear rise in absorbance at 500 nm from 0 to 0.200 as the amount of heparin was increased from 0 to 5 μg.

Assay of Anticoagulant Activity. The anticoagulant activity of the unfractionated heparin preparation was assumed to be equivalent to the U.S.P. unitage cited on its label. The potency of all fractionated heparin samples was determined by comparison with this starting material. To construct a standard titration curve, 50 μl of antithrombin-heparin cofactor (50 μg/ml) were added to 20-μl aliquots of various dilution of the reference sample. The resultant mixtures were incubated for 1–2 minutes at 37° C. Then 280 μl of 0.135 M NaCl in 0.05 M Tris-Imidazole (pH 8.3) was admixed with the latter solution prior to the addition of 50 μl of human thrombin (~60 NIH units/ml or ~25 μg/ml). After 30 seconds of incubation at 37° C, 300 μl of substrate were introduced and the reaction mixtures were incubated for an additional 60 seconds at 37° C. The substrate consisted of Benzoyl-Phen-Val-Arg-*p*-Nitroanilide. HCl (AB Bofors, Nobel Division, Molndal, Sweden) and polybrene dissolved in H_2O with each component at a final concentration of 0.33 mg/ml. Finally, 300 μl of glacial acetic acid was added to quench the action of thrombin upon the tripeptide and the extent of amidolysis was quantitated by measuring the absorbance of samples at 405 nm. All determinations were performed in triplicate. The titration curve of the heparin reference standard exhibited a linear decline in absorbance from ~0.8 to ~0.2, when heparin concentrations ranged from 0 to 1 unit/ml. To measure the anticoagulant activity of a fractionated heparin sample, it was diluted to approximately 0.5 units/ml, and assayed with the above technique by comparison with the reference standard.

Fluorometric Assay of Protein Concentration.[19] Fifty μl of a sample

(0–100 μg of antithrombin-heparin cofactor) was added to 250 μl of 0.2 M sodium borate buffer (pH 9.0). Then 100 μl of a solution containing fluorescamine dye (0.1 mg/ml in acetone) was injected while vortexing the solution, and the final volume of the resultant mixture was brought to 2 ml with the buffer described above. The fluorescence of this solution was read at 475 nm after excitation at 390 nm. A standard titration curve exhibited a linear increase in relative fluorescence from 0 to 1000 as the level of antithrombin-heparin cofactor was varied from 0 to 100 μg. Concentrations of heparin below 140 μg/ml have essentially no effect on this assay of protein concentration.

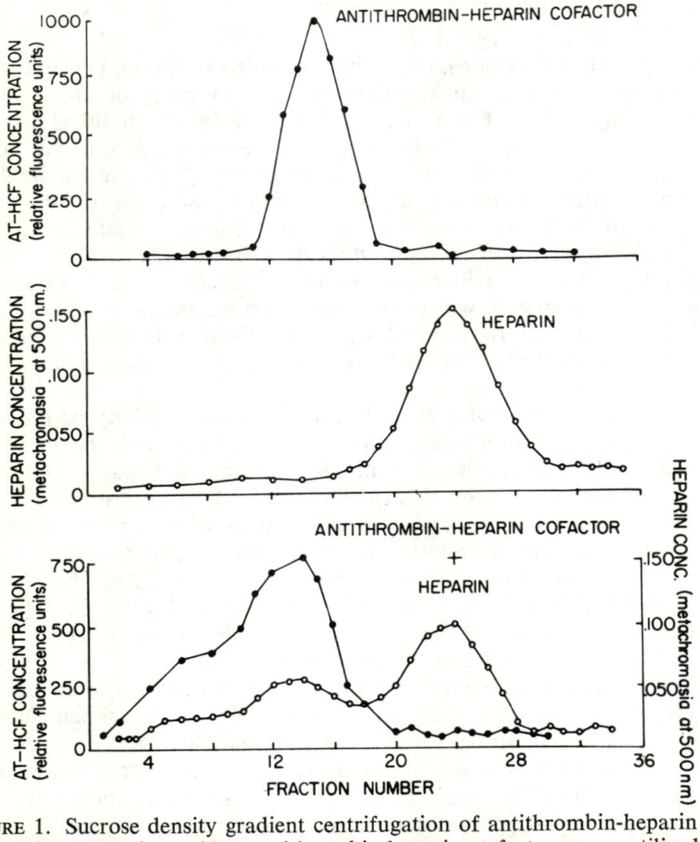

FIGURE 1. Sucrose density gradient centrifugation of antithrombin-heparin cofactor and heparin. Heparin and/or antithrombin-heparin cofactor were utilized at final concentrations of 33.3 μg/ml and 333 μg/ml, respectively. Each component had previously been extensively dialyzed against 0.15 M NaCl in 0.01 M sodium phosphate (pH 7.5). Approximately 300 μl of these solutions were overlayed on 4.7 ml of 10%–15% (w/v) sucrose density gradients in which the solvent was 0.15 M NaCl in 0.01 M sodium phosphate (pH 7.5). After centrifugation at 224,000 × g for 20 hours, 4° C, the bottom of each tube was punctured and fractions of ~120 μl were collected for analyses. See MATERIALS AND METHODS for additional details. (Adapted from Reference 14.)

TABLE 1

SPECIFIC ANTICOAGULANT ACTIVITY OF HEPARIN SAMPLES (ANTICOAGULANT ACTIVITY PER MG OF HEPARIN)

Experiment	Unfractionated Heparin	Heparin Bound to Antithrombin-Heparin Cofactor	Heparin Unable to Bind to Antithrombin-Heparin Cofactor
1	155	388	19
2	155	365	52
3	155	348	43

RESULTS

Samples containing 100 μg of antithrombin-heparin cofactor or 10 μg of heparin were examined separately by sucrose density gradient centrifugation. As shown in FIGURE 1 (upper and middle panel), single, narrow, nonoverlapping peaks of either protein or heparin were apparent. When both components were mixed together at the final concentrations and the solvent conditions previously employed, two major alterations in the pattern of component distribution were noted (FIGURE 1, lowest panel). First, the profile of the antithrombin-heparin cofactor concentration revealed a significant degree of polydispersity with large amounts of protein present at high sedimentation velocities (fractions 2–11). In addition, a shift in the sedimentation velocity of the antithrombin-heparin cofactor peak to a slightly higher value was apparent, and this subtle finding was noted during many centrifugation analyses. Second, heparin is no longer present as a discrete peak but is distributed throughout the density gradient. Approximately ⅓ of this component is located under the antithrombin-heparin cofactor peak, suggesting that it has been drawn into this region because of strong interactions with the inhibitor. Approximately two-thirds of the heparin is present at its original position in the density gradient and therefore does not appear to be capable of forming a stable complex with antithrombin-heparin cofactor. This is surprising, since a twofold-to-threefold molar excess of the inhibitor was present in the original reaction mixture. The data suggested that heparin bound to the inhibitor might represent an active species, whereas heparin unable to complex with antithrombin-heparin cofactor could signify a chemically similar but inactive form of this mucopolysaccharide.

To validate this hypothesis, it was necessary to quantitate the anticoagulant activity of each of these heparin species. Therefore, fractions were collected either from areas of the density gradient free of protein (fractions 21–28) or from regions in which heparin was bound to antithrombin-heparin cofactor (fractions 3–15). In order to accumulate sufficient material for analyses, it was necessary to obtain fractions from six to twelve individual density gradients. Heparin fractions unable to bind to antithrombin-heparin cofactor were pooled, extensively dialyzed, and assayed for anticoagulant activity as well as for heparin content. As shown in TABLE 1, the average specific activity (anticoagulant activity per mg of heparin) obtained during three separate experiments was 38 units/mg. Heparin fractions that had bound to antithrombin-heparin cofactor were also pooled and extensively dialyzed. Prior to quantitating the anticoagulant activity of these samples, it was necessary to free them of protein. This processing was necessary so that significant amounts of antithrombin-heparin cofactor were not introduced into the assay system, since this would invalidate the measurements obtained. To this end, samples containing ~0.6 mg of antithrombin-heparin cofactor and ~25 μg of heparin were adsorbed to a DEAE-cellulose column (0.85×1.8 cm); the chromatographic matrix was washed with 5 ml of 0.25 M of LiCl to elute protein differentially, and the mucopolysaccharide was harvested with 2 M LiCl. Approximately 70% of the heparin could be recovered by this procedure with only ~1% of the initial antithrombin-heparin cofactor present in these fractions. Additional experiments demonstrated that the specific activity of heparin was not altered by the above technique.

After elution from DEAE-cellulose, the samples were extensively dialyzed and assayed for anticoagulant activity as well as for heparin content. As shown in TABLE 1, the average specific activity obtained during three separate experiments was 367 units/mg. This is considerably higher than the specific activity of the unfractionated heparin (155 units/mg). Fractionation of these two heparin forms was dependent upon the presence of antithrombin-heparin cofactor. Attempts to duplicate this isolation procedure with bovine serum albumin, a plasma protein similar in size to antithrombin-heparin cofactor, were unsuccessful. Indeed, as judged by sucrose density gradient centrifugation, heparin does not interact with this plasma component.

DISCUSSION

In summary, our data would indicate that the heparin preparation examined consisted of two distinct forms that differ greatly in their ability to bind to and activate antithrombin-heparin cofactor. The first form constituted approximately two-thirds of the chemical mass of the unfractionated heparin and did not bind to antithrombin-heparin cofactor under the condition of these experiments. This fraction was responsible for only ~15% of the total anticoagulant activity of the starting material. The relatively low anticoagulant potency may be an intrinsic property of this molecular species or could be due to residual contamination with the more active form of heparin. The second form, comprising one-third of the remaining chemical mass of unfractionated heparin, bound tightly to antithrombin-heparin cofactor and contained approximately 85% of the total anticoagulant activity of the starting material. The heparin utilized in these studies was indistinguishable from preparation employed by other investigators, as judged by susceptibility to enzyme degradations and elution from DEAE-cellulose. We therefore suspect that other heparin products will exhibit similar inactive and active forms. Indeed, we have recently analyzed heparin obtained from a variety of sources and have obtained identical data. At the present time, we have no knowledge of the specific features that distinguish the biologically active from the relatively inactive heparin species. However, we do know that molecular size is not a critical parameter. Previous attempts to define the precise chemical structure of heparin responsible for its anticoagulant action have been unsuccessful. We suspect that these difficulties may have been due to the inability of prior investigators to fractionate this family of chemically related components and obtain the biologically active species. Indeed, we suggest that when appropriate heparin fractions are examined, unique structural features will emerge that are related to their anticoagulant activity. These pertinent heparin species may, of course, require even more highly refined separation procedures than those described in this communication.

It is known that platelets, white cells, blood proteins, and so on, can accumulate on "heparinized" surfaces. We believe that these phenomena may be responsible for reducing the nonthrombogenic properties of such surfaces. Effects of this kind may be caused by the inactive heparin species that have minimal anticoagulant activity. Therefore, we propose that "heparinized surfaces" be fabricated with only the active species of mucopolysaccharide bound to the matrix. This type of surface may well have dramatically improved nonthrombogenic properties.

References

1. Brinkhous, K. M., H. P. Smith, E. D. Warner & W. H. Seegers. 1939. Am. J. Physiol. **125:** 683–687.
2. Seegers, W. H., E. R. Cole, C. R. Harmison & F. C. Monkhouse. 1964. Can. J. Biochem. **42:** 359–364.
3. Damus, P. S., M. Hicks & R. D. Rosenberg. 1973. Nature. **246:** 355–357.
4. Highsmith, R. F. & R. D. Rosenberg. 1974. J. Biol. Chem. **249:** 4335–4338.
5. Rosenberg, J. S., P. McKenna & R. D. Rosenberg. 1975. J. Biol. Chem. **250:** 8883–8888.
6. Rosenberg, R. D. & P. S. Damus. 1973. J. Biol. Chem. **248:** 6490–6505.
7. Silva, M. E. & C. P. Dietrich. 1975. J. Biol. Chem. **250:** 6841–6846.
8. Taylor, R. L., J. E. Shively, H. E. Conrad & J. A. Cifonelli. 1973. Biochemistry **12:** 3633–3636.
9. Nieduszynski, J. A. & E. D. T. Atkins. 1973. Biochemistry **135:** 729–733.
10. Laurent, T. C. 1961. Arch. Biochem. Biophys. **92:** 224–231.
11. Hovingh, P. & A. Linker. 1970. J. Biol. Chem. **245:** 6170–6175.
12. Danishefsky, I., H. Steiner, A. Bella & A. Friedlander. 1969. J. Biol. Chem. **244:** 1741–1745.
13. Cifonelli, J. A. & J. King. 1973. Biochim. Biophys. Acta **320:** 331–341.
14. Lam, L. H., J. E. Silbert & R. D. Rosenberg. 1976. Biophys. Res. Commun. **69:** 570–577.
15. Rosenberg, R. D. & P. S. Damus. 1976. Methods in Enzymes Vol. 45. Academic Press. New York, N.Y.
16. Lewis, R. G., A. F. Spencer & J. E. Silbert. 1973. Biochem. J. **134:** 455–463.
17. Bitter, T. & H. M. Muir. 1962. Anal. Biochem. **4:** 330–334.
18. Jaques, L. B., F. C. Monkhouse & M. J. Stuart. 1949. J. Physiol. (Lond.) **109:** 41–48.
19. Udenfriend, S., S. Stein, P. Bohlen & W. Dairman. 1972. Science **178:** 871–872.

PERMEABLE SURFACES

John M. Ketteringham and Terrence J. Driscoll

Arthur D. Little, Inc.
Acorn Park
Cambridge, Massachusetts 02140

Introduction

In a variety of medical devices presently in clinical use or in development, material is selectively transported to and from blood through a synthetic permeable surface. The permeable surface or membrane separates the blood from the medium carrying the transported species, while ideally causing minimum trauma to the blood components.

The challenge of producing a relatively blood-compatible surface is clearly a formidable one; the complexity of the interaction of synthetic materials with blood components and the progress in its understanding have been discussed at length at this conference. When we add the additional requirement that the overall permeability must be high enough so that devices of reasonable size may be used and that the material has the appropriate selectivity, very few materials are candidates for use in practical devices. No ideal combination of these properties has been found, but considerable progress has been made in the last few years in improving blood compatibility, permeability, and selectivity of membranes, and in the proper hemodynamic design of devices to optimize performance.

The purpose of this paper is to draw attention to the way in which the interaction of the transport processes in the blood and in the membrane influence the performance of such devices. This is illustrated by experience with the membrane lung and the artificial kidney.

In those membranes which are essentially nonporous such as those fabricated from homogeneous polymers, flow of permeant material is generally via a mechanism of solution—diffusion. Transport occurs by dissolution of the permeating species on the high concentration side followed by diffusion down a thermodynamic activity gradient, and resolution on the low concentration side. As the structure of the membrane becomes more porous, bulk flow of water and other species, particularly those of small molecular weight, may occur. Bulk flow of the permeant occurs through the intersticies in the material's matrix due to hydraulic or osmotic pressure gradients. Diffusive contributions are usually small in comparison with the bulk flow.

In both the cases of porous and nonporous materials, the resistance to flow of a given species is the sum of the membrane resistance and interfacial resistances; one or the other resistance may dominate under different conditions and for different species. The mechanism of transport and the nature of the resistance controlling the rate of flow of a given species is of critical importance to the performance characteristics of the two devices under consideration: membrane lungs and hemodialyzers.

The requirements for membranes of hemodialyzers and membrane lungs share the needs of high flux and good blood compatibility, but these two factors have different relative priorities. This is best illustrated by comparing the normal operating parameters for these two devices (TABLE 1).

Membrane lungs involve a much greater blood flow rate over a larger permeable interface, emphasizing blood compatibility and mass transfer to minimize blood-contact area and priming volume. The lower flow rates and membrane areas in hemodialyzers place less emphasis on these factors, and research interest is directed more toward the control of the relative rate of transport of water and various other species across the membrane. This is influenced by an interaction of the transport properties in the blood interface and the membrane itself.

MEMBRANE LUNGS

Although the membrane lung has been in clinical use for over 20 years, recent developments in hardware and in clinical experience have increased the demand for new and improved membrane materials. Membrane lungs are now being used more frequently in cardiopulmonary bypass for open-heart surgery, successful protocols for use in prolonged respiratory support are being developed, and implantable lungs are undergoing preliminary research.

The membrane lung itself has recently been improved in two fundamental ways. Better hemodynamic design has reduced the normally limiting resistances to oxygen diffusion at the blood side of the blood-membrane interface so that membrane areas and priming volumes may be made smaller. Additionally, new membrane materials have been developed that have greater gas permeabilities to match the performance potential of these new devices, and in some cases superior blood compatibility as well.

TABLE 1

COMPARISON OF NORMAL OPERATING PARAMETERS FOR HEMODIALYZERS AND MEMBRANE LUNGS

	Hemodialyzers	Membrane Lungs
Priming Blood Volume	65–500 ml	500–1500 ml
Membrane Area	0.5–1.5 M^2	2–4 M^2
Blood-Flow Rate	~0.2 litres/min	~5 litres/min

The choice of polymers which have gas permeabilities in a range where they can be considered for membrane lungs is limited. To be permeable enough, they must, in general, have low crystallinity, limited cross linking, and a mobile polymer backbone.[1] Silicone rubber, which has only moderate permeability and is difficult to fabricate into thin, pinhole-free membranes, has a gas permeability some seven times greater than other available polymers and three times greater than its polycarbonate copolymer, which has superior physical properties. TABLE 2 summarizes the specific bulk permeabilities of materials currently being used or considered for use in membrane oxygenators.

Porous membranes, such as those made of porous polypropylene (Celgard®—Celanese Corporation) and expended polytetrafluorethylene (Gortex®—Gore Corporation) have significantly higher gas permeabilities than their solution-diffusion counterparts. This advantage, however, must be balanced with the

TABLE 2

SPECIFIC PERMEABILITY OF MEMBRANE MATERIALS

Homogeneous	cm³, cm/cm², sec, cmHg * $\times 10^{10}$ O₂	CO₂
Silicone Rubber	490	3240
Silicone Rubber/Polycarbonate Copolymers	160	970
Polyalkysulfone	60	250
Ethylcellulosı Perfluorobutyrate	45	225
Tetrafluoroethylene (Film)	4	12
Porous		
Polypropylene	high	
Expanded Teflon®	high	

* Volume of gas permeated per second for a 1-cm-thick membrane of area 1-square cm under a partial pressure driving force of 1 cmHg, otherwise known as the Barrer unit.

problems of fluid entering the gas space, possible bubble formation on the blood side caused by too high a gas pressure, and greater water-vapor permeability than desirable. Of necessity, these materials must be hydrophobic to prevent intrusion of blood. Large-scale production of such membranes is difficult because of the need for a narrow distribution of pore sizes over the entire piece of material and an absence of pinholes.

The requirements for gas permeability of membranes used in membrane lungs is revealed by examination of the gas-transfer performance of various designs that have been described in the literature. TABLE 3 lists the gas-transfer performance of various membrane lung configurations using a variety of membrane materials. The values of oxygen and carbon dioxide transfer rate are compared to the limiting gas-to-gas permeability of a silicone rubber membrane under typical partial pressure gradients. In the conventional flat sheet, hollow fiber, or spiral coil configurations, values of oxygen-permeation rate are far below the intrinsic permeability of the silicone rubber or other membrane material used, since oxygen transport is limited by the blood-film boundary layer at the surface of the membrane. Carbon dioxide permeation rate more closely approaches the intrinsic membrane permeability but in most cases comfortably exceeds the metabolic ratio of carbon dioxide released to oxygen absorbed (0.8). Increasing the membrane permeability to oxygen or carbon dioxide has little advantage in most of these devices. Only in the folded flat-plate membrane lung configuration using high blood shear rates does the permeability of conventional silicone rubber membranes begin to compromise the performance of the device, and a porous Teflon® membrane is used.

Recent developments in the augmentation of secondary blood flow at the membrane interface by shearing the blood with a rotating disk or by use of pulsatile flow across a transversely ridged membrane have also increased the oxygen-transfer efficiency of the blood film beyond the capability of conventional silicone rubber membranes. These devices can therefore use higher permeability membranes to advantage. Porous membranes give higher gas permeability, but they have problems of high water-vapor flux leading to condensation within the pores and deterioration of carbon dioxide clearance,[2] no better blood compatibility than silicone rubber,[3] and the risk of gas emboli. This has led to the development of composite nonporous membranes constructed by forming ultrathin layers of blood-compatible and moderately permeable polymers on porous substrates suitable for use in these new high-performance membrane lungs.

Although early attempts to coat polytetrafluoroethylene[4] and microporous cellulose[5] with a silicone rubber film were promising, two new approaches have been developed recently. The polyalkylsulfones, which are copolymers of straight chain α-olefins and sulfur dioxide,[6] have been developed in our laboratories,[7] and ethylcellulose perfluorbutyrate has been developed at the North Star Division of the Midwest Research Institute.[8] In both cases two-to-ten micron layers of the polymer are solvent cast onto a porous polypropylene substrate; the molecular size of the polymer is too great to enter the 10–100 Å porous structure of the substrate.

Extremely smooth, uniform coatings of polyalkylsulfone have been formed by this method. The gas-permeation rates for these membranes are summarized in TABLE 4. The ultrathin polyalkylsulfone membranes have a permeation rate some three to five times greater than conventional 100-μ silicone rubber membranes.

A membrane chosen for a given device must have adequate oxygen permeability for proper performance, but CO_2 permeability must be such that physiological requirements are met. Whereas the former is primarily controlled by the hemodynamics of the device, the CO_2 transfer is almost wholly membrane-limited. Plotting the ratio of CO_2 to O_2 flux versus increasing O_2 flux for various metals, FIGURE 1 illustrates that for a CO_2 flux fixed by the membrane properties, increased O_2 transfer will rapidly reduce the ratio of CO_2 to O_2 flux. At

TABLE 3

GAS-TRANSFER PERFORMANCES OF MEMBRANE LUNGS

Type	Membrane	Gas-Exchange Rate cc/min m^2 at Rated Blood Flow O_2	CO_2	CO_2/O_2
Conventional				
Flat Sheet	silicone rubber *	25–63	40–50	0.8–1.2
Hollow Fiber	silicone rubber *	30	45	1.5
Kolobow-Type Spiral	silicone rubber *	50	55	1.1
Porous Membrane	Teflon®, cellulosic	25–75	40–120	1.2–1.7
Augumented Secondary Flow				
Sheared Blood Film	porous	360	NA	NA
Pulsed Blood Film	silicone rubber	130	comparable to O_2	1.0
Reinforced Silicone Rubber 100 μ Flat Sheet Membrane-Limiting Gas Resistance under Typical Gradients		208	70	0.34

* And copolymers.

TABLE 4

GAS PERMEATION RATES FOR VARIOUS MEMBRANE MATERIALS (37° C)

	cc/meter²Flux, minute	
	O_2*	CO_2†
Polysiloxane/Polycarbonate (MEM 213)	129	38
Silicone Rubber (100 μ thick)	261	76
Ultrathin Silicone Rubber (40 μ thick)	653	190
Ultrathin Ethylcellulose Perfluorobutyrate	312	100
Ultrathin Polyalkylsulfone	1400	281

* Under 67 cmHg driving force, computed from gas-to-gas determinations.

† Under 4.3 cmHg driving force, computed from gas-to-blood and gas-to-gas determinations.

levels below the normal respiratory coefficient the membrane size must be increased to provide adequate CO_2 removal.

The performance of several commercial membrane lungs and one filming device [9] illustrates that to achieve gas fluxes as high as those with a direct contact device with an acceptable CO_2 and O_2 flux ratio, thin, composite membranes are at present the only acceptable materials.

Recent improvements in the blood compatibility of membrane materials used in membrane lungs have been equally dramatic. The use of filler-free silicone rubber has been shown to increase platelet survival [10] compared to conventional silica-filled materials. Recently ethylcellulose perfluorobutyrate has demonstrated comparable properties to filler-free silicone rubber.[11]

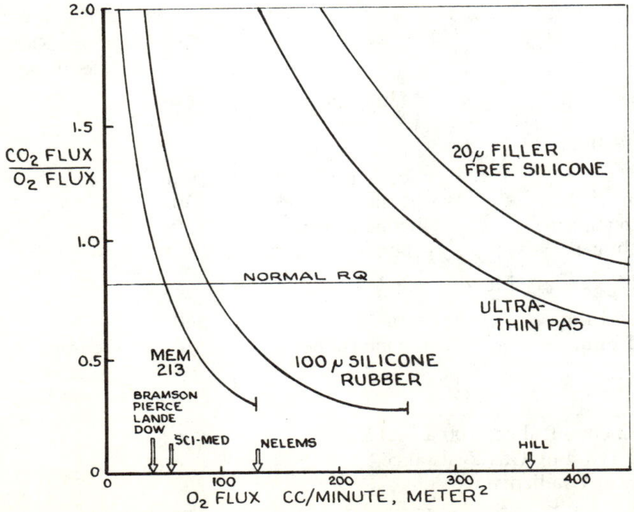

FIGURE 1. Ratio of CO_2 to O_2 flux for membrane lung materials.

Artificial Kidneys

As we have discussed, in the membrane lung high blood flows emphasize improvements in blood compatibility and mass transfer; in the artificial kidney the relative mass transfer of water and a variety of molecular species across the interface are the primary parameters of interest. A complex combination of operational parameters and membrane characteristics influences this process; the ultimate performance of the device is the result of a complex interaction of mass transport processes in the blood and in the membrane.

Specifically, the fundamental goals in continued membrane development and the evolution of artificial kidneys are:

1) controllable ultrafiltration rate;
2) high permeability to all species to minimize membrane area and dialysis times;
3) an enhanced permeability to middle molecular weight species relative to low molecular weight species.

Ultrafiltration rate is determined primarily by the membrane structure—mean pore size, tortuosity, proportion of mobile phase compared to dense phase, and so on—and the hydraulic or osmotic pressure gradients across it. The diffusion of low molecular weight species across conventional membranes is limited by diffusion at the blood side interface but may be augmented by bulk ultrafiltration flow. As the molecular weight of the diffusing species increases, the membrane resistance to flow becomes relatively more important compared to these interfacial resistances; the permeation rate of these middle molecules is almost entirely defined by the membrane characteristics—structure, thickness, and area.

The achievement of optional permeation characteristics of the combined device/membrane system may be approached by varying a number of membrane parameters:

1) dialysis membranes manufactured from different materials and by different methods but having substantially similar effective pore size and ultrafiltration rate;
2) use of membranes of more open structure with less diffusion-resistance to high molecular weight species but requiring careful pressure or other control devices to control potentially high ultrafiltration rate and diffusion rate of low molecular weight components;
3) use of thinner membranes to reduce membrane-limited resistance to flow of high molecular weight materials;
4) use of membranes of larger relative areas to enhance high molecular weight transport at a given total blood flow rate.

Table 5 gives typical permeability properties of two conventional dialysis membranes Cuprophan® and a viscose material.[10-12] Little variation in permeation properties is observed, or indeed with any other candidate membrane materials. The so-called ultrafiltration membranes of cellulose acetate and polyacrylonitrile, however, have a more open structure and have considerably higher water permeabilities. Compared to the dialysis membranes they restrict the flow of higher molecular weight species such as vitamin B_{12} relatively less than low molecular weight species. Thus the permeability ratio of B_{12} to urea increases from 0.1 to 0.05 for conventional dialysis membranes and to 0.2 for ultrafiltration membranes.

TABLE 5

TYPICAL PROPERTIES OF COMMERCIAL ARTIFICIAL KIDNEY MEMBRANES

Membrane Dialyzer	H_2O ml/min,m², mmHg	Permeability Urea cm/min	Creatinine cm/min	B_{12} cm/min	B_{12}/Urea
Cuprophan®	0.0004	0.09	0.06	0.008	0.09
Viscose	0.0009	0.08	0.05	0.004	0.05
Ultrafiltration					
Cellulose Acetate	0.003	0.09	0.06	0.017	0.18
Polyacrylonitrile	0.008	0.13	0.09	0.024	0.18

FIGURE 2 shows the ratio of permeability for different molecular species between a Cuprophan® dialysis membrane and a cellulose acetate ultrafiltration membrane.[13] Whereas, as expected, the ultrafiltration rate of the cellulose acetate membrane is eight times that of Cuprophan®, the permeability of low molecular weight materials is of comparable magnitude, since it is controlled by fluid-phase interfacial diffusion. As the molecular weight increases, the relative permeability of the particular species increases as the relative importance of membrane resistance increases in the overall diffusion process.

TABLE 6 shows the effect of membrane thickness on selectivity. The ratios of the permeabilities of several species for three membrane thicknesses is

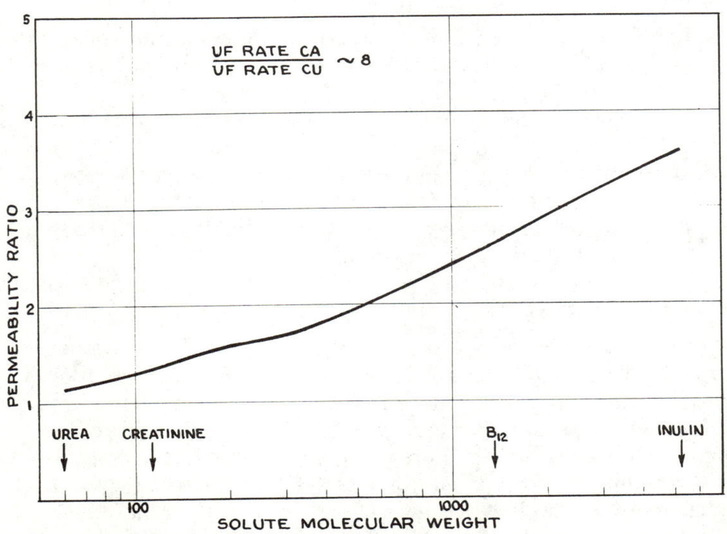

FIGURE 2. Comparison of Cuprophan® (CU) and cellulose acetate (CA) membranes.

TABLE 6

MEMBRANE THICKNESS AND MEMBRANE SELECTIVITY

Thickness (mils)	Ratio of Permeability		
	Urea	Creatinine	Raffinose
1.4	1.0	1.0	1.0
1.0	1.1	1.2	1.5
0.5	1.7	2.1	3.6

shown.[10] For a species of given molecular weight, decreasing the membrane thickness increases the relative permeabilities. But in addition, as the membrane is made thinner, the ratio for the high molecular weight species increases more rapidly than that for the low molecular weight species. This is clearly a consequence of a greater degree of membrane control over the permeation rate for larger molecules, as opposed to blood interfacial resistance control for the species of smaller molecular weight.

TABLE 7 shows the effect of increasing the membrane area in a device operating at a given blood-flow rate.[14] As the area of membrane is increased from 0.64 M^2 to 1 M^2, the permeation rate of urea actually decreases because the blood-flow rate per unit of area decreases and increases the blood interfacial resistance.[16] On the other hand, the permeation rate of the higher molecular weight species increases because the limiting membrane resistance is reduced in proportion to the membrane area. The ratio of permeability of high molecular weight species to low molecular weight species therefore increases dramatically as the membrane area is increased at a given blood-flow rate.

Thus a performance parameter of primary interest in artificial kidneys—the ratio of high molecular weight to low molecular weight permeation rate—can be changed by making use of the interaction between the membrane transport properties and the blood side diffusion resistance. The ratio increases with a more open membrane structure and also with use of thinner membranes or larger membrane areas at a given blood-flow rate.

TABLE 7

RELATIVE PERMEATION RATES OF DIALYZERS WITH DIFFERENT MEMBRANE AREAS

Membrane Area m^2	Blood Flow Rate ml/min	Relative Permeation		
		Urea	Creatinine	B_{12}
0.64	200	1.00	1.00	1.00
1.0	100	0.87	0.89	1.2
1.0	200	0.95	0.92	1.2
1.0	300	1.07	0.96	1.25

Conclusion

In both the membrane lung and the artificial kidney the ultimate mass-transfer performance of the device is the result of the interaction of the transport properties in the blood and in the permeable surface. Both the hemodynamics of the device and the properties of the membrane may be changed to alter the characteristics of the device, although the performance priorities are of a different nature in each case.

References

1. Crank, J. & G. Park. 1968. Diffusion in polymers. Academic Press. New York, N.Y.
2. Murphy, W., L. A. Trudell, L. I. Friedman, M. Kakvan, P. O. Richardson, K. Karlson & P. M. Galletti. 1974. Laboratory and clinical experience with a microporous membrane oxygenator. TSAIO **20:** 278.
3. Bartlett, R. H., S. W. Fong & C. McArthur. 1975. Prolonged extracorporeal circulation (ECC) with microporous membrane oxygenators: hematologic effects. TSAIO abstr.
4. Dantowitz, P., A. S. Borsanyi, M. C. Deibert, M. T. Snider, M. H. Lipsky & P. M. Galletti. 1969. A blood oxygenator and pre-formed membrane-lined capillary channels. TSAIO **15:** 138.
5. Lautier, A., P. Rey, J. Bizot, A. Faure, A. Sausse & D. Laurent. 1969. Comparison of gaseous transfer through synthetic membranes for oxygenators. TSAIO **15:** 144.
6. Crawford, J. E. & D. N. Gray. 1971. Preparation and properties of some poly (alpha-olefin sulfones). J. Appl. Polym. Sci. **15:** 1881.
7. Ketteringham, J. M., W. Zapol, J. Birkett, L. Nelsen, A. Massucco & C. Raith. 1975. A high permeability, nonporous, blood compatible membrane for membrane lungs: in vivo and in vitro performance. Vol. XXI. TSAIO: 224.
8. Peterson, R. J. & L. T. Rozelle. 1975. Ethylcellulose perfluorobutyrate: a highly non-thrombogenic fluoropolymer for gas exchange membranes. TSAIO Abstract.
9. Hill, J. D., A. Iatridis, R. O'Keefe & S. Kitrilakis. 1974. Technique for achieving high gas exchange rates in membrane oxygenation. TSAIO **20:** 249.
10. Ketteringham, J. Unpublished data.
11. Klein, E. 1973. Membrane and materials evaluation: permeabilities, physical and mechanical properties of hemodialysis membranes. Celanese Research Corporation Cellulose Acetate Membrane, Annual Report AK–1–72–2221, Artificial Kidney—Chronic Uremia Program, NIH, Bethesda, Md. July 16.
12. Klein, E. 1974. Membrane and materials evaluation: permeabilities, physical and mechanical properties of hemodialysis membranes. Rhone Polenc Polyacrylonitrile membrane. Annual Report AK–1–72–2221, Artificial Kidney—Chronic Uremia Program, NIH, Bethesda, Md. July 29.
13. Miller, J. H., J. H. Shinaberger & F. E. Martin. 1974. Dialysis membranes: cellulose acetate compared with other membrane materials. Medical Instrumentation **8**(3): 214.
14. Klein, E. 1973. Membrane and materials evaluation: permeabilities, physical and mechanical properties of hemodialysis membranes. Bemberg Cuprophan PT–150 Membrane. Annual Report AK–1–72–221, Artificial Kidney—Chronic Uremia Program, NIH, Bethesda, Md. July 16.

CELL-LINED, NONWOVEN MICROFIBER SCAFFOLDS AS A BLOOD INTERFACE *

William E. Burkel and Raymond H. Kahn

Department of Anatomy
University of Michigan
Ann Arbor, Michigan 48104

In order to provide blood-compatible interfaces for artificial vascular prostheses, technology has proceeded along several lines, including the use of (1) synthetic materials such as neutral, ionic and polarized polymers and pyrolytic carbons; (2) additive containing materials such as heparin; (3) hydrogels; (4) woven and nonwoven fiber scaffolds lined with cells or fibrin; and (5) composites of the above.[1,2] Although fiber scaffolds (in the form of porous woven or knitted fabrics) have been in use for many years, healing is somewhat capricious and is always preceded by the formation of a fibrin coagulum that subsequently undergoes organization and may or may not give rise to a healed endothelium. The use of porous prostheses permits flexion of the vessel as well as adherence of the fibrin coagulum and the potential for transinterstices growth of tissue, which, it is hoped, will lead to a healed pseudointima. Since adherence of the pseudointima (whether cellular or fibrin) and healing depends to a great extent on the surface characteristics and porosity of the prosthesis,[3-11] many types of surfaces have been developed (woven, knitted, velours, flocks, lattices, etc.) to promote better healing. Emphasis recently has been on the production of prostheses with smaller fibers and pores such as "Weavnit,"[9] "Microknit,"[10] and "Warpknit"[11] for clinical application. On the experimental side, in recent years nonwoven microfiber scaffolds have been produced[12-14] as an alternative to woven and knitted prostheses.

Heart-assist devices must of necessity be nonporous, given the nature of the pneumatic pumps. Since blood pumps have large surfaces exposed to the blood, the potential for thrombus, degradation of blood proteins, and hemolysis is great. To circumvent these problems, fabric-lined pumps have been developed.[15-20] However, such nonporous prostheses or pumps permit no growth of cells except from the natural vessel at the anastomotic line. Since this neointima comes only from the intima or media of the vessels at the suture line in both heart assists or in arterial grafts,[21] production of cellular pseudointimas before implantation of the devices would be beneficial.

Various methods of pseudointima production have been attempted, including: (1) the use of tissue fragments,[16,19,20] (2) trypsinization of organs, viscera, and so on, followed by immediate seeding of prostheses with dispersed cells,[20] (3) derivation of cells from tissues followed by cultivation *in vitro* and seeding of subcultured cells.[20,22-34] Numerous cell sources for culture-derived pseudointimas have been tried, including skin,[17,20] kidney,[20,24] arteries,[20] veins,[19,20,22] subcutaneous tissue,[19,20] lung,[16,20] pleura,[22] fascia,[22] granulation tissue,[19,20,22,28] bone marrow,[19] macrophages,[13] pericardium,[20,22] fibro-

* Supported by contract no. NIH–NO1–HB–2054 from the National Heart and Lung Institute, National Institutes of Health, Bethesda, Md. 20014.

blasts,[23, 24, 28] buffy coat,[25] endothelial cells,[18, 22, 25, 26, 30, 32, 33, 35] smooth muscle,[35] skeletal muscle,[16, 19, 20] ascitic cells,[19] epidermis,[26, 29, 31–33] WI-38 cells,[25–29, 31–33] and urothelium).[29]

This paper reports some of our experiences on the development of pseudointimas on nonwoven microfiber scaffolds with cells derived from human tissue, namely, WI-38, epidermal, endothelial, and urothelial cells.

Materials and Methods

Cell Sources

Diploid WI-38 cells derived from embryonic human lung were obtained from Professor L. Hayflick of Stanford University at approximately the twelfth passage. These cells were used to screen microfabrics for biocompatibility and to develop techniques for producing pseudointimas. Human epidermal cells were obtained from split-thickness skin explants obtained from the University of Michigan Dermatology Clinic. Endothelium was surgically derived from stripped veins, aneurysmectomy, and normal veins of kidney-transplant cadavers. Urinary tract epithelium, which we have referred to as urothelium, was obtained from biopsies of urethra, bladder, and renal pelves.

Epidermal, endothelial, and urothelial cells were isolated by treatment of the corresponding explants with 0.25% trypsin and 1% EDTA in balanced salt solution (Earle's calcium and magnesium-free, 1X, Grand Island Biological Company). After incubation of the explants for 15–20 minutes at 37° C in the above solution, the epithelial layer was gently teased off from the underlying connective tissue and transferred to growth medium in Falcon plastic tissue culture flasks. Growth medium consisted of Eagle's Basal Medium (BME, cat no. G13, Grand Island Biological Company) buffered with 0.10 M HEPES[36] (N-2 hydroxyethyl piperazine sulfonic acid, California Biochemical Corp.),

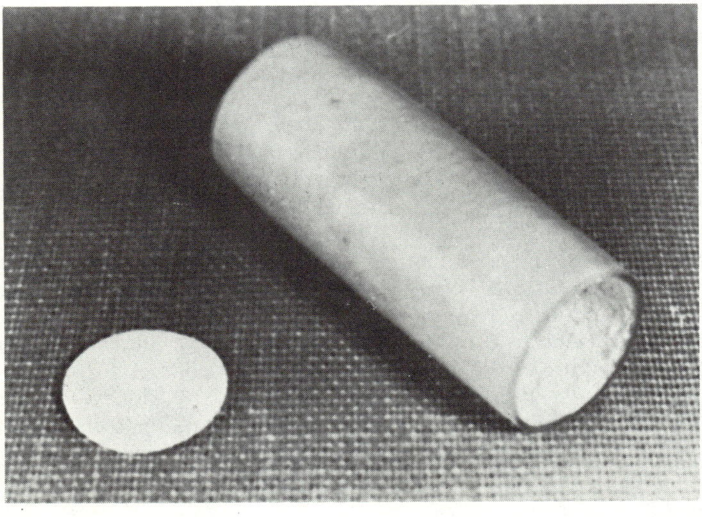

FIGURE 1. Tube and disc of the type used for compatibility testing and pseudointimal development. ×1.5.

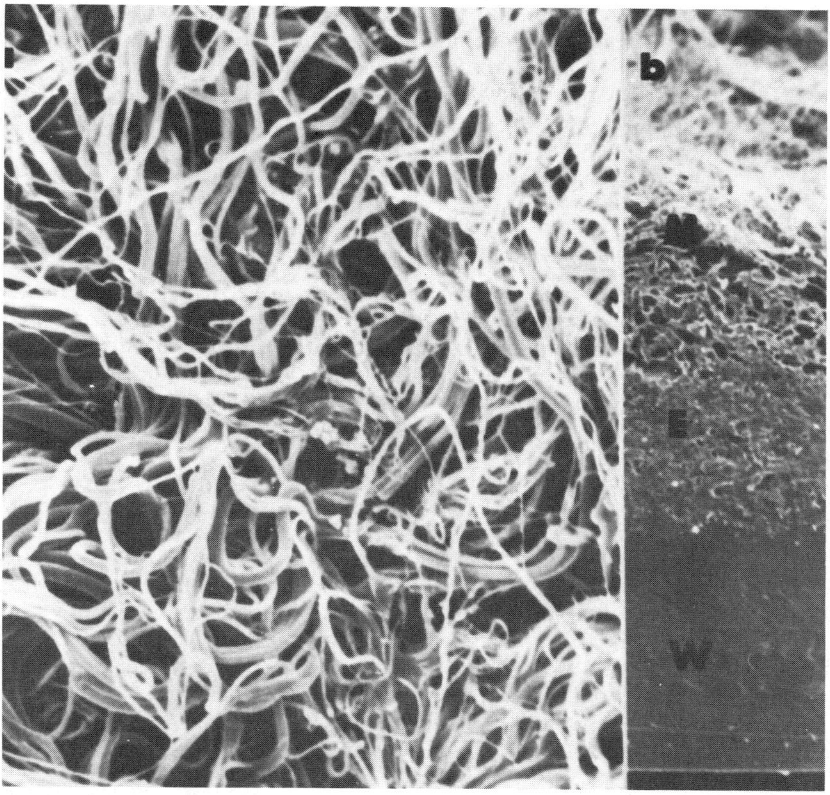

FIGURE 2. Polyester (polytetramethylene terephthalate) microfiber scaffold produced by hot-melt extrusion. a=Microfabric surface (×380); b=cross section of tube showing embeddment (E) of microfibers (M) into nonporous estane wall (W) (×130).

buffered to pH 7.4 at room temperature. The medium was supplemented with 10% bovine serum and 50 μg/ml Aureomycin Chlortetracycline HCl (Lederle Division, American Cyanimide Corp.)

Microfabrics

Polyurethane (5714-F1 estane) tubes (18 × 50 mm) and discs (15 mm in diameter) lined with microfiber scaffolds of nylon 6,6, carbon-coated nylon, polyester(polytetramethylene terephthalate), and polypropylene were used in these studies (FIGURE 1). Nylon 6,6 and polyester microfibers were produced by hot melt extrusion to give a nonwoven microfiber mesh of 0.2–2 μm fibers bonded to the nonporous estane by a negative casting procedure [12] by Abcor Corporation, Cambridge, Mass. (FIGURE 2). Some of the nylon was coated with a 3000 Å layer of pyrolytic carbon [36, 37] by Gulf Atomic Corporation, San Diego, Calif. or Parylene-C,[14, 39] and microwave discharge-treated. Polypropylene (Union Carbide, Inc., Boundbrook, N.J.) microfibers were produced by coextrusion of polypropylene and acrylic copolymers followed by extraction of the acrylic component and stretching or horizontal drafting of the extruded tape.[14, 40] The resulting fibers were 0.2–2 μm in diameter and were supplied in two configurations, a nonvertically drafted fiber mat produced by horizontal drafting only, and a vertically drafted fiber mat produced by horizontal and vertical drafting (FIGURE 3). These were attached to estane tubes and discs[41] and were coated with a 5000 Å layer of Parylene-C. All tubes and discs were sterilized by beta radiation.

Preparation of Pseudointimas

Pseudointimas were produced by a four-step process[27, 29, 32] which included (1) washing and degassing of fabric, (2) seeding of cells, (3) stabilization, and (4) static or perfusion culture. Prior to seeding with cells, the tubes or discs were washed and degassed in media at low negative pressures (10–15 mm Hg). The cell sources, propagated as monolayer cultures, were trypsinized (0.25% in balanced salt solution), washed in balanced salt solution, and seeded with an appropriate number of cells to give approximately 2000–10,000 cells/mm^2 of fabric surface. Seeding of tubes and discs was accomplished by centrifugation of cells into the fabric at about $50 \times g$ for approximately one minute. Emigration of the cells from the fabric was prevented by "stabilization" of the tube or disc in a confined environment for about 12 hours. After stabilization, the tubes were placed in a modified New Brunswick Rollacell perfusion apparatus and cultivated for six days. Tubes were rotated at 11 revolutions per hour and perfused for 5–10 seconds every hour, depending on the glucose content of the effluent medium. Discs were cultivated under static conditions in T-75 Falcon tissue-culture flasks for a corresponding amount of time, with media changes every two days.

Evaluation

Tubes and discs were evaluated by light microscopy and scanning and transmission electron microscopy. Samples were fixed in 2.5% glutaraldehyde and 0.1 M cacodylate buffer at pH 7.4 followed by postosmication and dehydration in a graded series of alcohols. Samples for light microscopy and transmission electron microscopy were embedded in Epon, cut at 1 μm and stained with methylene blue. Selected samples were thin-sectioned and stained with uranyl acetate and lead citrate for transmission electron microscopy. Corresponding samples were prepared for scanning electron microscopy by freeze- or critical-point drying followed by gold or gold-paladium coating. Pseudointimas were evaluated by estimating the percentage of surface area of the tube or disc covered with cells when observed with the scanning electron microscope. Penetration of fabric by cells and cell-fabric relationships were studied by light and transmission electron microscopy.

RESULTS

Pseudointima Appearance

Throughout our experiments we have emphasized the use of human cells, since the ultimate usefulness of pseudointimal lined tubes lies in man. The WI-38 cell line, derived from fetal human lung, has been widely used for biological testing and in studies of population dynamics and aging.[42–45] We have

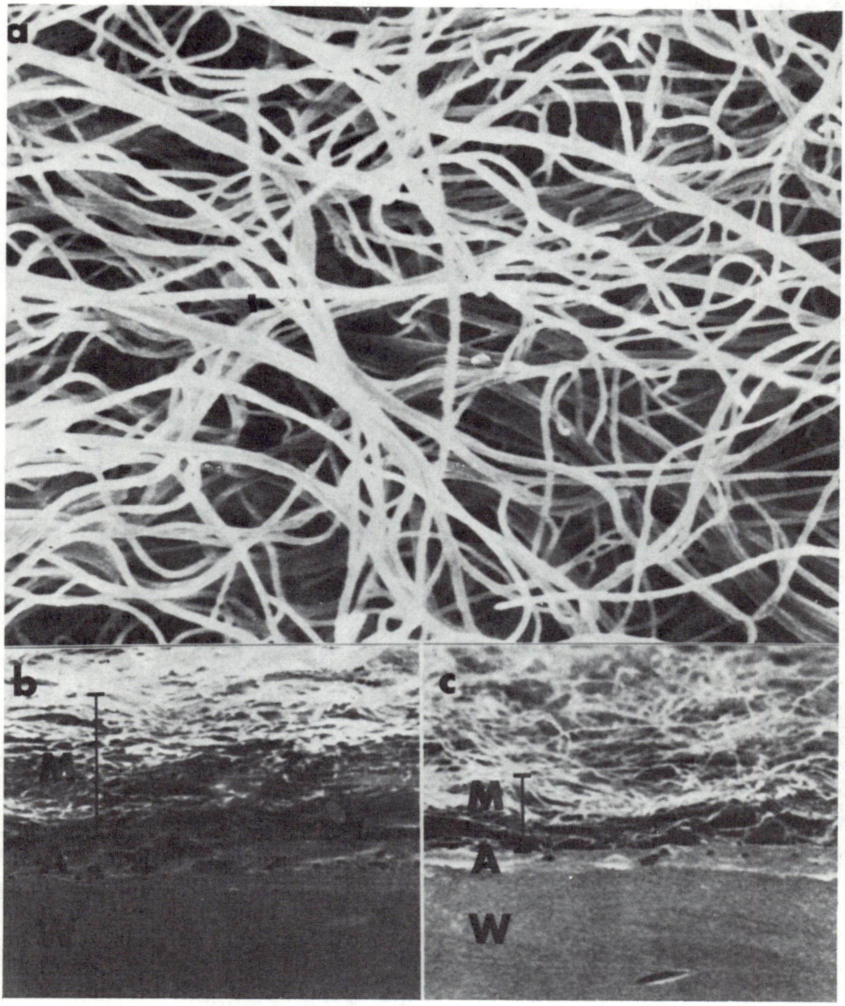

FIGURE 3. Parylene-C coated polypropylene microfiber scaffold. a=Surface (×1400); b=cross section of nonvertically drafted mat showing thickness of microfiber mat (M) and attachment to the impermeable estane backing (W) by adhesive (A) (×140); c=cross section of a vertically drafted microfiber scaffold (×140). Note the thinner fiber mat (M) and relative looseness of fibers in comparison to the nonvertically drafted mat.

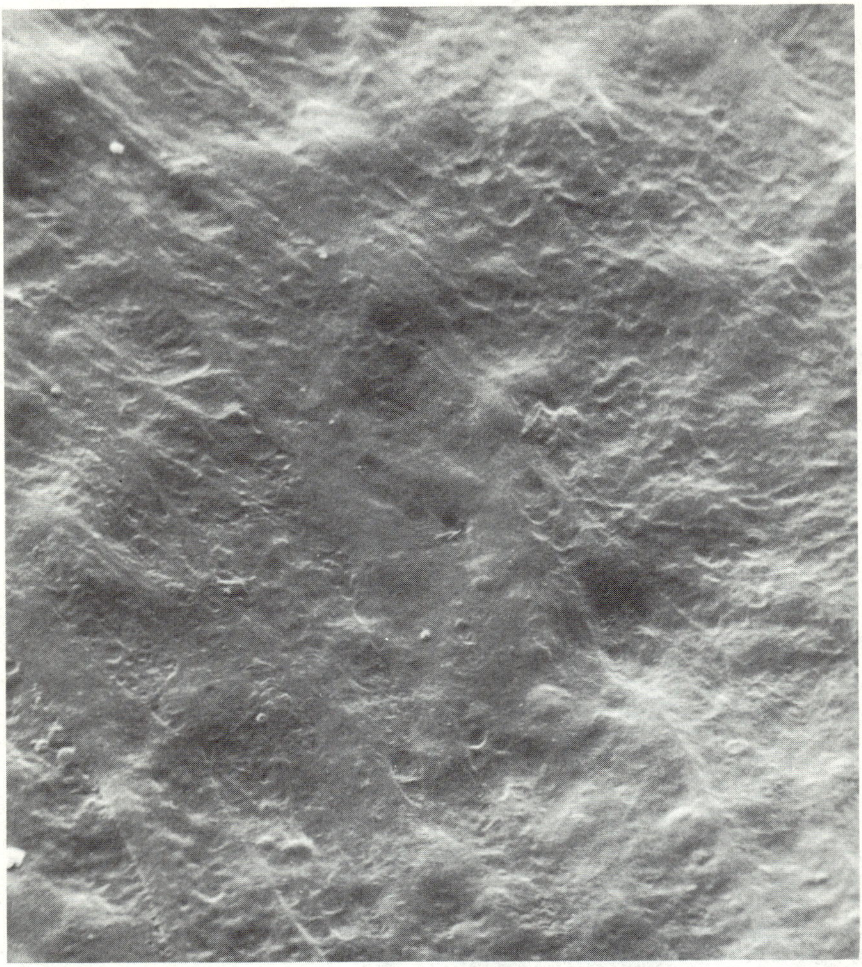

FIGURE 4. Pseudointima produced by WI–38 cells on polyester microfiber scaffold (×2600).

found this cell line very useful for testing biocompatibility of materials and for developing techniques.[25-27] Technically, WI-38 cells produced excellent, complete pseudointimas when seeded into microfiber scaffolds (FIGURE 4). However, the immune reaction of the recipient against such a cell line mitigates against its use in clinical situations. We therefore experimented with three relatively easily obtained, potentially autologous human cells for the production of pseudointimas, namely, epidermis, endothelium, and urothelium.

Because of the ease of acquisition and their abundance, epidermal cells represent perhaps the most potentially useful cells for lining prostheses. Like WI-38 cells, human epidermally derived cells produce excellent pseudointimas *in vitro* (FIGURE 5). They are smooth, confluent, and usually consist of one to four layers of cells (FIGURE 6), after seven days in culture.

Theoretically, endothelium would appear to be the most desirable for lining prostheses because of its inherent blood compatibility. These cells produce excellent pseudointimas (FIGURE 7). The difficulties in rapidly propagating sufficient cells from adult human endothelium, however, limits their potential usefulness at this time.

Although urothelium (particularly from bladder) is available in limited quantities, it can be obtained in amounts adequate to seed small vessels if cultivation time is sufficient. The limited number of experiments that have been done with this cell source seems to indicate that these cells will also produce confluent cell layers on prostheses if enough cells are seeded (FIGURE 8).

Microfiber Compatibility

Compatibility of microfiber scaffolds was evaluated by seeding various fabrics with the WI-38 cells and assessing the percentage of the surface area covered with cells after seven days *in vitro*. As can be seen from TABLE 1, nylon 6,6 fabric (Abcor) gave better pseudointimas (69% coverage) without

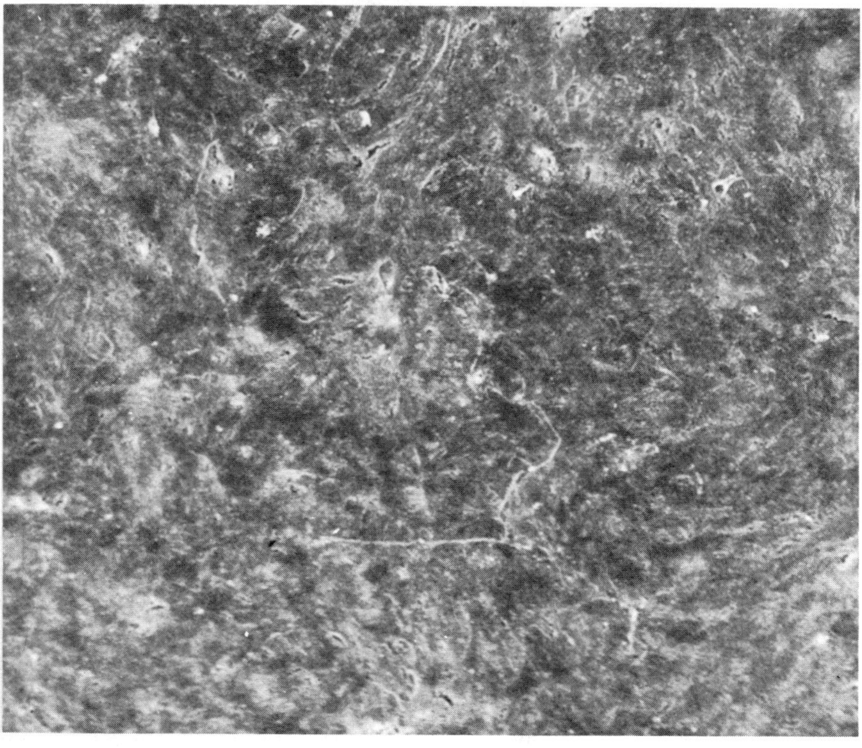

FIGURE 5. Surface of a pseudointima produced by human epidermal cells on polyester microfabric (×180).

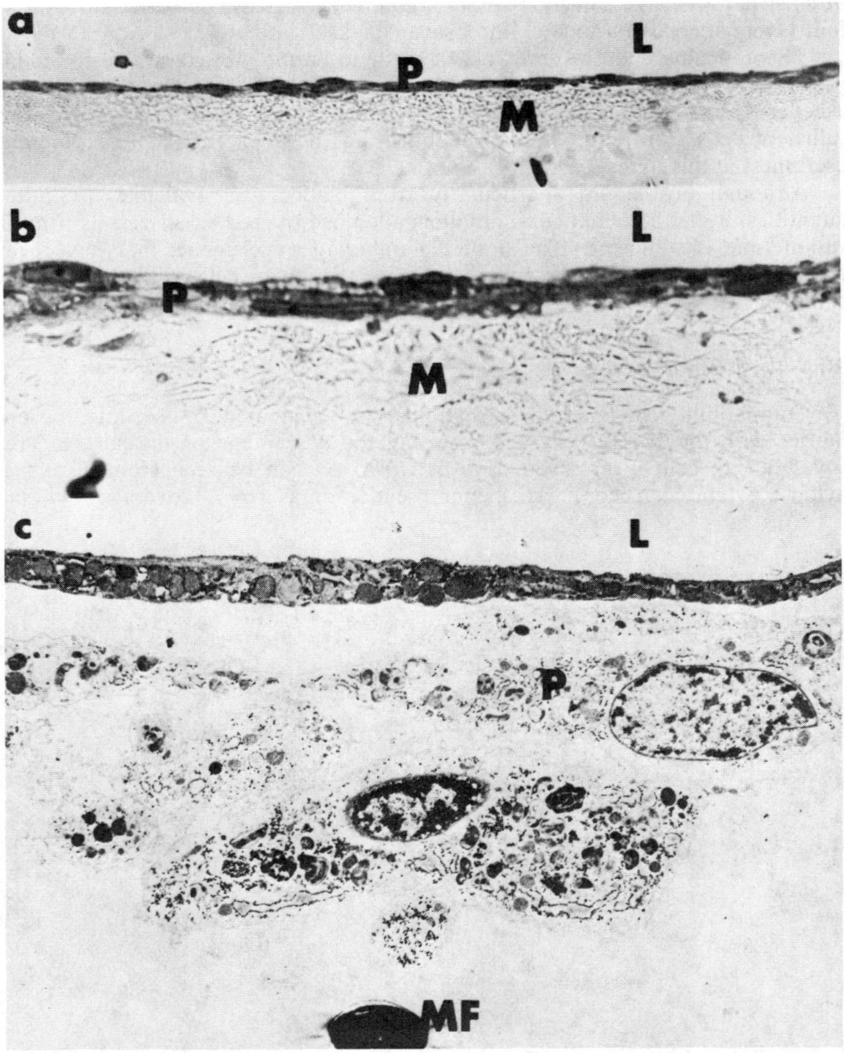

FIGURE 6. a+b=Cross section of a pseudointima (P) produced by human epidermal cells on nonvertically drafted polypropylene microfibers (M) (×150;500); c=electron micrograph of a portion of a similar pseudointima. Note that cells at the luminal surface (L) are flattened, whereas the deeper cells near the microfiber (MF) are polygonal (×3500).

a negative surface charge imparted by microwave discharge treatment. Carbon or Parylene-C coating of nylon (FIGURE 9) gave a dramatic improvement in coverage (100% and 93%, respectively). Parylene-C coated polypropylene fibers, whether vertically (71% coverage) or nonvertically drafted (71% coverage) gave slightly poorer results, but still produced good pseudointimas. The polytetramethylene terephthalate fabric with no special treatment or coating gave 77% coverage. It was apparent from these early experiments that carbon-coated nylon was the best pseudointimal substrate. However, transmission electron microscopy showed the carbon coating to be brittle (FIGURE 10) and subject to phagocytosis. Coupled with the known, limited life span of nylon *in vivo,* these findings led to the exclusion of all of the nylon fabrics for studies with potentially autologous cell lines.

Fabric coverages with epidermal, endothelial, and urothelial cells are shown in TABLE 2. Epidermal cells grew well on all of the fabrics tested, whereas endothelial and urothelial cells did considerably worse on the Parylene-C coated polypropylene. From the results of these and of the WI-38 experiments it is

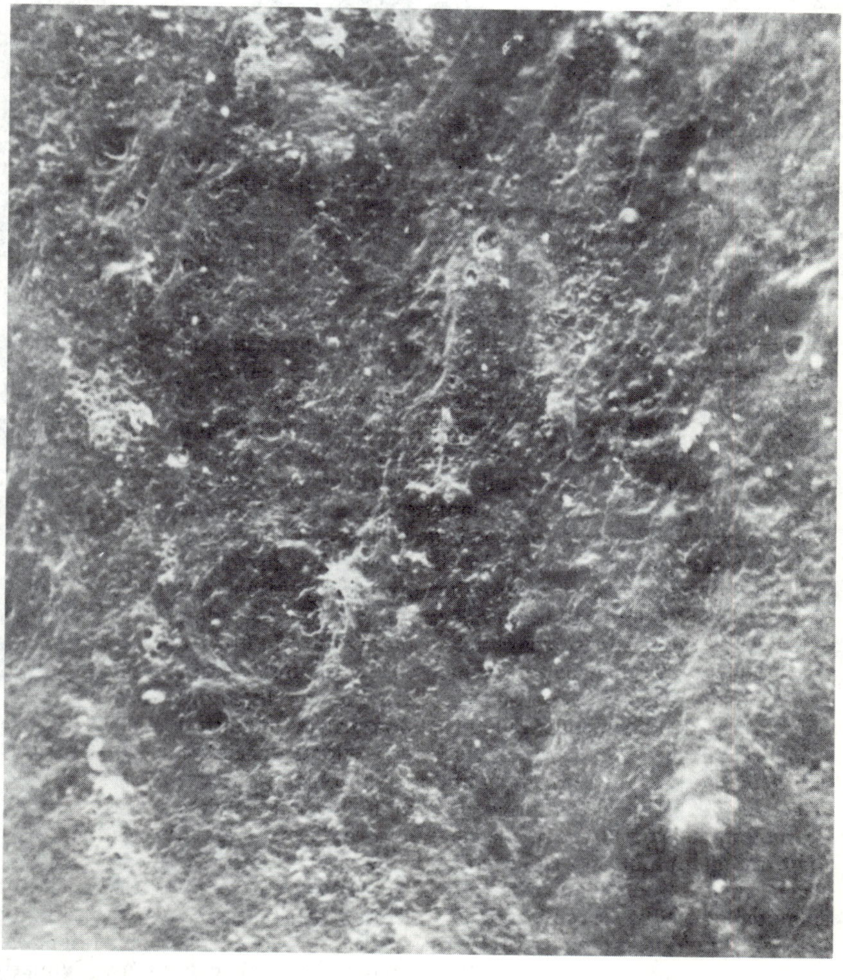

FIGURE 7. Surface view of a pseudointima produced by human endothelial cells on a polyester microfiber scaffold (×1400).

apparent that the polytetramethylene terephthalate microfibers offered the best substrates for pseudointimal development with the cell lines which we have tested. These microfiber scaffolds have the additional advantage of being firmly embedded (FIGURE 2b) in the estane backing and therefore are resistant to shearing forces.

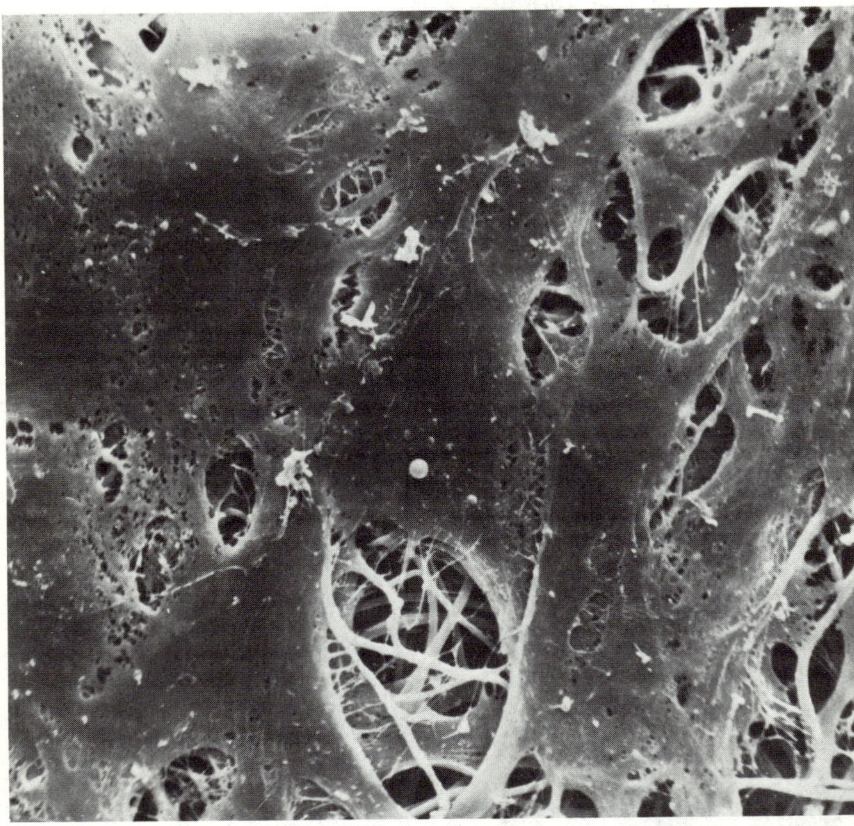

FIGURE 8. Pseudointima produced by urothelium on polyester microfibers. The cell layer is incomplete in this specimen because not enough cells/mm² were seeded (×1100).

Also important in the development of pseudointimas *in vitro* was the culture system used (TABLE 3). Devices cultivated in roller bottles by perfusion require significantly fewer cells/mm² ($p < .05$) to give 80–100% coverage within seven days when compared to static cultures under the same conditions. Similarly, perfusion culture requires the least number of cells/mm² to give the same coverage.

TABLE 1

MICROFIBER COMPATIBILITY WITH WI–38 CELLS

Fiber Type	Coating or Treatment	Number of Experiments *	Mean % of Surface Area Covered	
Nylon 6,6 †	—	(30)	69	30.9 ¶
Nylon-6,6 †	Microwave	(18)	54	47.7 ¶
Nylon-6,6 †	Parylene-C ‡	(13)	93	8.5 ¶
Nylon-6, 6 †	Pyrolytic Carbon	(6)	100	0.0 ¶
Polytetramethylene Terephthalate †	—	(48)	77	28.9 ¶
Polypropylene- Non-Vert. Draft ‡	Parylene-C ‡ Microwave	(90)	71	34.6 ¶
Polypropylene Vert. Draft ‡	Parylene-C ‡ Microwave	(75)	71	37.8 ¶

* ( ) = Number of cases.
† Abcor, Inc.
‡ Union Carbide, Corp.
§ Gulf Atomic, Inc.
¶ Standard deviation throughout column.

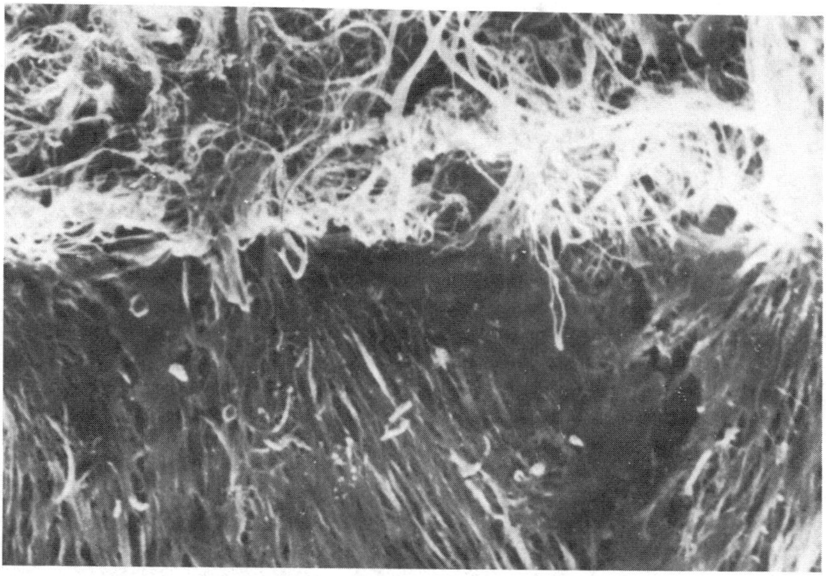

FIGURE 9. Pseudointima produced by WI–38 cells on a nylon 6,6 fabric only partly coated with carbon. The carbonized portion (below) is very compatible to, and almost completely covered with cells which are almost totally absent on the bare nylon above (×200).

TABLE 2

COMPATIBILITY WITH AUTOLOGOUS CELLS

Fiber Type	Coating	Epidermis % Cover *			Endothelium % Cover			Urothelium % Cover		
Polypropylene (Non-vertically drafted)	Parylene-C Microwave	(66) †	78	28.8 ‡	(3)	28	20.2 *	(2)	63	17.7 ‡
Polypropylene (Vertically drafted)	Parylene-C Microwave	(61)	66	37.5 ‡	(2)	75	35.4 *	(2)	25	35.4 ‡
Polyester (Polytetramethylene Terephthalate)	—	(39)	87	24.6 ‡	(7)	94	9.3 *	(2)	95	3.5 ‡

* % Cover = mean % of surface area covered with cells.
† ( ) = Number of cases.
‡ Standard deviation.

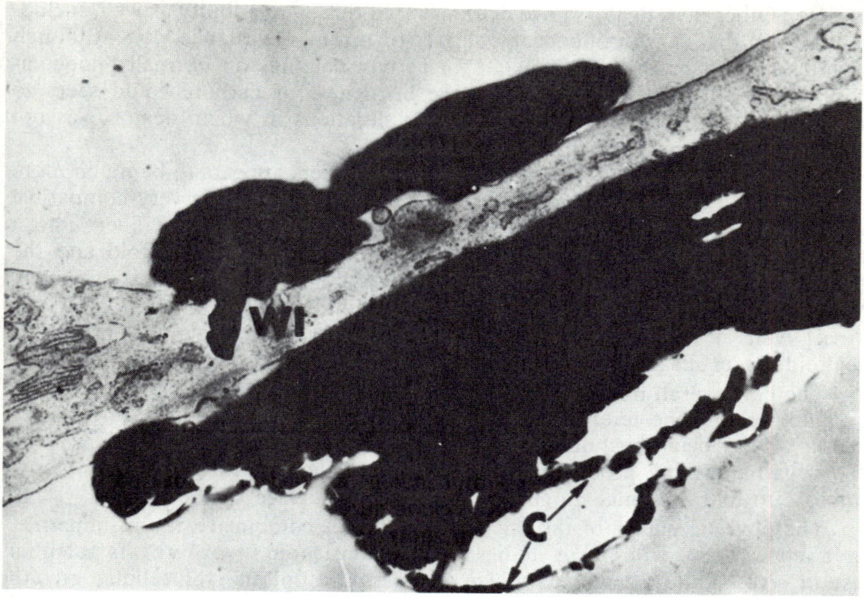

FIGURE 10. Transmission electron micrograph of carbon-coated nylon fibers on either side of a WI-38 cell (WI). Note that the carbon layer (C) has become fractured at the surface of the microfiber (×13,000).

DISCUSSION

The use of cell-lined microfiber scaffolds as blood interfaces depends upon (1) microfibers that are compatible with cells and durable *in vivo:* (2) the availability of nonthrombogenic, nonantigenic cells to line prostheses and the (3) tissue culture technology capable of cultivating suitable cells and producing reliable pseudointimas.

The present study demonstrates that tissue culture can provide a rapid and inexpensive procedure to screen materials and that there are wide differences in the biocompatibility of microfiber scaffolds to cultured cells *in vitro*. Carbon-coated fabrics are without question the best surface for cell growth encountered

TABLE 3

COMPARISON OF CULTURE METHODS

Cell Type	Mean number of cells/mm² yielding 80–100% coverage		Minimum number of cells/mm² yielding 80–100% coverage	
	Static	Perfusion	Static	Perfusion
WI–38	(119)* 11980	(64) 9146	(119) 5100	(64) 2480
Epidermis	(50) 9108	(44) 5267	(50) 5600	(44) 1840

* ( ) = Number of cases.

to date. Other investigators have demonstrated this compatibility as well, including the fact that carbon offers some degree of thromboresistance.[37, 38] Although it is possible to produce extremely thin carbon coatings on normally noncompatible microfibers (i.e. nylon 6,6), the brittleness of carbon would seem to preclude its use; the exception being those situations in which flexion was not required, such as in heart valves.

The use of Parylene-C as a coating for microfibers appears to be much more satisfactory in terms of flexibility than carbon. Moreover, it is very compatible with cells and has the additional advantage of binding all of the fibers into a continuing web, thereby providing structural integrity of the scaffold and the backing. The long-term durability of this material *in vivo,* however, is unknown. We have some concern that these microfiber scaffolds might separate from the vessel wall at the point of adhesion (FIGURE 3) or between layers of the scaffold, under shearing forces encountered at systole.

The best overall microfiber scaffold tested so far appears to be the polyester (polytetramethylene terephthalate). This material gives excellent cell growth, requires no special treatment, and is firmly embedded into the vessel wall by the negative casting procedure. The only drawback of this type of material appears to be occasional roughness of the inner surface of the fabric.

The physical nature of the microfiber scaffolds combined with an impermeable estane wall used in these studies must be considered in terms of its potential use *in vivo.* The fiber and pore size appear to be optimal for cellular growth and penetration. The nonporous outer wall has direct applicability to blood pumps but is less useful in arterial or venous replacement because of its relative inflexibility and exclusion of transinterstices growth. Ideally, it may be useful to produce a vessel with a microfiber scaffold attached to a biodegradable outer wall. This wall would prevent hemorrhage after implantation but would subsequently permit gradual replacement with connective tissue cells and ingrowth of blood vessels to the pseudointima. Ultimately, only the microfiber scaffold would remain as a supporting skeleton for the pseudointima and the connective tissue wall.

Cell sources for nonthrombogenic, nonantigenic pseudointimal linings must take into account ease of acquisition, numbers of cells available, adaptability to the *in vitro* environment, rapidity of growth, and their *in vivo* behavior. From a technical point of view, the WI-38 cells used for establishing biocompatibility form excellent pseudointimas *in vitro* and are very durable in simulated vascular systems.[31, 32] Yet, they would not be useful *in vivo,* since they are allogenic and, most likely, thrombogenic. While other investigators have used a variety of connective tissue cells,[19, 20, 46] they all required a fibrin coagulum. In one series of experiments Bernhard *et al.*[46] were able to use allogenic fetal fibroblasts to produce pseudointimas in calves without rejection. It is doubtful, however, that such allogenic cells would survive in other species or in adult cattle, for that matter. Rapidly growing fetal cells for pseudointimas would be useful only clinically if they were found to be nonthrombogenic and the immune response were lacking or could be suppressed without threat to the host. Since this is unlikely at the present time, potentially autologous cell lines seem to be the more reasonable approach.

The ease of acquisition and abundance of epidermis makes this a useful cell type for pseudointimal production. Skin fragments were used by Adachi *et al.*[20] to produce pseudointimas, but they found that fragments yielded rough surfaces and an irregular distribution of cells. Their attempts at producing pseudointimas from subcultured skin were unsuccessful. In these studies, cultivated epidermal cells produce excellent pseudointimas of one to four layers of cells *in vitro*. While demonstrating structural differences depending upon their position, epidermal cells appear to modulate in their new environment and have never exhibited any keratinization. The question, however, remains as to whether these pseudointimas are nonthrombogenic. Preliminary studies indicate that the epidermal cells we have used are less thrombogenic than fibroblasts.[47] However, further studies are required and are currently under-way with canine epidermis.

Although a natural endothelium would appear to be ideal because of its natural nonthrombogenicity and relative ease of acquisition from subcutaneous veins, culture of these cells is beset with technical problems. The first problem relates to the derivation of cells and the second to their slow growth *in vitro,* which appears to be only slightly faster than *in vivo.* Numerous investigators have cultivated fetal endothelial cells from human umbilical cord[48-54] and have used these cells extensively to study the properties of endothelium. These cells, however, are far different from adult endothelium in their adherence to underlying connective tissue and their growth characteristics.[55] To be sure, adult endothelium grows very slowly in man, as is shown by healing rates of prostheses.[4, 56] Moreover, arterial and venous endothelium differ structurally from each other, as does the endothelium of either of these vessels in different parts of the same animal.[57]

Although cells derived from adult human endothelium do produce confluent pseudointimal linings for prostheses (FIGURE 7), their ultimate use in clinical situations will depend upon the ability to enhance their proliferation. Perhaps adult endothelium requires a mitotic stimulant such as the "tumor angiogenesis factor,"[58] for, to our knowledge, no one has successfully cultivated adult human endothelial cells in quantity. Other investigators[19, 20, 22] have used pieces of blood vessels to produce pseudointimas, but whether the linings produced were of endothelial, smooth muscle, or connective tissue origin is unknown. Mansfield *et al.*[34] has shown excellent pseudointimas produced *in vitro* with calf endothelial cells, and this work holds some promise. Whether it can be extrapolated to human tissue, however, remains a question, since calf endothelium is relatively easy to propagate *in vitro* and calves are known to coat naked prostheses quite rapidly.[4] Clearly, the calf is not the closest experimental model for man.[4]

The use of urothelial cells to produce pseudointimas is questionable at this time. That these cells will line prostheses *in vitro* is apparent. These cells proliferatae quite rapidly, but their usefulness is limited by the small amounts of tissue that may be obtained for culture. Consequently, they would be useful to line small prostheses, and then only if they are found to be nonthrombogenic.

The advantages of perfusion over static cultures have been consistently demonstrated in this investigation. In all experiments we were able to produce comparable pseudointimas by perfusion culture with only 70% of the cells required to seed materials cultured under static conditions. These results corroborate those of Kruse *et al.*[59-61] in the production of multiple-layered populations of cells. The improvement in results in perfusion culture relate not only to the steady state of the media nutrients, but also to the periodic exposure of the pseudointimas to air as the tubes rotate, thus providing oxygenation.

The quality and completeness of pseudointimas produced also varies with the method of seeding the cells into the fabric. Various techniques have been employed, from simply pouring cells onto the surface of flat or concave devices,[35] to culturing tubes in a closed container with cells for a few hours,[46] to the elaborate seeding devices of Ghidoni *et al.*,[62] to the centrifugation and stabilization methods which we have employed.[27, 32] Even more complicated techniques will be necessary to seed and culture irregular shaped prostheses such as bifurcated tubes and specialized heart pumps.

It must be emphasized that tissue culture technology applied to the production of cellular blood interfaces varies with the type of prosthesis and the cell line used. Different cell types will have specific requirements for their optimal derivation and cultivation *in vitro*. Equally important, the effects of culture media, nutrient turnover, temperature, osmolality, gaseous environment, water quality, and materials used in cell handling will all influence viability, growth, and pseudointima development.[32]

Summary

In an attempt to develop blood-compatible interfaces, cells were cultivated *in vitro* on microfiber scaffolds lining nonporous vascular prostheses and discs. The scaffolds were fabricated as nonwoven meshes of nylon and polyester (polytetramethylene terephthalate) (Abcor, Inc.) or polypropylene (Union Carbide, Inc.). Microfibers ranged from 0.2 to 2 μm in diameter. The fibers were left bare, microwave discharge-treated, coated with carbon, Parylene-C, or combinations of these. WI-38 cells were used to test biocompatibility and potentially autologous human cell lines (epidermal, endothelial, and urinary tract epithelium) were used to produce pseudointimas. Tubes and discs were washed and degassed, seeded with cells by centrifugation, stabilized in a confined environment, and cultivated by roller bottle perfusion or in Falcon tissue culture flasks. WI-38 cells produced 54–100% coverage, depending on the microfiber composition. Epidermal cells yielded excellent pseudointimas with the polyester microfibers as the best overall substrate and nylon microwave-treated fibers as the least effective. Adult human endothelium produced coverages of 28–94%, while urothelium provided the poorest pseudointimas.

Acknowledgments

The authors wish to express their appreciation to Mrs. Ruth Sell, Mrs. Irene Loo, Ms. Rosalie Beer, Mrs. Maxine Chapo, and Mr. Richard Klann for their valuable assistance.

References *

1. Bruck, S. D. 1972. Macromolecular aspects of biocompatible materials—A review. J. Biomed. Mater. Res. **6:** 173–183.
2. Bruck, S. D. 1972. Biomaterials in medical devices. Trans. Am. Soc. Artif. Intern. Organs **18:** 1–7.
3. Wesolowski, S. A., C. C. Fries, K. E. Karlson, M. DeBakey & P. N. Sawyer. 1961. Porosity: primary determinant of ultimate fate of synthetic vascular grafts. Surgery **50:** 91–96.
4. Fry, W. J., M. S. DeWeese, R. O. Kraft & C. B. Ernst. 1964. Importance of porosity in arterial prostheses. Arch. Surg. **88:** 836–842.

* References identified as "Annual Reports" can be obtained from the National Technical Information Service, 5285 Port Royal Road, Springfield, Virginia 22151.

5. WESOLOWSKI, S. A., W. M. GOLASKI, L. R. SAUVAGE, J. D. MCMAHON & Y. KOMOTO. 1968. Consideration in the development of small artery prostheses. Trans. Am. Soc. Artif. Intern. Organs **14:** 43–47.
6. WESOLOWSKI, S. A., C. C. FRIES & J. D. MCMAHON. 1968. Arterial prosthetic materials. Ann. N.Y. Acad. Sci. **146:** 325–344.
7. SAUVAGE, L. R., K. E. BERGER, S. J. WOOD, S. G. YATES II, J. C. SMITH & P. B. MANSFIELD. 1974. Interspecies healing of porous arterial prostheses. Observations, 1960 to 1974. Arch. Surg. **109:** 698–705.
8. BENSON, R. W., D. D. PAYNE & J. A. DEWEESE. 1975. Evaluation of prosthetic grafts of different porosity for arterial reconstruction. Am. J. Surg. **129:** 665–669.
9. WESOLOWSKI, S. A., C. C. FRIES, J. D. MCMAHON & A. MARTINEZ. 1966. Evaluation of a new vascular prosthesis with optimal specifications. Surgery **59:** 40–56.
10. SAUVAGE, L. R., K. BERGER, S. J. WOOD, A. A. SAMEH, A. S. WESOLOWSKI, W. M. GOLASKI, M. DEMONENICO & J. R. HARTMANN. 1969. A very thin, porous knitted arterial prosthesis; experimental data and early clinical assessment. Surgery **65:** 78–88.
11. BUXTON, B. F., D. C. WUKASCH, C. MARTIN, W. J. LIEBIG, G. L. HALLMAN & D. A. COOLEY. 1973. Introduction of a new bifurcated graft. Am. J. Surg. **125:** 288–293.
12. NUWAYSER, E. S., S. BONACCI, J. KNUDSEN, R. TUELINGS & S. DAVIS. 1969. Research on materials compatible with blood. *In* Proc. Artificial Heart Program Conference : 153–168. U. S. Government Printing Office. Washington, D.C.
13. NUWAYSER, E. S. 1971. Microfiber substrate development. Ann. Rpt. Contract no. NIH–71–2047, National Heart and Lung Institute, Bethesda, Md. PB 206 758.
14. BYCK, J. S., W. A. MILLER, M. A. SPIVACK, L. J. GONSIOR, V. Z. WILLIAMS, JR., B. P. BARTH, H. D. BASSETT, R. K. DEARING, J. F. GAASCH, D. L. SCHOBER, D. D. STEWART & F. R. TITTMAN. 1970. Polymeric materials for circulatory assist devices. Ann. Rpt. Contract no. PH–43–68–1388, National Heart and Lung Institute, Bethesda, Md. 20014.
15. LIOTTA, D., C. W. HALL, A. VILLANUEVA, R. M. O'NEAL & M. E. DEBAKEY. 1966. A permanent autologous lining for implantable blood pumps: A pseudoendocardium. Cardiov. Res. Cent. Bull. **4:** 69–80.
16. GHIDONI, J. J., D. LIOTTA, C. W. HALL, R. M. O'NEAL & M. E. DEBAKEY. 1968. *In Vivo* culture of tissue fragments which produce viable cellular linings covered by endothelium (neointimas) in impermeable, velour-lined arterial prostheses, bypass pumps, and valvular prostheses. Trans. Am. Soc. Artif. Organs **14:** 69–72.
17. GHIDONI, J. J., D. LIOTTA, C. W. HALL, J. G. ADAMS, A. LECHTER, M. BARRIONUEVA, R. M. O'NEAL & M. E. DEBAKEY. 1968. Healing of pseudointima in velour-lined impermeable arterial prostheses. Am. J. Path. **53:** 375–383.
18. GHIDONI, J. J., D. LIOTTA, C. W. HALL, R. M. O'NEAL & M. E. DEBAKEY. 1968. Production of cellular linings in impermeable velour-lined cardiovascular prostheses: Growth from implanted tissue fragments. Surgery **65:** 70–77.
19. ADACHI, M., M. SUZUKI & J. H. KENNEDY. 1970. Preoperative coating of velour-lined circulatory assist devices with fibrin coagulum membrane (FCM). Trans. Am. Soc. Artif. Int. Organs **16:** 7–11.
20. ADACHI, M., M. SUZUKI & J. H. KENNEDY. 1971. Neointimas cultured *in vitro* for circulatory assist devices: I. Comparison of cultured cells derived from autologous tissues of various organs. J. Surg. Res. **11:** 483–491.
21. NOMURA, Y. 1970. The ultra-structure of the pseudointima lining synthetic arterial grafts in the canine aorta with special reference to the origin of the endothelial cell. J. Cardiovas. Surg. **11:** 282–291.
22. MANSFIELD, P. B. AND A. WECHEZAK. 1968. Tissue cultured cells as an endo-

thelial lining of prosthetic materials. Organ Perfusion & Preservation. J. C. Norman, Ed.: 189–201. Appleton-Century-Crofts, New York, N.Y.
23. SCHULTZ, L., R. GROBSTEIN, B. S. BULL & N. S. BRAUNWALD. 1969. Reconstruction of differentiated tissue layers from dissociated cells: Use of tissue culture techniques to develop nonthrombogenic autologous cell surfaces for use as cardiac linings. Ann. Rpt no. PB 43–68–1378–02. National Heart Institute, NIH, Bethesda, Md. 20014.
24. SCHULTZ, L., B. S. BULL & N. S. BRAUNWALD. 1971. Use of tissue culture techniques to evaluate new materials developed to serve as artificial heart linings. Surgery **69:** 557–562.
25. KAHN, R. H. 1971. Multiple-layered intimal linings by perfusion. Annual Rept. no. NIH 71–2054–01, Medical Devices Applications Program, National Heart and Lung Institute, NIH, Bethesda, Md. 20014.
26. KAHN, R. H. & W. E. BURKEL. 1972. Multiple-layered intimal linings by perfusion culture. Ann. Rpt. no. NIH 71–2054–02, Division of Technological Applications, National Heart and Lung Institute, NIH, Bethesda, Md. 20014.
27. KAHN, R. H. & W. E. BURKEL. 1973. Propagation of pseudointimal linings of vascular prostheses. *In Vitro* **8:** 451–458.
28. NUWAYSER, E. S., P. B. MANSFIELD, A. WECHEZAK, R. H. KAHN, W. E. BURKEL & J. B. BOATMAN. 1973. Cultured linings for vascular assist devices. Trans. Am. Soc. Artif. Int. Organs. **19:** 168–174.
29. KAHN, R. H. & W. E. BURKEL. 1973. Multiple-layered intimal linings by perfusion culture. Ann. Rpt. no. NO–1–2054–7, Biomaterials Program, Thrombosis and Hemorrhagic Diseases Branch, Division of Blood Diseases and Resources, National Heart and Lung Institute, NIH, Bethesda, Md. 20014.
30. WECHEZAK, A. R. & P. B. MANSFIELD. 1973. Isolation and growth characteristics of cell lines from bovine venous endothelium. *In Vitro* **9:** 39–43.
31. KAHN, R .H. & W. E. BURKEL. 1974. Multiple-layered intimal linings by perfusion culture. Ann. Rpt. no. 1–HB–2054–4, Biomaterials Program, Division of Blood Diseases and Resources, National Heart and Lung Institute, NIH, Bethesda, Md. 20014.
32. KAHN, R. H., W. E. BURKEL & V. P. PERRY. 1974. Homeostatic and mass culture technology. J. Nat. Cancer Inst. **53:** 1471–1477.
33. KAHN, R. H., W. E. BURKEL & J. C. STANLEY. 1975. Development and testing of pseudointimal-lined vascular prosthetic devices. Ann. Rpt. NIH no. 1–HB–1–2054, Biomaterials Program, Division of Heart and Vascular Disease, National Heart and Lung Institute, NIH, Bethesda, Md. 20014.
34. MANSFIELD, P. B., A. R. WECHEZAK & L. R. SAUVAGE. 1975. Preventing thrombus on artificial vascular surfaces: True endothelial cell linings. Trans. Am. Soc. Artif. Int. Organs. **21:** 264–272.
35. ESKIN, S. G. & L. TREVINO. 1976. Aortic endothelial cells and smooth muscle cells cultured on cardiovascular biomaterials. 9th Ann. Scanning Electron Microscopy Symp. Illinois Institute of Technology Research Inst. Chicago, Ill. In press.
36. MEDZON, E. L. & A. GEDIES. 1971. Substitution of 4-(2-hydroxyethyl)-1-piperazine-ethane sulfonic acid (HEPES) for bicarbonate in protein-free animal cell culture medium: application to vaccinia virus quantitation and fluorogenic acetylesterase assay in living LM cells. Ca. J. Microbiol. **17:** 651–653.
37. LAGRANGE, L. D., V. L. GOTT, J. C. BOKROS & M. D. RAMOS. 1969. Compatibility of carbon and blood. Proc. Artificial Heart Program Conference R. J. Hegyeli, Ed.: 47–58. National Institutes of Health, Bethesda, Md. U.S. Government Printing Office, Washington, D.C.
38. BOKROS, J. C., E. DALLE-MOLLE, B. D. EPSTEIN, F. J. SCHOEN & D. P. SNOWDEN. 1971. Biocompatibility of carbon. Ann. Rpt. Contract no.. PH43–67–1411, National Heart and Lung Institute, NIH, Bethesda, Md. Ann. Rpt. PB 198–404.
39. LOEB, W. E., F. R. TITTMAN & M. GOLDIN. 1969. U.S. Pat. 3,429,739, Feb. 25, 1966.

40. Gorham, W. F. 1966. J. Polymer Sci. **4:** 3027; U.S. Pat. 3,288,728, Nov. 29, 1966; U.S. Pat. 3,342,754 Sept. 19, 1967.
41. Byck, J. S., L. M. Baker, S. W. Chow, L. J. Gonsior, W. A. Miller, W. P. Mulvaney, L. M. Robewon, M. A. Spivack & V. Z. Williams, Jr. 1969. Polymeric Materials for Circulatory Assist Devices. Ann. Rpt. Contract no. 43–68–1388, National Heart and Lung Institute, NIH, Bethesda, Md. 20014.
42. Hayflick, L. 1965. The limited *in vitro* lifetime of human diploid cell strains. Exp. Cell Res. **37:** 614–636.
43. Hayflick, L. 1968. Human Cells and Aging. Sci. Am. **218:** 32–37.
44. Slonim, D . 1973. Study of the population dynamics of human diploid cell strain WI–38. I. The number of cells seeded. J. Biol. Stand. **1:** 305–311.
45. Slonim, D. 1974. Study of the population dynamics of human diploid cell strain WI–38. II. The composition of the medium. J. Biol. Stand. **2:** 51–58.
46. Bernhard, W. F., M. Hussain, J. B. George & G. W. Curtis. 1969. Fetal fibroblasts as a substratum for pseudoendothelial development on prosthetic surfaces. Surgery **66:** 284–290.
47. Pitlick, F. Personal communication.
48. Pomerat, C. M. & W. C. Slick. 1963. Isolation and growth of endothelial cells in tissue culture. Nature **198:** 859–861.
49. Maruyama, Y. 1963. The human endothelial cell in tissue culture. Zeit. Zellf. **60:** 69–79.
50. Fryer, D. G., G. Birnbaum & C. N. Luttrell. 1966. Human endothelium in cell culture. J. Atheroscler. Res. **6:** 151–163.
51. Jaffe, E. A., R. L. Nachman, C. G. Becker & R. C. Minick. 1972. Culture of human endothelial cells derived from human umbilical cord veins. Circulation **46:** 253–256.
52. Gimbrone, M. A., R. S. Cotran & J. Folkman. 1974. Human vascular endothelial cells in culture. Growth and DNA synthesis. J. Cell Biol. **60:** 673–684.
53. Haudenschild, C. C., R. S. Cotran, M. A. Gimbrone, Jr. & J. Folkman. 1975. Fine structure of vascular endothelium in culture. J. Ultra. Res. **50:** 22–32.
54. Henriksen, T., S. A. Evensen, R. F. Elgjo & A. Vefling. 1975. Human fetal endothelial cells in culture. Scand. J. Haematol. **14:** 233–241.
55. Blose, S .H. & S. Chacko. 1975. *In vitro* behavior of guinea pig arterial and venous endothelial cells. Dev. Growth Differ. (Nagoya) **17:** 153–165.
56. Berger, K., L. R. Sauvage, A. M. Rao & S. J. Wood. 1972. Healing of arterial prosthesis in man: its incompleteness. Ann. Surg. **175:** 118–127.
57. Buss, H. 1976. Endothelial surfaces of kidney, coronary and cerebral arteries: A comparative SEM and light microscopic study. Proc. 9th Ann. Scanning Electron Microscopy Symp. Illinois Institute of Technology Research Institute. Chicago, Ill. In press.
58. Folkman, J. E. Merler, C. Abernathy & G. Williams. 1971. Isolation of a tumor factor responsible for angiogenesis. J. Exptl. Med. **133:** 275–288.
59. Kruse, P. F., Jr. & E. Miedema. 1965. Production and characterization of multilayered populations of animal cells. J. Cell Biol. **27:** 273–279.
60. Kruse, P. F. M. Jr., W. Whittle & E. Miedema. 1969. Mitotic and nonmitotic multilayered perfusion cultures. J. Cell Biol. **42:** 113–121.
61. Kruse, P. F., Jr., L. N. Keen & W. L. Whittle. 1970. Some distinctive characteristics of high density perfusion cultures of diverse cell types. *In Vitro* **6:** 75–88.
62. Ghidoni, J. J., D. Liotta, J. G. Adams, R. M. O'Neal & C. W. Hall. 1968. Implantation of autologous tissue fragments in velour fabric used to line cardiovascular prostheses: An *In vivo* culture system to produce cellular blood-prosthesis interfaces. J. Biomed. Mat. Res. **2:** 201–208.

DISCUSSION

DR. VROMAN: Dr. Brash, I have wondered if you could get some useful information by looking at the receding contact angle and under a microscope. Micro-unevenness may be shown by a kind of feathering in the tail of the drop. Also, we found that on rather mobile surfaces, if you let water vapor condense and then let it evaporate and condense again, drops form in exactly the same spots. I think the advancing edge, for example of a condensing drop, will scoop up matter.

DR. BRASH: I'm sorry I really can't comment on contact angles. I haven't used the method.

DR. TURITTO: You mentioned you realized that if your system were diffusion-controlled, you wouldn't be observing differences between surfaces, and you mentioned something about your system not being diffusion-controlled. Why did you think it might not be?

DR. BRASH: We believe it was not diffusion controlled: we don't have any direct evidence for this, but we have characterized the flow patterns in the cell, and the sheer rates are extremely low. We feel that the red cell motion effects would be minimal in this kind of situation.

DR. YASUDA: You had some data there on polar groups and charged groups on the surfaces of rings for the Gott test. Would you summarize that as a general rule, sulfonate groups on the surface seem to be more effective than acholate groups as far as resisting thrombus formation is concerned?

DR. BRASH: I think there is a general belief in the research community in this area that sulfonate or negatively charged surface groups are beneficial, but there is evidence that in some situations they are, and in some they are not.

DR. J. BROWN (*General Electric Co.*): You reported that albumin showed very little adsorption on collagen-coated glass. It is a sharply divergent result from what we see for adsorption of albumin on elastin. I wonder how you made that collagen-coated glass.

DR. BRASH: An acid-soluble bovine tendon collagen was poured onto the glass at acid pH and then neutralized to reconstitute the collagen into fibers. Probably, albumin is adsorbed onto glass spaces in between the collagen fibers, and there is no adsorption onto the collagen itself.

DR. BLACKSHEAR: I'd just like to point out that the ratio of concentrations of platelets that you observed at hematocrit 40 and at zero hematocrit is the same ratio that we observed sucking platelets into the Cuprophane membrane, where the boundary condition is a reversible adhesion; this is, we think, simply the concentration of platelets that you'd expect to have on the surface and the way it increases when hematocrit increases, so that the two things that the red cells could do is one) promote diffusion, but two) push the platelets to the peripheral layer of the system and increase their concentration.

DR. BRASH: If this means that you agree with us, I'm very happy to hear it.

DR. BAIER: Dr. Hoffman, you used silastic as the control on most of the systems. There are, I think, a number of complications with an intrinsically hydrophobic material like silicone rubber; there might be some bubble entrapment and poor wetting. There should be some way to guarantee that the blood in fact wets out, fills all of the voids, crevices, and micro-roughnesses of an implant, as it automatically does on the hydrogel surfaces. Problems we have attributed to the surface texture or to hydrophobicity or to intrinsic materials differences may all have resulted from the poor scavenging of the little air bubbles, the niduses for fibrinogen denaturation and platelet adhesion that exist on the intrinsically nonwettable surfaces.

DR. HOFFMAN: An air bubble might well be a problem on the surface. We have surfaces that just don't wet.

DR. BAIER: The terms "wettable" and "nonwettable" mean different things to different people. What is the water contact angle, versus the contact angle for some other fluid?

DR. HOFFMAN: I don't believe in contact angles measured in air: it's the aqueous interface that matters, and these surfaces will change from what they are in air to what they are within the aqueous phase.

DR. E. NYILAS (*AVCO Everett Research Laboratory, Everett, Mass.*): Is water shed by the hema-hema copolymer? And how about glycerol or any other polar solvent? Contact angles between ice and water show that the water structure in the two faces may not necessarily be the same, although they are composed of the same molecules. Second, I would elaborate on that entropy-driven difference you referred to as far as protein adsorption is concerned.

DR. HOFFMAN: Obviously, the structure of the water is a much better way to describe wettability than by just dipping it in water; unfortunately, we haven't any measure of that. But insofar as entropy is concerned, the interfacial energy essentially is an excess interfacial energy. If it is high, there is a driving force for adsorption to lower it; and it is often high at hydrophobic water interfaces because of the local organization of water (call it structuring, if you like) at that interface. It is less at hydrophilic interfaces because there is more gradual transition into the normal water structure.

DR. SALZMAN: Dr. Haubold, can you give us some information about the blood compatibility of your materials in quantitative terms which would allow us to compare them to other materials? Can we get some idea about how they work?

DR. HAUBOLD: The vena cava and renal embolism tests were used. Dr. Bruck mentioned the results. Other test data shows that albumin adsorbs very quickly to the surface; platelet adhesion has been shown to be only moderate.

DR. BAIER: I'd like to make a comment on Dr. Salzmans' question. I believe that the biocompatibility demonstrated in the cardiovascular system for the pyrolytic carbons is a result not of thromboresistance in the classical sense, but of physiologic tolerability in the way I tried to describe in my opening talk the other day. The pyrolytic carbon does support the same initial events most other biomaterials do: protein adsorption, platelet adhesion and microthrombus generation, but at a very uniform rate. These small-sized aggregates are carried off and coped with very well on a continuous basis physiologically.

DR. HAUBOLD: They are not coped with that well, because after valve replacement I think most people continue on anticoagulants, especially if the aortic valve was replaced.

DR. VROMAN: I would like to point out that, under our experimental conditions, plasma deposits fibrinogen on your carbon surfaces, and does not convert it quickly, so that platelets in whole blood have a good chance of finding it and sticking to it. Yet, a so-called monolayer of platelets, forming on a valve in a high-flow area may be good instead of bad; we just don't know so far.

DR. HAUBOLD: But we do know that albumin is adsorbed on these surfaces rapidly.

DR. S. W. KIM (*College of Pharmacy, University of Utah, Salt Lake City*): We studied adsorption both out of plasma and out of protein mixtures, and found in both systems that onto most polymers, fibrinogen is adsorbed quite rapidly, but onto the carbon surfaces, albumin is adsorbed more rapidly than fibrinogen.

DR. HOFFMAN: What was the effect of support material surface texture and composition on the vena cava ring test results?

DR. HAUBOLD: I did 19 tests in the last three years with carbon on polyetherurethane and with carbon on stainless steel that had been polished well and not so well. Of those 19 tests, I think three were not valid, seven were of the X category and nine were of the doubtful category.

DR. DANIELS: For *in vivo* tests in the vena cava, extreme smoothness—of which the carbons from your company may be the prime example—tends to be a strong factor, probably related to what Dr. Baier suggested about the ease of sloughing off very small thrombi that have no physiological effects. We find that the vena cava tests on extremely smooth surfaces tend to split: we either get immediate clotting if the material is overtly chemically thrombogenic, or else the materials stay essentially clean after two weeks. This bimodal distribution of test results is caused by the interaction of the chemical properties of the material and its mechanical finish.

UNIDENTIFIED SPEAKER: Dr. Falb, is there any evidence that heparin coming off the surface initially might be inactive if, say, put back onto another polymer surface? Is this heparin partially degraded in the processing, so that the degraded heparin does not stick?

DR. FALB: There is some evidence from the *in vitro* column work. The heparin was radioactively labeled to assess the amount coming off. It did have enough activity to anticoagulate the eluted blood.

UNIDENTIFIED SPEAKER: I think that even the most homogenous polymer may be affected locally during casting or when forcing it into a mold so that hydrophobic groups get reoriented, for example, at edges; so even at this stage it may be impossible to characterize the surface.

DR. R. I. LEININGER (*Battelle Memorial Institute, Columbus, Ohio*): Several years ago we separated heparin—more crudely than did Dr. Rosenberg—chromatographically, and found the higher molecular weight material to have a higher specific activity. On quaternized surfaces this material performed better than did the unfractionated heparin.

DR. R. D. ROSENBERG (*Beth Israel Hospital, Boston, Mass.*): We can prepare various sized fractions and show that in each of the areas of the chromatogram, a good deal of the material is inactive. Also, the activity change in relation to size is largely a function of the source and of the preparation of heparin one is using.

UNIDENTIFIED SPEAKER: Does the high-potency heparin with the ability to bind purified antithrombin III also bind it when added to whole plasma, or does it show the same binding characteristic that Dr. Ewa Marciniak published?

DR. ROSENBERG: I suspect that the problem with Dr. Ewa Marciniak's experiments—showing in essence that only a small fraction of heparin added to plasma can be shown to be bound to antithrombin—is caused by most of the heparin's being inactive. We do have some preliminary data in that regard. I should like to point out that once heparin activates antithrombin, the antithrombin neutralizes activated Hageman factor almost instantaneously. This is a plausable mechanism for protecting surfaces against contact activation.

DR. YASUDA: Dr. Ketteringham, you showed that often when thickness is changed, permeability changes as well, particularly when the membrane has a tendency to form heterogeneous anisometric structures. Are you really only observing a thickness effect?

DR. KETTERINGHAM: Most membranes are indeed not homogeneous and do have a skin defect, so that one would not find a proportionate relationship between change in permeability and in thickness. Nevertheless, there is an effect that is significant and that is used clinically.

DR. HARKER: Dr. Kahn, do you have any experience in implanting your devices *in vivo?*

DR. KAHN: We are now doing that, but since most of these materials are of human source, we ran into a problem with the Human Use Committee, so we have gone back to the dog as our model system. We naively assumed that the technology we had developed for human skin and human materials would be quickly adaptable to the dog. In reality, however, we ran into many problems; the dog epidermal cells are much more tenacious than human epidermal cells, so that when you initiate a population in cell culture you have a hard time getting them off the surface, be it plastic or glass. We also were trying to genuflect to Science by using a specific species. We started off by using beagle dogs only, to remove one variable. It turned out that the beagle has some endogenous organism that I can demonstrate in scanning EM and TEM.

DR. KOLFF: I like the paper very much. I thought it was fascinating; but aren't you afraid that that skin will grow nails, or horns, or something?

DR. KAHN: No, that's exactly the point I was trying to make, sir, that in all our experience (and we've carried these in culture for 28, 30 days) we've never seen any evidence of keratinization. I think it's important. We, as anatomists, tend to define things when we say "This is skin, therefore it keratinizes," and "This is, shall we say, bladder, and it's a transitional epithelium." I think a cell is what it is because of where you put it; skin is skin and keratinizes because it's on a surface exposed to a gaseous environment. Given that same cell it has much, much more capability of modulating—a word that Paul Weiss devised a number of years ago—and adapting to its environment. If I may use an analogy: if you and I were thrown out on the classic Pacific Island with a single palm tree, you and I would be earning our living in a different way. And I think that's what happens to cells.

DR. KOLFF: I hope we'll be on the same island. It will be fun. I hope that you will test these membranes that you grow on a flexing surface, because that is where the trouble is going to come in.

DR. KAHN: That's exactly what we have done for the last year. We are growing them on surfaces and flexing them concomitantly and also exposing them to shear forces similar to systole. We've exposed these tubes to shear forces ranging from 100 to 250 mm pressures. Below 200 mm, we have no evidence of shear.

DR. KOLFF: Dr. Ketteringham, one of your slides gave the impression that you get less urea transfer at higher blood flow rates. If true, I would suspect there is another limiting factor, or else the chemistry is wrong.

DR. KETTERINGHAM: The numbers were correct, but referred to permeation rates for a given device; the blood flowing into the device was actually passing over membrane areas that were larger in one case than in another, so the shear rate on the 1 sq m membrane was lower than the shear rate on the 0.64 sq m membrane. Despite that, at the higher molecular weights there is an increased transfer—of B-12, for example. The numbers given should be a function of permeability times membrane area.

Dr. Haubold: I should like to point out that the particular carbon used in Dr. Kahn's paper was not pyrolytic carbon, but rather a vapor phase-deposited carbon, which we have already abandoned, since it always came out anisotropic.

BLOOD AT ARTIFICIAL ORGAN SURFACES: PROGRESS TO DATE AS STEPPING-STONES FOR THE FUTURE *

W. J. Kolff and Fritz Stellwag

University of Utah
Division of Artificial Organs
Salt Lake City, Utah 84112

OXYGENATORS

To make membranes for oxygenators compatible with blood, the surface has been treated in many ways, such as: [1]

(1) Binding of hydrogels to the surface;
(2) chemical attachments of urokinase;
(3) use of Chicago acid (related to Evans Blue)
(4) heparin (Merker attaches heparin to the silicone filler with APTES, Leininger uses TDMAC complex);
(5) streptokinase; and
(6) other membranes such as Avcothane, which is a compound of polyurethane and siloxyane (Kolobow eliminates the silica filler).

The multitude of choices seems to indicate that there is no ideal method yet. Bubble oxygenators are now generally considered to be bad,[2] which reminds us of the old experience of Clark and Golan, who worked with oxygen dispersion, extremely fine dispersion of oxygen bubbles in the blood, so fine that one could not possibly see them, but one could see the gradual change of the color of the blood from dark blue (venous) to bright red. If the dosage was correct, no oxygen bubbles ever appeared on the surface, but gas samples taken from the top of the oxygenator, which consisted of a blood repellent porous disc, had a very high content of CO_2. Some good things have fallen by the wayside for lack of some kind of appeal.

Why are microporous membranes so much better, as far as blood damage is concerned, than the bubble oxygenators? [3] According to Bartlett *et al.,* bubble oxygenators have surface areas of 10–15 square meters—many times larger than those of the microporous membranes. Moreover, the pores of the membranes have a size between .1 and 5 microns and seem to be actually filled with a protein-containing layer, so that the surface that faces the blood is no longer gas but some kind of a hybrid.

So long as we do not have the perfect surface, preperfusion with heparin improves the results considerably.[4] Even if you have heparinized surfaces, heparinized as well as J. T. Watson and coworkers can do it, then you still don't have a guarantee that you will not get clotting.

It helps to make the transit time extremely short. With transit times less than 20–25 seconds, one sees on the heparinized surface only a protein layer covered with some platelets and red cells. If the transit time becomes longer, extensive thrombosis, fibrin formation, and so on, takes place.[5]

* TDMAC=tridodecylmethyl ammonium chloride; MTCAC=methyltricapryl ammonium chloride; and APTES=amino propyltriethoxysilane.

The clinical results of long-time oxygenation by Hill and coworkers [6] indicates that one can get clinical results even if the ideal surface is not yet available. They point out that the platelet drop that occurs is relatively quickly restored after the procedure. We find it hard to believe that the platelets are stored in various places in the body to be released later, yet this is what was thought at one time.

Leininger and his group at Batelle have custom-coated with TDMAC heparin complex heart valves, arterial grafts, membrane oxygenators, artificial kidney, AV cannulas, balloon pumps, and caval umbrellas. None of these methods, however, has found general application.[7] C. A. Ward, at the University of Toronto, and others have stressed the necessity to remove small residual gas nuclei because they form the nidus around which platelet adhesion may start, even on an otherwise good surface.[8]

The removal of the silica, which is present in all commercially available Silastic, or rather the grafting of silica-free silicone on top of a silastic surface in the hands of Kolobow and coworkers at the NIH, results in a greatly improved compatability of the silicone surface.[9] Unfortunately, radiation grafting may influence the strengths of the silicone substrate.

It is possible to use membrane oxygenation without sytemic heparinization. This has been done by several groups—one of which is Rea and coworkers in Dallas. They went as long as 48 hours in 1972.[10]

In summary, there is promise for better blood compatability of membrane oxygenators, but compromise and combination of various techniques are still required in order to get clinical results.

Artificial Blood Vessel Walls

E. W. Salzmann [11] says that platelets adhere to damaged endothelium, particularly when collagen is exposed. Stemerman and Spaet [12] agree that there is a deleterious effect of the subendothelial tissue to which platelets adhere. When the wall itself is important, the flow, as Leonard [13] points out, is also important. The initiation and the propagation and the fate of the thrombus is largely determined by the local flow.

A large number of papers describe attempts to create small blood vessels with a multitude of different materials, more or less porous. Velour, which is a warp-knitted cloth resembling velvet, with loops of yarn extended perpendicularly from the surface, cannot be used for blood vessels of a diameter smaller than 8 mm.[14] Berkowitz *et al.*[15] believe that the attachments of the neointima is better when a polyurethane lattice is provided on the inner surface of knitted Dacron® grafts, yet he cannot get to a diameter smaller than 8 mm. Sawyer, of course, has been the champion of the importance of a negatively charged endothelial blood interface since he was a medical student. By now, everybody believes him. He and Srinivasan [16] point out that a negative charge of 1–2 mV measured against the surrounding fluid is what is needed, and say that neointima on Dacron and Teflon® grafts also becomes negatively charged and that anticoagulant drugs tend to potentiate this negative charge.

It is a little difficult for us to understand that an electrically conducted artificial blood vessel wall would also result in a negative charge on the inside. Miller and coworkers,[17] comparing foams, velour, flock, and other fabrics, found that knitted Dacron, when electrically conductive, was superior. Electrolour championed by Sharp and coworkers [18] since 1968, is a Dacron or nylon velour made electrically conductive with carbon-loaded polyurethane (28%). In carotid grafts in dogs they are now able to go down to 4 mm diameter and have 85% patency, but the material is difficult to handle.

Grafts of the same small diameter can be kept open when made of expanded polytetrafluoroethylene, patency 78%. There are two kinds of this expanded polytetrafluoroethylene. One is the original Gortex, made by Gore Associates, with which we had experience in our own laboratory;[19] the other is made by a company in Phoenix.[20] The same material has been used for creation of the portacaval shunts in human recipients and has apparently stayed open.

Wesolowski and coworkers[21] have pursued the perfection and application of grafts made of very fine knits. They speak of a milliknit (meaning 40 needles/inch) and a microknit (meaning 50 needles/inch). In 1975 they summarized their experience[21] and said they could keep 4-mm-diameter grafts open for four years. These grafts are commercially available from Golaski Laboratories, Inc., in Philadelphia, Pa. They require careful preclotting.

Lyman and coworkers,[38] at the University of Utah, are able to maintain patency of arterial grafts made of Lyman-blocked polyurethane. Contrary to all the other materials, this is a nonporous membrane; yet, 4-mm-diameter grafts stay open in dogs. The material is pleasant to suture, and Lyman and colleagues believe that the increased success of their method depends on the fact that the modulus—that is, the elasticity—of their grafts is the same as that of the blood vessel, so that when the blood vessel extends during pulsation, the graft extends in a similar way. This is a new concept that we have not encountered before.

Sharp and coworkers,[22] known for their work on electrolour, conclude that the neointima must be less than 500 μ thick to survive for any length of time, since it can no longer rely on nutrition from the blood flow on the inside of the vessel, when it becomes thicker than 500 microns.

Seeded or cultured cells on the inside of artificial organs in general have been plagued with difficulties. When successful, it was often very difficult to prove that the seeds themselves were the reason for the success.

Mansfield and coworkers,[23] having showed earlier that embryonic lung cells and fibroblasts do not work, said in 1975 that thrombosis could be prevented when the seeds themselves were taken from autologous endothelium scraped from the inside of the carotid artery.

Notwithstanding the outstanding clinical success, sometimes for many years, with Dacron grafts from the aorta to the femoral arteries or even further, the statement has been made by Berger *et al.*,[24] by Sauvage *et al.*,[25] and by others that they have never seen a complete healing of the graft in humans. There is only a pannus of tissue that looks like endothelium growing for about 10 mm from the suture lines, and the rest of the Dacron graft is either raw or covered with fibrinous material.

There seems to be a difference between grafts that are harvested a few months after implantation and those that are harvested after a few years. The latter ones are practically always raw. In 1975, however, Sauvage and coworkers published a report entitled "First Report of Complete Healing" of an auxiliary-femoral graft of knitted Dacron which was harvested 20 months after implantation. The fact that they published this in the *Annals of Surgery* seems to indicate that this is indeed a rare occurrence.

Talking about raw, irregular aortas, we must assume that new thrombi form almost continuously on the inside of the raw intima. Apparently, they are taken care of by the body without causing major insult. There must be a continuous formation and resolution of the thrombi.

Look at the pathological specimens as we know them from people who die from other causes but who have extensive atherosclerosis in the aorta, or review the inside of an aneurysm of the aorta filled with a large, irregular thrombus which may have been there for many years. We then realize that this process of continuous formation and resolution is compatible with life. When, however, the area where the thrombus forms pulsates, as does the pumping diaphragm of an artificial heart, then chunks of thrombus that come off may be larger than the body can cope with.

Sparks [26] had maintained all along that the intima of most Dacron grafts are raw, and it was reason for him to pursue the concept of the living graft, which is truly his. After many years of experimentation, the technique that resulted was that he put a long silicone mandril in the future recipient of a graft. If possible, it was made in the approximate location where the graft was to be used later. The very fine double Dacron stockings that surround the mandril serve as a skeleton for the living tissue that then forms the wall of the graft. After six weeks, the silicone rod is withdrawn and a smooth tube results. Dr. Spark's publication in *Annals of Surgery* (1973) is, unfortunately, his last one, because of his death. His work forms a beautiful example of self-supported, independent research, which, despite its excellence, has been largely ignored. Sparks does not speak of neointima, but of a smooth, living lining of his grafts.[26] It is generally believed that these grafts cannot be transposed from one part of the body to another, but Sparks has shown, and in our laboratory we have confirmed, that they can be transposed, which makes them useful for use as aortic to coronary bypass grafts or for blood access vessels in patients with artificial kidneys.

A gluteraldehyde-treated bovine mesenteric artery coated with natural rubber can also be punctured, and is self-healing.[27]

Preclotting done on the operating table is a source of chagrin, complications, and defeat. Therefore, Ruderman and coworkers [28] have developed a partially biodegradable vascular prosthesis which is composed of Dacron and alternate fibers of poly(DL-lactide). The prosthesis becomes more porous with gradual resorption of the lactide component and then allows ingrowth of tissue from the periphery. Everybody seems to agree that this ingrowth is an important factor in the longevity of the patency of grafts.

Artificial Hearts and Assist Devices

Only recently have we in Utah begun using anticoagulants in our calves sustained with artificial hearts. The calf, Burk, that lived for 94 days, did not have anticoagulants (Figure 1). When we did begin to use them, we followed the recipe propagated by Mansfield and coworkers,[29] who indicated that the combination Coumadin, Persantine (dipyridamole), and aspirin is superior to any other combination he has tried, and he does not seem to use Dextran any more. Indeed, this regimen has reduced the occurrence of thromboembolism in our animals considerably. Pierce and coworkers,[30] Boretos *et al.*,[63] and Pierce [64] use heparin for the first five days and then go over to a similar regimen.

There have been very few attempts to grow living intimas on artificial hearts the way Sparks did for arteries, but Volder and Kolff [31] made one such attempt. The worry, of course, is about the flexing surface and how that can be vascularized from the outside. Bruck[32] has summarized the present beliefs for the intima of artificial organs as: (1) negative charge, (2) low surface free energy, and (3) hydrophilicity. Ideally, one should not have to use any heparin or anticoagulants in an artificial organ. The work of Wakabayashi and others[33] shows that this can be done. They perfused dogs for 30 hours with a bypass system the inside of which was coated by a variation of Gott's old recipe of graphite-benzalkonium heparin. He recently reported the heparinless left-heart bypass for resection of thoracic aneurysms in 23 patients, using a refined bypass unit.

Sawyer, the original champion of negative surface charge[34] has stressed, with his coworkers, the importance of ultraclean surfaces. Anybody working

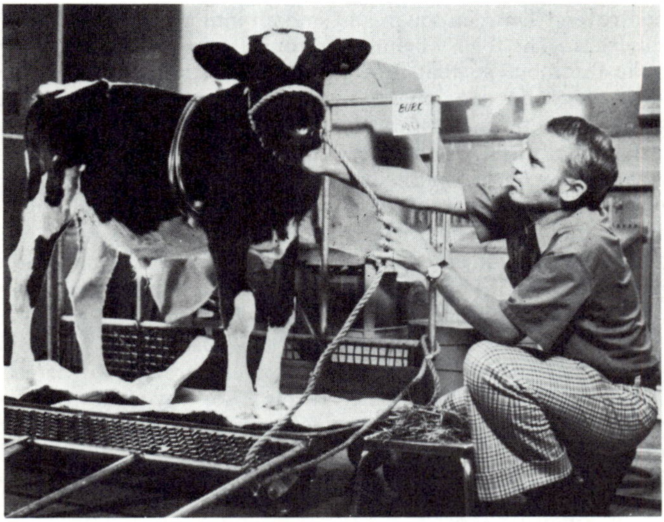

FIGURE 1. Burk lived for 94 days after removal of its natural heart. The artificial heart had a smooth intima of Biomer (a polyurethane made by Ethicon). This picture was taken at 41 days. The cause of death was *not* thromboembolism, but infection along the drivelines. This can now be avoided. Burk did not receive anticoagulants.

in this area would agree with him, notwithstanding the difficulties that it entails. Sawyer particularly pleads for electrochemical cleaning. Our coworker Lee Smith champions glow-discharge, which also activates the surface and makes it eager to adsorb the first substance that it encounters, which may be oxygen or perhaps albumin.

Grafting of hydrogels, pursued for years by our coworker Andrade, has been brought to further perfection by radiation grafting by Hoffman and associates.[35] From the same medical center, The University of Washington in Seattle, comes the remarkable work by Schmer,[36] which first proved that heparin is active only when it is part of a larger molecular complex. It is bound to heparin substrate. Schmer, however, can also bind heparin to a polyvinylpyrrolidon complex. This can be brought in solution in a solvent such as chloroform. This, in contact with silicon rubber, causes the rubber to swell. If the chloroform is removed, the heparin complex stays behind.

Schmer has treated the left auxiliary ventricle for us, and we have high hopes that it will remain free of thrombi. Excellent theoretical work has been done by Kim *et al.*:[37] protein adsorbed on a surface greatly determines how it is going to behave in regard to platelet adhesion and thrombogenicity. Adsorption of albumin is good; adsorption of fibrinogen and globulin is bad.

Andrade was actually the first one who successfully coated albumin on surfaces, and Lyman and coworkers[38] pointed out that the copolyether-urethane urea virtually adsorbs no other protein than albumin; therefore, it has antithrombogenicity. Of course, the albumin in many instances can come off.[39] It is no wonder, then, that we try to cross-link it *in situ,* which can be done with gluteraldehyde.[40]

The controversy between rough and smooth intimas for the inside of artificial organs still exists. The theory behind the rough intima, of course, is that it tries to retain the thrombus so that it will not form an embolus. A rough intima combined with a conductive polyurethane subsurface was used with considerable success by Kantrowitz in dogs and in a patient who lived for 96 days with a pulsating dynamic aortic patch. Yet Kantrowitz indicates that not the entire surface is covered with neoepithelium and that the fibrin layer may be from 1 to 2 mm thick. In a series of 65 long-term experiments in dogs, only five instances of emboli in the kidneys were found.[41-43]

Dacron fibrils are still, in the eyes of some, the preferred coating for the inside of an artificial heart or an auxiliary ventricle. Indeed, the results obtained in calves by Bernhard and coworkers[44] and by Norman[45] are enviable. In a combined paper with Keiser[46] they indicate that Dacron fibers should be glued to the polyurethane with Tecothane A polyurethane, which seems to be the same as Adiprene L 100 polyurethane. If this is so, why is the company (Teko) that is making their hearts now using another technique, which is the negative imprint of a velour or cloth on the inside of their polyurethane left auxiliary ventricle? We have always maintained that the Dacron fibrils come off, and that you will see them if you look for them with polarized light[47] (FIGURE 2).

The left auxiliary ventricle, which by some is called L.V.A.D. is advocated as a temporary assist to the circulation in the hope that the ailing heart will recover so that the L.V.A.D. then can be removed. We believe that the same left ventricular support can be obtained by a far simpler method—the Transapical Left Ventricular Bypass. This was first indicated by Chardack and has been explored in our laboratory by Peters *et al.*,[48] who recently brought it to experimental perfection (FIGURE 3).

A simple tube inserted in the apex of the left ventricle sucks the blood from the left ventricle through a commercially available roller pump and pumps it back into the aorta or a side branch of the aorta via a Pall filter. If you look at a Pall filter, the amount of thrombi, large and small, and other objectionable material (including air, sometimes, and particles from the pump tube) is quite amazing. We are aware of the fact that at the last meeting of the American Heart Association in Anaheim, Calif., the opinion was voiced that a filter in the use of heart lung machines is useful for no longer than ten minutes. In our experience, however, we found that in most instances the filter can remain in place for 14 days. If it has to be changed, this need can be easily detected by measuring the gradient across the filter. This Transapical Bypass, we believe, is

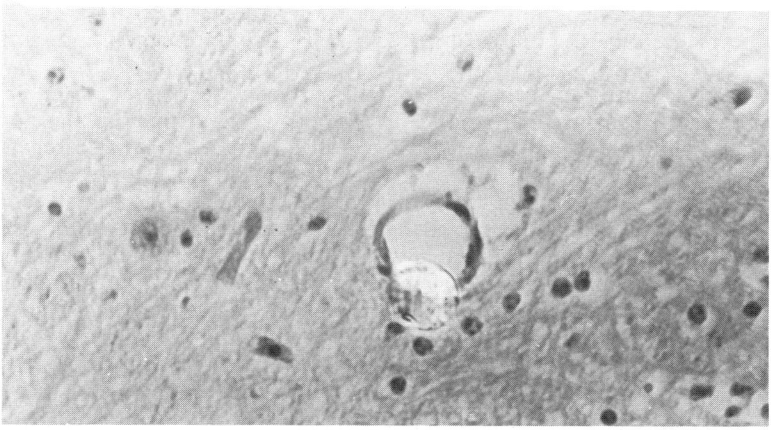

FIGURE 2. Dacron fibrils when shed from the intima of an artificial heart are hard to see, unless one looks for them with polarized light. Their birefringent property makes them stick out. Dr. Don Olsen found as many as 19 fibrils in one section of a calf's brain.

now ready for widespread clinical application—particularly in those patients who cannot be weaned of a heart lung machine.[48-50]

Once more returning to the rough surfaces and comparing them with the smooth surfaces, the rough surfaces enabled us to sustain calves with artificial hearts up to 36 days. The smooth surfaces, even without anticoagulation, allowed survival time of 94 days. We feel that this is only the beginning.[51, 52]

When it became clear that the rough surfaces formed ever-increasing layers of fibrin on the flexing diaphragm, which began to calcify in time, we felt that as far as we were concerned, this was the end of the rough surfaces. In one instance, some sharp, hard calcium perforated the pumping diaphragm. This observation seems to have been confirmed in the experience of Dr. Navratil[53] and his associates 4,000 miles remote from Salt Lake City, in Vienna, Austria.

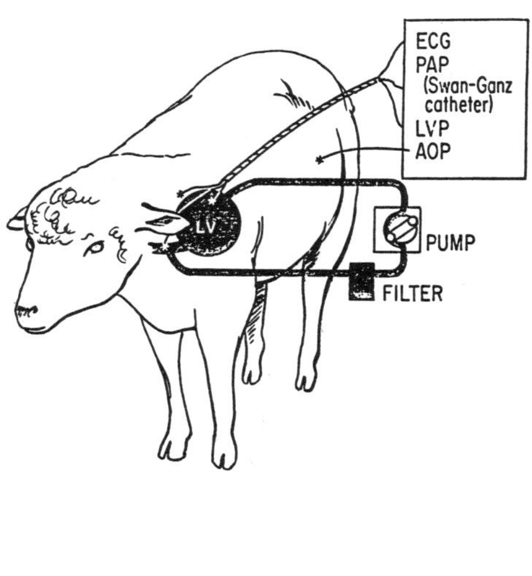

FIGURE 3. Diagram of Transapical Left Ventricular Bypass as presently used at the University of Utah. The use of a Pall's filter in the circuit for 14 days which can be replaced, and is probably responsible for the uncomplicated course of those experiments. Heparin is now used.

Although they had one calf live for 131 days, they found layers from 3 to 9 mm thick formed on the Dacron fibril surfaces (these are not Dacron fibril surfaces on a conductive matrix such as Kantrowitz [43] and Sharp [18] used).

In between the rough and the smooth surfaces are the so-called biolized membranes of Nosé and his group [54] in Cleveland. They treat animal pericardium with glutaraldehyde and bind it to purified natural rubber and segmented polyurethane. They also use heterologous human dura-mater glycerol-treated valves and homologous aortic valves. All these surfaces seem to be covered with an extremely thin layer of material that looks like fibrin but does not seem to have the tendency to grow. They have been less successful with their Hexsyn (Goodyear Polyoliphin) flexible membrane, which they coat with Dacron and gelatin.[54] The newest thing is that they make the Hexsyn porous with salts.

The Shape of the Heart

We believe that a few years from now it will not matter very much of what kind of intima the artificial heart will be made of as long as the flow conditions in that heart are such that thrombus formation is avoided. A visual way of demonstrating this is with computer graphics based on Navier-Stoker and other equations (FIGURE 4).[55] Greenfield and colleagues (at the University of Utah) has produced convincing pictures of the turbulence on presently used valves and on some parts of artificial hearts.

We see, in our artificial hearts, that there are definite predilection places for the formation of thrombosis. One of those is in the junction between the pumping diaphragm and the housing. In this area there is a narrow slit, and in part of the circumference you can almost count on the thrombus formation. The time when it comes off determines the fate of the animal. Needless to say, we are now designing the heart so that these prediliction places are avoided.[56]

Smooth Surfaces on the Inside of Artificial Hearts

From the above it is clear that even without the help of anticoagulants, we favor smooth surfaces inside of the artificial heart. With anticoagulants, the results in our hands, seem to be even better. It is remarkable that Atsumi and associates [57] have been able to get long-time survival in goats when they use PVC artificial hearts as bypass for both the right and left ventricle. Akutsu, presently in Houston, has championed for a long time the use of silicone rubber artificial hearts coated on the inside with a silicon gel that is free of silica. Indeed, he was able to get survivals up to 24 days, and he held a world record with that for a while. It was also obvious that the thrombus always occurred in the same place in his beautifully designed hearts, and that was somewhere on the middle of his inflow valve.[58, 59] In his book, among many other things, he points out once more that the thrombus in artificial organs or in artificial aortas causes trouble when it grows from the living tissue toward a smooth surface in the aorta, clearly on the inflow end and never on the outflow end. He has, therefore, suggested the use of a porous material between the natural tissue and the device.[60] Indeed, we have done the same by applying felt atria between the natural atrium and the inlet valve of our artificial heart (see Olson [61]).

Pierce consistently over many years has used a polyurethane, Biomer made by Ethicon for the intima of his artificial hearts and assist devices (see Boretos *et al.*[62]). They have had their Biomer tethered sack-type pump assisting the left ventricle for as long as 35 weeks. In their earlier experiences, thrombus would form in the tip of the sac when the sac was too long, once more emphasizing the prime importance of design. They claim that there is no lipid adsorption on the Biomer, and SEM (Scanning Electron Microscope studies by Baier)

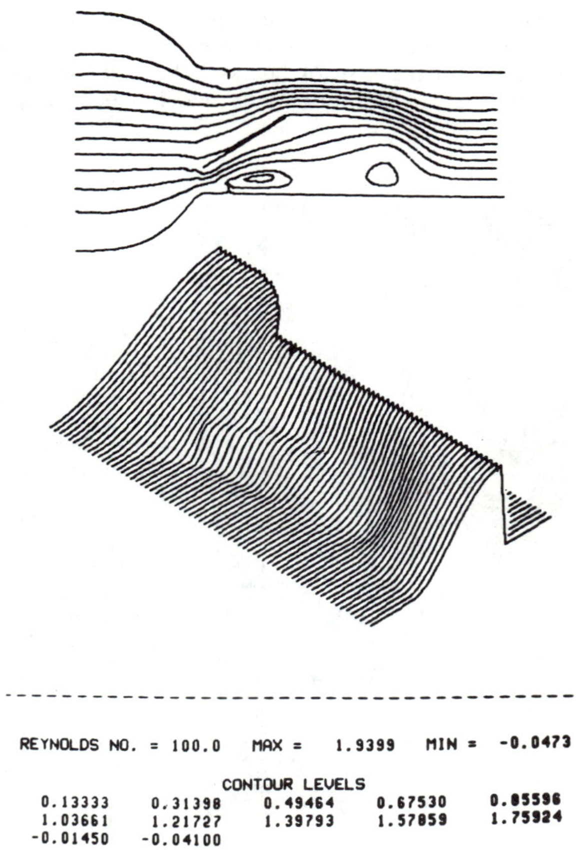

FIGURE 4. A drawing never touched by human hands made by Harvey Greenfield and coworkers by computer graphics at the University of Utah. The turbulence around a popular clinically used heart valve is obvious. The occurrence of thrombosis in the valve coincides with areas of stagnation.[55]

showed that the platelets distributed on the surface of the Biomer look remarkably normal.[63]

The remark that there is no lipid adsorption is at variance with the experience by Lyman and Knudsen [64] at the University of Utah, who found that there can be lipid adsorption in polyurethanes, and it is believed that this may be one of the reasons why they show a decrease in strength. This is presently under investigation (ERDA Contract).

We can end with a happy note. The intra-aortic balloons made of Avcothane have been used without any heparinization in calves up to eight hours, and in three patients up to 72 hours. Small fibrin flecks have been observed from time to time on the surface of the balloons; they are believed to originate from imperfections. These balloons pulsate all the time.[65] Once again, it is important to remember that in the living organism small thrombotic phenomenon occur but are not necessarily detrimental. The thrombus simply disappears, as was shown years ago by Gott when he implanted swords in the atria of dogs and showed that a large thrombus would grow around the sword immediately and could be detected within the first 24 hours. When the swords were removed 14 days later, nearly all of the thrombotic material had disappeared without any evidence of thromboembolism in the kidneys or elsewhere in the dog.[65, 66]

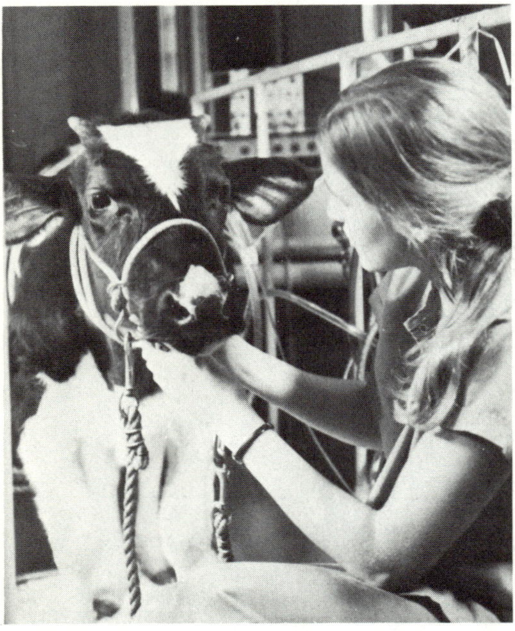

FIGURE 5. Aopa had its heart removed 93 days before this picture was taken. The intima of the heart is smooth Avcothane. Inflow valves are Bjork-Shiley valves. Outflow valves are Aopa's own. Our surgeons, Don Olsen and Jack Kolff, can save the animal's natural valves when they cut the natural heart out. Thus, the animal has only two artificial heart valves, reducing the risk of thromboembolism.

Using an artificial heart made of Avcothane Elastomer 51 (a compound of polyurethane and Siloxane made by Dr. E. Nyilas of Avco Everett), and using anticoagulants aspirin, persantin and coumadin, we have, at the time of writing, a calf, Aopa, that is going strong 116 days after implantation of an artificial heart (FIGURE 5).†

† A review of the state of the art for artificial organs in the United States was given by W. J. Kolff in the ASAIO, 1975,[67] and a book entitled, "Artificial Organs,"[68] about the experiences in Dr. Kolff's laboratory was published by John Wiley & Sons, New York, N.Y.

Summary

With oxygenators for long term use, it is more dangerous to use too little heparin than too much. Surfaces treated with silica free silicone greatly reduce clotting. Although few long-range aortas in man have an acceptable intima, the raw surface does little harm. The living grafts of Sparks are better. Most grafts of 4 mm ID are still fraught with failure, but when they have a smooth intima, with the wall as compliant as the artery, there is some promise. The use of a (Pall) filter in left ventricular bypass circuits in heparinized animals has facilitated this procedure for up to 14 days.

Artificial hearts and auxiliary ventricles have worked for many weeks or several months whether made of Silastic coated with silica-free silicone, PVC, biolyzed (gluteraldehyde treated) epicardium, or such polyurethanes as Biomer and Avcothane. Rough surfaces build up more and more fibrin when they move. Fibril surfaces shed. Thrombi form at predilection places inside artificial hearts, which are predictable. When artificial hearts are designed properly, nearly any surface goes. The correct use of Coumadin, Persantin and aspirin improves the result. The current record of survival with a total artificial heart is 122 days.

References

1. Petersen, R. J. & L. T. Rozelle. 1975. Ethylcellulose perfluorobutyrate: a highly non-thrombogenic fluoro polymer for gas-exchange membranes. ASAIO **21:** 24.
2. Hill, D. G., P. de Lanerolle, T. C. Kosek, M. J. Aguilar & J. D. Hill. 1975. The pulmonary pathophysiology of membrane and bubble oxygenators. Trans. ASAIO **21:** 165–170.
3. Bartlett, R. H., S. W. Fong, C. Woldanski, E. Hung, D. Styler & C. MacArthur. 1975. Hematologic responses to prolonged extracorporeal circulation (ECC) with microporous membrane devices. Trans. ASAIO **21:** 250–256.
4. Ward, B. D., A. G. Hood & E. J. Hershgold. 1975. Pathophysiology and mechanics of membrane lung performance deterioration. Trans. ASAIO **21:** 206–213.
5. Hagler, H. K., W. M. Powell, J. W. Eberle, W. L. Sugg, M. R. Platt & J. T. Watson. 1975. Five-day partial bypass using a membrane oxygenator without systemic heparinization. Trans. ASAIO **21:** 178–185.
6. Hill, J .D., M. R. de Leval, C. H. Mielke, M. L. Bramson & F. Gerbode. 1972. Clinical prolonged extracorporeal circulation for respiratory insufficiency: hematologic effects. Trans. ASAIO **18:** 546–552.
7. Leininger, R. I., J. P. Crowley, R. D. Falb, & G. A. Grode. 1972. Three years experience *in vivo* and *in vitro* with surfaces and devices treated by the heparin-complex method. Trans. ASAIO **18:** 312–315.
8. Ward, C. A., B. Ruegsegger, D. Stanga & W. Zingg. 1974. Reduction in platelet adhesion to biomaterials by removal of gas nuclei. Trans. ASAIO **20:** 77–84.
9. Kolobow, T., E. W. Stool, P. W. Weathersby, J. Pierce, F. Hayano & T. Suaudeau. 1974. Superior blood compatiblity of silicone rubber free of silica filler in the membrane lung. Trans. ASAIO **20:** 269–276.
10. Rea, W. T., D. Whitley & J. W. Eberle. 1972. Long-term membrane oxygenation without systemic heparinization. Trans. ASAIO. **18:** 316–320.
11. Salzmann, E. W. 1972. The events that lead to thrombosis. Bull. N.Y. Acad. Med. **48:** 225.
12. Stemerman, M. B. & T. H. Spaet. 1972. The Subendothelium and thrombogenesis. Bull. N.Y. Acad. Med. **48:** 289.

13. LEONARD, E. F. 1972. The role of flow in thrombogenesis. Bull. N.Y. Acad. Med. **48:** 273.
14. LINDENAUER, S. M., T. R. WEBER, T. A. MILLER, S. P. KAHN & R. S. WOJTALIK. 1974. Velour vascular prosthesis. Trans. ASAIO **20:** 314–319.
15. BERKOWITZ, H. D., L. J. PERLOFF & B. ROBERTS. 1972. Pseudointimal Development on microporous polyurethane lattices. Trans ASAIO **18:** 25–28.
16. SAWYER, P. N. & S. SRINIVASAN. 1972. The role of electrochemical surface properties in thrombosis at vascular interfaces: cumulative experience of studies in animals and man. Bull. N.Y. Acad. Med. **48:** 235.
17. MILLER, B. G., K. A. DYER, B. C. TAYLOR, J. I. WRIGHT & W. V. SHARP. 1974. Electrical conductivity: effect on intravascular performance of foams, velour, flock and fabric. Trans. ASAIO **20:** 91–100.
18. SHARP, W. V., D. L. GARDNER, G. T. ANDERSEN & J. WRIGHT. 1968. Electrolour: a new vascular interface. Trans. ASAIO **14:** 73–77.
19. VOLDER, J .G. R., R. KIRKHAM & W. J. KOLFF. 1973. New ways to create A. V. fistulas. Trans. ASAIO **19:** 38–42.
20. CAMPBELL, C. D., D. GOLDFARB, D. D. DETTON, R. ROE, K. GOLDSMITH & E. B. DIETHRICH. 1974. Expanded polytetrafluoro-ethylene as a small artery substitute. Trans. ASIAO **20:** 86–90.
21. WESOLOWSKI, S. A., Y. KOMOTO & H. UCHIDA. 1975. The small-caliber knitted arterial prosthesis. *In* Coronary Artery Medicine and Surgery. Appleton-Century-Crofts. New York, N.Y.
22. SHARP, W. V., B. C. TAYLOR, J. I. WRIGHT, E. NUWAYSER, B. G. MILLER, G. R. HAMPTON & C. L. WILSON. 1972. Neointimal survival—a function of attachment and thickness. Trans. ASAIO **18:** 232–237.
23. MANSFIELD, P. B., A. R. WECHEZAK & L. R. SAUVAGE. 1975. Preventing thrombus on artificial vascular surfaces: true endothelial cell linings. Trans. ASAIO **21:** 264–271.
24. BERGER, K., L. R. SAUVAGE, A. M. RAO & S. J. WOOD. 1972. Healing of arterial prostheses in man: its incompleteness. Ann. Surg. **175:** 118–127.
25. SAUVAGE, L., K. BERGER, L. BEILIN, J. C. SMITH, S. J. WOOD & P. B. MANSFIELD. 1975. Presence of endothelium in an axillary-femoral graft of knitted dacron with an external velour surface. Ann. Surg. **182:** 749.
26. SPARKS, C. H. 1973. Silicone mandril method for growing reinforced autogenous femoro-popliteal artery grafts in situ. Ann. Surg. **177:** 293.
27. NOSHINO, I., P. MALCHESKY, R. T. KIRALY, M. NAKAZONO, K. KOISO & Y. NOSÉ. 1974. Ziological puncturable shunt. Trans. ASAIO **20:** 320.
28. RUDERMAN, R. J., A. F. HEGYELI, B. G. HATTLER & F. LEONARD. 1972. A partially biodegradable vascular prosthesis. Trans. ASAIO **18:** 30–33.
29. MANSFIELD, P. B., L. R. SAUVAGE & J. C. SMITH. 1975. Factors influencing thrombus generation in artificial hearts. *In* Coronary Artery Medicine and Surgery. Appleton-Century-Crofts. New York, N.Y.
30. PIERCE, W. S., J. A. BRIGHTON, W. O. BANNON, J. H. DONACHY, W. M. PHILLIPS, D. L. LANDIS, W. J. WHITE & J. A. WALDHAUSEN. 1974. Complete left ventricular bypass with a paracorporeal pump: design and evaluation. Ann. Surg. **180:** 418–426.
31. VOLDER, J. R. & W. J. KOLFF. 1974. Induced growth of connective tissue in cardiovascular prostheses. Trans. ASAIO **20:** 521–526.
32. BRUCK, S. D. 1972. Biomaterials in medical devices. Trans ASAIO **18:** 1–8.
33. WAKABAYASHI, A., W. DIETRICK & J. E. CONNOLLY. 1969. Closed chest left heart bypass without anticoagulation. J. Thorac. Cardiovasc. Surg. **58:** 811–815.
34. SAWYER, P. N., B. STANCZEWSKI, S. SRINIVASAN, J. STEMPACK & G. W. KAMMLOTT. 1974. Implantation characteristics of metal-backed polymer coated heart valves: biophysical scanning and transmission electron microscopic studies. Trans. ASAIO **20:** 692–699.
35. HOFFMANN, A. S., G. SCHMER, C. HARRIS & W. G. KRAFT. 1972. Covalent bind-

ing of biomolecules to radiation-grafted hydrogels on inert polymer surfaces. Trans. ASAIO **18:** 10–16.
36. Schmer, G. Personal communication.
37. Kim, S. W., R. G. Lee, H. Oster, D. Coleman, J. D. Andrade, D. J. Lentz & D. Olsen. 1974. Platelet adhesion to polymer surfaces. Trans ASAIO **20:** 449–455.
38. Lyman, D. J., L. C. Metcalf, D. Albo, Jr., K. F. Richards & J. Lamb. 1974. The effect of chemical structure and surface properties of synthetic polymers on the coagulation of blood. III. *In vivo* adsorption of proteins on polymer surfaces. Trans. ASAIO **20:** 474–478.
39. Brash, L. L., S. Uniyal & Q. Samak. 1974. Exchange of albumin adsorbed on polymer surfaces. Trans. ASAIO **20:** 69–76.
40. Coleman, D. 1976. Platelet retention on albuminated glass and polystyrene beads. In preparation.
41. Schraut, W., I. Kiso, P. Freed, C. Baechler, M. Barnhart, J. Riddle, E. Mammen, G. Mandell & A. Kantrowitz. 1976. Permanent in series cardiac assistance with the dynamic aortic patch: blood-prosthesis interaction in long term canine experiments. In press.
42. Kiso, I., W. Schraut, W. Wajszczuk, M. S. Moskowitz, P. Freed & A. Kantrowitz. 1974. Long term *in vivo* testing of an auxiliary ventricle. Trans. ASAIO **20:** 637–642.
43. Kantrowitz, A., J. Krakauer, M. Rubenfire, D. Jaron, P. Freed, W. Welkowitz, P. Cascade, W. Wajszcauk, M. Lipsius, M. Ciborski, S. Phillips & M. Hayden. 1972. Initial clinical experience with a new permanent mechanical auxiliary ventricle: the dynamic aortic patch. Trans. ASIAO **18:** 159–167.
44. Bernhard, W. F., V. Poirier, C. G. LaFarge & J. C. Carr. 1975. A new method for temporary left ventricular bypass. J. Thorac. Cardiovasc. Surg. **70:** 880–892.
45. Norman, J. C. 1975. An intracorporeal (abdominal) left ventricular assist device cardiovascular diseases. Bull. Texas Heart Inst. **2:** 425–437.
46. Keiser, J., J. Norman & W. Bernhard. 1975. Left ventricular assist device: preclinical evaluation of temporary assist pumping. Annual Tech. Progress Rpt.
47. Olsen, D. B. 1976. Personal Communication.
48. Peters, J., J. McRea, H. Fukumasu & W. J. Kolff. 1976. Transapical left ventricular bypass (TALVB) without an auxiliary ventricle. Trans. ASAIO. **22:** 357–366.
49. McRea, J., J. Peters & H. Fukumasu. 1976. Continuous blood filtration for successful prolonged extracorporeal left ventricular bypass. Abstr. ASAIO. In preparation.
50. Fukumasu, H., J. Peters, J. McRea & J. Kolff. 1976. Use of the biomedicus blood pump (BMCP) for left ventricular bypass. Abstracts ASAIO. In preparation.
51. Olsen, D. B., F. Unger, H. Oster, J. Lawson & T. Kessler. 1975. Thrombus generation within artificial heart. J. Thorac. Cardiovasc. Surg. **70:** 248–255.
52. Lawson, J., D. B. Olsen, E. Hershgold, J. Kolff, C. Hadfield & W. J. Kolff. 1975. A comparison of polyurethane and silastic artificial hearts in 10 long survival experiments in calves. Trans. ASAIO **21:** 368–372.
53. Fasching, W., M. Deutsch, W. Haider, U. Losert, K. Polzer, A. Schlick, F. Stellwag, H. Thoma, F. Unger, E. Wolner & J. Navratil. 1975. Body reaction to long term blood pumping with a ventricular-aortic servo pump (VASP) implanted intrathoracically. Trans. ASAIO. **21:** 405–411.
54. Nosé, Y., R. Kiraly, G. Jacobs, C. Arancibia, K. Nakiri, G. Picha, H. Kambic, N. Morinaga, Y. Mitamura & T. Washizu. 1975. Development and evaluation of cardiac prostheses. Ann. Rpt. to NIH. May, 1975.
55. Greenfield, H., A. Au, S. Kelsey & W. J. Kolff. 1974. Simulation of assumed detriments. to prosthetic heart function. Trans. ASAIO **20:** 673–679.

56. JARVIK, ROBERT. 1976. Personal communication.
57. ATSUMI, K., Y. SAKURAI, I. FUHIMASA, K. IMACHI, T. NISHIZAKA, I. MANO, H. OHMICHI, J. MORI, N. IWAI & A. KOHNO. 1975. Hemodynamic analysis on prolonged survival cases (30 days and 20 days) of artificial total heart replacement. Trans. ASAIO **21:** 545–553.
58. HONDA, T., J. V. COCKRELL, Y. KITO, H. GIBSON & T. AKUTSU. 1975. Refinement in application of total artificial heart, with improvement in survival and histopathological findings. J. Thorac. Cardiovasc. Surg. **70:** 214–222.
59. AKUTSU, T. 1976. Personal communication.
60. AKUTSU, T. 1975. Artificial heart. Excerpta Medica. Amsterdam, The Netherlands.
61. OLSEN, D. B. 1976. Trans. ASAIO. In preparation.
62. BORETOS, J. W., W. S. PIERCE, R. E. BAIER, A. F. LEROY & H. J. DONACHY. 1975. Surface and bulk characteristics of a polyether urethane for artificial hearts. J. Biomed. Mat. Res. **9:** 327–340.
63. PIERCE, W. S. 1975. Personal communication.
64. LYMAN, D. J. & K. KNUDSEN. 1976. Degradation of polymers in a biological environment. In press.
65. DE LARIA, G., E. NYILAS & E. BERNSTEIN. 1972. Intra-aortic balloon pumping without heparin. Trans. ASAIO **18:** 501–504.
66. JACOBS, L. A., E. KLOPP & V. L. GOTT. 1968. Studies on the fibrinolytic removal of thrombus from prosthetic surfaces. Trans. ASAIO. **14:** 63–67.
67. KOLFF, W. J. & J. LAWSON. 1975. Status of the artificial heart and cardiac assist devices in the United States. Trans. ASAIO **21:** 620–638.
68. KOLFF, W. J. 1976. Artificial Organs (1) Cardiac Assist Devices, (2) The Artificial Heart, (3) The Artificial Kidney. Keter Publishing Company. Jerusalem and Halstead Press. New York, N.Y. In press.

Part IX. Evaluation of Artificial Interfaces

A. *In Vitro* Evaluation

BLOOD ELEMENTS AT FOREIGN SURFACES: *IN VITRO* EVALUATION OF BIOMATERIALS IN A SPINNING DISC APPARATUS *

Shaul Kochwa, Robert S. Litwak, and Richard E. Rosenfield

Mount Sinai School of Medicine
City University of New York
New York, New York 10029

Edward F. Leonard

Artificial Organ Research Laboratory
Columbia University School of Engineering
New York, New York 10027

Introduction

A large number of possibilities for assessing the magnitude and manner of interaction of plasma proteins with foreign surfaces was considered in our paper presented earlier in this conference.[1] Because many different candidate thromboresistant materials are available, it is essential to emerge from a world of abstract possibilities and generate a compact set of data by which these materials may actually be compared with each other with respect to their performance as blood boundaries. Initially, such a data set must be a compromise between the knowledge in depth that is necessary to understand the complex process of plasma protein adsorption, with subsequent participation in thrombus formation, and the need for simplicity, conciseness, and applicability of the data analysis to a wide range of materials. Thus, to date a simple, two-step hypothesis was proposed and tested on some seventeen candidate biomaterials furnished by contractors of the Biomaterials Program of the National Heart, Lung, and Blood Institute, NIH. The hypothesis stipulates that thrombogenesis is consequent to platelet adhesion and that platelet adhesion is related to antecedent adsorption of plasma proteins. In this paper are described the methods used for studying protein adsorption and platelet adhesion, including an explanation of critical choices made in the design of the test procedures. Steady state and time-varying data for the adsorption of human albumin, gamma globulin, and fibrinogen are presented and discussed. Corresponding data for the adhesion of canine platelets are presented and compared with protein adsorption results, from which a partial justification of the hypothesis is obtained. Then, the extent of nonuniformity of protein adsorption and platelet adhesion is tested and shown to be considerable. Finally, refined procedures and hypotheses for future testing are suggested.

Materials and Methods

The steady state uptake of each of the three plasma proteins—fibrinogen (Fibrinogen Human MSD, Merck Sharp and Dohme, West Point, Pa.), im-

* Supported by Contract NO1–HB–3–2910 from the National Heart, Lung, and Blood Institutes, NIH.

munoglobulin G (Gamma globulin human Fraction II, ICN Pharmaceuticals Inc., Cleveland, Ohio), and albumin (Normal serum Albumin (Human) 25% solution, Merck, Sharp and Dohme, Philadelphia, Pa.)—was studied by exposing discs of test material (1 cm in diameter) to solutions containing 1 mg/ml of one of the three repurified proteins in physiological saline. Freshly ^{125}I- (the Radiochemical Center, Amersham, England) labeled [modification of [2]] homologous protein was added to give a specific activity of about 3×10^5 cpm/mg. Discs were wetted with physiological saline before insertion in the protein solution, remained in the latter for one hour, and were then removed, washed with physiological saline, and were allowed to stand in saline overnight before counting. When only one side of a material was to be tested, the irrelevant side was covered with two layers of identical area, consisting of double-sided pressure-sensitive tape, backed on one side with a plastic cover. Discs were cut from this sandwich. The cover was assumed to have adsorbed labeled protein and was discarded prior to counting. In calculating, the net counts observed were converted to micrograms and expressed as μg per cm^2 by dividing by the area of test surface actually exposed.

Identical protein solutions and discs, the latter always backed as just described, were used in the studies of time-varying adsorption. The time-varying process was also dynamic in the sense that the discs were mounted on the end of a shaft and continually spun in the protein solution at a speed of 756 rpm. For this purpose, a series of special apparatuses have been constructed.[3-5] The one used in this investigation is shown in FIGURE 1. It consisted of a drive mechanism, chamber, and shaft that was capable of being moved up and down,

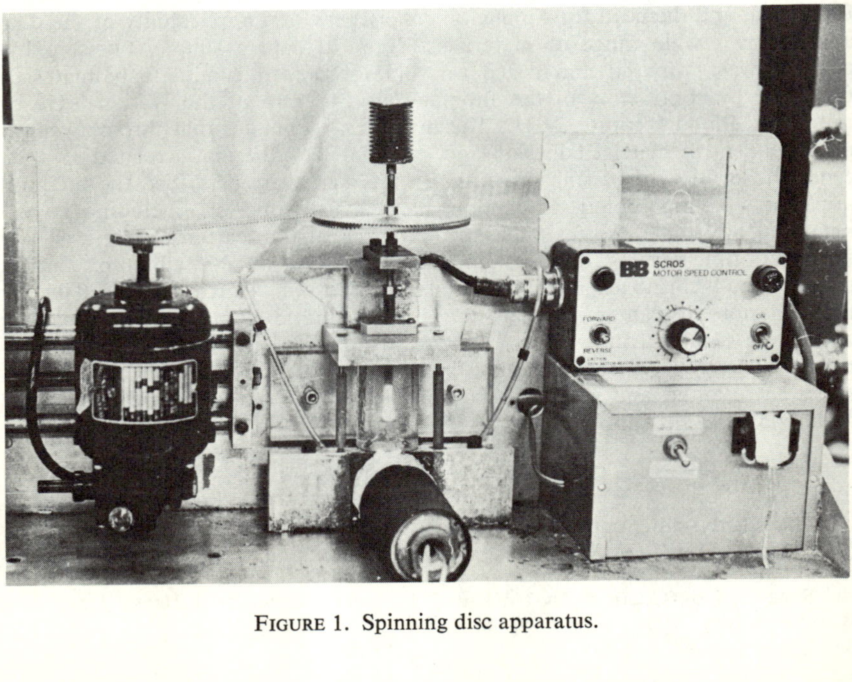

FIGURE 1. Spinning disc apparatus.

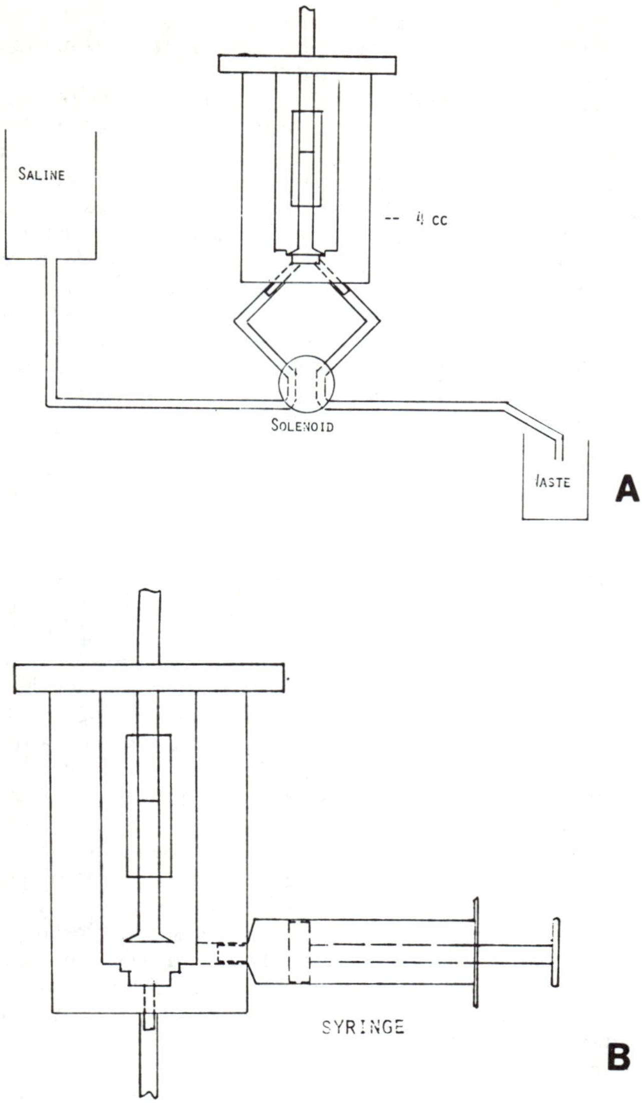

FIGURE 2. Schematic representation of the operation of the spinning disc. A: disc at the bottom of the reservoir, permitting washing and introduction of a sample; B: disc in spinning position after the sample was introduced through a syringe.

and of a reservoir. The method by which discs were exposed is shown in FIGURE 2. Before an exposure was begun the disc was lowered so as to serve as the cover of a well in the bottom of the reservoir (A). The well was flushed with saline through ports in the bottom of the reservoir. Protein solution was then injected via a syringe into the reservoir over the disc, and saline flow was stopped. The run was commenced by raising the disc and promptly starting rotation (B). At the end of the run, rotation was stopped; the disc was returned to the position shown in A, and saline flushing was recommenced. After washing, the disc was removed and counted.

An identical procedure was followed in the platelet adhesion experiments, except that the protein solution was replaced by freshly drawn blood from a heparinized canine having a chronic carotid-jugular shunt.[16] Platelet densities were obtained by counting under the light microscope and were recorded as platelets per 900 μm^2. Counts were obtained at four different radii and the surfaces were inspected at low power to test the uniformity of coverage.

In the time-varying experiments, exposures as short as 15 sec were made hence the importance attached to commencing and terminating contact of the test surface with protein solution in a prompt and reproducible manner.[5] It was also considered important to bring the test surface into the protein solution from saline without an intervening air interface and to return it to saline in a similar manner, because of the known generation of denatured protein layers at air-liquid interfaces.[7]

Discussion of Experimental Design

Flow and diffusion jointly determine the rate of delivery of protein molecules to an interface. Near the boundaries of aqueous systems, diffusion can be divided into that which occurs between the bulk solution and the neighborhood of the surface, through disordered water, and that which occurs over the last several hundred Ångstroms of solution before the surface is encountered, through water that is more or less ordered.[8] Diffusion through the latter part of the pathway (near the surface) is difficult to measure and is unaffected by the rate of bulk fluid movement. Its effects are usually lumped with the actual protein-foreign surface reaction. Transport through the more distant and more extensive layer of disordered water is affected by the rate of bulk fluid movement. This observation is important for three reasons: first, it suggests that when different surfaces are to be compared the observations must be made under identical conditions of fluid movement; second, rates of uptake from static solutions may, for dynamic reasons (in addition to other factors), be different from those that occur on prostheses exposed to flowing blood; and third, apart from the rates of uptake themselves being different, the final configuration and amount of adsorbed material may be different because low rates of arrival permit more time for irreversible reactions on the surface to occur before the advent of saturation, whereas high rates of arrival allow the surface to become quickly saturated, preventing further surface reaction.

We and others have presented the mathematical theory for this situation elsewhere.[9-13] For present purposes, it suffices to note: (1) that diffusion to the surface of a spinning disc will be uniform, specifically that it will not vary with either radial or angular position on the disc as shown by Levich,[9] and (2) that the diffusion-layer thickness ($x = 1.61\ (D/_v)^{1/3}\ (v/_w)^{1/2}$) was found at 756 rpm to be 4.9 μm for fibrinogen and 6.18 and 7.12 μm for IgG and albumin, respectively.†

† x=layer thickness in cm, v=kinematic viscosity of water (0.01 cm^2/sec), w=spinning rate in radians/sec, (79.17) D=diffusion coefficient in cm^2/sec (fibrinogen: 1.98×10^{-7}, IgG: 4.0×10^{-7}, albumin: 6.1×10^{-7}). (Modified from Ref. 4.)

At saturation a typical surface is covered with about 2 $\mu g/cm^2$ of fibrinogen. This amount is equal to that contained in a 20-μm layer of fibrinogen solution at the 1 mg/ml concentration used in this work. Such thickness is substantially greater than the 4.9-μm thickness of the fibrinogen diffusion layer calculated above for a stirred system. Thus, adsorption kinetics will be different in stirred and unstirred systems, even though the total quantity sorbed is similar. It can be shown [14] that the expected time of sorption from the stirred system will be on the order of 1 sec vs. about 20 sec in a stagnant system.

The observed adsorption times are long, compared to both of these times, suggesting that reaction phenomena at or near the surface occur with characteristic times of the order of minutes. Our time-varying results are available for the dynamic studies; only the extent of adsorption after one hour was observed in the static studies.

Results

In these studies, a type A segmented polyether urethane material supplied by the Stanford Research Institute was used as a reference material to insure the reproducibility of the test methods. Figure 3 shows protein adsorption for this material with error bars representing plus or minus the standard deviation of results taken from ten complete runs. The standard deviations are about 15% of the mean. Corresponding data for platelet uptake are also shown on this figure. Here the standard deviations are slightly more than for proteins. The adsorption data appear qualitatively to suggest two adsorption processes, one of which occurs instantaneously, relative to our measurement times, and another that occurs with a characteristic time of several minutes. For fibrinogen, the instantaneous adsorption corresponds to about 1 $\mu g/cm^2$, and rises over several minutes to more than twice this value. For μ-globulin, the instantaneous adsorption is of the order of 0.5 $\mu g/cm^2$; again the value more than doubles over a time course very similar to that of fibrinogen; for albumin the results are similar, except that the initial value is about 0.2 $\mu g/cm^2$. Adsorption curves approach the amount adsorbed statically after one hour of exposure for fibrinogen and albumin, but the dynamic asymptote for γ-globulin is much higher. Platelet adhesion is slow for about thirty seconds, rises rapidly for the next minute, and then continues to climb more slowly over the period of observation.

Because these observations are typical of what is observed of many, but not all, other materials, we shall consider their meaning before proceeding. The native fibrinogen molecule can be considered to have a cylindrical shape about 60 Å in diameter and 500 Å long.[5] If it adsorbs on its side, without distortion, it would occupy about 30,000 $Å^2$ and a monolayer would correspond to 0.19 $\mu g/cm^2$; if it is assumed to adsorb on its end, it would occupy about 3,000 $Å^2$ with a corresponding tenfold increase in the weight of the monolayer. The values observed approach this extreme. For γ-globulin, the area for undistorted side adsorption may be taken as about 6,000 $Å^2$,[5] giving a monolayer density of 0.42 $\mu g/cm^2$; the observed static steady state is comparable to this value; the dynamic results are higher. For albumin, with use of a spherical radius of 35.5 Å, the density of an undistorted monolayer can be calculated as 1.2 $\mu g/cm^2$; the observed values are generally lower.

Other materials that we have tested may be compared with the reference data for SRI polyurethane (Figure 3). Figure 4 summarizes the performance

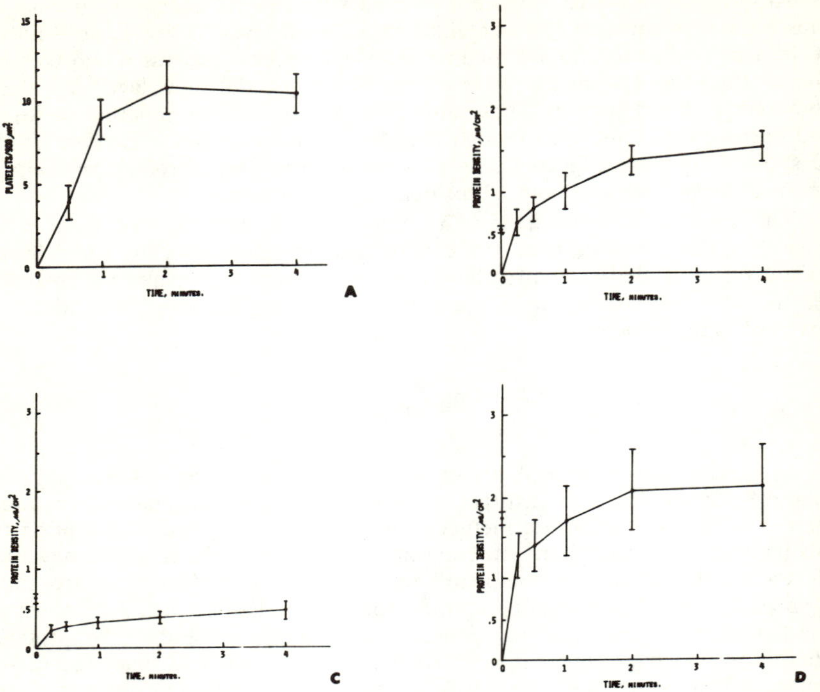

FIGURE 3. Time-varying studies of the uptake of human fibrinogen (A), human IgG (B), human albumin (C), and canine platelets (D) by discs of segmented polyurethanes SRI $3-\frac{1000}{425}-\left(\frac{70}{30}\right)-1-\times$ from Stanford Research Institute, Palo Alto, Calif., in spinning disc apparatus. Bars represent standard deviation of 10 experiments.

of a polycarbonate dialysis membrane (National Institute of Scientific Research) (A), and two other films proposed as gas exchange surface: polysulfone (A. D. Little Co.) (B) and ethylcellulose perfluorobutyrate (North Star Research Institute) (C). In each instance, the fibrinogen levels rise at a rate and to a level (between 1 and 2 $\mu g/cm^2$) similar to that for SRI polyurethane. The γ-globulin uptakes are also similar to polyurethane with a plateau value in excess of 1 $\mu g/cm^2$, except for the polycarbonate material, where the final level is halved. The albumin curves, which are the lowest of three proteins, are similar in all cases. All the data available for platelet uptake show responses similar to that of SRI polyurethane.

In FIGURE 5 (A & B) are compared two surfaces grafted onto polyurethanes by glow-discharge techniques. All the protein adsorption profiles are very similar, and the platelet uptake curves seem to be higher than that seen on the reference material.

In FIGURE 6 is shown the response of three heparinized materials. Battelle's TDMAC-heparin on silicone rubber (A) and Carnegie-Mellon's heparinized polyurethane (B) are very similar to SRI material in protein uptake. TDMAC-heparin on polyvinylchloride (C) shows generally higher protein uptake. The platelet data are different from those for polyurethane in two cases (A and C): the adhesion is delayed by two to four minutes and is apparently not related to protein uptake. For the heparinized polyurethane (B) the adhesion is similar to that on the reference material (FIGURE 3).

FIGURE 7 compares data from two carbon films. The General Atomic Company's vacuum deposited carbon (A) material shows platelet adhesion generally lower than that of the polyurethane standard. The IBD carbon furnished by Whittaker Corp. (B) shows reduced protein uptake, especially of fibrinogen, and slightly delayed platelet adhesion, although these values continue to rise over the period of observation to final values comparable to that of polyurethane.

A number of hydrophilic organic films (hydrogels) showed behavior significantly different from that of the reference polyurethane. Test results from two of these vinyl acetate-crotonic acid polymers prepared by Union Carbide Corp. are shown in FIGURE 8. (These differ in the amount of radiation crosslinking applied: A = 0.17 Mrad, B = 0.10 Mrad). The more highly irradiated

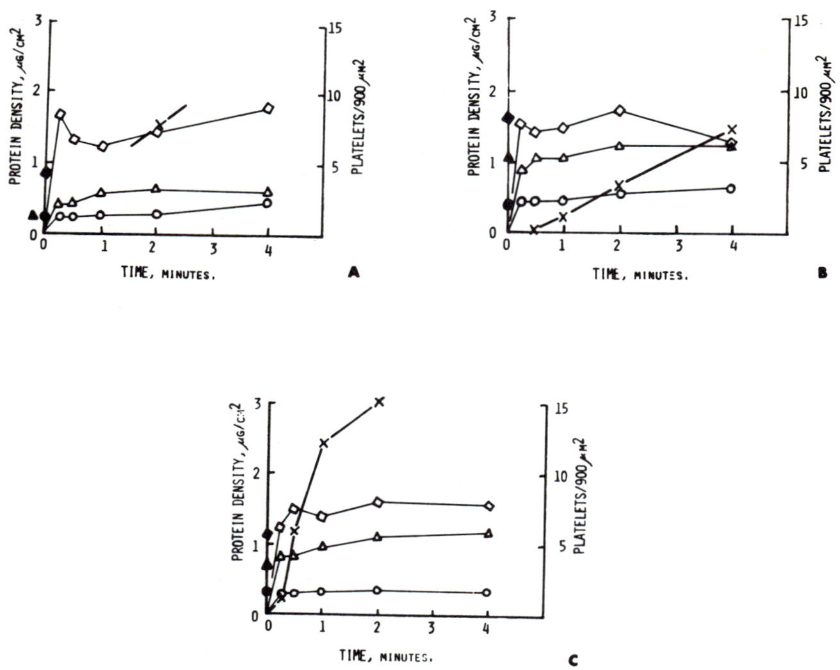

FIGURE 4. Time-varying studies of the uptake of human fibrinogen (◇—◇), human IgG (△—△), human albumin (○—○), and canine platelets (X—X) by A: polycarbonate dialysis membrane from National Institute of Scientific Research, Los Angeles, Calif. B: polyalkylsulfone membrane from Arthur D. Little Inc., Cambridge, Mass.; C: ethylcellulose perfluorobutyrate membrane from North Star Research and Development Institute, Minneapolis, Minn. Results of static experiments; exposure for 1 hr given on the y axis: fibrinogen ◆, IgG ▲, albumin ●. Protein concentration = 1 mg/ml.

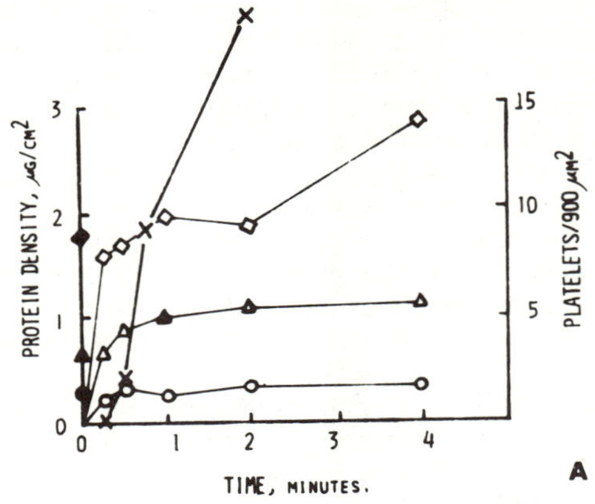

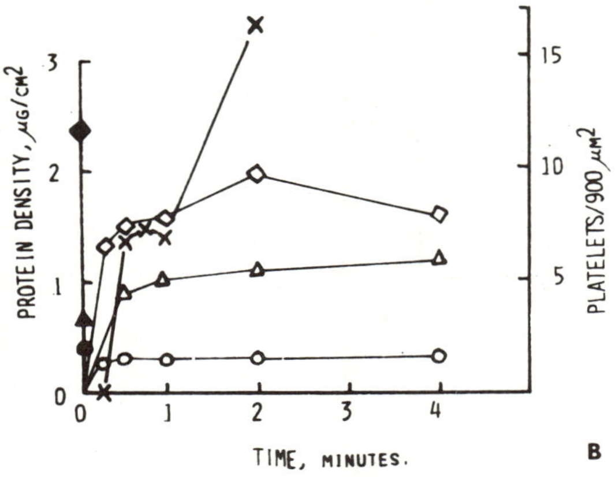

FIGURE 5. A: glow discharge in acetylene/N_2/H_2O, deposited on mylar; B: glow discharge in detramethyldisiloxane deposited on mylar both from Research Triangle Institute, Research Triangle Park, North Carolina. For explanations, see FIGURE 4.

crotonic acid polymer (A) shows fibrinogen uptake rates typical of other materials, but to a lower asymptote, and a corresponding intermediate level of platelet adhesion.

Three different formulations of acrylamide hydrogels coated onto polyurethane films have been tested (Polysciences Inc., Warrington, Pa.); two hydrogel formulations (uncross-linked and cross-linked by 1% methyl bisacrylamide) and two films, SRI types A and B, 3—(1000/425)—(70/30)—1—x, and 3-2000-1-E, respectively, were involved. Materials 707 and 709 comprised uncross-linked acrylamide on types A and B film, respectively; material 708 comprised cross-linked acrylamide on type A film. Three separate samples of material 707, designated 707, 707A, and 707B, and two separate samples of materials 708, designated 708 and 708A, were tested. Available static adsorption data are given in TABLE 1. Protein adsorption on material 707A was studied only via the uptake of specific antibodies to preadsorbed layers of protein.[1] All of these samples that were tested show lower protein adsorption than most films, both in static and kinetic studies. Three of the samples (707, 708, and 709), all received at the same period in 1973, also deviated from the order of protein adsorption seen in all materials (fibrinogen > gamma globulin > albumin), primarily by showing sharply reduced fibrinogen adsorption. These results were not confirmed in other samples of the same materials, either in static or kinetic adsorption studies. Material 707A showed very low platelet adhesion, whereas 708 showed lower adhesion than the bare type A polyurethane film used as control throughout this study. The data show strong variations from lot to lot (e.g., 707, 707B; 708, 708A), a fact that could not be explained by the manufacturer. Overall, these data suggest that low values of fibrinogen adsorption are a sufficient but not necessary condition (viz. the behavior of the heparinized surfaces) for the reduction of platelet adhesion.

As noted in our earlier paper,[1] protein adsorption has proved to be nonuniform on polyurethane discs. This nonuniformity has been investigated by autoradiography of several of the materials for which quantitative adsorption data are reported in this paper.

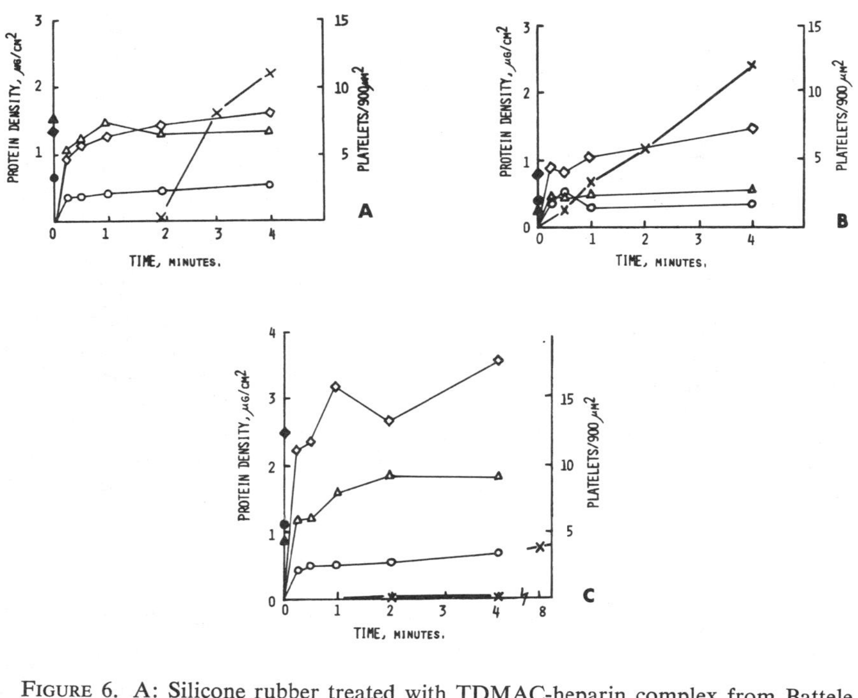

FIGURE 6. A: Silicone rubber treated with TDMAC-heparin complex from Battele Memorial Institute, Columbus, Ohio; B: ionically bound heparin on silastic (20 mil) from Carnegie-Mellon Institute of Research, Pittsburgh, Pa.; C: polyvinylchloride treated with TDMAC-heparin complex from Battele Memorial Institute, Columbus, Ohio. For explanations, see FIGURE 4.

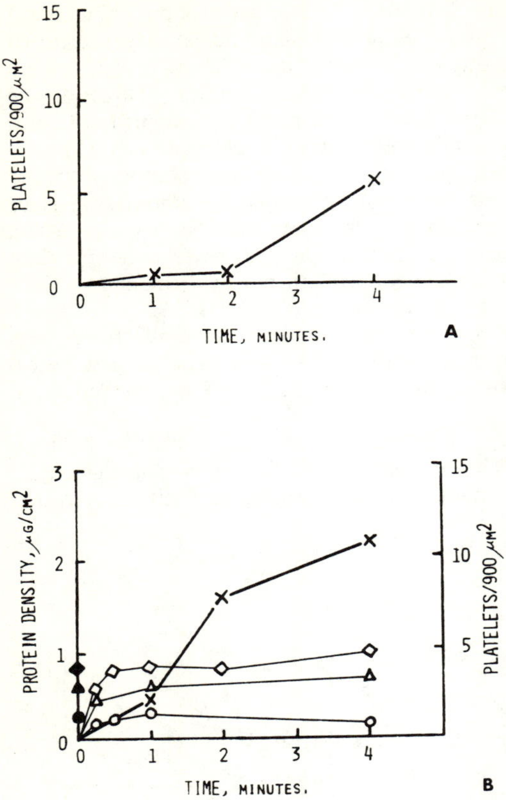

FIGURE 7. A: LTI carbon-coated glass cover slips from General Atomic Company, San Diego, Calif.; B: IBD carbon coated on SRI polyetherurethanes from Whittaker Corp., Waltham, Mass. For explanations, see FIGURE 4.

In all cases the discs were spun at 756 rpm in a solution of one of the three proteins used in the quantitative adsorption studies at the same concentration used in those studies, 1 mg/ml. The autoradiography procedure was that reported in our previous paper.[1] In FIGURE 9 are shown discs of poly (vinyl acetate Co-2% crotonic acid) grafted onto a polypropylene base with 0.17 Mrad Co^{60} radiation (cf FIGURE 8A). Those shown in the top row were exposed to fibrinogen, those in the middle row to albumin, and those in the

TABLE 1

UPTAKE OF HUMAN PLASMA PROTEINS BY DIFFERENT HYDROGEL FORMULATION

	707	707B	708	708A	709
Albumin	.26	.30	.19	.24	0.97
Fibrinogen	.04	.72	.18	.49	0.11
Gamma globulin	.29	.17	.29	.05	0.09

* For details see text.

bottom row to γ-globulin. In each case, exposures were (left to right) 15, 30, 60, and 240 sec. For each protein, the average density seems to increase with time. Nonuniformity of deposition is apparent on each disc.

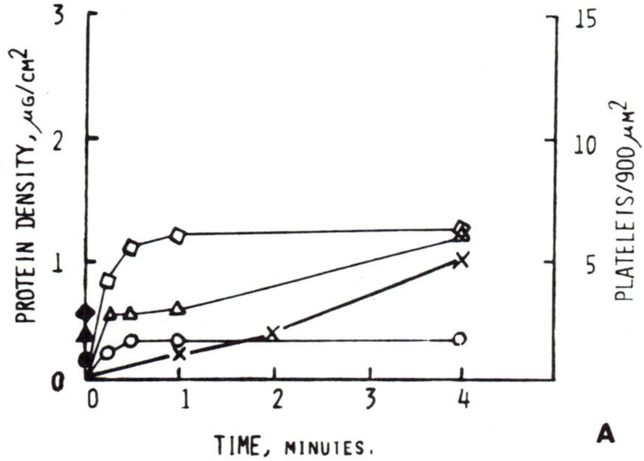

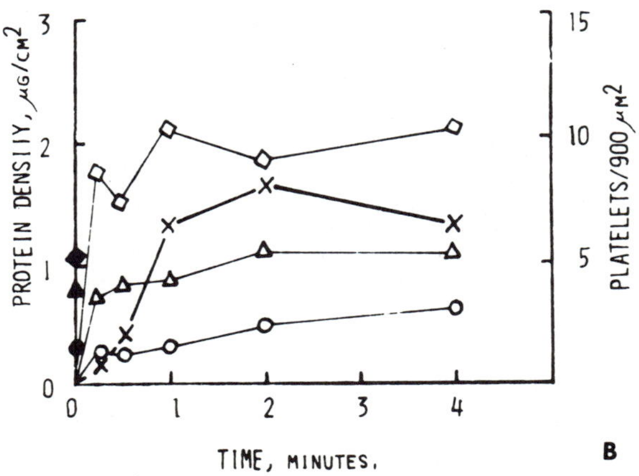

FIGURE 8. A: poly(vinylacetate—Co—2% crotonic acid) grafted onto polypropylene with 0.17 Mrad ^{60}Co. from Union Carbide Corp., Bound Brook, N.J.; B: as A, but grafted with 0.1 Mrad ^{60}Co. For explanation, see FIGURE 4.

Further discussion must be predicated on two facts: (1) that the quantitative relationship between intensity of shading of the photograph and protein density on the film has not been determined for these discs, and (2) that each disc is a separate sample of the film so that comparisons among them must be on the basis of the frequency of occurrence of certain features and not on a point-by-point comparison. Fibrinogen adsorption shows both intense specks and millimeter-sized cloudlike areas of denser coverage, both against a uniform

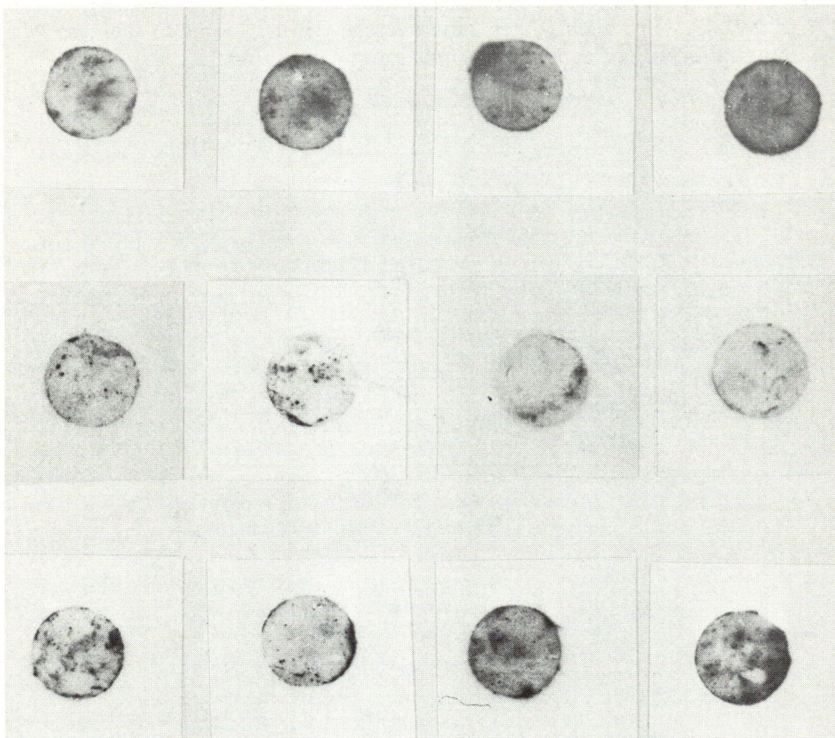

FIGURE 9. Autoradiography of discs from poly (vinylacetate—Co—2% crotonic acid) grafted onto polypropylene with 0.17 Mrad ^{60}Co. from Union Carbide Corp., Bound Brook, N.J. Time-varying studies in spinning disc apparatus. *From left to right:* 15 sec, 30 sec, 1 min, and 4 minutes. *Top:* ^{125}I human fibrinogen; *middle:* ^{125}I human albumin; *bottom:* ^{125}I human IgG. Protein concentration = 1 mg/ml.

background whose density increased with time. These features are also seen in the albumin sequence, except that more specks are seen and large intensely black areas develop over time. The γ-globulin sequence is also similar, except that extensive areas of intense blackness are seen at all times. Occasional bare spots of millimeter size are seen (fibrinogen at 30 sec and albumin at 240 sec).

It is possible that the areas of intense darkening are caused by protein aggregates, the number and size of which could increase during spinning, but the most significant areas of these discs may be those that show least adsorption, as suggested by information presented in the third paper of this series.[15]

In FIGURE 10 are shown autoradiographs of discs that were made after exposure to labeled fibrinogen. The materials from which the discs were cut were prepared by exposing Mylar film to a glow-discharge in one of two atmospheres (top row: acetylene, nitrogen, and water; bottom row: tetra methyl disiloxane) (cf FIGURES 5A, 5B). For each material, the discs have been exposed, inspecting from left to right, for 15, 30, and 60 seconds. The material presented in the top row shows a higher average density than that of the material in the bottom row, according to the studies reported earlier in this paper, and the density of the photographs given here is correspondingly higher for the top row. Both materials contain intense black spots as well as somewhat larger areas that are relatively light. The black spots show no consistent increase in number or size with time, as would be expected if they were associated with aggregates formed by the shear field induced by the spinning disc. The disc in the bottom row that was exposed for 30 sec is remarkably uniform, both in comparison to others in this series and to most that have been autoradiographed in this laboratory.

In FIGURE 11 are shown autoradiographs of discs from two other materials, also after exposure to labeled fibrinogen. The materials were: an ethylcellulose perfluorobutyrate membrane, NS-332–42 (top row) (cf FIGURE 4C) and a polyalkylsulfone oxygenation film, A. D. Little Co. (bottom row) (cf FIGURE 4B). For each material the times of exposure were, left to right, 60 and 240 seconds. A substantial "edge effect" associated with cutting or mounting of the disc is seen in the top left of the figure. Again intense black spots are apparent, but, again, there is no consistent indication of an increase in their number or size with time. The average density of adsorbed fibrinogen plotted against time, as reported earlier in this paper, is nearly identical for these materials. On close inspection, a considerable variation in density is seen over all of these discs, even when the intense black spots are ignored.

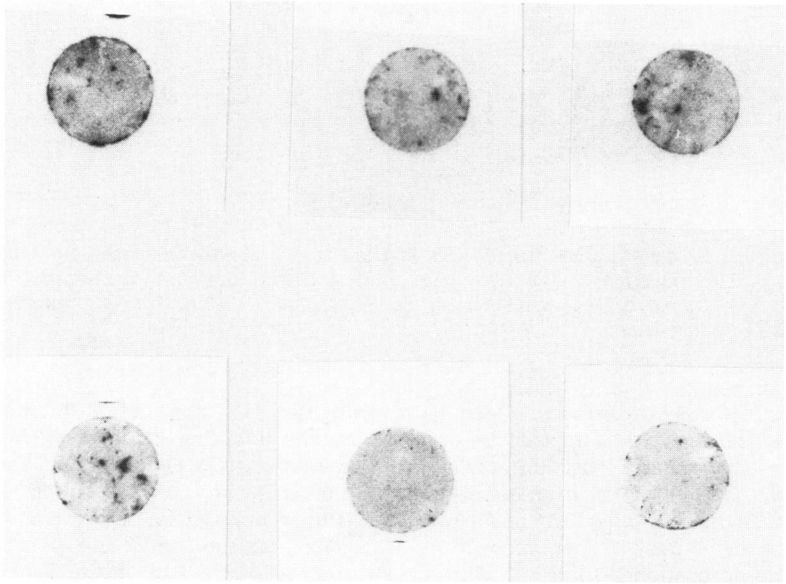

FIGURE 10. Autoradiographs of discs exposed to ^{125}I fibrinogen for 15 sec (left), 30 sec (middle), and 60 sec (right). *Top row:* glow discharge in acetylene/N_2/H_2O deposited on mylar. *Bottom row:* glow discharge coated in tetramethyldisiloxane deposited on mylar. Both materials from Research Triangle Institute, Research Triangle Park, North Carolina.

While the nonuniformity of these surfaces is apparent, it is difficult to objectivize what is seen. Not only are the patterns complex, but, as noted above, the analysis must be fundamentally statistical, since each disc in a time series or each among a set exposed to different proteins is a different sample. The consistent nonuniformity among the different proteins used and between the static exposures reported in the accompanying paper [1] and the kinetic studies reported here suggests that inhomogenities in the surface at the time of testing are responsible. Another paper in this series [15] reports the results of preliminary efforts to correlate these patterns with those seen for platelets and to develop methods for quantification of these observations.

We have no illusions that the test results reported here have proven rele-

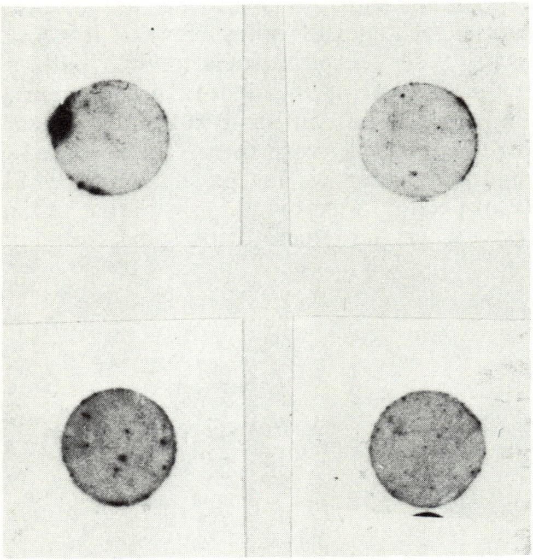

FIGURE 11. Autoradiographs of discs exposed to ^{125}I-labeled fibrinogen for 60 sec (left) and 4 min (right). *Top row:* ethylcellulose perfluorobutyrate membrane from North Star Research Development Institute, Minneapolis, Minn. *Bottom row:* polyalkylsulfone membrane from Arthur D. Little, Inc., Cambridge, Mass.

vance to thromboresistance. Over the range of materials considered, decreased fibrinogen adsorption appears to decrease platelet adhesion. Considered as a whole, the materials are, insofar as these observations are concerned, more similar than different in protein uptake. Nonuniformity of adsorption and platelet adhesion is present in all materials studied and, so far as we can tell, is not an artifact of our procedures, being apparent in static and dynamic protein adsorption studies and with a scale similar to that seen in the platelet-adhesion studies.

Materials-testing in controllable *in vitro* and *ex vivo* environments needs to penetrate farther into the thrombus-forming process. We cannot get platelets from fresh human blood to adhere to biomaterial surfaces as a monolayer. They appear to aggregate in bulk and then adhere later.[15] We are concerned with the meaning of adhesion for later events. On different surfaces, perhaps surfaces distinguishably different in terms of protein adsorption, a fixed amount of platelet adhesion leads to profoundly different sequellae. Additionally, irregularities of surfaces as revealed by autoradiography may give us a clue to the nature of the surface that does not adsorb protein or platelets if, by some ingenious chemical or physicochemical method, this difference could be analyzed.

The work reported in this paper accurately establishes two simple time-varying functions for a wide range of synthetic materials: the amount of protein they adsorb from single protein solutions and the amount of platelet adsorption from heparinized canine blood. We hope that to this modest but firm base, the complexities of competitive adsorption, configurational change, and finally, nonadhesional platelet behavior can be logically added.

Summary

In the interactions of artificial surfaces with blood, protein adsorption is widely believed to be the first step that is significant for thrombogenesis. Separate adsorptions of fibrinogen, gamma globulin or albumin by various artificial surfaces having different chemical and physical characteristics have been measured under static and various flow conditions. Hydrogels adsorb less protein than other solid surfaces, but large variations occur between different types and batches. Other solid materials also adsorb varying amounts of proteins. Platelet adhesion to these surfaces from fresh heparinized canine blood has been studied under flow conditions identical to those used for kinetic uptake of proteins. High levels of fibrinogen adsorption correlate with high levels of platelet uptake. Protein distribution on all surfaces studied was not uniform, and autoradiography revealed variations among surfaces prepared from the same batch of material.

Acknowledgment

The authors gratefully acknowledge the excellent technical assistance of Estelle Makuku in performing the protein adsorption and autoradiographic procedures.

References

1. Kochwa, S., R. S. Litwak, R. E. Rosenfield & E. F. Leonard. Blood elements at foreign surfaces: A biochemical approach to the study of the adsorption of plasma proteins. This volume.
2. McFarlane, A. S. 1958. Efficient trace labeling of proteins with iodine. Nature **182:** 53.
3. Hare, J. 1973. A spinning disc apparatus for the study of the interactions of blood with an artificial surface: initial experiments. M.S. thesis. Columbia Univ. New York, N.Y.
4. Truritto, V. T. & E. F. Leonard. Platelet adhesion to a spinning disc. Trans. Am. Soc. Artif. Intern. Organs **18:** 348.
5. Adler, M. A. 1975. Protein adsorption to artificial biomaterial surfaces, an in-

vestigation involving the spinning disc apparatus. M.S. thesis. Columbia Univ. New York, N.Y.

6. Benis, A. M., M. Anthony, M. L. Nossel, L. M. Aledort, R. M. Koffsky, J. F. Stevenson, E. F. Leonard, M. Shiang & R. S. Litwak. 1975. Extracorporeal model for study of factors affecting thrombus formation. Thromb. Diath. Haemorrh. **34:** 27.
7. Lee, W. H., Jr., O. Krumhaar, E. W. Fonkalsrud, O. A. Schjeide & J. W. Maloney, Jr. 1961. Denaturation of plasma proteins as a cause of morbidity and death after intracardiac operations. Surgery **50:** 29.
8. Hagler, A. T. & H. A. Scheraga. 1973. Current status of the water-structure problem: application to proteins. Ann. N.Y. Acad. Sci. **204:** 51
9. Levich, V. G. 1962. Physicochemical hydrodynamics. Prentice Hall, Inc. Engelwood, N.J.
10. Riddiford, A. C. 1966. The rotating disc system. Adv. Electroch. Eng. **4:** 47.
11. Lehmkuhl, G. D. 1968. Flow and mass transfer near a rotating disc. Ph.D. thesis. Univ. Illinois. Urbana, Ill.
12. Serad, G. 1964. Chemical hydrodynamics with a rotating disc. Ph.D. thesis. Univ. Pennsylvania. Philadelphia, Pa.
13. Butruille, Y. A., E. F. Leonard & R. S. Litwak. 1975. Platelet-platelet interactions and nonadhesive encounters on biomaterials. Trans. Am. Soc. Artif. Int. Organs **21:** 609.
14. Butruille, Y. A., S. Savitz & E. F. Leonard. 1976. Transient diffusion effects in the study of early platelet adhesion. J. Biomed. Mat. Res. **10:** 145.
15. Leonard, E. F., Y. A. Butruille, S. Puszkin & S. Kochwa. This volume.

IN VITRO EVALUATION SYSTEMS: A BIOLOGICAL APPROACH

Leo Vroman

Interface Laboratory
Veterans Administration Hospital
Brooklyn, New York 11209

The primary problem becoming most apparent during the Workshop session on this subject was: What is the purpose and meaning of our *in vitro* tests? Many of us have recently become aware, I believe, of the danger in first developing a theory on the basis of a rather arbitrarily chosen test system, and then limiting ourselves to the same test system in efforts to prove the theory. Dr. Silberberg pointed out that the limitations imposed by specific techniques upon the way in which surfaces are to be prepared often appear unrelated to planned medical application. I stressed my own position: in our laboratory we promise no more than data that indicate what proteins are adsorbed under our conditions onto more or less flat material surfaces out of plasma, what reactions these adsorbed proteins may be subjected to by the plasma, and what effects the resulting film may have on the adhesion of platelets and white blood cells. We are not testing for thrombogenicity. Those who claim they do have a predictive test for *in vivo* behavior will have to correlate much *in vitro* and *in vivo* data for many biomaterials to prove their claim. This does not relieve any of the work load resting on those now occupied with true (namely, *in vivo*) thrombogenicity testing. Yet, the original purpose of *in vitro* testing must have been to provide such relief.

Let us presume, then, that the primary purpose of studying the blood/material interface reactions *in vitro* now is to understand how certain chains of events—especially those no longer than a few hours—are set in motion by certain surface properties. Removed as far away as possible from the living organism, we replace its complex and therefore confusing homeostatic system by a different, lifeless, and therefore more controllable kind of constancy. If, however, its isolation renders plasma subject to scrutiny so close that single molecular films can be observed, then the biomaterial substrate must be studied at least as closely. At this initial point of study we are already blocked by the nonbiological problem that sample surfaces, especially of many polymers, are nonuniform beyond description, as Dr. Yasuda, Dr. Brash, Dr. Chawla, Dr. Stromberg, and others pointed out at this session. The variability of these surfaces requires handling history as well as preparation of samples to be reproducible.

Why can even the most minute surface discontinuities have such profound effects upon the behavior of blood that they will determine the fate of an implant? Perhaps it is because blood must have the ability to defend itself against surface accidents by means of its molecular contact-sensitive system. The sensitivity of this system provides a biologically amplified image of the material's physical and chemical surface properties, as soon as the blood "sees" this surface. The roughness described by Dr. Merrill earlier as either being of a scale of about 1000 Å—and significant to protein molecules—or of a scale of about 100 microns—and significant to cells—is only one example where mere size of an imperfection could trigger very different responses in the contacting blood.

Most subjects of this conference have been arranged in a sequence that suggests one amplification of initial surface properties after another: selection of only certain proteins for adsorption out of plasma, and orientation of the adsorbed protein; effects of this orientation upon certain interactions with the plasma, as described by Dr. Kochwa, Dr. Morrissey, Dr. Ratnoff, Dr. Kaplan, and Dr. Hemker as well as by us, probably provide an image of surface properties translated into a mottled carpet hundreds of Angstroms thick. The carpet's pattern may be either an exaggerated or a muted reproduction of the underlying solid pattern.

Our own work, combined with that of others reported during this conference in papers and in the Workshop, provides new details of some mechanisms responsible for the biological amplification or deamplification ("passivation") of the man-made surface image. If the surface adsorbs fibrinogen out of plasma, it does so within about two seconds. The conformation of fibrinogen being adsorbed depends on the substrate surface (Morrissey) and changes with increased adsorption (Cuypers). It competes well with other plasma proteins (Kochwa, Brash, Vroman); it can be replaced by proteins in serum (Vroman *et al.,* this volume, and Cuypers), and is not desorbed spontaneously but is removed by plasma (Kochwa, Vroman). The rates at which intact normal plasma converts and then removes part of the film depend on certain incompletely known surface properties (Vroman *et al.*). The first layer of platelets to be deposited requires fibrinogen (Zucker) to be present on the solid in unconverted condition (Vroman); but the arrival rate of these platelets depends on the effects of surface geometry upon flow (Leonard, Goldsmith, Turitto) as well as on porosity (providing a force normal to the wall: Blackshear). Subsequent platelet-to-platelet adhesion and aggregation require von Willebrand factor rather than fibrinogen (Zucker); substances released by the first adhering platelets will encourage this aggregation, probably at a rate reflecting some effect of substrate through adsorbed fibrinogen on the rate of shape change suffered by these firstcomers.

If the rate of first platelet adhesion is a product of surface-determined fibrinogen conversion and surface geometry-determined platelet arrival, this product will in itself be another amplifying step, unless the two events are well separated in time. Dr. Silberberg suggested that any material might be pre-exposed to plasma and become passivated in this fashion (allowing all adsorbed fibrinogen to be rendered harmless by conversion). Another way of rendering a device acceptable, suggested by Dr. Sawyer at another meeting, would be to implant it first in a high flow (arterial) region, then in the demanding low flow (venous) position. For example, we have found that most carbon surfaces of the kind used on heart valves adsorb fibrinogen out of plasma, do not convert it quickly, and do cause deposition of platelets out of whole blood, yet these materials perform well (Haubold) in high flow regions. The main task of those doing *in vitro* studies therefore should be to understand rather than to predict performance of biomaterials. With this in mind, the *in vitro* tester need not mind that materials may fail or succeed in many diverse ways. We found platelets deposited on hemodialyzer surfaces only in certain areas, and granulocytes in most others. We do not yet know whether these deposits mean failure or success. We do know that globulins deposited *in vitro* on a hydrophobic surface (rather than on a hydrophilic one) cause granulocyte adhesion. Our next task is, therefore, to see whether this *in vitro* finding helps to explain the *ex vivo* events in real life. If we find, for example, that prekallikrein is involved *in vitro,* we must see if adsorption of this protein onto cuprophane during dialysis precedes deposition of granulocytes.

If minute local surface properties can indeed be the cause of large local differences in blood/interface reactions, other initial local conditions must often have great consequences as well. At least several of these occur as blood enters a device; surface temperature, variable washout times of priming solution, flexing of material surface during or after first contact with blood (intended or not) can all create early events with later consequences, and can all be imitated *in vitro.* When they are, an alarmingly great set of such variables may be discovered that the surgeon cannot help introducing, and that the *in vitro* tester must reproduce. Methods for such studies are now available. Some were discussed during the workshop; others, omitted for lack of time, are also briefly mentioned below.

It was felt that, thus far, attenuated total reflection in the infrared can detect but cannot identify adsorbed proteins. Dr. Lyman, however, believed Fourier transform techniques will soon allow recording of spectra in sufficient detail to be specific for certain proteins. I proposed that less sophisticated equipment also be used to identify adsorbed proteins by exposing the films to antisera and observing intensification of spectra when antibody is adsorbed.

We have discussed some simpler ways of both detecting and identifying proteins adsorbed onto relatively flat surfaces (this volume). One of these, the method of using condensing water vapor to detect the highly wettable antibody/antigen complex surface, though only qualitative, is quite sensitive. It also allows detection of surface nonhomogeniety, but, like Dr. Baier's contact-angle measurements, it creates advancing air/liquid/solid interfaces that may be somewhat destructive.

Other methods, including those identifying adsorbed clotting factors, were discussed by us elsewhere (this volume). Dr. Stromberg and Dr. Morrissey, Dr. Hemker and Dr. Cuypers, and our own group all use ellipsometry as a means of observing protein adsorption; in addition, we use it as a means of recording rate and quantity of antibody adsorption and thus of estimating the surface concentration of identifiable proteins. From discussions at the present conference as well as from earlier conversations, I have gained the impression that automation of the instrument does yield data indicating that protein orientation or conformation at the interface varies with time, concentration, and kinds of protein and of interface. However, the more specific we want our conclusions to be, the more adventurous must be our presumptions. For example, we are not sure on what basis to assume that, in the spaces among sparsely deposited protein molecules, a lightbeam will "see" either a film of water (with a lower-than-protein refractive index) or the bare substrate (usually with high refractive index).

Several investigators have measured the loss of specific proteins suffered by plasma passed through a column of pulverized biomaterial. Flow and surface conditions in these experiments are quite unlike those required *in vivo,* although, as Dr. Baier pointed out, they do allow—as in chromatography—recovery of adsorbed protein. We agreed, however, that the most firmly bound proteins may never be detected and identified this way and yet may be exactly the ones responsible for specific blood/interface reactions, such as fibrin formation and platelet and granulocyte adhesion.

These grossly or at least microscopically visible events are handy tools for measuring our own limitations; the larger any biological event, the more complex it must be and the harder to understand both its origin and its consequences. Certainly the time it takes under very artificial conditions for fibrin to form or for platelets to adhere bears only a very indirect relationship to thrombogenicity. We have found surfaces that retard clotting and yet appear to activate factor XII or the reverse, and surfaces that cause fibrinogen deposition and no platelet deposition, or the reverse. To us, this means that more, rather than less study is required; most of all, sequences of a surface's interactions with plasma constituents must be separated in time from those with the blood's formed elements. Until differences among biomaterials can be explained rather than merely listed and grouped, no laboratory must be asked to judge surfaces on the basis of *in vitro* tests.

B. *Ex Vivo* AND *In Vivo* EVALUATIONS

A TECHNIQUE FOR THE ELUCIDATION OF VIRCHOW'S TRIAD

William A. Morton * and Robert D. Cumming

Avco Everett Research Laboratory, Inc.
Everett, Massachusetts 02149

INTRODUCTION

As first enumerated by Virchow,[1] hemodynamics, surface chemistry, and blood chemistry are the primary factors influencing thrombus formation. The study of the effects of any one of these parameters on thrombogenesis is complicated by the interdependence of the other two.

A test system, developed at this Laboratory and referred to as the Stagnation Point Flow Experiment (SPFE), provides a technique for the control and/or systematic variation of each of the factors defined in Virchow's triad. This experimental technique and its applications have been described in the literature.[2-9] In the SPFE, blood flows directly from the carotid artery of an anesthetized dog into a test chamber under controlled and reproducible flow conditions. The chamber is designed to assure that only blood having no prior foreign-surface contact impinges upon the surface forming the top of the chamber. Steady-state blood flow, which may be electively pulsatile or nonpulsatile, is maintained through the chamber. The blood then flows out into a collecting cylinder and is not returned to the animal. The primary advantage of the SPFE is that, on transparent test surfaces, the interaction of the cellular blood elements, fibrin formation, and thrombosis can be directly observed *in situ* by light microscopy and recorded by cinematography. The effects of surface chemistry or the thrombogenic properties of various materials under well-defined hemodynamic conditions can be studied by placing test surfaces having the proper dimensions into the chamber. Opaque or translucent materials can also be studied with an experimental protocol in which test surfaces are exposed to blood flow for specified periods of time, removed from the flow chamber, and fixed or stained for detailed examination by scanning electron or light microscopy.

For hemodynamic studies in which the chemical structure of the contact surface is of secondary importance, the magnitude of flow over the test surface can be controlled or systematically varied at the discretion of the investigator. The formation of recirculating flow regimes within the stagnation point area can also be performed by changing the shape of the test surface.

It is generally desirable to minimize the blood loss by the animal. This is accomplished through the use of several flow chambers with the same general flow configuration but with slightly different dimensions. As a result, different shears can be induced at the test surface with a constant rate of flow adjusted to yield maximum utilization of the blood supply that can be safely withdrawn from a particular experimental animal. In this manner, experiments of up to

* Present address: Avco Medical Products, Inc., 9 Plymouth St., Everett, Mass. 02149.

three hours' duration are possible without a substantial decrease in the animal's blood volume and without induction of hypovolemic shock.

In hemodynamic studies and in the hemocompatibility evaluation of various materials, experimental animals whose hematologic parameters have been established to fall within normal ranges are used. The animal's hematology is also continuously monitored during the course of these experiments. However, to study the effects of the third factor of Virchow's triad, viz., those of altered blood chemistry, experimental animals having either congenital or drug-induced hematologic abnormalities can be used in the SPFE.

As a result of the control afforded, the SPFE provides a short-term *ex vivo* investigative technique that is adaptable to such studies as biomaterials evaluation, geometric considerations in the design of prosthetic devices, evaluation of the effects of drugs or hematologic variations on the rate or degree of thrombosis, and basic studies, i.e., kinetics of thrombosis.

Experimental Concept

A schematic diagram of the SPFE flow chamber is presented in Figure 1. As illustrated, blood enters the chamber directly from the carotid artery of an anesthetized dog. Only blood flowing through the center of the artery and having had no prior foreign-surface contact impinges upon the test surface to form a stagnation point. From this domain, the blood flows radially outward along the test surface into a collecting trough. The blood flowing alongside the walls of the entrance hole proceeds alongside the bottom of the chamber and does not contact the test surface. A withdrawal port in the outer region of the chamber draws the blood from the peripheral collecting trough and directs it to the withdrawal system-holding cylinder. Thus, no activated blood contacts the stagnation point and the blood is not returned to the animal.

Stagnation points occur on the front side of all blunt objects placed into a fluid stream. The flow fields associated with stagnation points have been extensively studied.[10, 11] A description of the stagnation point flow field as it relates to the SPFE has been previously published.[4] For the sake of continuity, however, a similar discussion is presented here.

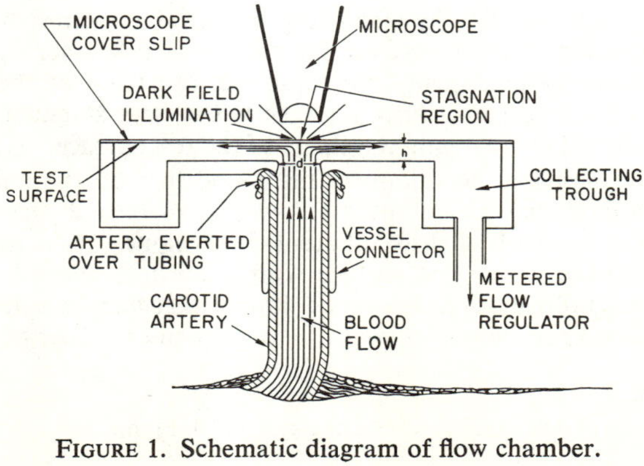

Figure 1. Schematic diagram of flow chamber.

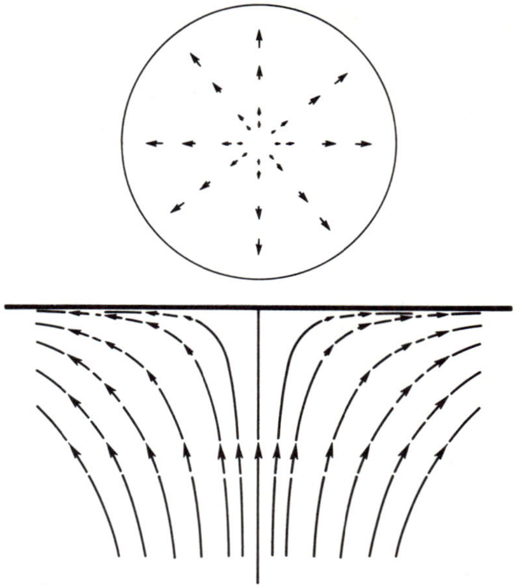

FIGURE 2. Streamline pattern for a stagnation point flow-neglecting viscosity.

FIGURE 2 shows the streamline pattern for a stagnation point flow neglecting the effects of viscosity. The arrows indicate the direction of flow and their lengths indicate the relative magnitudes of velocity. The velocity component toward the surface gradually decreases as the fluid approaches the surface. In the vicinity of the surface, the velocity is predominantly along the surface and not toward it. The velocity component toward the surface, U_z, and its radial component along the surface, U_r, are given by the expressions

$$U_z = 2\ Az \tag{1}$$

and

$$U_r = Ar \tag{2}$$

where z is the distance from the surface, r is the radial distance from the central streamline, and A is the flow parameter describing the magnitude of the flow velocity outside of the viscous layer. The streamline shapes, shown in FIGURE 2, remain unchanged for all flow velocities. However, for higher flow parameters, the magnitude of the velocity vectors will be larger at all points on the diagram.

Viscosity effects are confined to a thin layer near the surface, the thickness of which can be expressed by

$$\delta = 2.8\ (\nu/A)^{1/2} \tag{3}$$

For a Newtonian fluid with a given kinematic viscosity, ν, the thickness of this layer decreases with increasing flow. Knowing the velocity near the surface, the shear force on the surface may be derived. The velocity profile in this thin viscous boundary layer can be approximated as a linear variation with the distance, z, away from the surface.

In the viscous layer

$$U_r\ (r,\ z) = U_r\ (r)\ (z/\delta) \tag{4}$$

so that when $z = \delta$ the velocity becomes the same as the inviscid value. Substitution from Equations 2 and 3 into Equation 4 gives

$$U_r = \beta\ rz \tag{5}$$

where

$$\beta = \frac{1}{2.8}\left(\frac{A^3}{\nu}\right)^{1/2} \tag{6}$$

The shear rate on the surface is the rate of change of radial velocity with distance from the surface

$$\partial\ U_r/\partial_z = \beta\ r \tag{7}$$

The shear stress on the surface, τ, is defined as

$$\tau = \rho\ \nu\ \beta\ r \tag{8}$$

where ρ is the density of blood.

For a Newtonian fluid, the shear at the surface can be shown to increase as the 3/2 power of the flow parameter, A, and to increase linearly with distance from the stagnation point. Thus, for a given flow parameter, the shear is zero at the stagnation point and increases as one moves outward. The shear at any given distance from the stagnation point is larger the higher the flow parameter. The radius at which a given shear is reached decreases as the 3/2 power of the flow parameter. Thus, for a situation in which local shear is the significant parameter, one would expect similar phenomena to occur at radii that decrease with increasing flow as the 3/2 power of the flow parameter. For some of the results to be described later, the departure of blood from a Newtonian viscosity is significant. In this case, the shear still increases with radial distance from the stagnation point, but its variation with distance is different. It can be shown, however, based on an analysis of non-Newtonian stagnation point flow, that the radius at which a given shear is reached still scales as the inverse 3/2 power of the flow parameter.

The parameter, β, is theoretically well defined only for the ideal stagnation point flow, in which the streamlines are hyperbolic in shape, as shown in FIGURE 2. Since the flow in the chambers does not correspond exactly to this ideal, the parameter, β, has been measured empirically for each chamber. This also allows the determination of an effective inviscid stagnation point flow parameter, A, for a given flow rate of blood through a given chamber.

This Laboratory uses five analogous flow chambers, each characterized by its flow parameter, β. Beta is a function of the mass flow rate of blood through the chamber, the distance, h, between the cover glass and the bottom of the chamber shown in FIGURE 1, and the diameter of the entrance hole, d. At a constant mass flow rate of 2 ml/min, the five test chambers have fixed β values ranging from 2.8 to 300 $(\text{mm-sec})^{-1}$. For comparison, a blunt No. 14 French catheter in a stream having a velocity of 20 cm/sec would have a corresponding β value of 200 $(\text{mm-sec})^{-1}$.

Experimental Methods

As a technique for the study of the effects of hemodynamics, surface chemistry, or blood chemistry on thrombosis, the SPFE requires the careful preparation of test surfaces, a variable rate withdrawal system, and surgical preparation and maintenance of a test animal.

Preparation of Test Surfaces

The primary criteria for any test surface employed in the SPFE is that it can be solvent cast or otherwise coated onto a 25-mm-diameter microscope cover glass, or fabricated into a disc suitable for mounting in the flow chamber. Flexible surfaces must be backed with a cover glass or other rigid material. To minimize the occurrence of nonrepresentative surface inclusions, all surfaces are prepared within a glove box that is pressurized with filtered nitrogen and maintained at a constant humidity and temperature.

For test surfaces such as polyurethanes, which may conveniently be solvent cast, both solvent and solute should be of high purity and dryness. Solutions of about 1-percent concentration have been found to be the easiest to cast, using two coats on each cover glass. Casting solutions are filtered with a fine or ultrafine fritted glass filter to assure a particulate-free solution. Prior to use of a new filter, a large volume of water is forced through it to remove any residual glass particles within the filter. The filter is then rinsed with ethanol and oven dried. All instruments or glassware to be used in the glove box are thoroughly cleaned and dried.

Cover glasses are freed of any adherent glass fragments and cleaned. Prior to placement in the glove box, each cover glass is passed through a pencil flame to remove residual moisture. If, in the process of solvent casting onto the surface, the glass does not wet completely, either the glass is improperly cleaned and should be subsequently discarded or recleaned, or the glass is not wettable by the solvent and a more suitable solvent should be selected.

The casting solution forced through the glass filter is collected in a cleaned and dried test tube or beaker. A large glass slide, also cleaned and dried, is used as a casting plane. Each cover glass is coated with the solution and placed coated side up on a stainless-steel pellet to assure even coverage and to facilitate handling. If the cast film is removable from the cover glass, annealing is required and the annealing temperature is dependent on the softening temperature for that material. After satisfactory coating of the surface, the cover glasses are placed in a stainless-steel annealing chamber that has an inlet and outlet port for the passage of nitrogen within the chamber during annealing. Should the surface being prepared firmly bond to the glass without annealing, it is packaged and labeled for later use in the SPFE. The packaging medium must not damage or otherwise alter the surface coating or structure. On exposure to native blood in the SPFE, should wedge thrombi develop at nonparticulate foci within three minutes of test time, uncoated glass may be showing through and additional coatings are required.

The material preparation discussed above is but one of many conceivable techniques. The specific procedure employed will depend upon the nature of the particular material, and the investigator should employ whatever technique affords the greatest ease and reproducibility. However, all reasonable precautions should be taken to assure (1) clean cover glasses, (2) properly prepared solvents and solutes, (3) inclusion-free surfaces, and (4) uniform surface structure, in order to yield reproducible and meaningful test results.

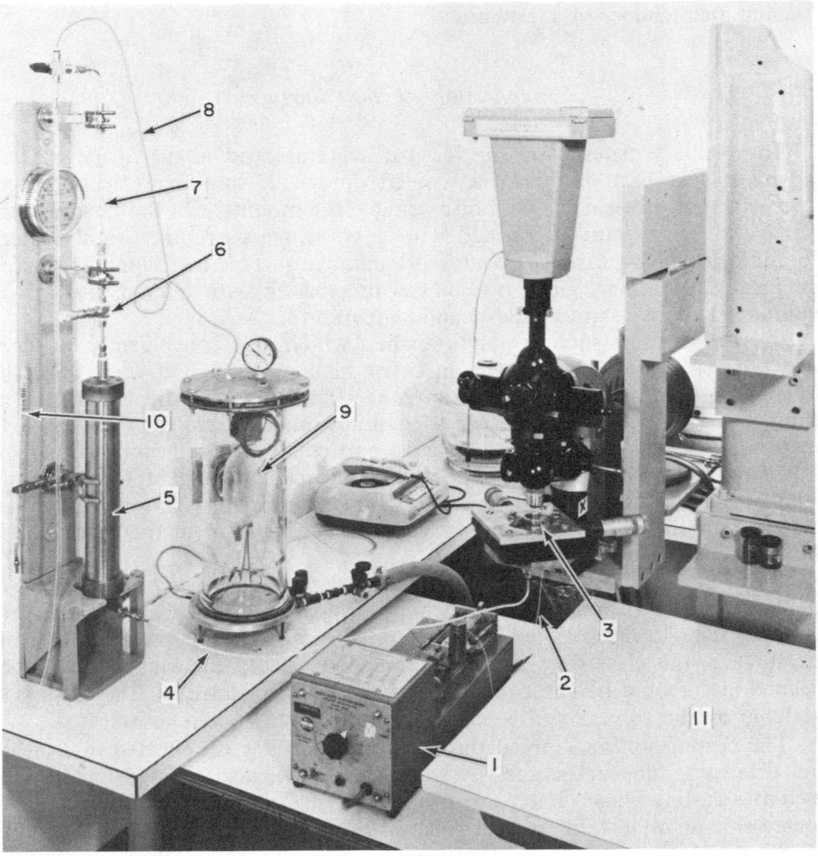

FIGURE 3. Assembled components of SPFE. 1=heparin infusion pump; 2=heparin infusion line; 3=flow chamber mounted on microscope stage; 4=chamber withdrawal line; 5=withdrawal system holding cylinder; 6=micrometer needle valve; 7=flow meter; 8=capillary tubing resistance line; 9=blood bag; 10=calibrating pipette; and 11=table on which animal support (not shown) lies.

Preparation and Setup of Flow System

It is of primary importance to accurately maintain a constant withdrawal rate of blood through each of the flow chambers. This is accomplished by means of the system shown in FIGURE 3. Although simpler withdrawal systems may be devised, this system allows for extremely precise flow control. A standard blood bag is modified so as to provide an evacuation port and an entrance port. A 20-gauge needle is placed at the entrance port, and a length of polyethylene capillary tubing is passed from the needle through the top of the bell jar and attached to another 20-gauge needle on a two-way ball valve on top of the rotometer assembly shown in FIGURE 3. The blood bag is evacuated and the bag withdrawal line is clamped. The bell jar is then evacuated, causing the collapsed blood bag to expand. Flow through the system is monitored by the rotometer. The desired withdrawal rates are achieved by varying either the length of capillary tubing or by adjusting the micrometer needle valve. Prior to an experiment, the withdrawal lines from the flow chamber and the holding cylinder are filled with saline and the flow rate is calibrated by means of a small volume-graduated pipette.

During an experiment, blood flows from the flow chamber through the withdrawal line and displaces the saline in the holding cylinder. The saline from the cylinder flows through the rotometer and capillary tubing and is drawn into the blood bag. In this manner, blood flows only into the holding cylinder and does not "contaminate" the flow-control system.

Since the removal of 30–40 percent of the total blood volume from a dog will begin to induce hypovolemic shock,[12] the total blood volume withdrawn from the animal is monitored. A 25-kg dog, for example, has an approximate blood volume of 2250 ml (90 ml/kg). For this size animal, the total volume withdrawn should be kept below 800 ml. To assure a reasonable margin of safety, the holding cylinder has a 400-ml capacity. At a withdrawal rate of 2 ml/min, this allows for three and one quarter hours of actual bleeding time.

Surgical Preparation and Maintenance of Test Animal

Conditioned or unconditioned dogs weighing 20–30 kg are fasted for 24 hours prior to surgery. For each experiment, the animal is anesthetized by the intravenous injection of sodium pentobarbital (Nembutal 50 mg/ml, Abbott Laboratories) into the radial vein at a dosage of 30 mg/kg. The use of any preanesthetic agent is avoided because of the undesirable additional decline in metabolic rate. If the animal becomes hyperactive while being anesthetized, it is returned to the kennel, and a second fasted animal is prepared.

The neck region of the anesthetized animal is shaved and the animal is intubated. Positive-pressure forced ventilation is used only when there are indications of hypoxia. An electrocautery is used to make a 10–15-cm sagittal incision in the neck. The right common carotid artery is dissected free from the carotid fascial sheath for a distance extending from the thyroid branches to the vicinity of the jugular fossa. Extreme care must be exercised in dissecting the vessel adventitia so as not to damage the vessel wall and induce hemorrhagic lesions. Three 1–0 silk ligatures are placed caudally, stagnant blood within the artery is pushed cranially, and the vessel is clamped. The artery is transected between the two most cranial ligatures. A section of tube gauze, presoaked in Ringer's solution, is pulled over this portion of the artery. The artery is then pulled through the stainless-steel connector and the vessel is carefully cut, everted, and tied over the portion of the connector that fits into the various test chambers. FIGURE 4 shows an artery everted over the chamber connector. Following the establishment of hemostasis, the vessel and connector are led out through the surgical incision, which is then sutured closed to minimize hemoconcentration due to evaporation from the exposed tissue to ambient.

During an experiment, blood flows from the carotid artery in a reversed direction from that of normal. Because of the arterial circle of the head, however, the blood reaching the test surface is arterial in oxygen content and composition. The purpose of this reversed cut is to minimize the pulsatile flow induced by the animals heartbeat and to reduce the fluctuations in arterial pressure due to blood loss during the course of an experiment. Should a pulsatile flow regime be desired, the ligatures are placed at the carotid bifurcation and the thyroid branches are ligated and transected from the artery.

The test animal is placed on a table beneath the microscope stage and covered with a large heating pad and a surgical drape. The animal's rectal temperature is monitored prior to each test, and the incidence of hypothermia is avoided by the use of the external heat source.

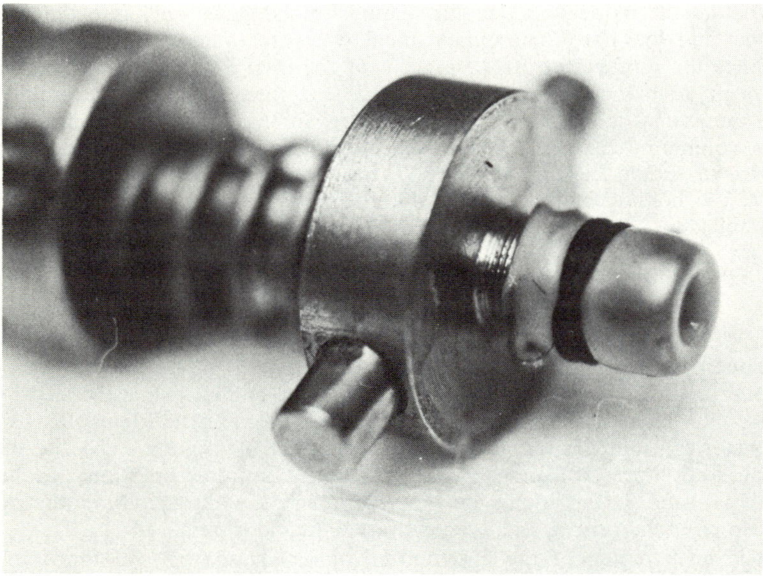

FIGURE 4. Artery everted over vessel connector.

TEST PROCEDURE

Exercising the utmost care to insure the absence of particulate debris that would alter the flow configuration and potentially lead to thrombogenic phenomena, the test surface is assembled into the selected flow chamber.

A typical chamber and its components are shown in FIGURE 5. FIGURE 6 shows the top view of an assembled flow chamber. Blood flows out of the hole in the center of the chamber as discussed earlier. The four supports outside of this region control the distance, h, between the contact side of the test surface and the chamber bottom. A silastic gasket is placed between the test surface and lucite ring. The stage mounting plate is screwed into place over the lucite ring, exerting slight compression on the silastic gasket.

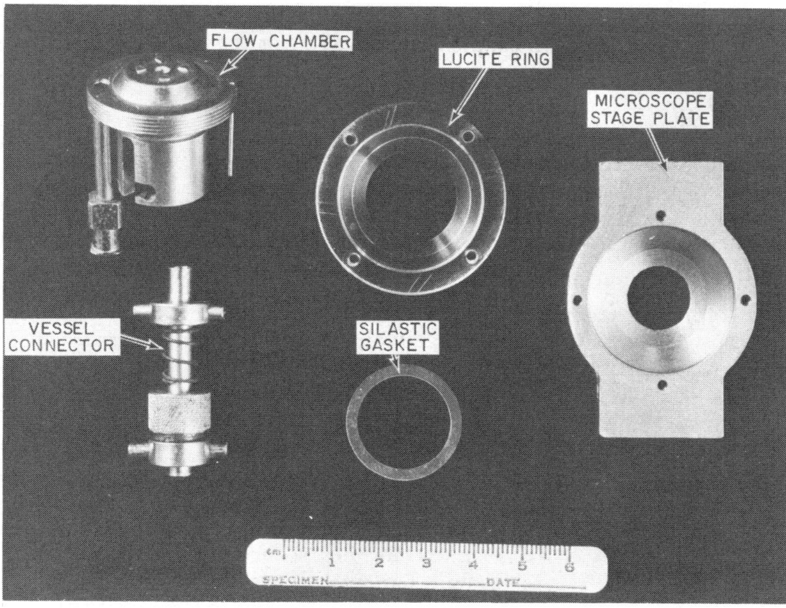

FIGURE 5. Typical flow chamber and its components.

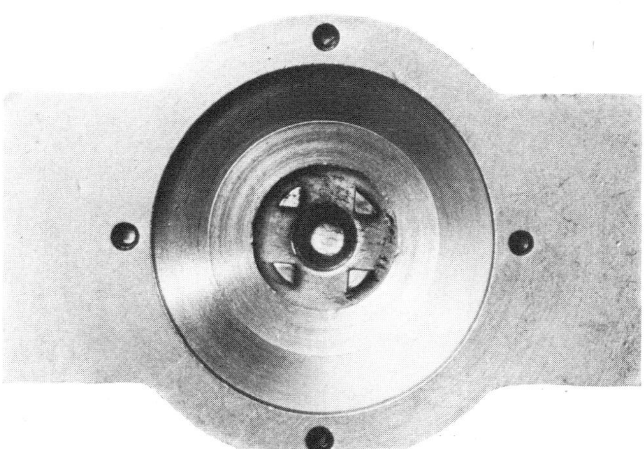

FIGURE 6. Top view of assembled flow chamber.

The chamber is primed with sterile saline to prevent the formation of an air-blood interface and the chamber is checked for leaks. The primed withdrawal line is then connected to the withdrawal port of the chamber. The chamber design also incorporates a port for the infusion of heparinized saline into the chamber trough to prevent coagulation of withdrawn blood within the holding reservoir.

Following assembly and inspection of the flow chamber, the vascular clamp is removed from the artery. Flow is controlled prior to connecting the artery to the chamber by digital pressure on the vessel. Approximately 10–20 ml of blood are allowed to flow from the vessel and discarded. An additional volume of blood is collected before each test for hematologic analysis including Lee-White Clotting Time, hematocrit, erythrocyte, leukocyte and platelet counts, mean corpuscular volume, leukocyte differential, prothrombin time, activated partial thromboplastin time, total protein, plasma hemoglobin, fibrinogen, serum albumin and globulin, total cholesterol, and calcium. Test results are considered valid only for those animals whose hematologic variables fall within the normal ranges of a cumulative data pool.

Following collection of the required blood samples, the vessel connector is joined to the flow chamber, and the withdrawal system is activated by opening the valve shown in FIGURE 3. Immediately following initiation of blood flow, the chamber assembly is mounted on the microscope stage and observation of the stagnation point flow is begun. Throughout the experiment the vessel is kept moist with Ringer's solution to prevent vasoconstriction and subsequent interruption of flow.

For transparent test samples, the stagnation point flow field is observed by dark-field reflected light microscopy with a high-intensity mercury lamp. The microscope is fitted with a triocular head designed for photomicroscopy. Polaroid and 35-mm SLR cameras as well as a 16-mm movie camera are available for photographic documentation of *in situ* test events. Phenomena occurring during the test (such as leukocyte adhesion, inclusion- or noninclusion-induced wedge thrombus formation, platelet aggregation, leukocyte or platelet aggregate embolization, or formation of a symmetric mural thrombus) are recorded chronologically.

Upon conclusion of each test, the vessel is carefully clamped and the connector is removed from the chamber. The chamber is gently flushed with saline to remove the stagnant blood, and disassembled. The test sample is removed from the chamber and either stained with Wright's stain or fixed in a glutaraldehyde solution for SEM examination. The stained samples are mounted on slides and placed in a slide box to avoid contamination until posttest examination is performed. The vessel is rinsed with Ringer's solution and the everted intima is examined for abrasions. If evidence of trauma is found, the damaged section is removed and the vessel is retied around the connector.

Observable Events and Evaluation Criteria

For the SPFE a general sequence of events leading to thrombus formation on a foreign surface has been identified.[4] This sequence of events, illustrated in FIGURE 7, provides several quantifiable parameters for the study of thrombogenesis. When a foreign surface is exposed to blood, proteins rapidly adsorb onto the surface[13,14] and may be denatured. During the first 30 seconds to

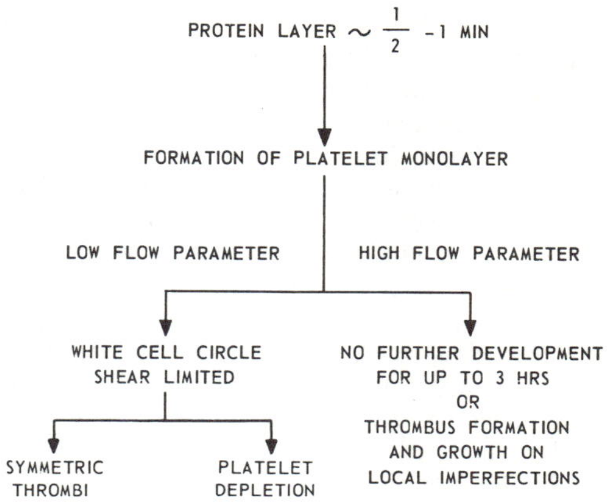

FIGURE 7. Sequence of events that may lead to thrombus formation.

one minute of exposure to blood flow in the SPFE, no formed elements adhere to the surface. The extent to which events proceed and their rate of occurrence are dependent upon blood chemistry, material surface properties, and hemodynamics.

Immediately following protein adsorption and denaturation, platelets begin to adhere to the surface to form a uniform layer. For "normal" blood the rate of adhesion will vary with the flux of platelets to the surface, as well as with the material surface properties. FIGURE 8 is a scanning electron micrograph of platelets adherent to two polyurethane surfaces having slightly different molecular surface structures. Both surfaces were exposed to five minutes of blood flow and clearly illustrate a different platelet surface number density and morphology.

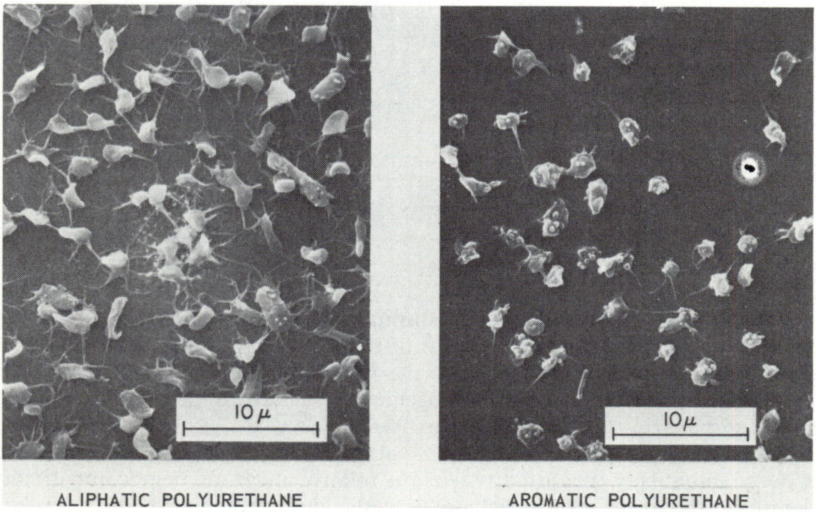

FIGURE 8. Scanning electron micrograph of platelets adherent to two analogous polyether-urethane surfaces.

At high flow rates on relatively nonthrombogenic surfaces, this layer of platelets remains intact, as observed during exposure periods of up to three hours. The only thrombi that form on such surfaces are those originating at surface imperfections, where wedge-shaped thrombi develop. An example of these is shown in FIGURE 9. On surfaces of moderate thromboresistance, or under lower flow conditions, leukocytes adhere to the test surface around the stagnation point. The polymorphonuclear neutrophil has been found to be the predominant leukocyte type within this white cell circle (WCC).

The diameter of this WCC has been shown to be shear-limited and is reflective of the surface forces attracting the leukocytes and the hydrodynamic forces trying to shear them off, the former being dependent on the surface chemical structure. For materials of different surface structure, tested at identical flows, the resultant diameter of a WCC is used as a quantitative measure of their hemocompatibility. FIGURE 10 is a photomicrograph of a small WCC.

Under extremely low flow conditions, or on relatively thrombogenic surfaces, white cells may adhere over the entire surface. Subsequently, large platelet aggregates or thrombi may form in a radially symmetric pattern around the stagnation point.

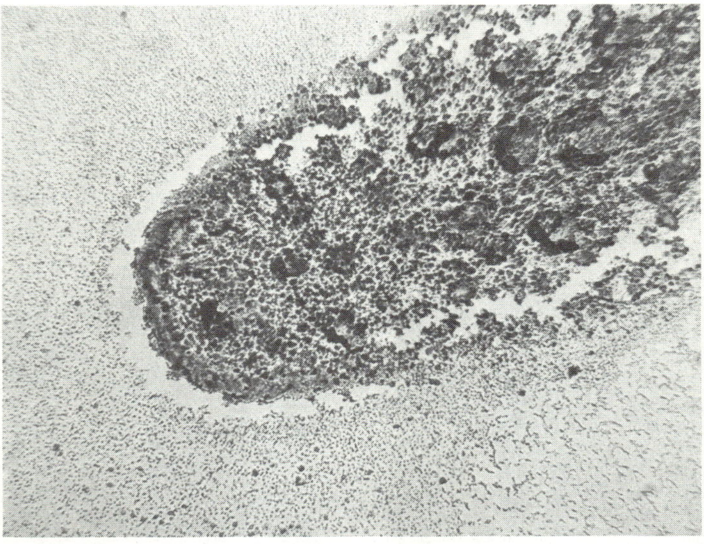

FIGURE 9. Typical wedge-thrombus.

In contrast to the wedge-shaped thrombi that form at localized imperfections, symmetric aggregation is a result of the inherent thrombogenic characteristics of the test surface. The higher the flow conditions at which symmetric aggregation occurs, the more thrombogenic the surface. FIGURE 11 is a micrograph of symmetric platelet aggregation.

As can be seen, this sequence of events provides several parameters which can be quantitatively measured to yield a relative index of hemocompatibility. Specifically, these parameters include: (1) the surface number density of platelets which become adherent to a surface after fixed periods of exposure to blood flow, (2) the diameter of a WCC or the maximum shear at which white cells remain adherent, and (3) the flow conditions below which symmetric platelet aggregation routinely forms.

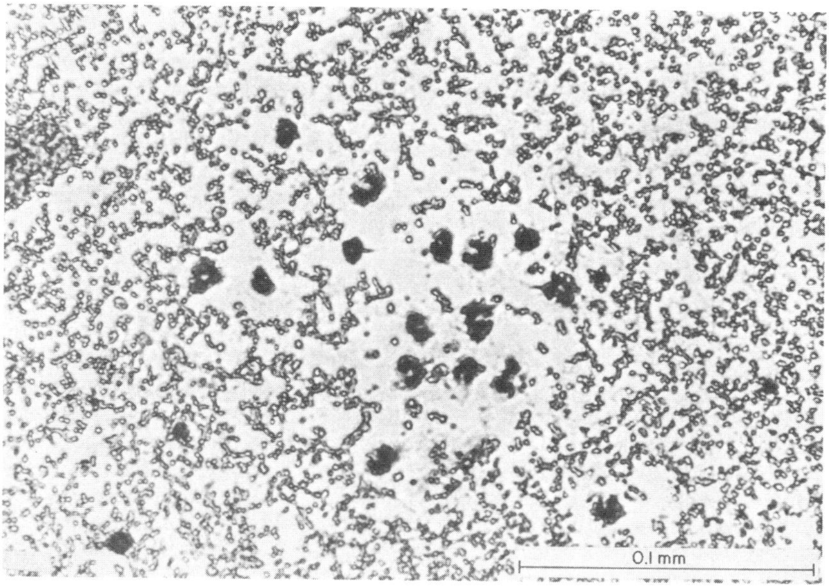

FIGURE 10. Small white cell circle.

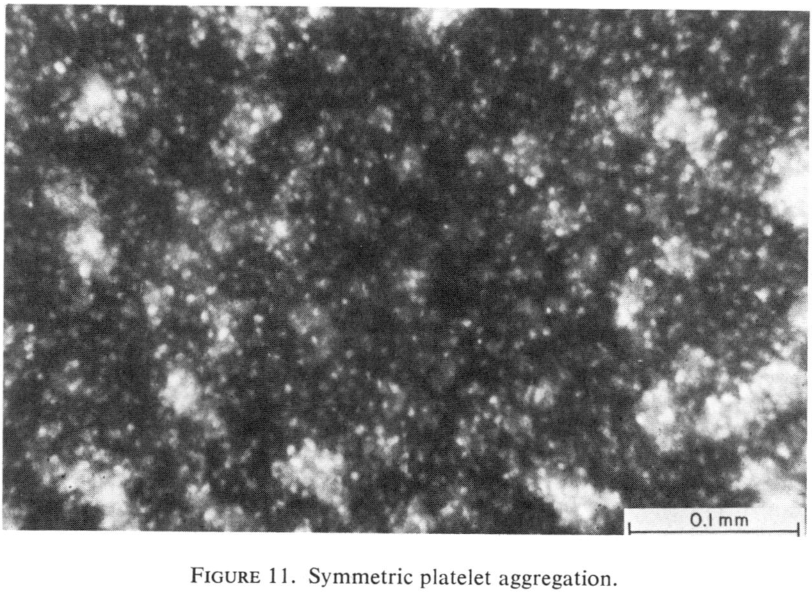

FIGURE 11. Symmetric platelet aggregation.

Applications

Since its development in 1968, the SPFE has been applied to a number of different types of studies, including: (1) effects of surface molecular structure on thromboembolic phenomena; (2) assessment of hemocompatibility of candidate biomaterials; (3) influence of hemodynamics on platelet aggregation, thrombosis, and embolization; and (4) protein/platelet/leukocyte interdependence in thrombogenesis with "normal" and "abnormal" canine blood. A summary of these applications of the SPFE is presented below.

Effects of Surface Molecular Structure

The correlation between surface molecular structure and the degree of thrombogenicity has been studied by exposing three sets of model materials to canine blood under the controlled conditions of SPFE.[6] The model materials included: (1) two analogous polyether-urethanes, (2) three homologous polyamides, and (3) two analogous siliconized glass surfaces. These model surfaces, having well-defined molecular structures, allowed for the introduction of incremental changes in their surface properties without alteration of the basic chemical nature of the surface. Each of the model surfaces was characterized by IRATR spectroscopy and its wettability spectrum.

With use of the criteria described above under Observable Events and Evaluation Criteria, the relative thrombogenicity of each set of model surfaces was evaluated. In terms of these evaluation criteria, quantitative differences were observed between the different types of model surfaces as well as between members of the same class. Figure 8 illustrates the difference in the surface number density of platelets which remained adherent to the two analogous polyether-urethane surfaces after five minutes of exposure under identical hemodynamic conditions.

Hemocompatibility Evaluation of Biomaterials

The SPFE requires that test specimens be ~25 mm in diameter for mounting in the various flow chambers and either solvent cast onto glass or fabricated into a disc. Transparent, translucent, and opaque materials may be tested in the SPFE with the only limitation that for the latter two, *in situ* phenomena are not observable. For materials of this nature, test protocols involve fixed-period exposure and subsequent staining or fixing for examination by light or scanning electron microscopy, respectively.

Although tests of up to three hours duration have been performed on a surface, it has been established throughout the application of the SPFE that tests of thirty minutes to one hour duration are usually sufficient to assess hemocompatibility of a given material. The SPFE has been used to evaluate the hemocompatibility of candidate biomaterials following an experimental protocol which results in a quantitative comparison between different materials.[9]

To assure the validity of each experiment a "control surface" of polymethylmethacrylate (PMMA) is tested at the beginning and end of each flow experiment. Using an intermediate flow chamber the PMMA control will induce a consistent, shear-limited, white cell circle for "normal" blood. Should symmetric aggregation occur on this control surface, the validity of other tests using that animal must be carefully assessed.

Hemodynamics

Several investigations have been performed to study the influence of blood flow on thrombosis. In one such study, a polyurethane surface was exposed to blood flow in each of the five different flow chambers.[4] A flow-dependent sequence of events that may lead to thrombus formation was identified and is illustrated in FIGURE 7. At low-flow parameters, gross symmetric platelet aggregation was observed, while at higher flows only a platelet layer or a shear-limited white cell circle formed on the test surface. Wedge-shaped thrombi were also observed to form at local surface imperfections even at relatively high flow conditions.

The formation of wedge-shaped thrombi provides a useful mechanism for the study of the kinetics of thrombus formation. The shape, size, and growth rate of these thrombi can be continuously monitored by cinematographic techniques. Considering the rate at which proteins can diffuse to and be convected

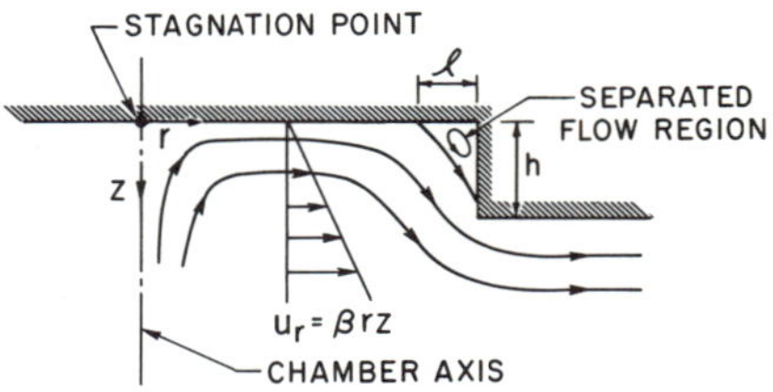

FIGURE 12. Streamlines of flow over step in stagnation-point flow.

from the thrombus, as well as the rate at which new platelets diffuse from the flowing blood to the surface, a model for thrombus growth was proposed.[3] This model suggests that the growth rate of a thrombus is primarily limited by the diffusion rate of platelets from the flowing blood, whereas the shape is controlled by the diffusion and convection of activated protein from the thrombus.

The SPFE can also be used to study other flow geometries.[5, 7] For example, by modifying the shape of the test surface to include a forward-facing step, as shown in FIGURE 12, it was possible to produce a region of separated flow. The step shown in FIGURE 12 was fabricated by bonding two cover glasses together, one having a 2-mm-diameter hole ultrasonically drilled through it. The bonded cover glasses were then coated with polyurethane. In all experiments performed with this flow configuration, symmetric platelet aggregation was observed immediately distal to the step. With the same polyurethane surface without a step, symmetric aggregation was observed only at the lowest flow condition.

Within the separated flow region, freely floating platelet aggregates were observed to form and grow. Under certain flow conditions, aggregates 30–45 microns in diameter would embolize from the separated flow region. The embolization phenomena may be similar to those occurring in extracorporeal circulatory devices.[15, 16]

Protein and Cellular Interaction

The microscopic *in situ* observability of stagnation point flow phenomena facilitates the investigation of thrombosis. The protein adsorption and platelet and polymorphonuclear neutrophil adhesion on any test surface appear to be transitive. The interrelationship of these components in "normal" or "abnormal" (clotting factor-deficient) blood can be studied by the SPFE. Pharmacological agents such as aspirin or dextran, known to affect the platelet-release reaction or platelet adhesiveness, respectively, may be used to study the platelet-PMN or protein-platelet interaction. The use of isotopically labeled fibrinogen or platelets could enhance the understanding of protein adsorption and platelet adhesion rates.

Summary

The intention of this article has been to explain the use of the SPFE as a technique to further the knowledge of the preventative and causative aspects of hemodynamics, surface chemistry, and blood chemistry on thrombosis. The experiment allows for several tests to be performed with one test animal and has applications to many areas of research.

Acknowledgments

The Stagnation Point Flow Experiment was developed by Dr. Harry Petschek, whose continued contributions and guidance are gratefully acknowledged.

References

1. Virchow, R. 1856. Gessammelte Abhandlungen zur Wissenschaftlichen Medzin. Meidinger. Frankfurt, Germany.
2. Petschek, H. E., D. Adamis & A. R. Kantrowitz. 1968. Stagnation flow thrombus formation. Trans. Am. Soc. Artif. Int. Organs **14:** 256–259.
3. Monsler, M., W. A. Morton & R. Weiss. 1970. The fluid mechanics of thrombus formation. AIAA paper 70–787. AIAA 3rd Fluid and Plasma Dyn. Conf. Los Angeles, Calif.
4. Madras, P. N., W. A. Morton & H. E. Petschek. 1971. The dynamics of thrombus formation. Fed. Proc. **30:** 1665–1676.
5. Morton, W. A. & H. E. Petschek. 1972. Hemodynamics of thrombus formation on foreign surfaces. *In* Proc. Symp. Blood Damage in Extracorporeal Circulation. II: Idealized Experiments. Am. Inst. Chem. Eng. 72nd Nat. Mtg. St. Louis, Mo., May 21–24.
6. Nyilas, E., W. A. Morton, D. M. Lederman, T-H. Chiu & R. D. Cumming. 1975. Interdependence of hemodynamic and surface parameters in thrombosis. Trans. Am. Soc. Artif. Int. Organs **21:** 55–69.
7. Morton, W. A., E. M. Parmentier & H. E. Petschek. 1975. Study of aggregate formation in region of separated blood flow. Thromb. Diath. Haemorrh. **34**(3)**:** 840–854.
8. Nyilas, E., W. A. Morton, R. D. Cumming, D. M. Lederman, T-H. Chiu & R. E. Baier. 1977. Effects of polymer surface molecular structure and force-

field characteristics on blood interfacial phenomena. I. Accepted for publication in J. Biomed. Mater. Res. **8**.

9. Lederman, D. M., W. A. Morton, T-H. Chiu & E. Nyilas. 1975. Improved test procedures for the hemocompatibility evaluation of biomaterials. PB 245874. National Technical Information Service. Springfield, Va.
10. Milne-Thomson, L. M. 1960. Theoretical Hydrodynamics. MacMillan. New York, N.Y.
11. Schlichting, H. 1960. Boundary Layer Theory. McGraw-Hill. New York, N.Y.
12. Schalm, O. W., N. C. Jain & E. J. Carroll. 1975. Veterinary Hematology. 3rd edit. Lea & Febiger. Philadelphia, Pa.
13. Dutton, R. C., A. J. Webber, S. A. Johnson & R. E. Baier. 1969. Microstructure of initial thrombus formation on foreign materials. J. Biomed. Mater. Res. **3**(1): 13–23.
14. Lyman, D., J. L. Brash & K. G. Klein. 1969. The effect of chemical structure and surface properties of synthetic polymers on the coagulation of blood. *In* Artificial Heart Program Conference Proceedings. Chap. **11:** 113–121.
15. Hill, J. D., M. J. Aguilor, A. Baranco, P. Delanerolle & F. Gerbode. 1969. Neuropathological manifestations of cardiac surgery. Ann. Thorac. Surg. **7:** 409–419.
16. Patterson, R. H., Jr. & J. B. Twichell. 1971. Disposable filter for microemboli use in cardiopulmonary bypass and massive transfusion. JAMA **215:** 76–80.

AN *EX VIVO* METHOD FOR THE EVALUATION OF BIOMATERIALS IN CONTACT WITH BLOOD *

Jerome S. Schultz,† Joe D. Goddard,† Arthur Ciarkowski,†
John A. Penner,‡ and S. Martin Lindenauer §

† *Department of Chemical Engineering*
‡ *Department of Internal Medicine*
§ *Department of Surgery*
University of Michigan
Ann Arbor, Michigan 48104

The use of extracoporeal (*ex vivo*) shunts for studying thrombus formation was given impetus by a number of studies from J. F. Mustard's laboratory.[1, 2] In these studies the essential problems of this method were recognized and the requirements for a reproducible system were delineated. The basic features are: 1) uniform blood flow, 2) a chamber that represents preferential region for thrombus formation, and 3) access to the thrombus for analysis. Murphy *et al.*[1] tried a number of flow chamber designs and finally settled on the use of a model bifurcation for their studies,[2] and other investigators [3, 4] have evaluated alternative flow chamber configurations. This type of *ex vivo* test with recirculation of blood should be distinguished from other *ex vivo* procedures in which animals are bled through a test chamber.[5, 6] In the latter cases chronic shunts are not used, which simplifies the procedure, but the loss of blood usually limits the duration of the experiment to less than one hour.

To develop an *ex vivo* method for the evaluation of the thrombogenicity of materials in contact with blood, a system was devised that exposes a test chamber to a dog's systemic circulation by means of a chronic arteriovenous shunt. The general aspects of this approach are shown in the flow diagram in FIGURE 1 and the schematic FIGURE 2.

Male dogs were selected after screening to ensure that they were normal with respect to weight and blood coagulation values. An arteriovenous shunt was implanted in accepted animals, and after surgery, coagulation factors and other physiological parameters were evaluated periodically to monitor the approach of the dog's coagulation system toward steady state. After about one week, labeled fibrinogen and platelets were introduced systemically, and after 24–48 hours the chamber containing the test material was introduced into the bypass system. The rate of thrombus formation was determined by monitoring the buildup of radioactive fibrinogen and platelets in the test chamber. Blood flow through the chamber was measured with an electromagnetic or Doppler flow meter and controlled at a constant value.

After a predetermined time the chamber was disconnected from the shunt, and any thrombus formed was removed and quantitated in terms of clot weight, moisture, fibrinogen, red cell, and platelet content. These values are used as indices of thrombus formation on a given biomaterial under defined flow conditions.

* Supported in part by the National Heart and Lung Institute, Contract No. 1–HB–4–2962, and a Research Career Development Award (to J. S. Schultz) from NIGMS no. 1KO46MO8271.

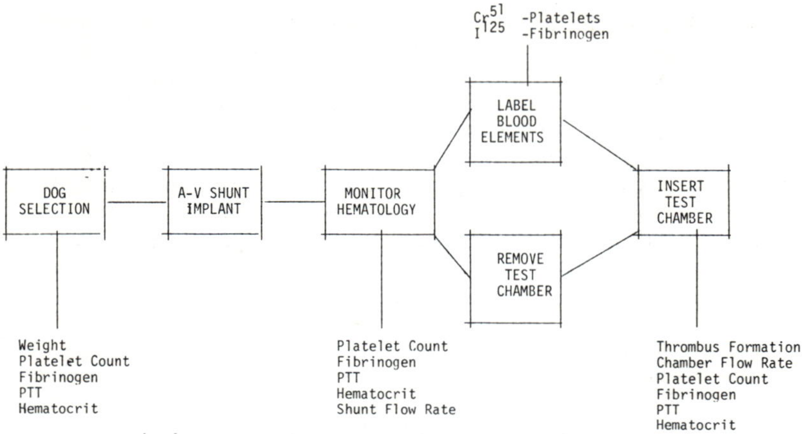

FIGURE 1. Schematic stages in biomaterials testing.

During exposure of the biomaterial to blood in the test chamber and subsequent to its removal, blood samples were taken and examined for possible systemic effects, as indicated by variations in hematocrit, fibrinogen, platelets, and other coagulation indices. The recovery of the animal from exposure to the test material was evaluated, and after a sufficient period of time, usually one week, the animal was used again in a similar study.

Ex vivo SHUNT

Chronic intermittent access to the vascular system is difficult to maintain because of several problems. Use of the venous circulation exclusively is un-

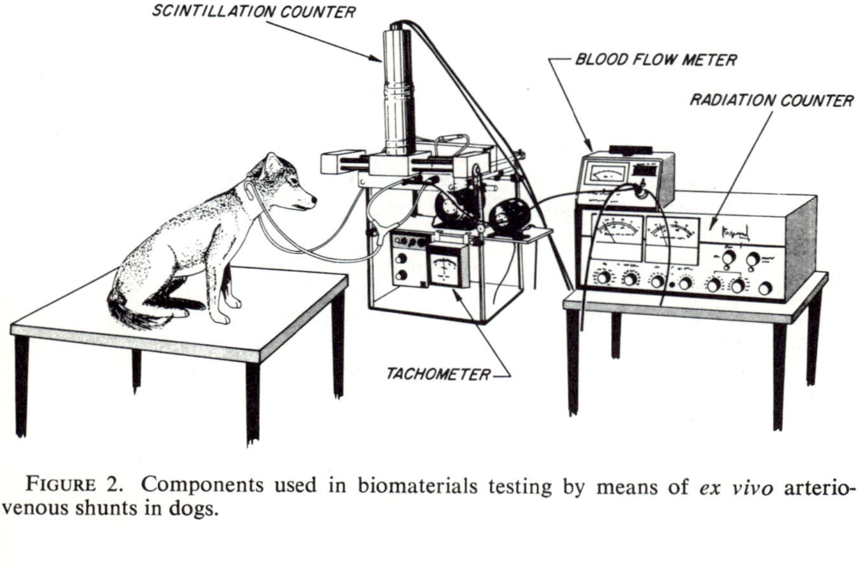

FIGURE 2. Components used in biomaterials testing by means of *ex vivo* arteriovenous shunts in dogs.

satisfactory because the venous flow rates are too low to prevent thrombosis. Although increased flow may be achieved in an exclusively intraarterial shunt, similar problems of thrombus formation are encountered. But in the case of an arteriovenous shunt, the capillary bed is bypassed and the blood is returned to the venous circulation with essentially no peripheral resistance, so that the volumetric blood flow is very large and may equal or exceed the normal total cardiac output. Although flow rates of such magnitude seem to inhibit thrombus formation in the access device, it is nevertheless essential that the shunt surface have compatibility with blood. One such material that is compatible and highly effective in maintaining shunt patency is Silastic † tubing, coated internally with a heparin complex.‡

In these experiments for the testing of biomaterials and study of the dynamics of thrombogenesis, the *ex vivo* arteriovenous shunt is surgically implanted in the neck, and when in place bridges the carotid artery and internal jugular vein. Two pieces of Silastic tubing (I.D. 3⁄16 inches and about 10 inches long) are sutured to the respective vessels, and their *ex vivo* ends tunneled through the neck subcutaneously and dorsally so as to emerge 1.5 or 2 cm dorsal to the vessel-tubing anatomosis. Thus the carotid branch meets the jugular branch on the dorsal aspect of the dog's neck, a few centimeters caudal to the ears; here they are joined to form the shunt by a Teflon® stent (3⁄16 inches I.D., ¼ inches O.D., 1.25 inches long). Between experiments the *ex vivo* portion of the shunt is wrapped in soft gauze for protection.

In order to obviate the problem of proliferation of intima at the junction of the vessel and the tubing, a process which gradually narrows the lumen and restricts flow, a porous prosthetic material is bonded to the end of the Silastic tubing, as illustrated in FIGURE 3. The material, Dacron® velour, constitutes about a 2-cm extension on the end of the Silastic tube, and the jugular vein anastomosis joins to this porous material. The arrangement for the artery is similar, except that because of the disparity between the smaller diameter of the carotid and the Silastic, it is necessary to interpose between the artery and the Dacron a 1.5-cm segment of autogenous jugular vein. Closure of the anastomoses is done with 5–0 cardiovascular suture in continuous fashion. Although standard surgical techniques are employed, extraordinary care must be exercised: in securing vessel-to-tubing junctions; in the stereoscopic placement of the shunt to avoid kinking with the movements of the head and neck in the recovered animal; and in adherence to scrupulous sterile technique to minimize risk of infection.

Emerging from the subcutaneous tunnel, the prosthesis crosses the cutaneous epithelial surface and can become a conduit for infection through the break in the skin. To combat this possibility, a sleeve of polyester felt (⅛ inch thick) is bonded around the Silastic, starting from the Dacron velour and extending about 10 cm, so that in the final placement, two or three centimeters of the felt-sleeved Silastic tube protrude beyond the skin surface. In the healing process, the soft tissue becomes densely adherent to the polyester, with excellent incorporation; a reliable seal is formed between the soft tissues and the shunt, effectively preventing ingress of bacteria from the skin surface.

The incisions are closed with subcuticular absorbable suture following closure of the muscle and fascia over the vascular anastomoses. For prophy-

† Dow Corning Medical Grade Silastic Tubing.
‡ Battelle Laboratories, TDMAC Process.

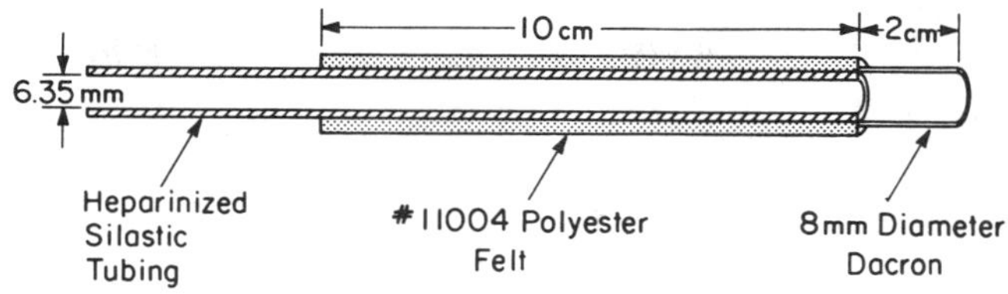

FIGURE 3a. Construction details of the arteriovenous shunt prosthesis; two are used in a complete shunt. Blood vessels are anatomosed to the Dacron velour.

laxis, kanomycin is administered for several days both intramuscularly and as an irrigant in the wound. No adverse cardiovascular effects were noted due to the shunt for periods of up to two months. Occasional shunt failures were attributed to kinking and/or infection. Usually, however, the dogs recovered with wounds healed sufficiently to permit postoperative testing within one week. Repeated access to the circulatory system for materials testing was easily accomplished, and volume flow rates in the range of 500–1000 ml/min were regularly obtained.

Dogs selected for these studies were preconditioned males of an average weight of 30.4 ± 6.4 kg. The hematological profile was as follows: platelets $309 \pm 95 \times 10^3$ (per mm^3), fibrinogen 276 ± 101 (mg/100 ml), hematocrit $44 \pm 4.4\%$, PTT 25.7 ± 7.3 (sec). The platelet and fibrinogen levels were depressed somewhat (about 30%) after surgical implantation of the shunt, but the levels returned to normal after a one-week recovery period.

Platelet survival studies with a modified Frasher preparation[7] indicated a much faster turnover rate than in normal animals; compare the solid line in FIGURE 4 with the normal values shown as the dashed line. It should be noted

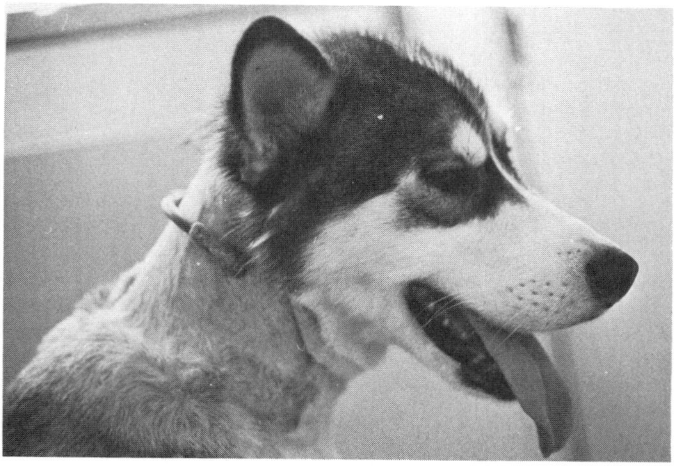

FIGURE 3b. Arteriovenous shunt in place between carotid artery and jugular vein.

that in these experiments the test chamber was inserted in the neck shunt for about three hours on the first day, and may have accounted for some of the acceleration in platelet turnover. However, the general pattern in FIGURE 4 of selective platelet consumption along with normal fibrinogen turnover is typical of Silastic arteriovenous cannulae as described by Harker.[8]

TEST CHAMBER DESIGN

In designing the test chamber several factors were given primary consideration.

1. A well-defined flow pattern was desired to allow for future analysis of the effects of flow on various rate phenomena, such as shear rate and diffusion rates.

2. Accessibility of the thrombogenic surface to measuring techniques was desired, along with the possibility of using a variety of methods, particularly radioisotopic methods, for evaluating the rate of thrombus formation.

3. Since there are a number of schools of thought as to which of these factors play the most significant role in the development of thrombi,[9, 10] a configuration that allows the separation of the effects of shear and convective mass transport is desirable. The separation or independent variation of these parameters allows the determination of the more important causative factors in thrombus development.

Based on these criteria a test chamber of the couette type was selected for the evaluation of materials in contact with blood. There is much background information available on couette-type flow geometries, and, in addition, some recent studies on platelet diffusion and platelet adsorption to surfaces have been carried out using this general configuration.[11, 12]

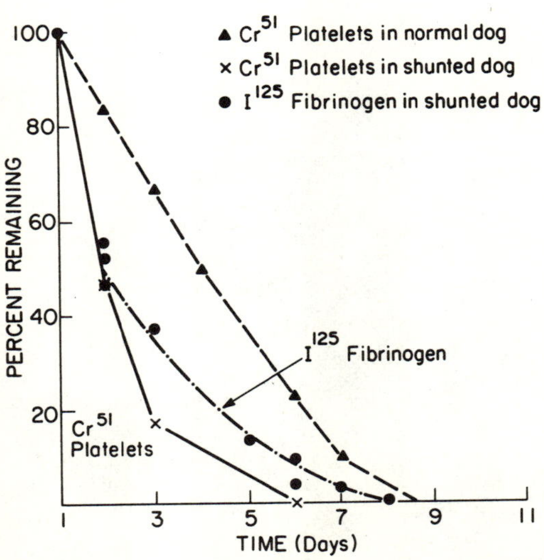

FIGURE 4. Turnover rates of labeled fibrinogen in shunted and labeled platelets in shunted and control dogs.

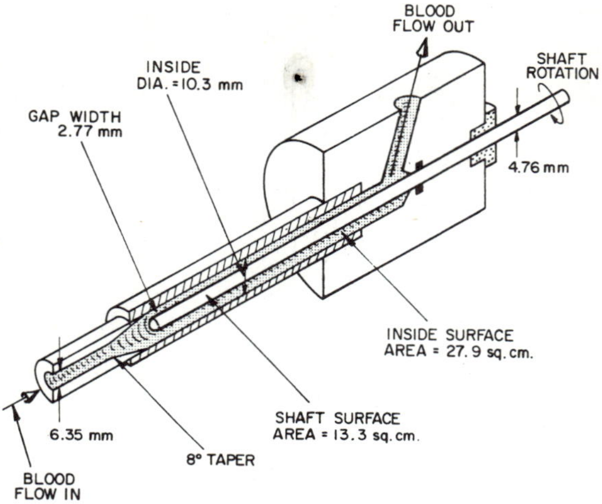

FIGURE 5. Biomaterials test prosthesis used in *ex vivo* arteriovenous shunt in dogs.

FIGURE 5 shows the configuration of the current prototype test chamber. Blood enters the chamber from the left through an expansion section and then flows down the chamber in a somewhat helical pattern to the exit port at the right, which comes off at approximately a 45° angle. The test material can be coated onto the surface of the central shaft (usually 303 stainless steel) and also onto the interior surface of the cylindrical shell.

Most of the *ex vivo* work was done with a chamber having a central shaft of 3/16 in diameter and an outer cylinder of 13/32 in internal diameter. The length of the chamber is approximately 4 inches. The inlet and exit ports are approximately 1/4 in I.D. The chamber presents an expansion in cross section from the inlet to the central region, and the effective (hydraulic) Reynolds number within the chamber is less than the Reynolds number in the inlet and exit tubes by a factor of about 1/2.§ Based on the rule of thumb that thrombi develop in "low-flow" regions, the chamber constitutes a preferential site for thrombus development relative to the connecting inlet and outlet tubes.

The principal fully developed flow regimes associated with this device are:

A. laminar-helical
B. laminar-cellular or Taylor-vortex
C. turbulent

At low axial flow rates and at low shaft rotation speeds of the shaft, the flow through the chamber is helical in pattern. The idealized fully developed helical flow pattern for constant flow in this device is shown in FIGURE 6(A). Under these circumstances, the flow in the axial direction and the tangential

§ $\dfrac{\text{Re (chamber)}}{\text{Re (entry tube)}} = \dfrac{R_T}{R_1 + R_2}$

R_T=radius of tube, R_1= radius of shaft, R_2=radius of cylinder.

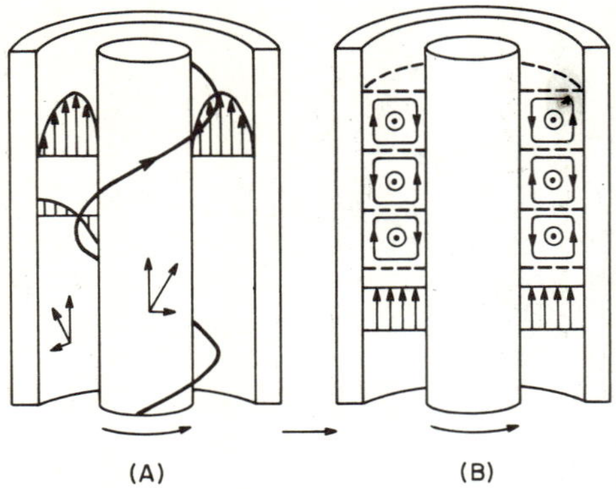

FIGURE 6. Flow regimes in couette biomaterial test chamber.

(or angular) flow in the circumferential direction are independent of each other (for Newtonian fluids), and the net flow is the vector sum of these two independent flow patterns. Shown in the figure is the axial parabolic flow pattern that exists between the central shaft and the coaxial cylinder. Above a critical shaft rotational speed the flow pattern changes to that shown in FIGURE 6 (B). But all biomaterial evaluations were made below this critical speed, i.e., in the laminar-helical regime.

The flow in the chamber is actually pulsatile in nature (see FIGURE 17 and below), but this pertubation does not drastically alter the transport behavior in the test chamber.

METHODS

Labeled Blood Elements

Measurements of the rate of thrombus development involved the use of radioisotope-labeled fibrinogen and platelets. Previous works by Olson *et al.*[13, 14] demonstrated the use of labeled blood elements for the determination of the amount and composition of a thrombus. It was shown that by labeling platelets with chromium-51, and fibrinogen with iodine-125, and by monitoring these simultaneously, the relative amounts of these blood elements in a thrombus is obtained.

Autologous platelets were labeled as follows.[15] One day prior to an experiment, blood (500 ml) was withdrawn from the animal; the platelets were separated, washed, labeled with ^{51}Cr and, along with the erythrocytes, were reinfused. The peak platelet radioactivity after infusion ranged from 100 to 1000 cpm/ml of whole blood.

Also, on the day prior to an experiment ^{125}I-labeled human fibrinogen ¶ was injected. The peak level of radioactivity in whole blood after infusion was about 10×10^3 cpm/ml.

A dual channel counter was placed over the test chambers to monitor the

¶ Amersham-Searle.

total amount of radioactivity (FIGURE 7). It can be seen in FIGURE 8 that ^{51}Cr gives some low-energy emission which interferes with the iodine counts; however, an energy window can be selected that minimizes interference in the ^{51}Cr channel from ^{125}I. There is a simple formula for the correction of spillover of ^{51}Cr into the ^{125}I channel.

The field of view detected by the sodium iodide crystal is shown in FIGURE 9. The crystal diameter is approximately 33 mm. A 1-mm "point" source of ^{51}Cr was placed at different lateral distances from the center of the crystal and

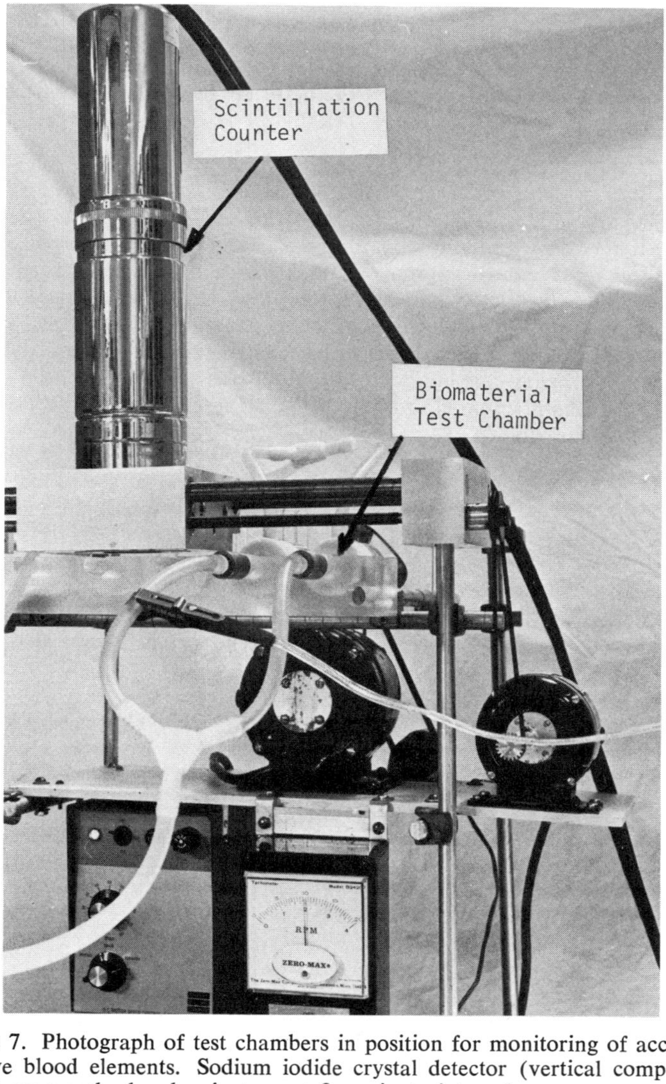

FIGURE 7. Photograph of test chambers in position for monitoring of accumulated radioactive blood elements. Sodium iodide crystal detector (vertical component) is translated over each chamber in turn at five-minute intervals.

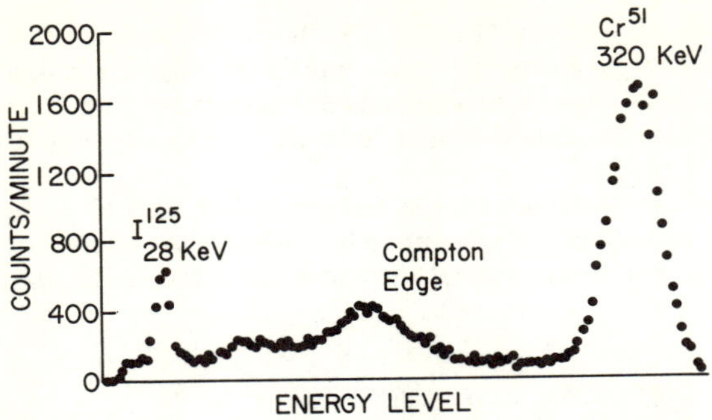

FIGURE 8. Energy spectrum of gamma-emitting isotopes used for labeling blood elements. Platelets were labeled with ^{51}Cr and fibrinogen was labeled with ^{125}I.

on two planes at different vertical heights from the crystal. The 4-mm height represents the closest approach of the test chamber to the crystal, and the 10-mm height represents the approximate distance of the shaft to the crystal. At the distance of the shaft from the crystal, 10 mm, the apparent field of view of the counter is approximately 25–30 mm to each side of center. This means that an approximate length of 60 mm of the shaft in the test chamber is counted at any time. Also, since the center to center distance of the adjacent chambers in our multiple chamber apparatus is 40 mm, there is very little interference from adjacent chambers.

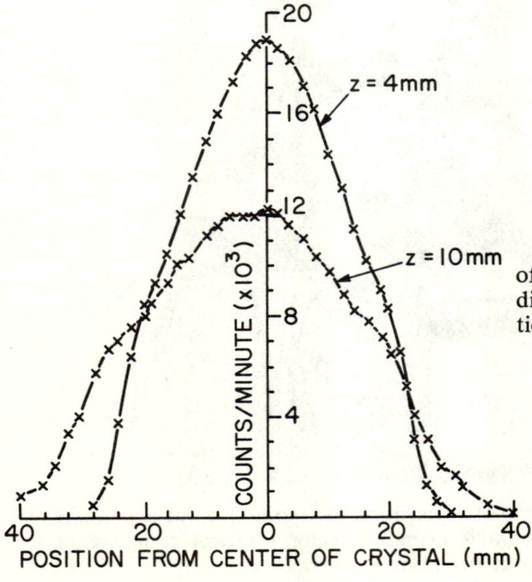

FIGURE 9. Calibration of sensitivity of NaI crystal to point sources of radioactivity placed in different positions.

Test Procedure

Chambers were assembled with new shafts and cylinders for each biomaterial test and connected into the A-V neck shunt by means of ¼ in I.D. Silastic tubing. The tubing and the chamber assembly were filled with saline and then attached to the clamped shunt; after making sure that there were no trapped air bubbles, the clamps were released to allow the blood to flow. Anticoagulants were not used except as noted below. The deposition of platelets and fibrinogen within the chamber was monitored at five-minute intervals with a dual-channel scintillation counter.

Blood flow rate through the chamber was controlled at 200 ml/min, and the shaft rotation speed was maintained at 200 rpm. Under these conditions the flow in the chamber is within a laminar flow regime.

Experiments were carried out for periods of one hour. After completion of each experiment, the chamber was flushed with saline; from the total monitored radioactivity, the individual contributions of shaft and wall deposits were determined. The thrombi were then removed from the shaft, blotted, and weighed. In many instances the thrombi were removed in four equal sections to determine the distribution of the deposit along the length of the shaft. Then the individual pieces were placed in counting vials and the total ^{51}Cr and ^{125}I isotope content determined with a well counter.

The fact that the shaft in this test-chamber configuration seems to be more thrombogenic than the shell is fortunate but cannot be explained by conventional notions as to the effect of flow and velocity profiles on rates of thrombus formation. Whatever the cause, the fact that the shaft represents a more thrombogenic environment than the cylinder wall ensures that the results will not be complicated by large amounts of thrombus formation on the shell. Therefore, it is expected that thrombogenicity comparisons of materials can be made by using shafts coated with different materials, whereas a single type of surface coating is used on the inner wall of the cylinder.

Results

Rate of Thrombus Formation

Typical accumulation patterns of platelets and fibrinogen within the test chamber are shown in Figure 10. Generally, the increase in either isotope was linear with time over the standard one-hour test period. The initial radioactivity values were related to the "background" volume of blood within the chamber. The radioactivity monitored over a control section of the return tubing remained at the same level during the course of an experiment, suggesting no major consumption of platelets or fibrinogen. However, samples taken for hematology showed about a 25% loss in platelets and fibrinogen. The appearance of a typical thrombus formed on the shaft is shown in Figure 11.

To evaluate the systemic effects of labeling platelets and of subsequent material tests, blood samples were taken before labeling, one hour after reinfusing platelets, before a material test (usually the next morning), and after each test period of about 90 minutes duration. A follow-up sample was taken on the next day to determine the extent of recovery.

The results of ten experiments are shown in Figure 12. The largest effect

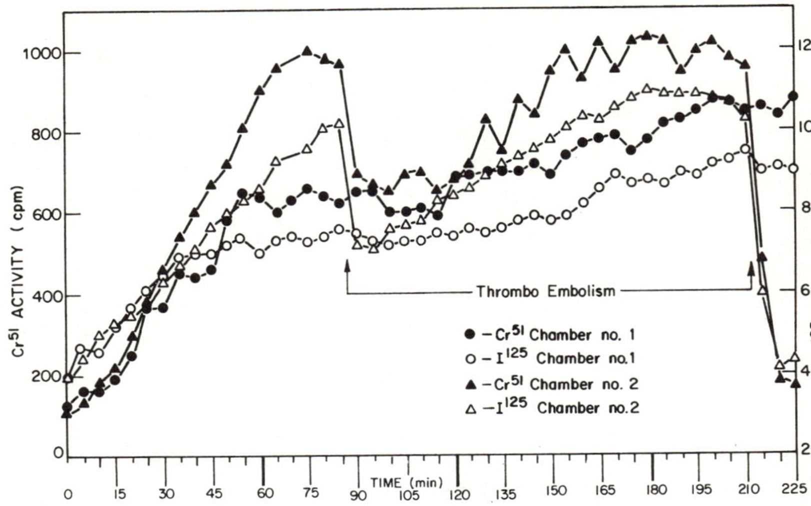

FIGURE 10. Accumulation patterns of radioactivity-labeled platelets (^{51}Cr) and fibrinogen (^{125}I) in biomaterial test chambers. Simultaneous reductions in platelet and fibrinogen radioactivity in chamber 2 are indications of thromoembolism.

of the test procedure was on platelet count, which dropped about 40% during three hours of testing. There was some indication that the platelet count is stabilized after this period and that it shows substantial recovery by the next day. On the other hand, fibrinogen levels were only mildly affected by the test apparatus, and the recovery was somewhat slower. An almost parallel pattern was found by counting the ^{51}Cr and ^{125}I content of whole-blood samples during the same periods, as shown in TABLE 1. This correlation provides further evidence that the labeled platelets and fibrinogen are reflecting the behavior of the total population.

PTT values showed some increase, indicating some depletion of clotting factors during the test period, but a full recovery of PTT by the next day was observed. These changes in the coagulation system may explain, to some extent, the observation that the amount of thrombus formed decreased with sequential tests. It should be recalled, however, that for the different animals used in these

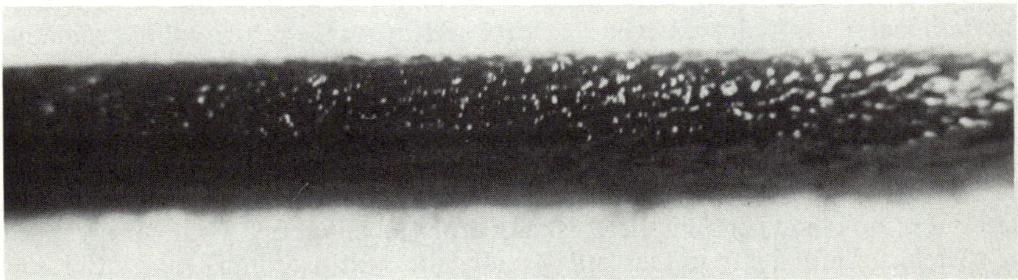

FIGURE 11. Close-up photograph of a typical thrombus formed on a stainless-steel rod.

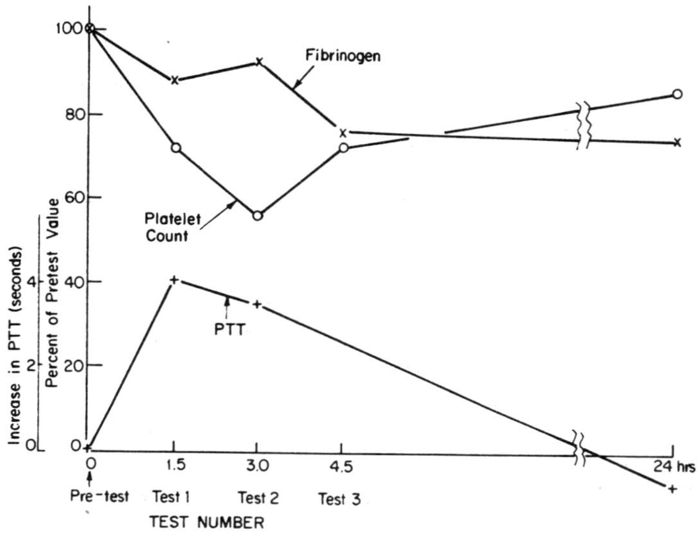

FIGURE 12. Systemic hemotology patterns in the dog during and after several sequential biomaterial testing procedures on the same day.

studies, the platelet count and fibrinogen levels varied by as much as 50% from animal to animal. And, although these variations influenced thrombus formation, the magnitude of the effect was less than that of sequential tests on the same animal.

Thrombus Composition

The average platelet and fibrinogen content of the thrombi formed on stainless steel shafts in the *ex vivo* test chamber are given in TABLE 2. These results, which are averages of 20 runs, are compared with some other published

TABLE 1

COMPARISON OF CLINICAL AND RADIOISOTOPE METHODS FOR PLATELET AND FIBRINOGEN CONTENT OF BLOOD DURING BIOMATERIALS TEST PROCEDURE

	Pretest	Run 1	Run 2	Run 3	24 hr
Method			Platelets		
Microscopic Counting	100%	72%	57%	72%	86%
^{51}Cr Count	100%	86%	72%	73%	
			Fibrinogen		
Fibrometer	100%	89%	93%	76%	75%
^{125}I Count	100%	95%	86%	90%	

TABLE 2

THROMBUS FORMATION AND COMPOSITION ON STAINLESS STEEL SURFACES IN FLOWING BLOOD

	Thrombus Radioactivity		Whole Blood Radioactivity		Thrombus		Enrichment Ratio (γ)	
	Platelets ^{51}Cr cpm	Fibrin ^{125}I cpm	Platelets ^{51}Cr cpm ml	Fibrinogen ^{125}I cpm ml	Wet weight (gm)	Thickness (nm)	Platelets †	Fibrin ‡
Stainless steel shaft	3953	85,127	146 *	9590 *	0.49	0.32	112	14.3
Stainless stel tube in artery [13]	—	—	—	—	0.21	0.99	68	2.0
Stainless steel tube in vein [13]	—	—	—	—	0.27	1.08	28	2.0
Quartz tube in vein [16]	3.06×10^4	—	1688	—	0.31	0.65	51	—

* Range platelet count $1–3 \times 10^5/mm^3$,range fibrinogen content 100–500 mg%.
† Number of platelets per gram of thrombus ÷ number of platelets per gram of blood.
‡ Weight fibrin per gram of thrombus ÷ weight fibrinogen per gram of blood.

experiments on thrombus formation in the absence of anticoagulants. The first two columns give the radioactivity values for the entire thrombus as determined by the well counter. The next two columns give the ^{51}Cr and ^{125}I counts per ml of whole blood taken from the animals before the test period. The fifth column gives the wet weight of thrombus accumulated on the shaft. By assuming a specific gravity of 1.0, an estimate of the mean thickness was obtained.

In order to compare results from different animals and different tests, it is useful to calculate the ratio of the specific activity of the thrombi divided by the specific activity of blood for the same experiment. These results, given in columns 7 and 8, show the relative concentration of platelets and fibrin in thrombi as compared to whole blood.

The platelet content of thrombi (platelets per unit volume) was up to 112 ± 105 times that of whole blood. This enrichment ratio compares with a value of 68 obtained by Olson *et al.*[13] for stainless steel tubes placed in the carotid artery, and with a value of 28 for tubes placed in the jugular vein after one hour of exposure time. Foster and Dobell[16] also determined the platelet content of thrombi formed on quartz tubes placed in the thoracic vena cava for two hours and found an average thrombus/blood ratio of 51. Considering the differences in these experiments, the values are remarkably similar.

The fibrin content of thrombi formed in our system averaged about 14.3 ± 7.3 times that of whole blood. Olson *et al.*[13] found a lower fibrin content in his implanted tubes, reporting an enrichment ratio of approximately two for both arterial and venous locations.

Some trends were observed with respect to the composition of thrombi as related to size. A regression analysis showed that the inverse relationship $\text{platelet content of thrombus} = \alpha \left(\frac{1}{\text{thrombus weight}} \right)$ is significant at the 0.002 level. This indicates that the larger thrombi have a proportionately larger amount of red blood cells and that the size of the thrombus may be the distinguishing feature between the so-called venous "red clots" and the arterial "white thrombi."

Based on enrichment ratios, an estimate of the ultimate sensitivity of the current monitoring system can be made. One can have reasonable confidence in a change detected by the scintillation counter if the radioactivity, due to the accumulated thrombus, increases more than twice the baseline level due to blood in the chamber initially. The approximate thrombus thickness, Δ, that can be detected for different values of the enrichment ratio γ is given by

$$\Delta = \left(\frac{R_2^2 + (\gamma - 2)\ R_1^2}{\gamma - 1} \right)^{1/2} - R_1 \qquad \textbf{(1)}$$

where R_2 and R_1 are the radii of outer cylinder and shaft, respectively. For our apparatus the relationship between the minimum detectable thrombus thickness, Δ, and thrombus radioactivity enrichment ratio, γ, is given in TABLE 3.

Based on our values of γ of about 110 for platelets and 15 for fibrinogen, an approximate minimum thrombus thickness of 0.05 mm by ^{51}Cr-labeled platelets and 0.3 mm by ^{125}I-labeled fibrinogen can be detected.

Discussion

The primary purpose of this study was to evaluate the thrombogenicity of different biomaterials in contact with blood. A number of other factors, however, were found to influence the rate and amount of thrombus accumulation in the test chamber, and these led to the concept of running parallel tests to obtain the best comparative information.

Effect of Biomaterial

In order to evaluate the response of the test procedure to different materials, a large number of runs were made with etched 303 stainless steel and Silastic**-coated shafts. Photomicrographs of these two surfaces, along with a comparative picture of a thrombus, are shown in FIGURE 13. Greater amounts of thrombus appear to form on the stainless steel surface. As shown in TABLE 4, data pooled from all runs at different flow rates, different shaft rotation speeds, and in different animals gave an average wet weight of 0.74 grams for thrombus formed on the stainless steel surface, in contrast to 0.48 grams formed on the silicone rubber surface. The significance of this difference is at the 95% level. If only those data for "standard" runs with a flow of 200 ml/min and a shaft speed of 200 rpm are considered, there still is greater amount of clot formed on the stainless surface, 0.49 grams vs. 0.39 grams. But the variability of the data does not permit assignment of statistical significance to this difference.

TABLE 3

SENSITIVITY OF RADIOISOTOPE TECHNIQUE FOR MEASURING THROMBUS THICKNESS

Thrombus Enrichment Ratio (γ)	Minimum Detectable Thrombus Thickness Δ (microns)*
5	920
10	447
25	176
50	88
100	44
150	29

* For R_1=0.238 cm. R_2=0.515 cm.

However, a comparison of parallel experiments in an animal at a given flow condition offers the most reliable evaluation. Values on the last line in TABLE 4 indicate that the size of thrombus formed on 303 stainless steel was about 70% greater than on Silastic when both materials are tested simultaneously. Also, the variance of the data obtained in this fashion, i.e. paired comparisons, is the lowest found in this study.

** Dow Corning Medical Grade Adhesive 819 was dispersed in toluene and the shafts were dip-coated in this preparation.

TABLE 4

COMPARISON OF THROMBUS FORMATION ON STAINLESS STEEL AND SILASTIC RUBBER SURFACES

	Thrombus Weight (grams)					
Test Conditions	Stainless Steel	Silastic Rubber	Difference	Ratio Weights	Number Observations	Significance Level
All runs	0.74±0.65	0.48±0.59	0.26	1.54	87	0.06 *
200 rpm, 200 ml/min runs	0.49±0.33	0.39±0.37	0.10	1.25	60	0.32
All paired runs	1.02	0.82	0.20	1.24	20	0.12 **
200 rpm, 200 ml/ min paired runs	0.63	0.38	0.25	1.66	9	0.05 *

* Highly significant.
** Moderately significant.

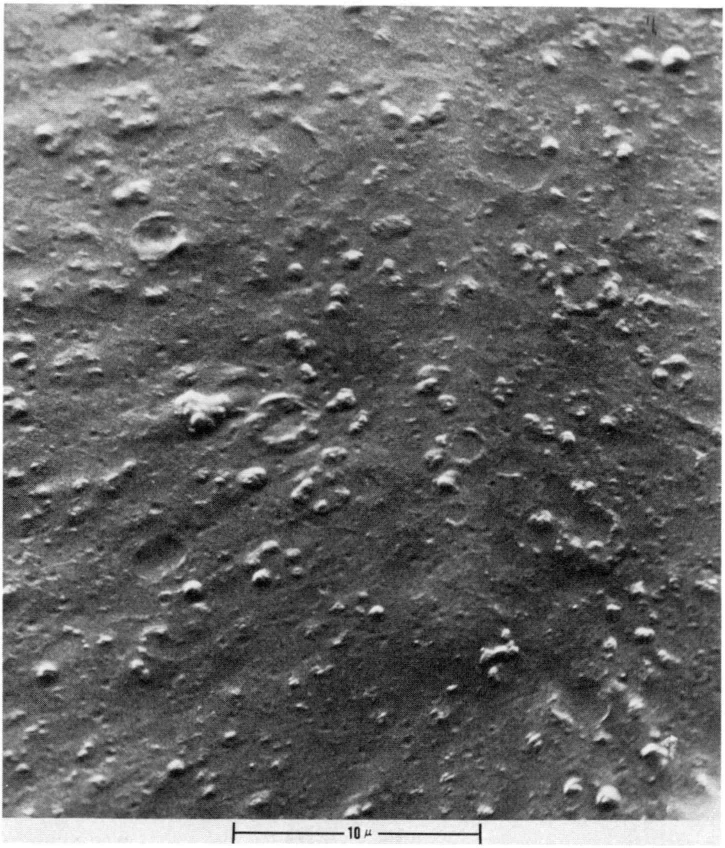

FIGURE 13a. Scanning electron micrographs of surfaces used in the evaluation of the *ex vivo* biomaterial testing procedure. Silastic rubber (coating made by dipping stainless-steel rod in a dispersion of Dow-Corning Silastic Medical Adhesive).

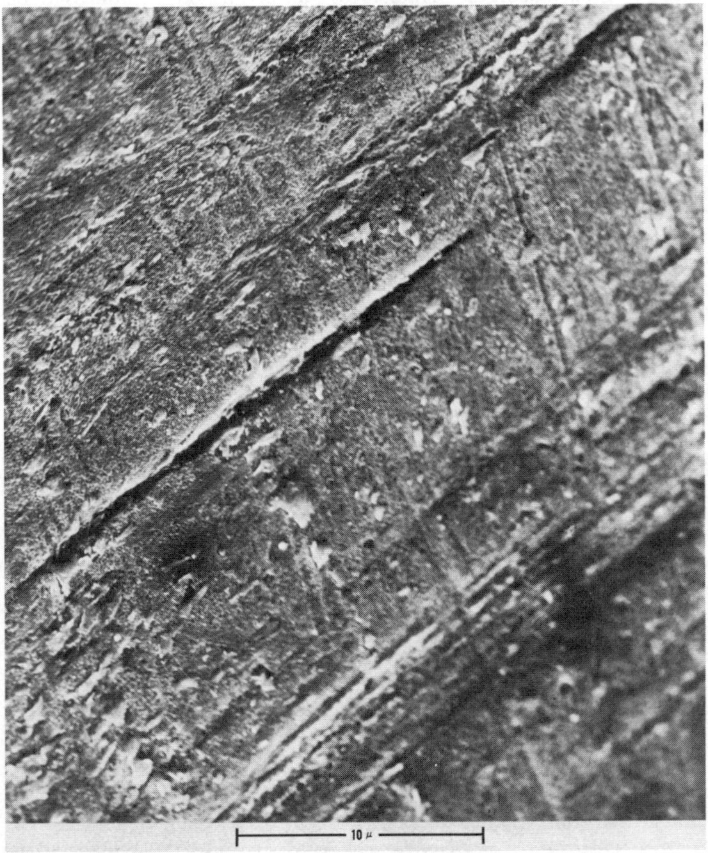

FIGURE 13b. Etched 303 stainless steel. (See FIGURE 13a legend.)

Effect of Anticoagulants

In a number of experiments, heparin at a level of 60 μ/kg was administered to the animal one half hour before initiating the biomaterial test procedure. Assays of systemic blood samples during the procedure showed that heparin disappeared from the circulation in about 45 minutes. Coincident with heparin disappearance, thrombus accumulation, as measured by the scintillation counter, began. The amount of thrombus adhering to the shaft surface was less after a dose of heparin, and the distribution was different, with some thrombus formed both on the inner surface of the cylinder and on the shaft surface.

Although the amount of thrombus formed on the shaft was slightly lower than for the tests conducted in the absence of heparin, the results were much more consistent from test to test. In addition, the difference in thrombus weight between Silastic and stainless was greater.

Embolization

One factor often considered important in evaluating biomaterials is the amount of embolization due to the presence of biomaterials in the bloodstream. These test procedures do not measure embolization except as indirectly reflected in an abrupt decrease in the amount of radioactivity in the chamber during the test. This type of decrease was not observed during our normal one-hour test period. In some cases where tests extended up to four hours, however, abrupt drops in radioactivity in the chamber were observed. An example is shown in FIGURE 10. The simultaneous abrupt changes in amounts of platelets and fibrin in the chamber indicate that some embolization took place with subsequent thrombus reformation, the amount of embolization being reflected by the differ-

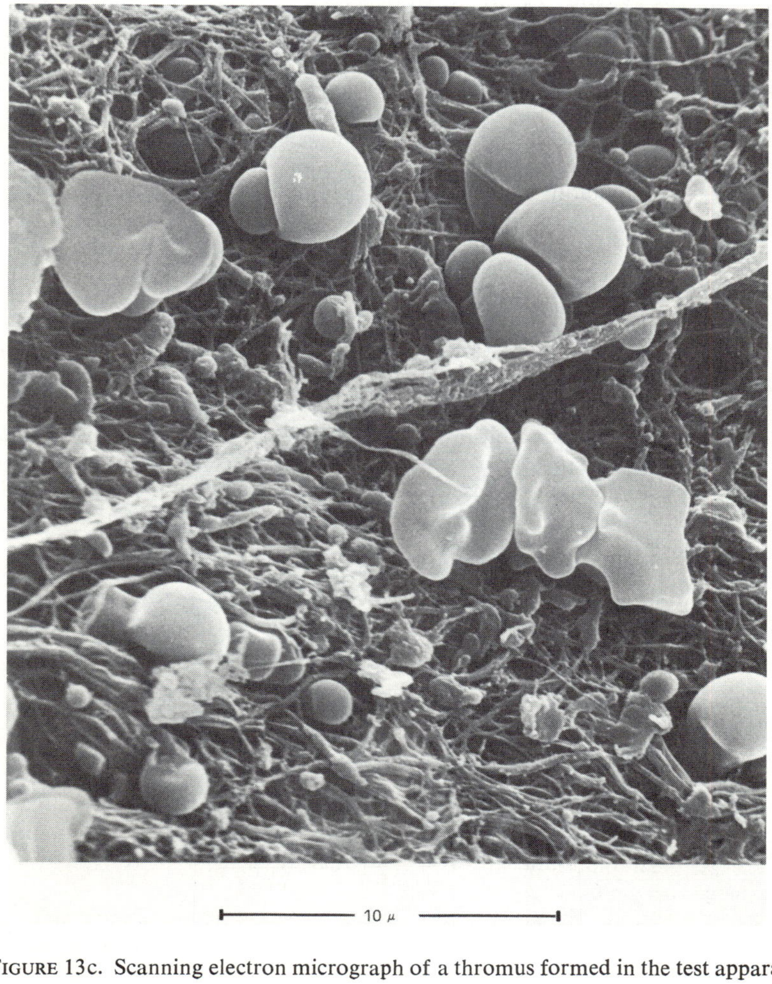

FIGURE 13c. Scanning electron micrograph of a thromus formed in the test apparatus.

ence in radioactivity after the abrupt change. The embolization in this particular animal did not cause any visible untoward effects after the test.

Effect of Sequential Tests

A most consistent observation was that the weight of thrombus varies with the order of testing in a sequential series of tests on the same day. Generally, the weight of the thrombus decreases from the first to last test. For example, in TABLE 5 the average weight of clots at a specific flow condition, 200 ml/min and 200 rpm, decreases from approximately 0.55 grams on the shaft for the first test to 0.21 grams of clot for the fourth test. An analysis of variance showed that this effect was significant at the 0.003 level.

The decreases in platelet and fibrinogen levels during the test period shown in FIGURE 12 appear to correlate with diminished thrombus formation. The variance of the observation for each test period decreases with time, an indication that the system becomes more stable or reproducible for tests carried out after one to two hours of testing and that the most variable observations are in the first hour of testing. In the last line of TABLE 5 there is a trend that suggests that the composition of the clot may be changing during sequential periods of testing. The relative fibrin content of the clot was lowest during the first period and increased for the last period of testing. This observation may reflect an increase in circulating coagulants that promote a more rapid rate of fibrin formation.

Flow and Transport Characteristics of the Test Chamber

In the laminar regime, the flow pattern of a Newtonian fluid in the annular space between a stationary cylinder and a rotating shaft is well known. The pertinent equations for velocities and shear rates are given in the appendix. The resulting flow pattern and direction of shear forces are given by the vector resultant of axial and angular components, as illustrated in FIGURE 6(A). Some typical values of shear rates based on fully developed flow and calculated for

TABLE 5

RESULTS FROM SEQUENTIAL BIOMATERIAL TESTS ON SAME DAY

	Run			
	A(First)	B	C	D(Last)
Thrombus weight (grams)	0.5±0.4	0.5±0.4	0.4±0.2	0.2±0.1
Platelet enrichment ratio $\left(\frac{\text{no. per gm thrombus}}{\text{no. per gm blood}}\right)$	120±100	100±70	100±50	140±30
Fibrinogen enrichment ratio $\left(\frac{\text{Fibrin per gm thrombus}}{\text{Fibrinogen per gm blood}}\right)$	11±6	12±7	13±6	18±3

Blood flow (ml/min) through test chamber 200 ml/min, shaft rotation speed 200 (rpm).

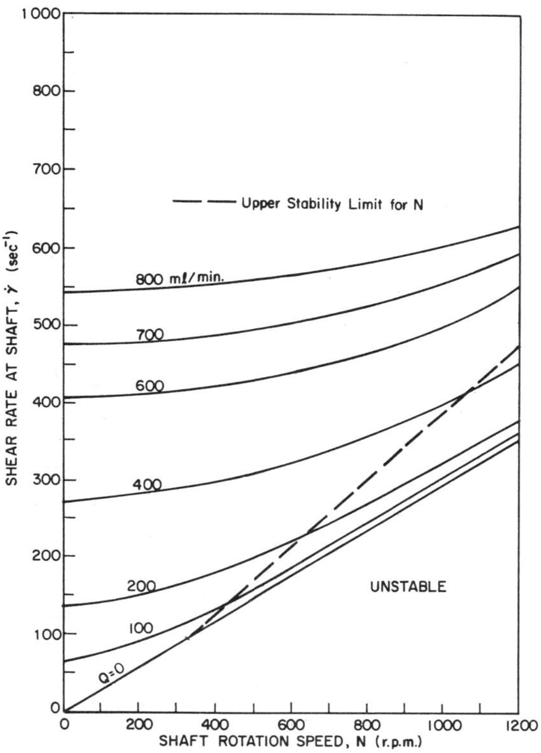

FIGURE 14. Effect of flow rate and shaft rotation speed on shear rate at the surface of the surface of the shaft. Dashed line indicates the boundary between the laminar helical-flow pattern regime and the unstable Taylor-vortex regime.

the chamber used in these experiments are given in FIGURE 14. As can be seen, the net shear on the central shaft is almost a direct function of the rotational speed. However, the shear on the shaft surface is also affected by axial flow rates through the chamber, so that at high axial flow rates the relative effects of rotational speed are, to some extent, diminished. The effect of rotational speed on shear stress at the shaft is more pronounced at either low axial flow rates or larger gap widths. There is very little effect of shaft rotation speed upon the shear stress on the outer cylindrical wall.

In the absence of density variations and before the onset of Taylor vortices, the mass transfer coefficients on the shaft and on the wall are independent of rotation. It is in this range, therefore, that it is possible to distinguish between the mechanical effects of shear and its effect on transport phenomena. Comparing FIGURE 14 with FIGURES 15A & 15B, for example, at an axial flow rate of 140 cc/min the mass transfer coefficient, as reflected in the Sherwood number (Sh), remains constant up to a shaft speed of 300 rpm, whereas the shear stress is increasing on the shaft.

Another factor to be considered is the axial dependence of mass transfer coefficients on the shaft and cylindrical surfaces. In the laminar flow regime

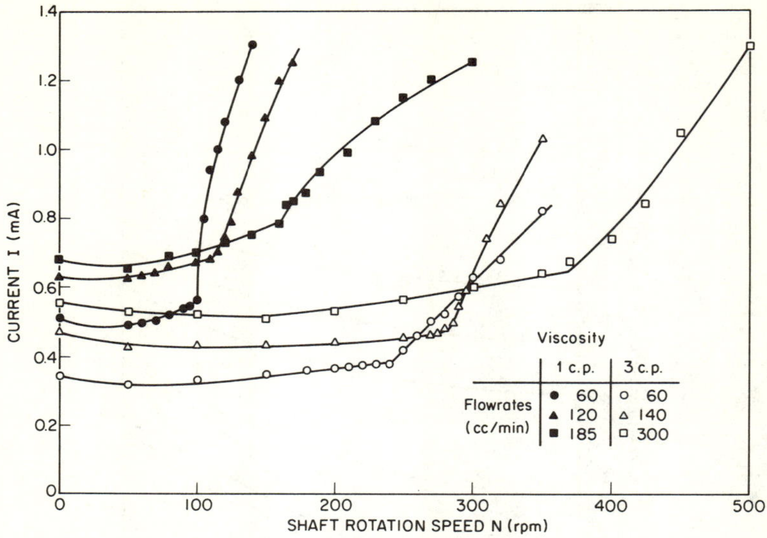

FIGURE 15a. Polarographic measurement of mass-transfer coefficients at the surface of the shaft as a function of rotation speed, flow rate, and viscosity. Measured current is directly related to mass transfer coefficients. Breaks in curves are a result of the onset of unstable Taylor-vortices.

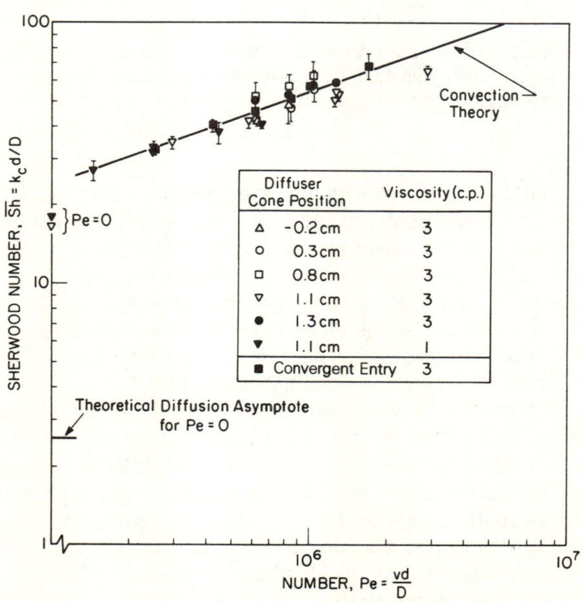

FIGURE 15b. Mass-transfer data from the laminar helical-flow regime correlated with dimensionless Pe number. (See FIGURE 15a.)

there is a developing concentration boundary layer from the tip of the shaft to the exit portion. If the flow field of FIGURE 6(A) is assumed, then a theoretical calculation of steady-state mass transfer coefficients can be made by a modification of the classical asymptotic Leveque formula [17] (see APPENDIX).

As the rotation rate is increased in the helical flow regime, a critical speed is finally attained where the flow becomes unstable. A new flow regime with radial motion ensues, and Equation 5 is no longer valid. In this regime, depicted on the right-hand side of the FIGURE 6, a cellular flow pattern with "Taylor vortices" emerges. These vortices have the appearance of smoke rings stacked one upon another, with the circulation in alternate rings opposing. This vortex regime persists to much higher rotational speeds, whereupon "wavy" vortices are formed, and finally turbulence is achieved. The flow pattern of the Taylor vortices is similar to that used by other workers to study thrombus formation such as the captured-vortex device of Leonard and Litwak [3] and the standing vortex in an expansion section, studied by Goldsmith.[18]

During blood flow through the chamber, thrombi may form on the internal wall of the cylinder as well as on the rotating shaft, and a significant gap width was considered necessary to avoid occlusion of the annular space during extended experimental periods. Therefore, our device falls into the "wide-gap" couette-flow category, where theoretical stability analysis has not been as extensive. Some mass transfer studies were done in order to characterize the transport rates or fluxes to the shaft surface as a function of rotational speed and axial flow rate and the critical speeds for the transition to Taylor vortices. These are described more extensively below.

Theoretical Prediction of Hydrodynamic Stability

The helical (Poiseuille-Couette) flow in the annulus between coaxial circular cylinders of a Newtonian fluid is characterized by two dimensionless parameters, an axial flow Reynolds number

$$\mathrm{Re} = \frac{\mathrm{Ud}}{\nu} = \frac{\mathrm{Q}}{\pi(\mathrm{R}_1 + \mathrm{R}_2)\nu} \qquad (2)$$

and a rotational Taylor number

$$\mathrm{Ta} = \frac{\Omega^2 \mathrm{R}_1 \mathrm{d}^3}{\nu^2} \qquad (3)$$

where

U = mean axial flow velocity in the annulus $= \mathrm{Q}/\pi(\mathrm{R}_2^2 - \mathrm{R}_1^2)$
Q = axial volumetric flow rate ($\mathrm{cm}^3/\mathrm{sec}$)
R_2 = outer cylinder (chamber) radius (cm)
R_1 = inner cylinder (shaft) radius (cm)
$\mathrm{d} = \mathrm{R}_2 - \mathrm{R}_1$ = annular gap width, (cm)
$\nu = \mu/\rho$ = kinematic viscosity of fluid $\left(\frac{\mathrm{cm}^2}{\mathrm{sec}}\right)$
Ω = angular velocity of outer cylinder (rad/sec) $= 2\pi\mathrm{N}$
N = rotational speed (rev/sec)

As mentioned above, the laminar helical flow becomes unstable at a critical shaft rotational speed N_c. This is properly characterized by a critical rotational Taylor number Ta_c, which depends on the axial flow Reynolds number Re.

To date, no complete stability theory exists for arbitrary radius ratios $\eta = R_1/R_2$ and flow Reynolds numbers. Theoretical results are, however, available for zero axial flow, Re = 0, at over an extended range of η, as well as for the thin gap limit, $\eta \rightarrow 1$, at moderate Reynolds numbers. TABLE 6 summarizes results given by Sparrow *et al.*[19] for the first case.

For the second case, the thin gap, several investigators (Chandrasekhar,[20] Datta,[21] Krueger and Di Prima,[22] and Hughes and Reid[23]) have made theoretical studies on the influence of Re. According to Hughes and Reid the theoretical results for Re < 500 appear to be reasonably well represented by a formula proposed by Datta[21]:

$$Ta_c = 1708 + 2.35\, Re^2 \quad \textbf{(4)}$$

which actually should be accurate only for very low Reynolds numbers. This relation can be empirically extended in the form

$$\frac{Ta_c}{(Ta_c)_o} = 1 + 1.38 \times 10^{-3}\, Re^2 \quad \textbf{(5)}$$

where $(Ta_c)_o$ denotes the critical Taylor number for zero axial flow, Re = 0, as given in TABLE 6.

TABLE 6

CRITICAL TAYLOR NUMBER AS A FUNCTION OF RADIUS RATIO η FOR NO AXIAL FLOW, RE=0 *

$\eta=R_1/R_2$	1.0	0.95	0.75	0.5	0.35	0.25	0.10
$(Ta_c)_o$	1708	1801	2453	4649	9097	18605	1.614×10^6

* After Sparrow *et al.*[19]

Verification of Chamber Mass Transfer and Stability Characteristics

To verify the applicability of the mass transfer theory for the stable helical flow and to detect the onset of unstable flow, experiments were done on a model chamber employing an electrochemical-mass-transfer technique. The model chamber had a slightly larger shell I.D. (½ inch) than that of the test chamber (13/32 inch).

Mass transfer rates to the shaft surface were measured by means of an electrochemical polarographic technique developed by Eisenberg *et al.*[24] (and also used for an annular geometry by Ross and Wragg[25]). An electrolyte was used that consisted of 0.001 M potassium ferri- and ferrocyanide (as the electroactive species) in 1 M aqueous NaOH.

FIGURES 15A and 15B give typical mass transfer data shown as limiting currents for the polarographic experiments as a function of flow rates, rotation speeds, and viscosity.††

†† Viscosity was adjusted with a cellulosic polymer (Natrosol®—Hercules, Inc.).

On theoretical grounds, it can be anticipated that the plateau currents and, consequently, the mass transfer coefficients are relatively independent of rotation speed for a given flow rate, at least up to a certain critical speed. At this speed, which is presumed to represent the onset of instability and Taylor vortices, the mass transfer coefficient begins to increase sharply.

Two pieces of information are extracted from such plots: (1) the mass transfer coefficient as a function of axial flow rate for rotation below the critical speed, and (2) the critical rotation speed as a function of axial flow rate.

Reduction of the data to the dimensionless form indicated in FIGURE 15B by the equation

$$\overline{Sh} = \frac{i}{2\ \pi R_1 L\ F} \frac{(R_2 - R_1)}{C_0\ D}$$

(where i = current, F = Faraday's constant, C_0 = concentration of ferricyanide, L = length of shaft) requires a knowledge of the effective diffusion coefficient D for the electroactive current-limiting species $Fe(CN)_6^{-3}$ in the electrolyte solution. For the 1 c p aqueous solution, the value reported by Eisenberg *et al.*[24] was used at 23° C, $D = 5.11 \times 10^{-6} \frac{cm^2}{sec}$; for the 3 c p solution a value of $2.92 \times 10^{-6} \frac{cm^2}{sec}$ was used to bring the data into coincidence.

FIGURE 15B gives a comparison of the corresponding values of mean Sherwood number for the whole shaft vs. the Peclet number, together with the theoretical relation of Equation 10 (Appendix). Also shown are data for zero axial flow, together with the theoretical estimate, Equation 3.

The data correspond to shaft rotation rates midway between zero and the critical rotation speed.

The agreement of the data with the convection theory of Equation 10 is considered satisfactory for $Pe > 0$ and tends to indicate the absence of severe hydrodynamic end effects. On the other hand, the data for zero axial flow, $Pe = 0$, lie far above the pure diffusion asymptote of Equation 11, which can probably be attributed to natural convection or unsteady-state diffusion effects.

The sharp breaks in FIGURE 15A represent the onset of Taylor vortices in the test chamber. According to the above stability theory, the relation between Ta_c (or N_c/ν) and Re (or Q/ν) should be independent of the viscosity of the particular Newtonian fluid used. FIGURE 16 summarizes the data for the solutions with viscosities of 1 c p and 3 c p. There is in the data evident scatter, which is thought to be due in large part to entry effects in the chamber.‡‡

There is no theory available for the wide gap used here, but the thin gap result of Equation 5 was modified by taking $(Ta_c)_0$ to be equal to the value 8,250 from TABLE 6, rather than its thin-gap value 1708. This modification is shown as the solid curve in FIGURE 16. Within the precision of the data, there appears to be agreement with our modified thin-gap theory for the Reynolds numbers up to about 60. This value of Re may correspond to the onset of higher order instability and the "wavy-vortex" regime predicted for $Re > 75$ by theory (Chandrasekhar),[20] but it may also involve hydrodynamic entry effects in the present device.

‡‡ See FIGURE 16 for a description of the entry positions.

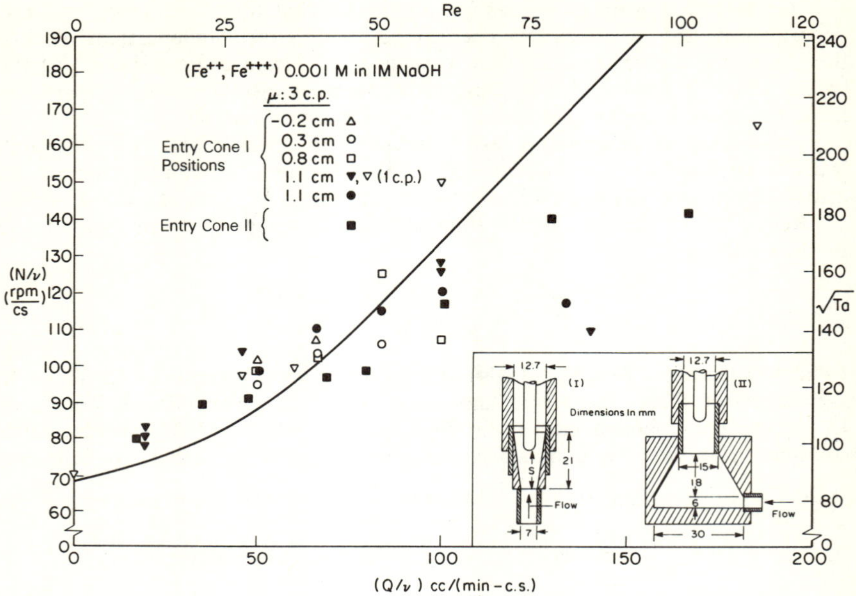

FIGURE 16. Shaft rotation speed (N) where onset of Taylor-vortex regime commences as a function of flow through the chamber (Q). Solid line is from the modified thin gap theory given in text.

These polarographic data give some confidence in our modified thin-gap theory, Equation 5, for the prediction of the critical rotation speed for blood flowing in the test chamber. Using a value of 3.5 cs for the kinematic viscosity of blood, the critical rotation speeds were calculated from Equation 5 and plotted as a dashed line in FIGURE 14.

Thus, in the stable laminar-helical flow regime, the blood flow rates between 50 and 800 ml/min and shaft rotation rates between 0 and 1000 rpm, it is

TABLE 7

SUMMARY OF SHEAR RATES USED IN PLATELET-ADHESION AND RELATED STUDIES

Flow Geometry	Investigators	* Approx. Shear Rate Range, Sec^{-1}
Stagnation point	Nyilas *et al.*[26]	0–25
Annular (Couette) rotational	Feuerstein *et al.*[12]	10–20
Tube (Poiseuille)	Grabowski, *et al.*[27]	10–100
Annular axial (Poiseuille)	Turitto and Baumgartner[28]	2–840
Rotating disc	Butruille, *et al.*[29]	0–1565

* As reported in the articles cited.

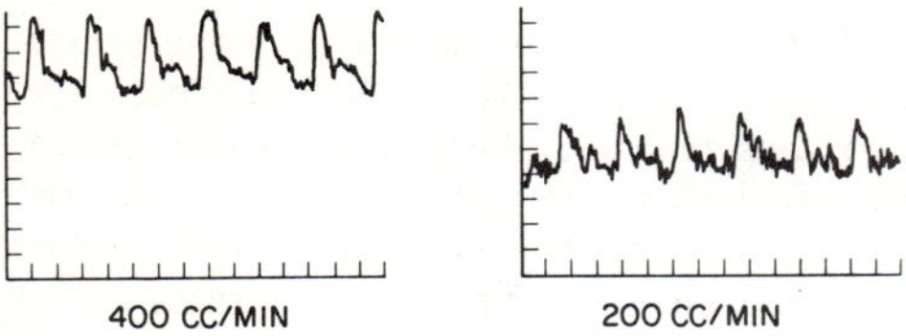

FIGURE 17. Pulsatile blood flow in *ex vivo* test chamber when connected to an A-V shunt at mean flows of 200 and 400 cc/min. Time marks on abscissa are at one-second intervals.

possible to attain a range of shear rates of 40–600 sec^{-1} on the shaft surface. This compares well with the shear rates employed in several other platelet adhesion studies, summarized in TABLE 7, and are comparable in range to those found in the larger vessels of the human vascular system.

To assess the effects of pulsatile flow on hydrodynamics and mass transfer, some polarographic studies were undertaken with fluctuating flow (±15%) to simulate the flow pattern found in the A-V shunt (FIGURE 17).

It appeared that pulsations of this magnitude do not have an appreciable influence on mean mass transfer rates nor on critical rotation speeds for transition to the Taylor-Vortex regime.

SUMMARY AND CONCLUSIONS

The flexibility of this test system allows for many different conditions and arrangements to be explored in the testing of biomaterials. The variables include flow rate, shaft rotation speed, sequential order and duration of test, single or parallel sample testing, and systemic anticoagulants.

Up to four test chambers can be run simultaneously. The major constraint on the number of parallel chambers is the blood flow available. Blood flow rates through the shunt without any chambers attached are on the order 800 ml to 1.3 liters/minute. When the test apparatus is connected, the available blood flow often decreases somewhat because of the flow resistance imposed on the system, so that the flow to the individual chambers is limited by the total shunt output. Four to five chambers in parallel would seem to be the most that can be run at one time.

Flow Conditions

In the choice of flow conditions for evaluating the different materials, there are some constraints on the flow rate that can be used in these parallel tests. If flow is reduced below 50 ml/min per chamber, there is a very high likelihood of getting a very rapid thrombus buildup to an extent that the chamber becomes

TABLE 8

VALUES OF CONSTANTS a(k) *

$\eta = 1/k$	0.2	0.3	0.4	0.5	0.6
a(k)	1.427	1.359	1.319	1.293	1.274

* After Lundberg *et al.*[17]

occluded during a normal test period of about one hour. Because of the limitations on total flow available from the shunt, it is unlikely that one could use above 250 ml/min per chamber if more than two chambers were used in a test.

Within the range of flow rates through the chamber of 50–200 ml/min, the maximum variation in shear rate that can be achieved within the laminar-flow regime is roughly a factor of three and is within the range of shear rates found in the normal vascular system. Although the shear rates in this regime may not be high enough to evaluate embolization, at speeds on the order of 800–1000 rpm the device does achieve the Taylor-vortex regime with concomitant high shear stresses.

Duration of Test

Our measurements of rates thrombus formation with time have indicated that thrombus accumulation is more or less linear with time, at least for the first 30–45 minutes. In some tests the formation rate began to decrease or to level off at about one hour, and in the tests that were conducted for longer periods of time there was a definite indication that thrombus formation had begun to level off completely. As a matter of practical importance, the ultimate deposition thickness may be a more important parameter than the initial rate of thrombus formation.

Based solely on the normal turnover of platelets and fibrinogen, there are limitations on the length of these chronic tests. Since the turnover time of these blood elements is on the order of four days, the label washes out of the system, and the radioactive detection system becomes less sensitive with time. A more practical procedure is to discontinue the test when, after a few days, the amount of circulating labeled platelets has decreased appreciably.

References

1. Murphy, E. A., H. C. Rowsell, H. G. Downie, G. A. Robinson & J. F. Mustard. 1962. Encrustation and atherosclerosis: The analogy between early *in-vivo* lesions and deposits which occur in extracorporeal circulations. J. Can. Med. Assoc. **87:** 259–274.
2. Downie, H. G., E. A. Murphy, H. C. Rowsell & J. F. Mustard. 1963. Extracorporeal circulation: A device for the quantitative study of thrombus formation in flowing blood. Circulation Res. **12:** 441–448.
3. Leonard, E. F. & D. S. Litwak. 1972. 5th Ann. Contractors Conf. Artificial Kidney Program. DHEW Pub. NIH **72–248:** 97.
4. Rembaum, A., S. P. S. Yen, M. Ingram, I. F. Newton, W. G. Frasher & B. H. Barbour. 1973. Platelet adhesion to heparin-bonded and heparin-free surfaces. Biomat. Med. Div. Art. Org. **1:** 99–119.
5. Dutton, R. C., R. E. Baier, R. L. Dedrick & R. L. Bowman. 1968. Initial thrombus formation on foreign surfaces. Trans. Am. Soc. Artif. Intern. Organs **14:** 57.
6. Petschek, H., D. Adams & A. R. Kantrowitz. 1968. Stagnation flow thrombus formation. Trans. Am. Soc. Artif. Intern. Organs **14:** 256.
7. Frasher, W. G. 1967. Blood sampling by a chronic artificial external arteriovenous shunt in dogs. J. Appl. Physiol. **27:** 348.
8. Harker, L. A. 1974. Hemostatis Manual. 2nd edit. F. A. Davis. Pa.
9. Mustard, J. F., R. L. Kinlough-Rathbone & M. A. Packam. 1974. Throm-

bosis: Pathogenesis and clinical trials. Thromb. Diath. Haemorrh. (Suppl.) **59**.
10. THOMAS, D. P. 1972. The role of platelets in arterial and venous thrombosis. Adv. Exp. Med. Biol. **34:** 23.
11. BAUMGARTNER, H. R. 1973. The role of blood flow in platelet adhesion, fibrin deposition and formation of mural thrombi: Microvascular Res. **5:** 167.
12. FEUERSTEIN, I. A., J. M. BROPHY & J. L. BRASH. 1975. Platelet transport and adhesion to reconstituted collagen and artificial surfaces. Trans. Am. Soc. Artif. Intern. Oragns **21:** 427.
13. OLSON, P. S., U. LJUNGQVIST & S. E. BERGENTZ. 1974. Analysis of platelet, red cell and fibrin content in experimental arterial and venous thrombi. Thromb. Res. **5:** 1.
14. OLSON, P. S., C. BUSCH & O. LINDQUIST. 1974. Thrombus formation in the arterial and venous circulation in thrombocytopenic dogs. Europ. Surg. Res. **6:** 54–64.
15. ASTER, R. H. & J. H. JANDL. 1964. Platelet sequentiation in man. I. Methods. J. Clin. Invest. **43:** 843.
16. FOSTER, E. D. & A. R. C. DOBELL. 1971. Evaluation of rigid prosthetic rings as *in-vivo* intravascular thrombogenic models. J. Surg. Res. **11:** 550.
17. LUNDBERG, R. E., W. C. REYNOLDS & W. M. WAYS. 1963. NASA Report: NASA-TND-1972.
18. GOLDSMITH, L. H. 1972. The flow of model particles and blood cells and its relation to thrombogenesis. Progress in Hemostasis and Thrombosis. Vol. 1. E. Spaet, Ed. : 97. Grune and Stratton. New York, N.Y.
19. SPARROW, E. M., W. D. MUNRO & V. K. JONSSON. 1964. Instability of the flow between rotating cylinders: The wide-gap problem. J. Fluid. Mech. **20:** 35.
20. CHANDRASEKHAR, S. 1961. Hydrodynamic and hydromagnetic stability. Oxford Clarendon Press. Oxford, England.
21. DATTA, S. K. 1965. Stability of spiral flow between concentric circular cylinders at low axial number. J. Fluid Mech. **21:** 635.
22. KRUEGER, E. R. & R. C. PRIMA. 1964. Stability of viscous fluid between rotating cylinders with axial flow. J. Fluid Mech. **19:** 528.
23. HUGHES, T. H. & W. H. REID. 1968. The stability of spiral flow between rotating cylinders. Proc. R. Soc. Lond. [Biol.] **A263:** 8.
24. EISENBERG, M., C. W. TOBIAS, C. R. WILKE. 1955. Mass transfer at rotating cylinders. Chem. Eng. Prog. Symp. Ser. **51**(16): 1.
25. ROSS, K. & A. WRAGG. 1965. Electrochemical mass transfer studies in annuli. Electrochem. Acta **10:** 1093.
26. NYILAS, E., W. A. MORTON, D. M. LEDERMAN, T. H. CHIU. & R. D. CUMMING. 1975. Interdependence of hemodynamic and surface parameters in thrombosis. Trans. ASAIO. **21:** 55.
27. GRABOWSKI, E. F., L. I. FRIEDMAN & E. F. LEONARD. 1972. Effects of shear rate on diffusion and adhesion of blood platelets to a foreign surface. Ind. Eng. Chem. Fund. **11:** 224.
28. TURRITTO, V. T. & H. R. BAUMGARTNER. 1975. Platelet deposition on subendothelium exposed to flowing blood: mathematical analysis of physical parameters. Trans. Am. Soc. Artif. Intern. Organs **21:** 593–600.
29. BUTRUILLE, Y. A., E. F. LEONARD & D. S. LITWAK. 1975. Platelet-platelet interaction and non-adhesive encounters on biomaterials. Trans. Am. Soc. Artif. Intern. Organs **21:** 609.

APPENDIX

For a Newtonian fluid the axial (z) velocity profile in an annulus is given by the following equation:

$$v_z(r) = 2U\left\{\frac{1 - r^2/R_1{}^2 + \dfrac{k^2-1}{\ln k}\ln(r/R_1)}{1 + k^2 + \dfrac{1-k^2}{\ln k}}\right\} \tag{6}$$

with

$r =$ radial position in annulus, $R_1 \leq r \leq R_2$
$k =$ radius ratio * $= R_2/R_1$

and the axial component shear stress on the shaft and the wall are given by the following equations:

$$\tau_z = \mu\gamma_z$$

where

$$\gamma_z = \frac{4U}{\alpha R_1}\left\{\frac{k^2-1}{\ln k^2}\right\} - 1, \text{ at } r = R_1$$
$$= \frac{4U}{\alpha R_2}\left\{\frac{k^2-1}{\ln k^2}\right\} - k^2, \text{ at } r = R_2 \tag{7}$$

and

$\tau_z =$ axial (rz) shear stress (force/area)
$\gamma_z =$ axial shear rate (time^{-1})
$\mu =$ fluid viscosity

$$\alpha = \left(1 + k^2 + \frac{1-k^2}{\ln k}\right).$$

The angular (θ) or tangential velocity and the corresponding angular components of shear stress are given by the following formula:

$$v_\theta = \left\{\frac{kR_1}{1-k^2}\frac{r}{R_2} - \frac{R_2}{r}\right\} \tag{8}$$

$$\tau_\theta = \mu\gamma_\theta$$

where

$$\gamma_\theta = \frac{2k^2\Omega}{1-k^2}, \text{ at } r = R_1$$
$$= \frac{2\Omega}{1-k^2}, \text{ at } r = R_2 \tag{9}$$

$v_\theta =$ angular-tangential velocity component
$\tau_\theta =$ angular ($r\theta$) shear stress (force/area)
$\gamma_\theta =$ angular shear rate (time^{-1}).

The resulting flow pattern with the shear direction and its magnitude are given by the vector resultant of the respective perpendicular components v_z, v_θ and τ_z, τ_θ, for the axial and angular directions. These are illustrated vectorially in the left-hand side of FIGURE 6.

* The notation $\eta = 1/k$ is used for the inverse gap ratio, which is that usually employed in the literature on hydrodynamic stability.

For the test chamber, the axial and angular shear rates on the shaft are

$$\gamma = 0.645Q$$
$$\gamma_\theta = 0.266N$$

Mass transfer coefficients to the shaft surface are most conveniently correlated by the dimensionless Sherwood number, Sh. In the mass transfer entry flow regime, the Sh number is given by:

$$\mathrm{Sh} = \frac{N_A(\bar{z})\, d}{(C_1 - C_0)D} = \frac{a(k)}{2}\, \bar{z}^{-1/3}$$

and

$$\overline{\mathrm{Sh}} = \frac{1}{L}\int_0^L \mathrm{Sh}\,dz = \frac{3}{4}\, a(k)\, (\mathrm{Pe_h}\, h/L)^{1/3} \qquad \textbf{(10)}$$

Sh = local dimensionless Sherwood Number (based on the gap width, d)
$\overline{\mathrm{Sh}}$ = average or overall value of Sh.
$N_A(\bar{z})$ = local molar diffusion flux of diffusing species, from shaft wall to fluid (moles/area-time)
C_1 = molar concentration of species (moles/vol) at shaft wall
C_0 = (chamber) inlet concentration of species
D = molecular diffusivity of diffusing species (cm^2/time)
h = hydraulic diameter of annulus
= 4 × cross section/perimeter = $2(R_2 - R_1) = 2d$
a(k) = dimensionless constant dependent on annulus radius ratio, $k = R_2/R_1$,

and with

$\bar{z} = z/h\, \mathrm{Re_h}\, \mathrm{Sc}$
z = distance from (mass-transfer) entry, $0 \leq z \leq L$
L = total length of mass transfer surface
$\mathrm{Pe_h} = \mathrm{Re_h}\,\mathrm{Sc} = Uh/\nu$, Peclet number based on h
$\mathrm{Re_h} = Uh/\nu$ = Reynolds Number based on h
$\mathrm{Sc} = \nu/D$ = Schmidt Number.

The relation **(10)** holds for uniform conditions on the surface of shaft, in which case the local mass transfer rate is independent of rotation rate, at least in the stable helical flow regime.

The functional form of the constant and numerical values of a(k) have been given by Lundberg *et al.*,[17] and TABLE 8 gives some select values in terms of $1/k = R_1/R_2$.

Their computations indicate that relative to an exact numerical solution the above asymptotic mass transfer relation should be accurate to about 5% for $\bar{z} < 0.05$. Of course, this equation will be valid only below the critical rotation speed.

We note that in the case of zero axial flow the mass transfer coefficient for radial steady diffusion in the annulus is given by

$$\overline{\mathrm{Sh}} = \mathrm{Sh} = \frac{(k^2 - 1)\,(k - 1)}{k^2\left[\ln k - \frac{1}{2}\right] + \frac{1}{2}}. \qquad \textbf{(11)}$$

AN INSTRUMENTAL APPROACH TO *IN VIVO* HEMOCOMPATIBILITY ASSESSMENT: DEVELOPMENT OF THE INTRAVASCULAR MAGNETIC SUSPENSION OF A TEST DEVICE *

D. M. Lederman, R. D. Cumming, H. E. Petschek, T.-H. Chiu, and E. Nyilas

Avco Everett Research Laboratory, Inc.
Everett, Massachusetts 02149

E. W. Salzman

Beth Israel Hospital and Harvard Medical School
Boston, Massachusetts 02215

The present paper describes the development of a new technique undertaken to advance the current state-of-the-art of the *in vivo* hemocompatibility evaluation of prosthetic materials using experimental animals. The characteristic feature of this technique is the support-free, coaxial, suspension of a test device within a large, canine blood vessel by means of electromagnetic forces. The test specimen has a blood-contact surface made of the material to be evaluated, while its geometrical configuration is variable to allow for the study of the effects on thromboembolic propensity of stasis, turbulence, and, in general, different flow patterns near its surface. The development of this method has recently reached the phase of preliminary acute *in vivo* trials. Since refinements and extensive testing of the system hardware are required to render this technique routinely employable, the present paper is limited to a description of the rationale, principles, and operational characteristics of this method.

Background

Compared to the variety of *in vitro* and *ex vivo* techniques currently in use or reportedly under development, there are essentially two methods that have found wide acceptance and are in routine use for the *in vivo* hemocompatibility assessment of prosthetic materials. These are the caval-ring-implant test pioneered by Gott and coworkers [1] and the renal embolus test system devised by Kusserow and associates.[2] Both of these methods can be utilized for short- as well as long-term exposures employing dogs as test animals. For evaluation by either one of these procedures, candidate materials are required to be in the form of ring-shaped samples having specified dimensions. In most cases, the test rings are usually made of polycarbonate (Lexan®) and subsequently coated with the material to be evaluated. The experimental animals employed in both procedures have to be within a specified size range, and preoperatively treated according to specified protocols.

* This work was supported by the Biomaterials Program, Division of Heart and Vascular Diseases, National Heart, Lung, and Blood Institute, under Contract NIH-N01-HB-4-2961.

In the method developed by Gott, the specimens are inserted into the inferior vena cava, resulting in the exposure of the test material under quite stringent conditions as far as flow is concerned. This implantation site represents, therefore, a challenge to the thromboresistance of a test surface under the low shear flow conditions prevailing in the vena cava. A modification of the caval-ring-implant test, introduced by Sawyer and Srinivasan[3] also employs ring-shaped specimens, but their length is greater than that of samples used in Gott's method. The extension of specimen length was reportedly introduced to increase the blood-contacting surface area in order to amplify the effects induced by the material under evaluation. It is noteworthy that this change in sample dimensions resulted in substantial changes in the relative *in vivo* hemocompatibility ranking of a number of materials exposed in both forms in the canine vena cava.[3] By contrast with the hemodynamic conditions prevailing in vena cava implantations, the renal embolus test system involves exposure of the candidate material under aortic flows. In this technique, test specimens are inserted into the canine abdominal aorta immediately above the renal arteries, following a partial infrarenal aortic constriction to force a relatively larger fraction of the exposed blood and potential emboli into the kidneys.

In the caval-ring-implant test, the assessment of *in vivo* hemocompatibility is based on evaluation criteria pertaining to the degree to which the lumen of implanted rings becomes occluded by thrombus in the course of specified periods of indwelling time, and the percentage distribution of specimens that either remain open or become partially or completely occluded during the same periods. In the renal embolus test system, the rings exposed for specified periods are also evaluated in terms of the degree of occlusion. In the latter, however, experimental animals are, in addition, routinely subjected to nephrectomy to assess the degree of infarction induced by emboli generated by the test surface.

Rationale and Basic Principles

In any particular method for assessment of *in vivo* hemocompatibility, the results obtained are obviously affected by a large number of variables inherent to such experiments. Since only some of the variables can be carefully controlled, the rest of other factors remaining uncertain proportionately affects the degree of reproducibility. In both caval-ring-implant and renal embolus techniques, for example, experimental uncertainties are attributable to factors that include, among others, complex mechanisms potentially induced by the abrasion of endothelium where the rigid test rings join the natural vessel wall or, the introduction of uncontrolled regions of flow separation conducive to the formation of junction thrombi.

An improvement of the capabilities of methods currently employed for the evaluation of *in vivo* hemocompatibility can be conceivably achieved if the exposure of test surfaces is accomplished under conditions that exclude a series of uncontrollable effects that may be induced by contact between the specimen and vascular intima.

To attain the desired support-free suspension of test specimens within suitably-sized canine blood vessels, a system involving a magnetically suspended test device (MSTD) has been designed. As schematically illustrated in Figure 1, the principles of this test procedure involve the maintenance of a coaxially suspended MSTD in a specified dynamic equilibrium position against the forces exerted upon it by the flowing blood. To meet this requirement, the fluid forces acting on the MSTD are continuously balanced by electromagnetic forces exerted on the MSTD by components of a Magnetic Housing (MH) placed externally around the otherwise intact vessel. Depending upon the hemocompatibility of the MSTD surface under the prevailing hemodynamic conditions, deposition of thrombi can occur to varying degrees on the specimen leading to corresponding changes in the effective magnitude of the fluid forces acting on the suspended device. These, in turn, are compensated by proportionate and instrumentally measurable changes in the servomechanically actuated electromagnetic forces required to hold the specimen in its equilibrium position. Conversely, should embolization of large thrombi from the MSTD occur, this phenomenon will manifest itself by a variation of the magnitude of the electromagnetic forces that hold the specimen against the flowing blood. Thus, at least in principle, the method of support-free magnetic suspension allows for a real-time recording of thromboembolic events taking place on a given test surface.

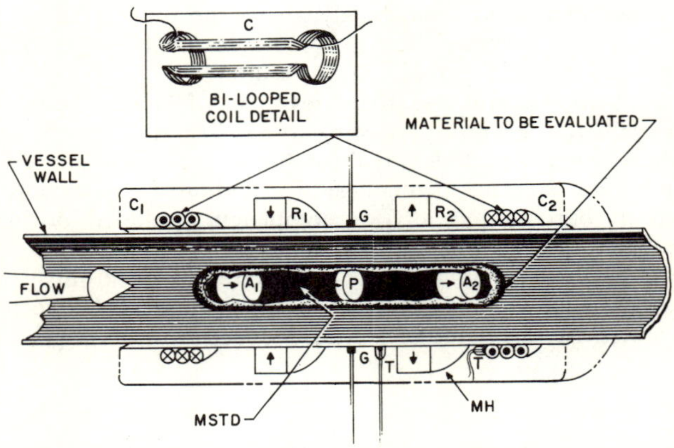

FIGURE 1. Schematic illustration of the intravascular magnetic suspension of a test device (MSTD).

Mechanism and Experimental Aspects of the Magnetic Suspension of a Test Device

The experimental implementation of the principles described above obviously requires the consideration of a number of factors including compatibility of the size of the device with anatomical dimensions of the selected experimental animal, the ease of access to appropriately sized blood vessels for the suspension of specimens, and the nature and potential side-effects of surgical interventions required for specimen implantation.

Within the context of these constraints, the MSTD was chosen to be a slender axisymmetric body of revolution, as schematically depicted in FIGURE 1, with an O.D. ~0.5 cm and a length ~5 cm. The exact dimensions of the

MSTD are a function of the overall weight of each selected geometry, because the device is required to be approximately neutrally buoyant in blood to eliminate variations in the magnitude of the component of the gravitational force acting in the direction of flow during the animal's normal changes in posture.

As shown in FIGURE 1, the MSTD specimen incorporates two axially magnetized cylindrical magnets (A_1 and A_2) placed in lateral positions, and one axially magnetized central disc magnet (P). All of these permanent magnets were chosen to be of a samarium/cobalt alloy ($SmCo_5$) that was found to be optimal because of its high specific magnetic moment, the constancy of its magnetic properties with time, and its commercial availability at reasonable cost.

To suspend the MSTD and to control its position, a MH consisting of separable sections is assembled and gently clamped around the freed but otherwise intact blood vessel selected for implantation. This involves first the placement, around the external vessel wall, of a bi-looped coil (C) which is then precisely encased by the MH. The other components of the MH include two radially magnetized permanent ring magnets (R_1 and R_2) selected to be of flexible barium ferrites; three high-sensitivity Hall Effect generators (G) positioned equidistantly on the inner circumference at the geometrical center of the MH; and two fast-response thermistors (T).

As indicated in FIGURE 1, magnets A_1 and A_2 in the MSTD have polarities opposed to those of the corresponding ring magnets, R_1 and R_2, in the MH. Compared to other possible magnetic polarity configurations studied, the arrangement depicted in FIGURE 1 was found to be optimal to passively stabilize the MSTD in a radial direction. When the concentricity of the rings, R_1 and R_2, and the cylindrical magnets, A_1 and A_2, is disturbed by a radial displacement of the MSTD, the magnetic repulsive force that arises in the region where the rings and cylindrical magnets are closest to each other is always greater than the force at the diametrically opposite direction.

However, when the MSTD is subjected to an axial deviation such as that caused by fluid forces acting in the direction of flow, a force develops that tends to make the deviation still larger. Thus, the equilibrium is unstable in the axial direction and hence, servo-controlled stabilization is required. This is achieved by means of the Gs which continuously sense the position and velocity of the MSTD and generate a corresponding Hall-voltage signal that is proportional to the change in the magnetic field intensity emanating from the positioning magnet, P. The signal from the Gs is then amplified and used to energize the bi-looped coil, C. In the situation shown in FIGURE 1, flow tends to displace the MSTD away from loop C_1 toward loop C_2. In this case, the signal from the Gs generates a current flowing through the bi-looped coil in a direction such that loop C_1 exerts an attractive force on magnet A_1 while look C_2 exerts a repulsive force on magnet A_2. This results in a net axially stabilizing magnetic force that acts in a direction opposite to the flow. Conversely, if a force disturbance acts on the MSTD in a direction opposite to that indicated in FIGURE 1, the flow of current through the bi-looped coil is generated in the reverse direction so that the net force arising between C_1 and A_1, and C_2 and A_2 always opposes the direction of force disturbance.

Thus, under this arrangement, radial stabilization for concentric support of the MSTD is achieved through passive magnetic repulsion providing an electronically uncoupled, self-centering suspension. Along the axis of symmetry of the vessel, independent electromagnetic control is provided to balance all forces expected to act on the MSTD including (1) hydrodynamic forces due to flow,

(2) magnetic instability forces resulting from the interaction between the permanent magnets placed in the MSTD and those incorporated in the MH, and (3) perturbation forces caused by disturbances in each of the above.

Depending upon the flow conditions under which the MSTD is suspended, the amount of heat dissipation at the bi-looped coil represents another potential constraint. Whereas the power requirements for operation under simulated venous flow conditions were found to be low enough to rule out the possibility of inducement of hyperbiological temperatures, suspension of the MSTD under aortic flows posed some difficulties due to the large power required during systolic acceleration. This limitation, however, was overcome by operating the system in a mode in which the mean aortic flow is balanced passively by means of the magnets in the MH while the bi-looped coil actively controls the time-varying components of the flow. This measure resulted in an average heat dissipation at an acceptable rate in the order of a few watts, excluding the possibility of reaching hyperbiological temperatures during aortic suspension. As a precautionary measure, however, fast-response precalibrated thermistors (T) are incorporated into the MH to monitor continuously the actual temperatures prevailing at the coil surface and outer vessel wall.

In FIGURE 2, a pair of MSTD prototypes are displayed to illustrate their actual size. FIGURE 3 shows a disassembled MH prototype, made from Plexiglas®, with all of the components described above. The same completely assembled MH is depicted in FIGURE 4. The dynamic *in vitro* testing of protoype MSTDs and MHs using the servocontrol system has been performed under both mildly and strongly pulsatile flows simulated in a Circulation Model. The photograph displayed in FIGURE 5 illustrates the support-free suspension of a MSTD prototype in a liquid contained within a tube around which a MH is positioned.

Although the electronic control system for suspension of MSTDs under venous flow conditions is substantially less complex than that required for opera-

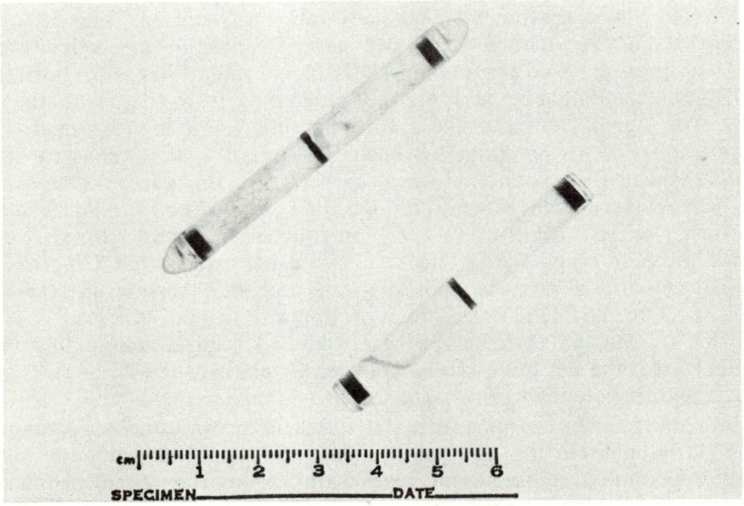

FIGURE 2. Actual size of MSTD prototypes displaying different geometri

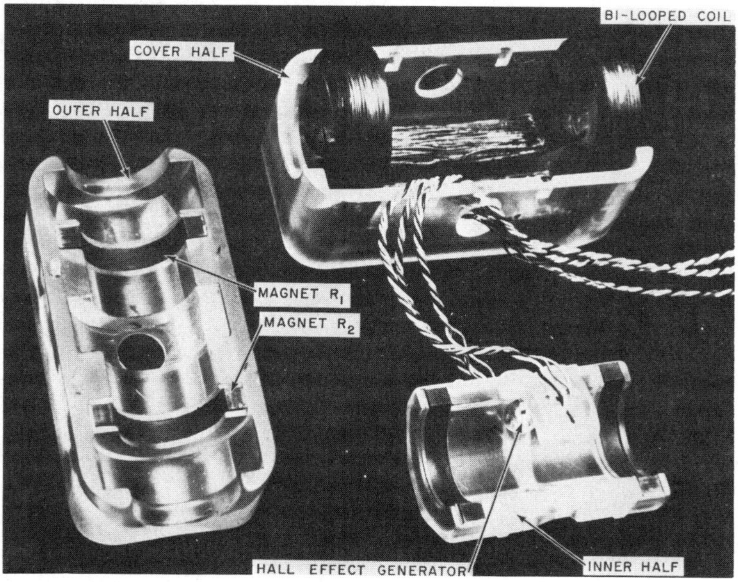

FIGURE 3. Magnetic housing (MH) components.

tion under aortic flows, application of this procedure in large veins is complicated by the relatively low internal pressures and the poor mechanical properties of venous walls. Both of these factors are liable to lead to collapse and/or kinking of the vessel unless external reinforcement is implemented. Exploratory surgeries performed on large St. Bernard dogs weighing in excess of 50 kg indicated that their external jugular vein is favorably positioned as a potential site for MSTD implantations. This vein provides a sufficient length of straight vessel, and it is accessible with minimal amount of surgical intervention. Neither the intrathoracic nor the abdominal portions of the cava were found feasible for eventual long-term implantations. However, preliminary studies, which involved the external placement of DeBakey single crimp Dacron® grafts as reinforcements around the external jugular vein of those animals have not as yet yielded conclusive results.

In view of the anatomical/surgical uncertainties potentially encountered on the venous side, the aortic implantation of MSTDs was emphasized particularly in terms of the required surgical techniques as well as the refinements needed in the electronic control system for routine operation under strongly pulsatile flow conditions.

For aortic MSTD implantations, large St. Bernard dogs were, again, selected as experimental animals because their aortic I.D.s are generally in the suitable range of 1.8–2.0 cm. Following a thoracotomy performed under standard sterile conditions, the thoracic aorta is dissected from surrounding tissues for a length of about 8 cm, and several pairs of intercostal arteries are located and tied off. The components of the MH displayed in FIGURE 3 are subsequently assembled over and around the exposed aortic segment, as schematically illustrated in FIGURE 6. The MH whose dimensions and contours are designed to provide a

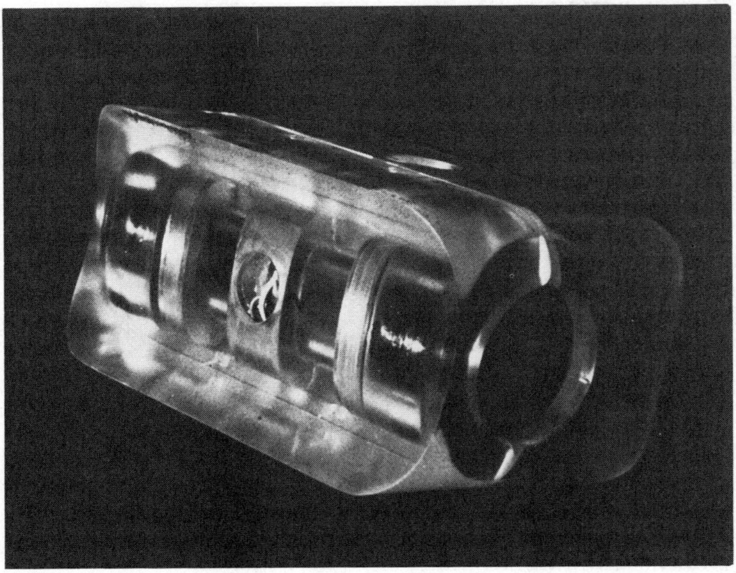

FIGURE 4. Assembled magnetic housing (MH).

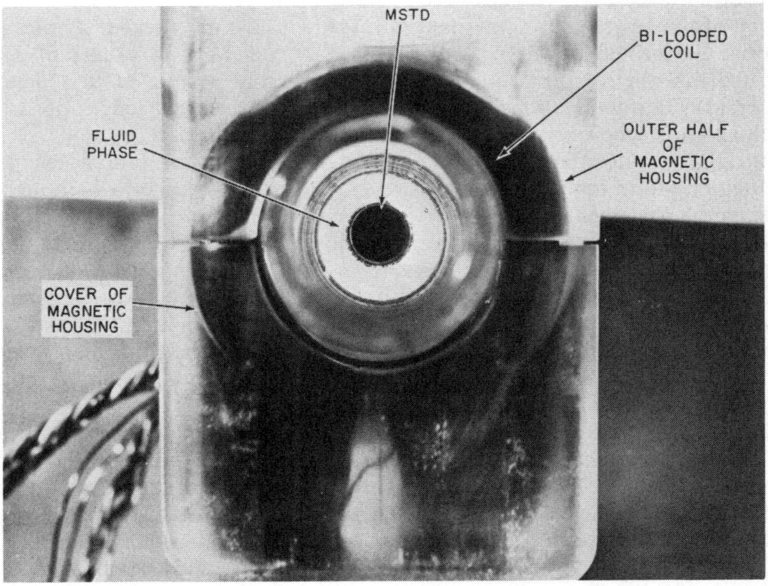

FIGURE 5. MSTD electromagnetically suspended in a liquid.

good fit when placed between the spinal column and the aorta is immobilized by being anchored to the ventral ligaments of the vertebrae by monofilament sutures. At a small distance downstream from the MH, a periarterial electromagnetic flow probe (not shown in FIGURE 6) is also implanted for the continuous monitoring of mean and pulsatile flow velocities. In the case of long-term tests, in which the animal is allowed to recover from the MH implantation, all connecting leads are expected to be exteriorized through a skin button with a tissue-facing side promoting ingrowth. Following an ample period of post-operative recovery, and after it has been established that its hematologic parameters have returned to normal preoperative levels, the experimental animal is ready for MSTD insertion. As indicated in FIGURE 6, this is accomplished via the right femoral and iliac arteries by moving the MSTD, which is enclosed in a hydraulically controlled catheter filled with normal saline, to the vicinity of the MH. The specimen is moved upstream toward the MH until a Hall-

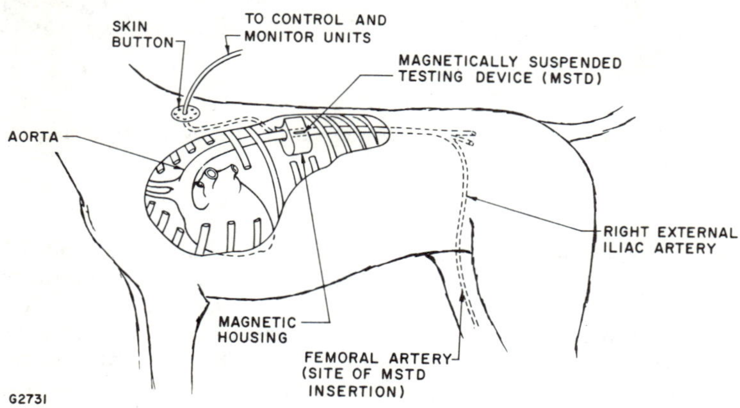

FIGURE 6. Schematic of MH implantation and MSTD insertion in an experimental animal.

voltage signal of prespecified magnitude is detected by the Gs indicating that it is sufficiently close to its operational region. At this point, the MSTD is gently dislodged and electromagnetically retrieved from the catheter by activation of power to the control system.

By means of the insertion technique described above, the test material constituting the surface of the MSTD becomes exposed only to native arterial blood. Since transfer of the MSTD from the catheter to the operational region is performed electromagnetically, contact with arterial intimae can be avoided. Surgical trauma and the release of thrombogenic tissue components occur at an insertion site far downstream from the test region. Results obtained during chronic implantations of nonoperational prototypes confirmed that the intima within the aortic segment externally surrounded by the MH remains completely free of thrombi and without any detectable evidence of trauma or lesions. This is exemplified in FIGURE 7, where a canine aortic segment around which a MH was positioned for 31 days is shown.

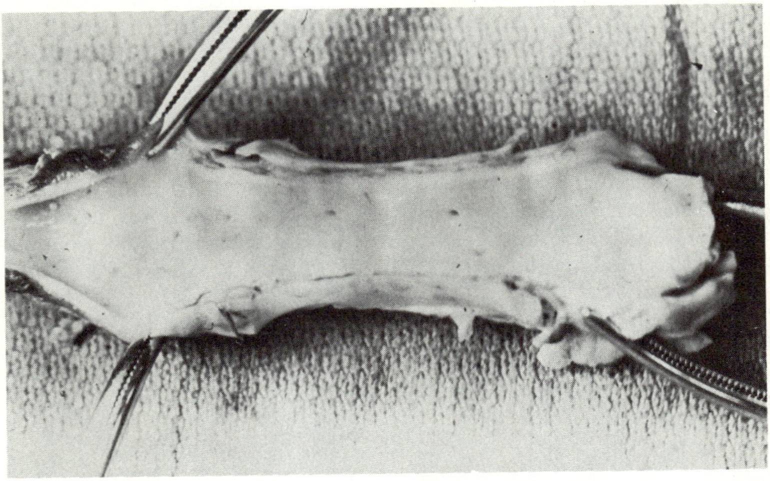

FIGURE 7. Canine aortic segment which was surrounded by a MH implanted for 31 days, showing no evidence of intimal lesions.

During a hemocompatibility test, the exact position of the suspended MSTD is continuously monitored, as are the mean and instantaneous controlcoil currents and the mean and pulsatile flow velocities. Since the magnitude of the coil current is proportional to the net electromagnetic force required to balance the fluid forces acting on the suspended specimen, the simultaneous measurement of currents and aortic flow velocities provides a real-time instrumental monitor of variations in the drag forces that occur as a result of the deposition of thrombus on the surface under evaluation. The degree of sensitivity for the detection of thrombus growth on a MSTD prototype of given geometrical configuration is primarily determined by the precision in the measurement of flow velocities.

The capability of the MSTD system to detect thrombus growth was simulated by the suspension of several MSTD prototypes of identical geometrical configuration but displaying incrementally increased outer diameters. Illustrative results obtained during *in vitro* testing of these prototypes under dynamic conditions corresponding to the velocity range typical of canine aortas are shown in FIGURE 8. The current required to balance the drag induced by two MSTD prototypes, differing by about 10% in diameter, is plotted as a function of the square of the flow velocity. As indicated, the 10% increase in diameter results in a drag increase of about 20%, which can be easily detected by measurement of the corresponding values of the coil current. These data also indicate that for MSTD specimens possessing the tip configuration depicted in FIGURE 8, uniform growth of thrombi can be expected to become instrumentally discernible from that point on when the thickness of the deposited layer exceeds a value in the order of 100 μ.

The drag forces acting on a suspended MSTD are obviously a function of its shape as well as the smoothness and uniformity of its blood-contact surface.

In addition to size, the only other geometrical constraint is that the specimen must be an axisymmetric body of revolution. Otherwise, test prototypes can be built to display variable degrees of streamlining, as has been illustrated in FIGURE 2, to assess the effects on thrombus growth, if any, of different flow patterns near the MSTD surface. For example, a specimen for suspension within the canine aorta can be shaped so as to present a large stagnation flow region on its forebody to evaluate the hemocompatibility of the blood-contact surface under flow conditions known to favor the formation of thrombi. The flat-ended MSTD prototype displayed in FIGURE 2 exemplifies this hydrodynamically unfavorable case. The performance of a material in this type of flow regime is of considerable importance in view of the fact that many prosthetic devices exhibit stagnation areas. Alternatively, MSTDs can be shaped into more favorable hydrodynamic geometries to assess the performance of their surface material under less stringent flow conditions. In these cases, however, the sensitivity in the measurement of drag changes associated with thromboembolic phenomena is correspondingly increased.

It is anticipated that ambiguities will arise in the interpretation of the continuously-recorded *in vivo* drag measurements since the shape and texture of thrombi depositing on the specimen are likely to vary. It is expected, however, that by means of extensive testing of appropriately designed MSTD models under simulated flow conditions as well as by the examination of specimens

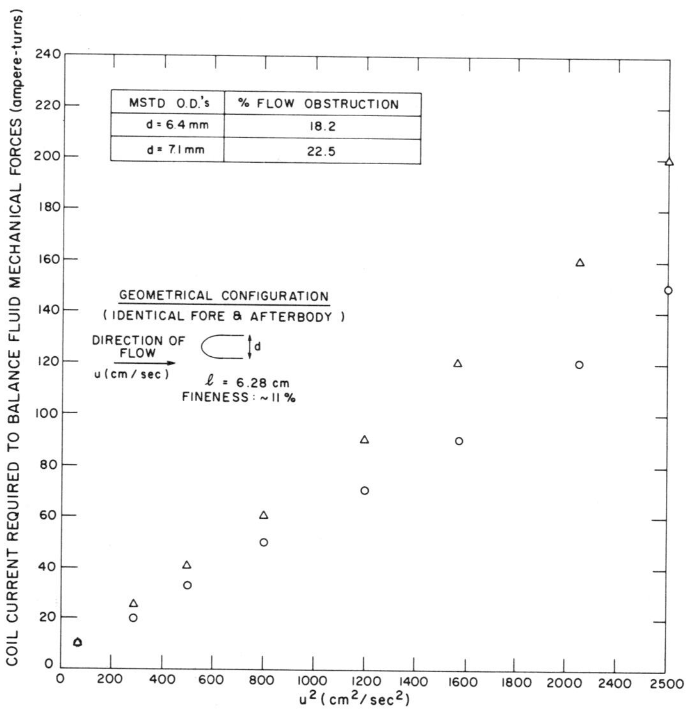

FIGURE 8. Calibrating measurements illustrating system sensitivity in the detection of simulated uniform thrombus growth.

recovered intact from *in vivo* experiments, information useful to the resolution of potential ambiguities will be obtained.

Following extensive testing of the MSTD system which, as noted earlier, involved use of a Circulation Model to simulate mildly as well as strongly pulsatile flows, short-term suspension trials were initiated with large St. Bernard dogs. The experiments performed to date were designed only to allow for an assessment of the system's performance capabilities under *in vivo* aortic flow conditions, and to reveal any operational difficulties that may not have come to light in the course of *in vitro* testing. In view of the preliminary acute nature of these *in vivo* trials, MSTD prototypes were inserted into the aorta immediately after implantation of MHs. While intermissions in the support-free suspension occurred in these experiments requiring external manipulations to reestablish the coaxial position of MSTDs, the *in vivo* operational feasibility of the system, including the catheter-guided specimen insertion procedure, was found to be satisfactory.

Summary

A system that is capable of the support-free, coaxial, suspension of test specimens in suitably sized canine blood vessels has been under development to advance the state of the art of the *in vivo* hemocompatibility assessment of prosthetic materials. The support-free suspension of the test device, whose surface is of the material to be evaluated, is accomplished by means of servomechanically controlled electromagnetic forces that continuously balance fluid forces acting on the specimen. The variations in drag that result from the deposition or embolization of thrombi are expected to be continuously monitored, yielding a real-time instrumental assessment of the evolution of thromboembolic phenomena on the test surfaces. The suspension of specimens in venous flows was found to be contingent upon the success achieved in the external reinforcement of the easily collapsible venous walls. Under aortic flow conditions, test devices with geometries displaying large stagnation flow regions are used initially. Although preliminary acute *in vivo* trials performed in the thoracic aorta of large St. Bernard dogs have experimentally verified the feasibility of the required surgical techniques and the adequate performance of the suspension system, additional refinements and extensive testing of hardware are actively pursued at present to reach the stage of routine applications.

Acknowledgment

The authors are grateful to Drs. R. E. C. Collins and N. P. Coe for their cooperation in the development of required surgical techniques and to Mr. R. A. Morgan for his assistance in the design and construction of the hardware components.

References

1. Gott, V. L., D. E. Koepke, R. L. Doggett, W. Zarnstoff & W. P. Young. 1961. The coating of intravascular prostheses with colloidal graphite—the relative im-

portance of electrical charge in the prevention of clot formations. Surgery **50:** 382.

2. KUSSEROW, B. K., R. W. LANOW & J. E. NICHOLS. 1970. Observations concerning prosthesis—induced thromboembolic phenomena made with an in vivo embolus test system. Trans. Am. Soc. Artif. Intern. Organs. **16:** 58.
3. SAWYER, P. N. & S. SRINIVASAN. 1969. New approaches in the selection of materials compatible with blood. Proc. Artif. Heart Program Conf. R. Johnsson-Hegyeli, Ed. : 243. U.S. Gov. Printing Office. Washington, D.C.

IN VIVO EVALUATION OF PROSTHETIC SURFACES

Philip N. Sawyer and Boguslaw Stanczewski

Electrochemical and Biophysics Laboratory
and Vascular Surgical Services
The Departments of Surgery and Surgical Research
State University of New York, Downstate Medical Center
Brooklyn, New York 11203

Basic ground rules must be established to permit the equivalent evaluation of various surfaces implanted in biologic systems. One notes that the dog, calf, and pig, as well as the lower primates, represent different opportunities in terms of the studies one may wish to carry out. This is illustrated in TABLE 1. The lower primates are the most satisfactory animals to use as physiological models of man. However, limited appropriate living space and cost make it very difficult to use large numbers of primates except in special care centers in the United States. Special primate centers have been established that have solved this problem only in part.

For this reason investigators tend to use dogs. A good equivalency has been established between man and dog in various experimental situations. In evaluating a prosthetic material, a number of criteria must be met in order to correlate prosthetic implantations carried out by various groups.

The materials to be tested must also be implanted in the form and shape in which they are to be used in man. The mechanical and rheological characteristics should, insofar as possible, be similar. The blood must be capable of seeing the prosthestic surface as it flows by. With respect to a tube prosthesis, the interface surface must be sufficiently long to have more than junctional inflow and junctional outflow potentials if one is to effectively evaluate the surface *per se*. This is one of the major problems of the Gott ring, which is very short.

Surfaces tested:

Must be electrochemically clean.

If positive in contact with blood, more than 250 mV with respect to the normal hydrogen electrode, these almost invaribly are thrombogenic.

If homogenously negative vs. NHE, the material is essentially worth testing in biological systems.

Shape and diameter: mechanical and rheological biological characteristics must be similar. Materials must be equivalent. The blood must be able to see the surface as it flows by.

Initial testing must involve both arterial and venous sides. The arterial side involves aortoiliac, femoral, and carotids, and the veins jugular and femoral in dogs.

Final evaluation must take place in the area of ultimate application.

Initial testing of any prothesis must involve evaluation in both the arterial and venous sites. Arterial implantations are usually done in the carotid, femoral, or aortic arteries. Venous implantations are usually done in the jugular and femoral veins or in the inferior or superior vena cava.

Within the matrix, if the conductive materials are homogeneously negative with respect to the normal hydrogen electrode in contact with blood, they tend to be nonthrombogenic (FIGURES 1 & 2). If nonconductive materials adsorb albumin or fibrinogen without subtracting an electron or denaturing the protein, this would normally tend to provide a less thrombogenic surface than is conventionally the case. We have never, however, seen a completely clean polymeric surface following implantation into any biologic system (see FIGURE 3).

The tissues removed are evaluated not only by gross inspection and photography, but should also have scanning electron microscopy, histology, histochemistry, and transmission electron microscopy evaluation to permit total visual examination of any interactions between the surface and blood at the interface.

Evaluating techniques should take the following into consideration.

Structural Integrity
How sterilized

TABLE 1. ANIMALS AS PHYSIOLOGICAL MODELS OF MAN

Choice of Animal	
Dog	No blood plasmin. One year followup is equivalent to three years of human life.
Calf	One year is equivalent to five years in humans. Healing rate, particularly fibroplasia, is approximately 5–10 times the adult human rate.
Pig	Genetically the pig is most like man, other than other primates. One year in a young pig approximates five years in the human. They are also very good for evaluating the effect of growth, if the implant is put in the pig when young
Lower Primates	The coagulation system is a good deal like that in man. One year approximates 2–3 years in man.

Observed changes or problems on removal. Inflammatory changes in the surrounding tissue which may be due to the reaction to polymer or to desorbed chemicals of the polymer itself
Histology
Histochemistry
Scanning electron microscopy to evaluate visual interreactions of surface with blood at the interface
Transmission electron microscopy for appropriate materials

If the prosthetic material is of biologic origin, porous, and/or tubular, one can also carry out electrokinetic and other electrochemical evaluations. We have recently completed the evaluation of a number of materials for potential use as catheters. The rules relating to utility described above also apply here. These studies included evaluation of sulfonated teflons, heparinized polypropylene, and polyethylene, native polypropylene, and polyethylene as well as ethylene acrylic acid (EAA) and its 60% ionized sodium salt. We found the latter to be least susceptible to thrombosis and periphlebitis when implanted in the

Metal or Alloy	Rest Potential in Blood mv/NHE: Before Pre-treatment	After 10/NHCl Cleaning	Post Mortem	THROMBOGENIC BEHAVIOR: Tube %Occlusion 0%. 100%	Valve %Occlusion 0%. 100%
Mg	-1500 to -1400	-	-		
Mg (Mg,Al,Zn)	-1110 to - 420	-1350 to - 500	-		
Al	- 750 to - 450	- 780 to - 540	- 560 to - 290		
Al (Al,Cu)	- 420 to - 390	- 530 to - 420	- 480 to - 280		
Al	- 760 to 630	Electro-polished	- 780 to - 730		
Al	- 485 to - 775	Glow discharge	- 560 to - 460		
Ti	- 250 to + 10	- 350 to - 200	- 190 to - 130		
Cd	- 250 to - 210	- 320 to - 280	-		
Co	- 240 to - 160	- 300 to - 260	-		
Ni	- 250 to - 230	- 300 to - 280	-		

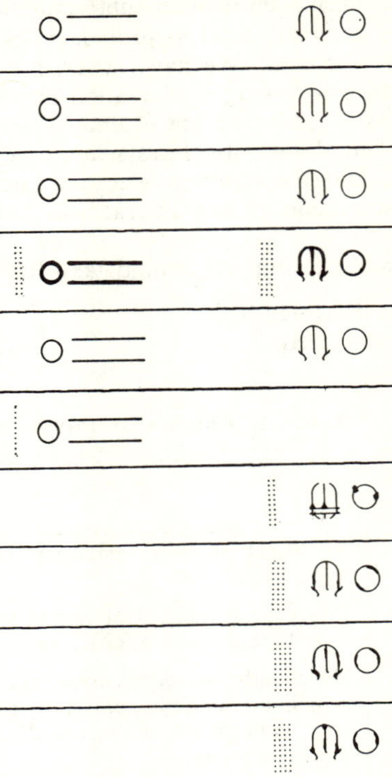

FIGURE 1. Materials from high in the electromotive series tend to be resistent to thrombosis in contact with blood. The numbers in columns two, three, and four refer to millivolts versus the normal hydrogen electrode in this figure. The materials most resistant to thrombosis are those which have the most negative corrosion potentials.

juglar and femoral veins and the right atrium of dogs. EAA 9500 catheters were next compared to commercially available intravenous catheters during long-term implantation in man for periods greater than three days (see FIGURE 4).

The Catheter Standards Committee of the Food and Drug Administration evaluates a catheter with respect to the following standards:

1) Toxicity
2) Radio Opacity
3) Thrombogenecity
4) Surface Properties
5) Physical Properties (thermal, chemical or mechanical, etc.)
6) Longevity

Metal or Alloy	Rest Potential in Blood mv/NHE Before Pre-treatment	After 10/NHCl Cleaning	Post Mortem	THROMBOGENIC BEHAVIOR Tube %Occlusion 0%. 100%	Valve %Occlusion 0%. 100%
Cu Cathodically polarized	+ 90 to + 150	- 10 to - 160	- 20 to + 40		
Cu Ac polarised 100,000/sec	+ 90 to + 180	+ 40 to + 90	+ 20 to + 80		
Cu	+ 120 to + 130	Glow discharge	+ 160 to + 165		
Cu	+ 90 to + 350	- 60 to + 140	+ 40 to + 70		
Ag	+ 800 to	+ 280 to	-		
Pt	+ 860	+ 320	-		
Au	+1500	+ 430			

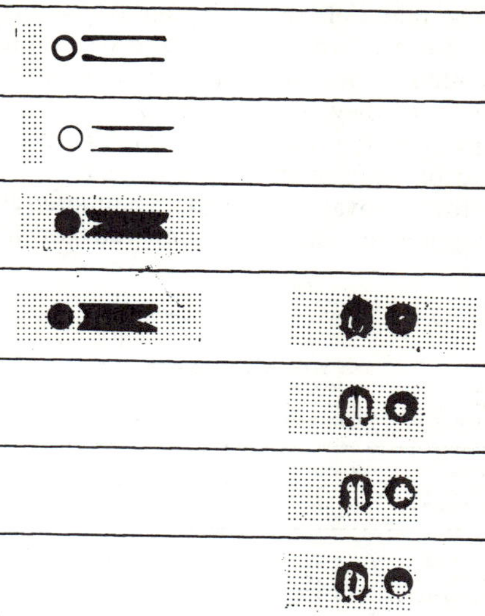

FIGURE 2. Normal metal tubes such as copper, silver, and platinum here illustrated are invariably thrombogenic. However, in the first two rows of this figure one can see cathodically polarized copper tubes that were maintained in a negative potential by use of a battery. Two types of negative charging were carried out; one DC and the other RF. The negative polarization in both instances tend to prevent thrombosis.

7) Identifiability
8) Pyrogenic Characteristics
9) Recommended use, sterilizing procedures
10) Contraindications.

The modern copolymer EAA 9500 has distinct advantages as an intravenous catheter in all the positions in which it was tested (FIGURE 4). EAA is biologically *minimally reactive* and relatively *nonthrombogenic* during long-term implantation.

It appears not to desorb oxidants and/or catalyzers, which produce both phlebitis and periphlebitis during long-term implantation in both experimental animals and man.

The materials now appear ready for general application in man. This group has tested more than 200 different materials in the past fifteen years. The various materials tested by all of us include Gott rings, Sawyer rings, tubes, catheters, heart valves, prosthetic heart chambers, and so on. The *in vivo* evaluation techniques, although increasingly expensive, are extraordinarily useful in the final evaluation of the materials considered for use in man. This is an integral component of the developing situation relating to the testing of prosthetic devices in man as applied by the Food and Drug Administration.

SUMMARY

The materials tested in this laboratory are implanted in the area of choice in the form in which they are to be evaluated. If they are heart valves they are implanted in one or another anulus in the heart of a satisfactory experimental animal. If they are tubular they can be placed into the arterial-venous tree of any one of a number of experimental animals. Implanted for an indicated period of time, they are left in place until the animal either dies or the elected time for removal is reached. The materials are then removed, grossly evaluated, photographed, and then prepared for the histological and scanning electron

Metal or Alloy	Rest Potential in Blood mv/NHE: Before Pre-treatment		Rest Potential in Blood mv/NHE: Post Mortem	THROMBOGENIC BEHAVIOR: Tube %Occlusion 0%. 100%	THROMBOGENIC BEHAVIOR: Valve %Occlusion 0%. 100%
Porous CARBON (Le Carbone)	+ 300 to + 320	Not treated	+ 300 to + 310		
Vitreous CARBON (Le Carbone)	+ 280 to + 970		+ 300 to + 90		
Porous CARBON (Gulf General Atomic)	+ 280 to + 220		+ 230 to + 180		
Pyrolytic CARBON (Gulf General Atomic)	+ 320 to + 570		+ 130 to - 280		
BIOELECTRIC POLYURETHANE (Goodyear Res. Lab.)	- 160 to - 140		- 160 to - 10		
ELECTROLOUR	+ 320 to + 360		- 460 to - 410		
TEFLON Coated Stellite-21 valves Untreated	-		-		
Sulfonated TEFLON (Coated Stellite-21) 1.3 to 0.6 moles/cm^2	- 140 to - 80		- 260 to + 60		
Carboxylated TEFLON (Coated Stellite-21 0.53 moles/cm	- 10 to + 40		+ 210 to + 180		
Untreated POLYPROPYLENE	-		-		
Sulfonated POLYPROPYLENE	-		-		

FIGURE 3. Certain types of polymer surfaces with an appropriate negative charge also are resistent to thrombosis. It is seen here that various types of carbon as well as specially modified Teflon ® in this instance sulfonated or "green" Teflon, also proved to be very resistent to thrombosis when in contact with blood.

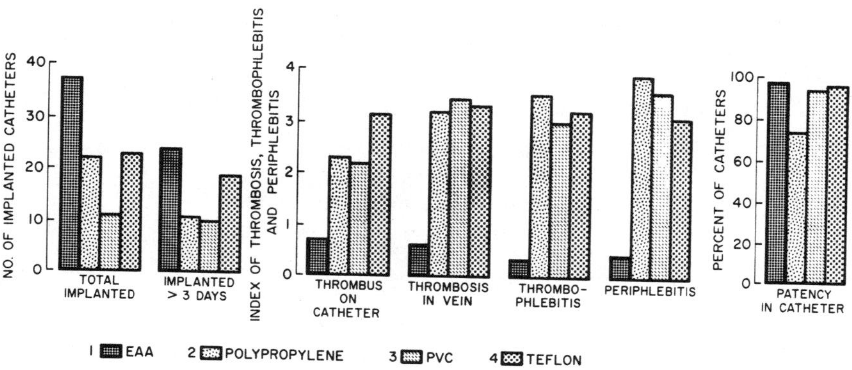

FIGURE 4. Evaluation of several catheter materials in man reveal that ethylene acrylic acid produces least thrombosis, thrombophlebitis, and periphlebitis.

micrographic analysis. When this is done, selected sections of the material are subjected to transmission microscopy. The resulting analysis is codified as tabular data with use of a distinctive analytic approach to the evaluation of the materials in question.

EVALUATION OF ARTIFICIAL INTERFACES WITH *IN VIVO* SYSTEMS

Robert S. Litwak, George Silvay, Howard Shiang

Department of Surgery
Division of Cardiothoracic Surgery
The Mount Sinai Medical Center
New York, New York 10029

Edward F. Leonard

The Artificial Organs Research Laboratory
Columbia University School of Engineering and Applied Science
New York, New York 10027

There is universal agreement that the adverse reaction which occurs when blood comes in contact with foreign surfaces is the dominant cause of mortality and morbidity associated with prosthetic valve and vascular replacement or protracted mechanical cardiorespiratory support. Thus, during the past two decades major efforts have been made to discover inert, thromboresistant—"biocompatible"—materials with durable and physiologically acceptable performance characteristics.

Evaluation of potential cardiovascular implant materials in the intact animal remains a complex task, since our knowledge of factors associated with *in vivo* compatibility is so incomplete. The ideal study method would be performed in an environment that would accurately reproduce the clinical conditions demanded of the material, permit controlled perturbation of each of all known variables, and, finally, allow continuous analysis of biophysical and pathophysiologic events associated with or caused by the material. Presently, there is no testing method—*in vitro, ex vivo* or *in vivo*—that satisfies the criteria of the ideal study method. Discussion of the former two methods will be found elsewhere in this volume. It is the purpose of this communication to consider progress and problems with *in vivo* systems employed in evaluating artificial interfaces.

In Vivo Testing Methods

In the absence of *in vitro* methods of established reliability and relevance to clinical situations, an obvious course open to investigators was the empirical placement of implants in the intact animal cardiovascular system to see "what would happen." During the past 16 years an extraordinary variety of implants of every conceivable description have been inserted into virtually every cardiac chamber, major artery, or vein. These include daggers, swords, discs, flaps, fiber loops, hollow tubes, solid tubes, and fabricated prostheses consisting of valves and tubular grafts. Gott's demonstration [1-3] that inferior vena caval implantation of varyingly treated molded tubes could be a screening method to test thrombogenicity soon led to its widespread use. The method continues to be used as a means of attempting to determine the nature, sequence, and severity of events at the cardiovascular material-flowing blood interface. Both Baier and Daniels and their respective colleagues have refined the Gott tube implantation method and have documented that careful engineering and handling of the tubes is essential (smooth nonflawed bores, precisely beveled ends, meticulous cleaning, improved surgical technique) so that more reliable results can be obtained.[4-5]

Information Developed by *In Vivo* Testing Methods

Thrombus Generation

Early studies performed with a variety of geometric forms (swords, flaps, etc.) placed in an area of the test animal's cardiovascular system did not predictably establish controlled conditions for variables such as fluid mechanics (flow rate, shear stresses), precise loci, area, and angular relationships of tissue-material contact, nor was the need for meticulous engineering and handling of the test implant properly appreciated. Thus, interpretation of these data is difficult.

The caval ring test of Gott[1-3] was the first attempt to systematically control some of these variables utilizing a carefully engineered geometric configuration. As suggested earlier, these important studies permitted screening of a large number of candidate materials and surfaces, some of them demonstrating significant thromboresistance as qualitatively defined by absent or minimal thrombus within the tubes when examined after two hours or two weeks of implantation. In subsequent studies Gott and associates[6] added a circumferential ridge within the tube (Figure 1) to adversely alter flow geometry in order to provide a more severe test of thromboresistance. It was observed that the amount of thrombus that developed in these "turbulent rings" was significantly greater when compared to the smooth rings coated with the same thromboresistant material. Moreover, the thrombus appeared to have a tendency to start on the exposed corner of the leading edge of the ridge.

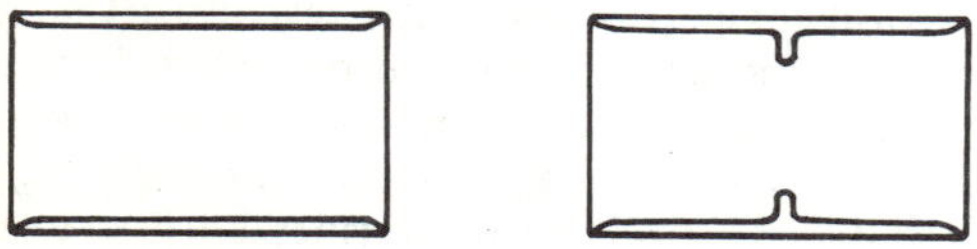

Figure 1. Illustration of two types of Gott vena caval ring implants. On the left is the more widely used smooth internal surfaced ring. On the right is the turbulent type, a later design with a circumferential ridge within the tube to alter flow geometry adversely.

Attempts have been made to study the rate of thrombus generation in tubes acutely implanted in the canine external jugular vein utilizing continuous flow measurements.[7] A correlation was demonstrated between the reduction of measured flow through the tubes and thrombus buildup (Figure 2). It is apparent, however, that moment-to-moment changes in cardiac output and venous return could significantly influence the flow measurements and potentially invalidate conclusions regarding the onset of thrombosis within the tube.

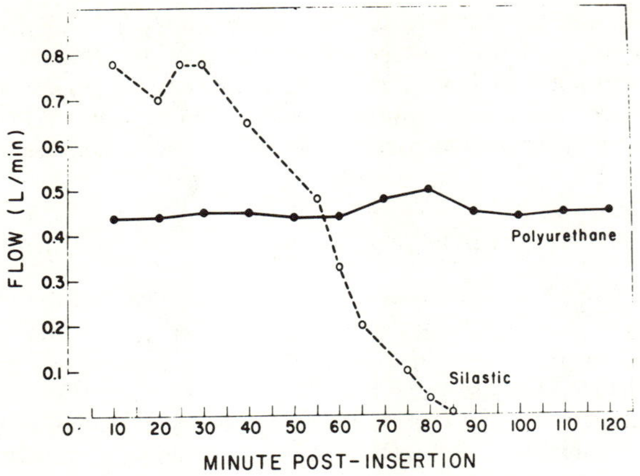

FIGURE 2. Flow measurements vs. time, after implantation of test rings in the external jugular vein of dogs. The study suggests substantial thromboresistance of polyurethane compared to "Silastic." (By permission of the publishers of Trans. Amer. Soc. Artif. Int. Organs.[7])

Thrombus Alteration: Fibrinolysis and Embolization

In vivo lysis of a coagulum is a well-recognized homeostatic response. Using implanted atrial "swords," each of which had an incorporated thrombus-detecting device operating on a thermal flux principle, Jacobs and associates[8] were able to detect the rate of thrombus growth and disappearance. The data suggested that thrombus formation on the "sword" occurred during the first two hours of implantation with a definite diminution of thrombus between 4 and 24 hours. It was suggested that the gradual fall of the curve (FIGURE 3) was more compatible with lytic mechanisms than thrombotic embolization off the "sword," which presumably would have been accompanied by a sudden sharp drop in the curve. No consistent alteration in euglobulin lysis time could be

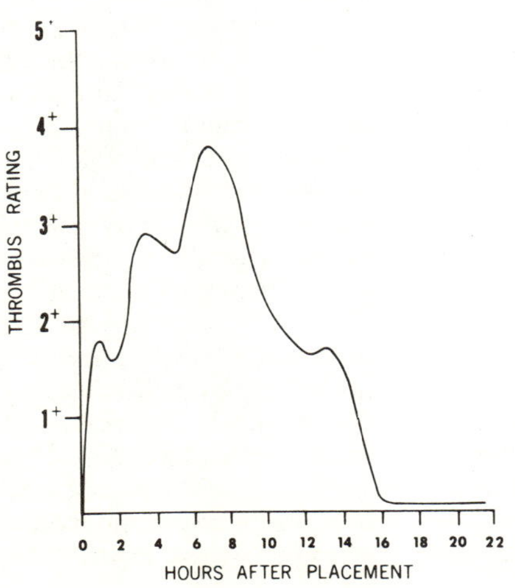

FIGURE 3. Thermal flux monitoring of thrombus present on an atrial "sword" over a 22-hour period. The gradual fall of the curve suggests lysis of the thrombus. (By permission of the publishers of Trans. Amer. Soc. Artif. Int. Organs.[8]

detected during sword implantation, suggesting that the process was a local one taking place in the immediate environment of the sword.

An obvious critical determinant of thromboresistance of any cardiovascular implant would be clear demonstration of absent or minimal embolic potential. Although the physical and biological events underlying embolization of all or a portion of an implant thrombus are still poorly understood, the major role played by fluid shear stresses is well recognized. A second mechanism, characterized as a consumptive coagulopathy, has been elucidated from studies with the artificial heart. Multiple small platelet and fibrin emboli are formed as a result of blood-foreign material contact, and a clinical picture analagous to that seen with disseminated intravascular coagulation (shock) ultimately develops.[9]

The late Bert Kusserow and his colleagues [10] attempted to develop a sensitive *in vivo* test system capable of detecting both thrombotic and embolic events. Conceptually, Kusserow reasoned, an organ with little or no effective collateral circulation through which there was an obligatory course of blood would, of

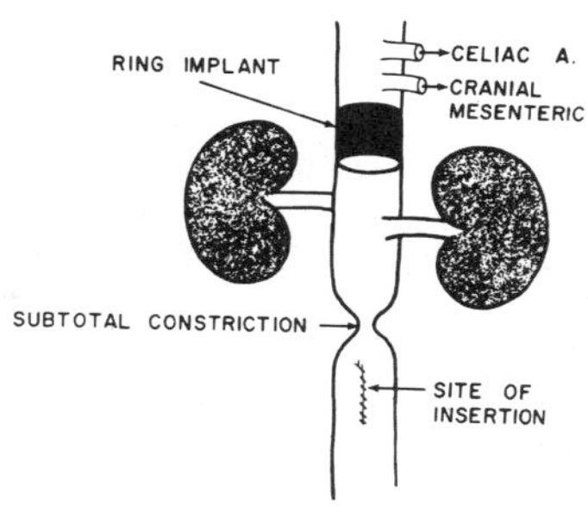

FIGURE 4. Renal embolus test system: *in vivo* test system utilizing downstream renal vascular bed and parenchyma as biologic indicators of embolic events. Subtotal occlusion of distal aorta results in renal perfusion of more than 90% of blood traversing the ring implant. (By permission of the publishers of Trans. Amer. Soc. Artif. Int. Organ.[11])

necessity, demonstrate the pathologic evidence of emboli (ischemic necrosis or degenerative changes) originating from an upstream implanted prosthetic device. Initial attempts involved experimental modification of the pulmonary circulation in such a fashion that the lung became increasingly susceptible to infarction by pulmonary emboli.[10] The model was abandoned because of the variability of the bronchial arterial collateral circulation in the dog. A second and more satisfactory indicator of embolic events involved use of the kidneys [11, 12] (FIGURE 4). The test prosthesis was implanted immediately above the origin of the renal vessels (for periods of two to five days) and the aorta below the renal arteries was constricted subtotally. Under these conditions it was demonstrated that more than 90% of blood that coursed through the implant perfused the kidneys. These important studies conclusively demonstrated the high incidence of embolization (as indicated by the presence of renal infarcts) that was associated with smooth-walled aortic ring implants. Further, the finding of multiple renal infarcts in circumstances where the implanted test ring was completely free of thrombus defined a key weakness inherent in contemporary *in vivo* testing methods by confirming that absence of thrombus on a test implant in no way eliminated the possibility of antecedent embolization.

Problems With *In Vivo* Testing Methods

A number of problems can be identified when evaluation of materials is conducted by an implant method in the intact animal.[13-15] Since the functional requirements and environments of different cardiovascular devices vary substantially, it is probable that no single *in vivo* test can be expected to yield across-the-board reliability and relevance. For example, we know that a knitted polyester tubular conduit placed in a high-flow, high-velocity vessel such as the aorta provides long-term satisfactory functional performance and is adequately thromboresistant in that environment. However, use of the same material as leaflet valves placed in areas of relative stasis and turbulence will be disastrous because of the greater propensity of thrombus formation in that environment. On theoretical grounds it could be argued that a single *in vivo* test would indeed suffice if a material was found which, when implanted as an experimental leaflet, functioned physiologically, was highly durable, and exhibited exceptional thromboresistance in that environment. Unfortunately the proposition must remain theoretical, since such a material would come close to satisfying requirements for the optimal cardiovascular biomaterial, an achievement that is nowhere in sight.

A critical deficiency that is characteristic of *in vivo* testing methods is the fact that each study yields but one conclusive datum at the end of the test. Thus, systematic analysis of transients is not possible. This problem has been clearly characterized in the pathological studies of Kusserow and his colleagues,[11, 12] who showed that a thrombus generated in a test system (ring implant) may well have totally embolized by the time the device is subsequently examined, leading to the erroneous conclusion that it possessed a high degree of thromboresistance (Figure 5). The criminal, so to speak, would have left the scene of the crime. Moreover, the evidence that a crime had taken place at all may be virtually nonexistent, since, given time, the remarkable fibrinolytic and reparative systems of the intact animal may have obliterated most or all of the evidence of prior thrombus generation in the device or subsequent embolization to downstream organs.

Biological variability from animal to animal poses a major problem, particularly differences in coagulation spectra. An example of this was observed in a

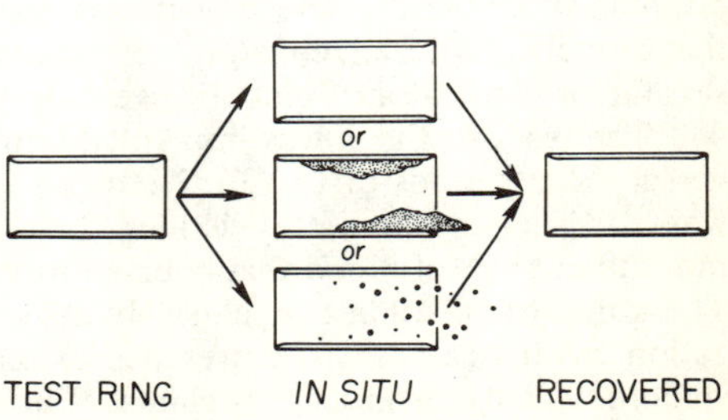

Figure 5. The problem characteristic of current *in vivo* testing methods in which only one observation is permitted at the end of the test. Three *in situ* possibilities are illustrated: consistent absence of thrombus or formation of either large or multiple small thrombi with embolization in the latter two circumstances. In two of the three possibilities, recovery of the device without evidence of retained thrombus could lead to an erroneous conclusion that the system was thromboresistant.

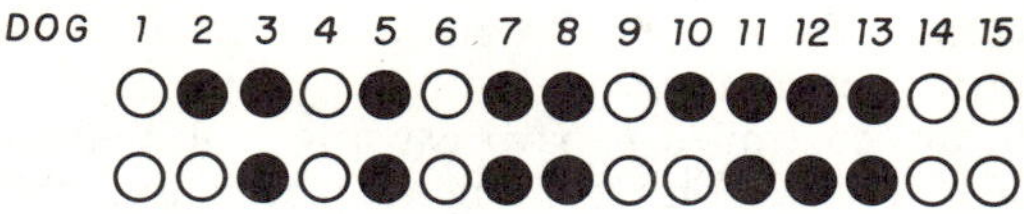

FIGURE 6. Two-hour tube implant test (duPont PR-241E). Biologic variability is suggested by the results of combined superior and inferior vena caval implants in 15 animals. Although the presence or absence of thrombus in the 30 rings yielded disparate results, the frequency of identical observations in both tubes (13 of 15) was statistically significant, implying that dog-to-dog systemic differences may account for these findings. Thrombus *in situ:* ○=absent in both (6); ●=present in both (7); in one (2).

series of combined inferior and superior vena caval ring implants performed in our laboratory. The rings were molded from a candidate fluoropolymer (Dupont PR-241-E). The results of the two-hour paired implant study are depicted in FIGURE 6. Seven animals had thrombus formation in both tubes, whereas in six dogs both tubes were free of thrombus. Only two dogs had thrombus in one tube but not the other. Thus, although the presence or absence of thrombus yielded largely disparate results (in that nine dogs had evidence of thrombosis in at least one ring and six dogs had none in both rings), the frequency of identical results in both implants observed in 13 of the 15 animals (i.e., both tubes either free of thrombus or both thrombosed) was statistically significant ($p < 0.01$). The conclusion is inescapable that dog-to-dog differences of coagulation and possibly hemodynamic transients must have played a significant role in the results. Although the data derived from the 30 rings in the 15 dogs were inconclusive regarding the relative thromboresistance of the fluoropolymer, the high degree of directional agreement of the paired-ring results in each animal is noteworthy.

Finally, in view of the fact that each *in vivo* study generally allows only one experimental observation period with little certainty that apart from the implant all variables are controlled, statistical requirements demand performance of a relatively large number of experiments, the cost of which is considerable.

DISCUSSION

Despite the seemingly superior relevance of *in vivo* material-blood-recipient locus evaluation, the control and analytical problems associated with existing test methods tend to raise more questions than provide answers. Indeed, at this time we really are not certain what it is that we should measure, much less how best to do it. Emil Fischer's admonition, "Die methode ist alles," comes to mind.

There is reasonable certainty that the notion of a "nonthrombogenic *surface*" is simplistic; there probably isn't such an entity. We should have inferred this, since, given the proper adverse set of conditions, thrombosis may occur in man on histologically normal left atrial endocardium or intima of a vessel. It is now generally agreed that thromboresistance is determined by an *environment.* While it is certainly true that the physical properties of a surface play a significant role in determining interfacial events, at least four other factors are involved: hematologic variables, flow geometry, flow rate, and exposure time.[16] It therefore seems unreasonable to expect that any *in vivo* test that does not permit systematic control and perturbation of each of these variables could yield precise information concerning the relative thromboresistance of a candidate material, surface, or geometric configuration.

Only when rigidly controlled *in vivo* experimental methods are developed will there be reliable information regarding the mechanism and, it is hoped, the time sequence of those three phenomena which presently limit design and wider application of prosthetic cardiovascular prostheses: consumption, thrombus formation, and embolization.

Five years ago at the New York Academy of Medicine *Symposium on Problems in Evaluating the Blood Compatibility of Biomaterials,* Dr. Vincent Gott concluded his remarks by stating ". . . at this time we have some rather crude methods for the evaluations of . . . materials, and I think it is time that we now apply the scientific method to this problem of determining the biocompatibility of intravascular test materials."[13] The goal still eludes us.

References

1. Gott, V. L., D. E. Koepke, R. L. Daggett, W. Zarnstorff & W. P. Young. 1961. The coating of intravascular plastic prostheses with colloidal graphite. Surgery **50:** 382–389.
2. Gott, V. L. 1966. The causes and prevention of thrombosis on prosthetic materials. J. Surg. Res. **6:** 274–283.
3. Gott, V. L. & A. Furuse. 1971. Antithrombogenic surfaces, classification and *in vivo* evaluation. Fed. Proc. **30:** 1679–1685.
4. Baier, R. E., V. A. de Palma, D. Goupil, S. Perlmutter, V. L. Gott & J. O'Riordan. 1975. Interfacial biophysics of materials in contact with blood. Ann. rpt. prepared for Biomaterials Program, Division of Blood Diseases and Resources, National Heart and Lung Institute. : 114–158.
5. Daniels, A. U. & J. D. Mortensen. 1975. Vena cava ring tests of biomaterials in dogs. Annual rpt. prepared for Biomaterials Program, Division of Heart and Vascular Diseases, National Heart and Lung Institute.
6. Gott, V. L., M. D. Ramos, F. B. Najjar, J. L. Allen & K. E. Becker. 1969. The *in vivo* screening of potential thromboresistant materials. Proc. Artif. Heart Program Conf. R. Johnsson Hegyeli, Ed. : 181–191.
7. Whalen, R. L., D. L. Jeffrey & J. C. Norman. 1973. A new method of *in vivo* screening of thromboresistant biomaterials utilizing flow measurement. Trans. Amer. Soc. Artif. Int. Organs **19:** 19–24.
8. Jacobs, L. A., E. Klopp & V. L. Gott. 1968. Studies on the fibrinolytic removal of thrombus from prosthetic surfaces. Trans. Amer. Soc. Artif. Int. Organs **14:** 63–68.
9. Devries, W., C. Kwann-Gett & W. Kolff. 1970. Consumptive coagulopathy, shock and the artificial heart. Trans. Amer. Soc. Artif. Int. Organs **16:** 29–36.
10. Kusserow, B., R. Larrow & J. Nichols. 1969. Analysis and measurement of the effects of materials on blood. An *in vivo* embolus test system. Proc. Artif. Heart Program Conf. R. Johnsson Hegyeli, Ed. : 233–242.
11. Kusserow, B., R. Larrow & J. Nichols. 1970. Observations concerning prosthesis-induced thromboembolic phenomena made with an *in vivo* embolus system. Trans. Amer. Soc. Artif. Int. Organs **16:** 58–62.
12. Kusserow, B. 1972. The use of pathologic techniques in the evaluation of emboli from prosthetic devices. Bull. N.Y. Acad. Med. **48:** 468–477.
13. Gott, V. L. 1972. The second decade of biomaterials development and evaluation: a time to apply the scientific method. Bull. N.Y. Acad. Med. **48:** 216–224.
14. Galletti, P. M. 1972. Discussion of paper by Bert K. Kusserow, M.D.: Use of pathologic techniques in the evaluation of emboli from prosthetic devices. Bull. N.Y. Acad. Med. **48:** 478–481.

15. SILVAY, G. 1972. Discussion of paper by Vincent L. Gott, M.D., and Akira Furuse, M.D.: Standardized methods for *in vivo* evaluation of artificial surfaces. Bull. N.Y. Acad. Med. **48:** 491–493.
16. BENIS, A. M., H. L. NOSSEL, L. M. ALEDORT, R. M. KOFFSKY, J. F. STEVENSON, E. F. LEONARD, H. SHIANG & R. S. LITWAK. 1975. Extracorporeal model for study of factors affecting thrombus formation. Thrombos. Diathes. Haemorrh. **34:** 127–144.

DISCUSSION

DR. DANIELS: Blood may be in contact with other surfaces before reaching the *ex vivo* test area. Do any of the speakers have comments on this major problem?

DR. HARKER: In trying to answer the question, we need some understanding of how matter moves in blood. Assuming laminar flow, one can make some calculations of the distance a particle or a molecule can move from the wall of a shunt to another spot in the shunt or on the device. For moderate flow rates, you will then find that a piece of tubing about 1000 cm long may not have a single molecule from the wall at the entrance reach the center line downstream. This means that in laminar flow, the shunt material would not affect the surface you are studying.

DR. LEONARD: There are two problems associated with answering that question. One is the local problem that Dr. Harker just talked about. The other is a systemic problem of the presence of the shunt creating some kind of general response in the animal. For example, the platelet counts that Dr. Schultz presented or the fibrinogen turnover rate may be changed. I believe there was about a 30%-reduction in platelet count as a result of shunting Dr. Schultz's animals.

DR. SCHULTZ: There are two phases, one acute and one chronic one. When the shunt was put in, there was a reduction of about 30% in platelets, representing about a 20% increase in turnover of platelets, while the other blood elements more or less leveled off after a week. After a testing procedure there was another drop in platelets and there was a consumption of fibrinogen amounting to another 10 or 15%. The question therefore is: what kind of blood are you testing even in an *ex vivo* system or an *in vivo* one?

DR. LEONARD: Either there can be a consumption coagulopathy so that you find an underresponse, or there may be a potentiation of certain enzymes and inactivation of others, so that you will find an overresponse. Though I do not think we know in detail yet which of these is likely to occur in which situation, I do think the shunted animal models are now known to be stable and to produce good relative results. Their responses are not contradictory to those gathered in other systems.

DR. S. AISENBERG (*Whittaker Corp., Waltham, Mass.*): The spatial resolution of ultrasonics—a technique that was proposed here to measure emboli—is limited by the wavelength of sound in the fluid. Several years ago we measured the size of emboli optically and found that we could get resolution down to 50 microns. I do not think ultrasonics will go down that far.

DR. LEONARD: True, but for particles smaller than 50 microns, one can get reflections without knowing the exact point of origin. Even smaller emboli may not be distinguishable from individual erythrocytes. Russell Patterson of Cornell University has used the noise from an ultrasonic flow meter in an extracorporeal circuit as a measure of embolus generation. The data are not quantitative.

We have been working on the creation of a uniform ultrasonic field through which the particles pass, so that the magnitude of the reflection will be a measure of particle size. I think the spatial resolution is not a key factor.

DR. AISENBERG: Another advantage of the optical method is that you can use several wavelengths, possibly to differentiate between red and white thrombi.

DR. BAIER: Dr. Kochwa, I believe you stated that protein adsorption and platelet adhesion are correlated with thrombogenesis, but we saw yesterday that platelet adhesion to the subendothelial lining does not cause thrombosis.

Second, I wonder if the inhomogeneity of your autoradiographs may be caused by peeling of the substrate. In the straight flow-through chamber I have seen such peeling, especially in the presence of heparin, rather than where no anticoagulants were used. The peeling was excessive on the lower energy surfaces such as polyalkyl sulfones, well siliconized, or very smooth surfaces. Your initial adsorptive events may have been uniform, but the film may have been disrupted by accumulation in the shear regime.

DR. KOCHWA: I presented data earlier (this volume) on static exposure—with no shear rate—of polyurethane, where we saw bare spots in about the same distribution as in this study. Also, this was pure protein solution and had nothing to do with peeling.

DR. BAIER: Dr. Vroman, in all of these *in vitro* systems, if dried for analysis, we are dealing with molecules that have been ripped out of context. Do you have a solution for this, such as a fixative?

DR. VROMAN: I think drying is always bad before most forms of testing. You, for example, should do your contact angles under water. We have a problem when applying antisera; we sometimes dry a flat surface with unknown adsorbed protein on it, so that we can then apply drops of different antisera on it simultaneously and identify the adsorbed protein quickly. However, a drop of antiserum on protein, or even a drop of protein on a clean surface, will spread and leave a "bull's eye"-shaped deposit. If we allow a drop of fibrinogen solution to fall and slowly spread on a clean, dry glass slide, then rinse it off and cover the slide with a platelet suspension, platelets will adhere also in a "bull's eye" pattern, with concentric densely and less-densely covered circles. I believe an advancing air/liquid/solid interface is especially damaging to adsorbate.

UNIDENTIFIED SPEAKER: Do any of these techniques allow the study of adsorbed protein conformation?

DR. BAIER: Rather than answer from our own work, I would like to report on a preprint from a coworker, Dr. James Mattson of the University of Miami, in Florida. He is using polarization-infrared spectroscopy, and found that with a change of surface potential on carbon, the unnatural form of adsorbed fibrinogen decayed back to the natural form. This situation can be reversed, so that one can create configurational changes of fibrinogen while it is at the interface.

DR. STROMBERG: We have observed similar, although not identical, kinds of changes; by means of ellipsometry we found that the applied potential caused conformational changes of adsorbed proteins.

DR. VROMAN: I would like to add, though, that at the moment the conformation of the adsorbed proteins we are discussing does not yet tell us much about their activity. We do not know yet, for example, what conformation of adsorbed fibrinogen is most attractive to platelets.

DR. BAIER: I think many of us believe that the best way to achieve biological compatibility of materials is to have the initially deposited material look as closely as possible like its state in solution. Many surfaces, such as those of polyether urethanes, have been modified on this basis. The very low surface free energy materials such as fluorocarbons and Teflon and the very high surface free energy ones such as metals and ceramics are both biologically intolerable to blood, because extremes of surface free energy probably cause unnecessary distortion in the deposited protein molecules. There is some happy middle ground of surface state—whether described by surface charge, surface chemistry, or some other parameter of the interface—that will correlate with deposition of undistorted matter.

DR. DANIELS: In efforts to overcome one of the problems that Dr. Litwak has described, we are in the process of exploring techniques for continuous monitoring of thrombus formation and embolization during *in vivo* experiments by two methods.

In addition, having looked at many dogs and many rings with and without clots on them, it strikes me, seeing Dr. Litwak's data as well, that often if a material is neither particularly thrombogenic nor particularly nonthrombogenic, the biological phenomena may dominate and create scattered results.

DR. LITWAK: I agree.

UNIDENTIFIED SPEAKER: One more difficulty to be remembered is that we are performing *in vivo* tests on animals, and cannot translate our data to human physiology.

DR. AISENBERG: It often takes two weeks per datum point of an *in vivo* study, so that it is extremely difficult to react quickly and do the parametric studies required. That is why I think we must concentrate on continuous *in vivo* tests. We have been developing one invasive and two noninvasive ones that could be very useful in animals, and in humans as well, to test patency of arterial grafts in legs. There is considerable concern in verifying the patency of these grafts. Ultimately, when biocompatible materials get to be used in humans, we will need such continuously monitoring equipment.

PART X. SUMMARY

A PHYSICAL SCIENTIST'S VIEW *

A. Silberberg

Polymer Department
Weizmann Institute of Science
Rehovot, Israel

It might seem that the most appropriate way to discuss the physical features of the interaction of blood with interfaces would be to deal, in the most general way, with the transfer of the various cellular and macromolecular components from the blood to the interface, and vice versa, and to consider the mechanical, rheological and fluid mechanical aspects of flow in this connection. To do so, however, would miss an essential point; that at the interface of most interest, the physiological cell lining, the blood/interface interaction is in a stable steady state, which is not normally realized under other circumstances. In fact, the question arises whether these physiological conditions are unique, whether any combination of purely physical circumstances can create a stable blood-flow situation in any other way, whether, in other words, only the physiological situation is and can be stable and all other cases are transient.

An important reason for these circumstances might be that in the normal physiological steady state an active, cellular process is coupled to the physical processes, a process which, involving perhaps the endothelial cell layer, cannot be reproduced in any other way.

Whether or not, however, a purely physical steady state is involved, it is of great advantage to discuss the blood/interface interaction from the point of view of its normal steady state, considering it as reference and treating departures from these conditions, i.e. destabilization, predominantly in its physical aspects.

DESTABILIZATION AS A PROBLEM OF PLATELET ACTIVATION

The blood component most prominently responsible for destabilization is the platelet. It responds in particular to high levels of adenosine diphosphate (ADP) in the blood and itself acts as a source of this material. When ADP level is sufficiently high, the platelets undergo aggregation and set off the whole chain of events that lead to blood coagulation.

ADP can be released from platelets undergoing change in particularly stressful flow situations, but under more physiological conditions, ADP-release generally follows platelet adherence to a surface. Although contact with the intact endothelial lining does not produce activation, contact with most artificial surfaces does, and so, in particular, does contact with the collagen fiber surface. In fact, this is generally believed to be the mechanism of *hemostasis*. Vessel injury exposes collagen, and platelet activation produces first a platelet thrombus and then a full-fledged fibrin plug as first and second lines of defense against blood loss from the injury.

* Some of the ideas expressed have evolved out of work supported by contract no. NO1–HB–5–2907 with the National Heart and Lung Institute. They have been influenced in particular by results, as yet unpublished, of Dr. F. A. Meyer and Dr. Z. Weisman.

We may thus sharpen up this discussion of the behavior of blood at interfaces by concentrating on the physical aspects of the platelet/interface interaction—what produces and what controls platelet adherence at a surface and what gives rise to platelet activation and ADP-release when it is adherent.

Events subsequent to ADP-release are mainly biochemical in nature and no longer are very dependent upon physical parameters. Events that lead up to ADP-release are not well understood and are strongly dependent upon the physical aspects of the blood/interface interaction, but they may, as already pointed out, involve coupling to an active process. It is nevertheless most certainly worth while to examine the physical aspects of platelet activation and to see if they are the only ones that matter. Even if suitable physical conditions by themselves cannot produce a stable steady state at an artificial surface, it may be possible to find conditions that will introduce a minimal degree of destabilization. The passage of the flowing blood through the locally destabilizing region at the site of the prosthesis may then be sufficiently rapid to be counterbalanced by the subsequent contact with the normal interface.

Let us therefore ask a series of questions.

How Do Platelets Get to the Surface?

This is, in the first stage, a fluid mechanical problem. Particles suspended in a viscous fluid do not easily make contact with the confining walls unless additional non-Stokes flow effects are superimposed. These could be jostling by other cells in confined situations, inertial or gravitational effects, long-range forces between interface and cell, and, of course, diffusion. In a given flow situation, however, in steady state it may be assumed that the rate of arrival of cells at the wall is a well-controlled effect even though this rate may vary considerably from place to place. It is obviously of advantage to have this flux reduced to a minimum near surfaces that are suspected of being capable of activating platelets.

What Makes Platelets Adhere?

Whether cells adhere or not depends upon what happens to the cell when it is within the range of the forces that could attach it to the surface or is in the range of the dimensions of the structural units that sterically and mechanically delimit the molecular contact that can be established. In this respect, diffuse macromolecular surface layers on the interfaces involved could act both as contact-inhibiting and as contact-facilitating agents, and so could a variety of long-range molecular forces. One could imagine, moreover, that some metabolically supported active element is present that mechanically attaches and then speeds up the adherence of the cell. This could be incipient pseudopod formation but could also be based on other mechanisms that produce cell-shape changes and thereby promote the preliminary adherence stage. Such mechanisms could also operate in the opposite direction and on physiologically stable surfaces could inhibit efficient contact. It is not at all unreasonable in the case of platelets to assume that mechanochemically coupled reactions could affect the efficiency of "capture" of the cells by the surface.

In this respect, however, we are very much in the area of speculation, and it is perhaps impossible as yet to detail in any way the processes that occur when a cell reaches a certain proximity of the interface and then either stays in that proximity and adheres or wanders away and does not adhere. What may happen to a large extent depends upon the next question we may ask.

What is the Nature of the Surface with which the Platelet Interacts and How Does it Affect Adherence?

Neither the endothelial lining nor any artificially prepared surface interacts directly with the cells. The presence of so many different proteins in the blood make it almost certain that some, at any rate, will attach to the surface, and that the surface/surface interactions that occur are via superimposed protein coats. As is well known, macromolecules are very surface-active, and it is the exception, rather than the rule, that a surface involved will not get coated. At a completely virgin surface suddenly exposed to plasma, the rate of protein deposition would exceed that of cell interaction and, except for a few early cell arrivals, the test surface seen is the protein-coated one. Moreover, the proteins on the surface may not be in the structure in which we know them in solution. They may undergo conformational rearrangement, slow or fast, and the surface after some period of exposure may react quite differently from the surface that has just completed its first protein layer.

Is the Platelet/Surface Interaction Specific?

When, therefore, we ask the question whether the platelet/surface interaction is specific, it is to the protein layer-modified interface that we should relate, rather than to the virgin surface. It is thus very probable that the chemical variability of the surfaces that are to be considered is confined to the nature of the plasma proteins present and is far more restricted than might otherwise be supposed.

Not only are differences between surfaces smoothed out by the common protein coat, but the protein coat may convey the specificity that makes platelets adhere so effectively to the majority of surfaces that acquire the coat, rather than to the exceptional surface that does not. For example, many hydrogel surfaces, even in the presence of plasma proteins, do not interact with platelets, and there is little adhesion of platelets to the endothelial or red cell surface even though both these latter are in contact with plasma.

The effects, however, could also go in the opposite direction, and some surfaces that do not take the protein coat may bind platelets more effectively than the surfaces that have acquired it. This is the case with the collagen fiber surface to which binding is much more extensive than to nonorganized collagen or to plasma protein-coated surfaces. We do thus suspect that binding may involve factors which can single out some surfaces and cause the platelets to adhere to them in very large numbers under otherwise comparable conditions.

Adherence, however, is only part of the story. Once on the surface, the platelets in some cases do and in some cases do not go into activation; i.e., release ADP into their vicinity so that other platelets still in suspension become activated and aggregate on top of the initiating platelet. Hence the act of adherence *per se* is not enough and further differences between the surfaces to which the platelets can attach must be looked for.

Is the Mechanical Character and the Structure of the Surface Important?

It could be argued that if a substrate is mechanically weak and binding to it is not very strong, no activation is to be expected. The platelet has to be strongly attached at several separate locations on its surface to a mechanically stiff object of adequate size for activation to result. Not only a suitable chemical composition is important but the sites on the substrate must also be well distributed and the support has to be mechanically stiff.

Observations with collagen seem to favor this kind of view. Whereas platelets are rapidly activated by collagen fibers, platelet interaction with soluble collagen does not cause activation until tropocollagen aggregates (fibrils) of adequate size have been produced by self-assembly. It is not enough to get platelet adhesion, but the platelet surface must become strongly attached at several rigidly connected points. Thus, adhesion to a gel-like surface is not only poor to start with but also ineffective when it does occur. Hence it could be argued that attachment of a platelet to a red cell, or to the endothelial surface, does not provide the needed mechanical features.

But how is the mechanical character of the substrate supposed to influence activation? This could be due, for example, to the deformation introduced into the adherent cell by flow.

Is Flow a Factor in Activation?

It should not be forgotten that platelets *in vivo* are almost always in relative motion to some surface. The normal surfaces the platelet sees are the endothelial lining and the erythrocyte membrane. With these, as we have already speculated, the interaction, if it occurs at all, is mechanically poor. The support surface would yield too easily.

But if the vessel is injured and the platelets come into contact with the basement membranes or the tissue fibers, strong attachment results and flow will tend to pull the adherent cells off the surface. This kind of pull could be the activation step.

Are Platelet-Shape Changes a Factor in Activation?

In addition, or as an alternative mechanism, the contractile elements in the platelets may spontaneously induce platelet-shape changes which, if strongly enough resisted, could be assumed to lead to release. Alternatively, the spreading of cells caused by a strong tendency to increase their area of contact with the surface could be the activation trigger. Hence, while flow may help, it may not be absolutely essential for the activation step.

Conclusions

We thus favor a picture in which platelets adhere to most surfaces with roughly equivalent intensity, since most surfaces will have become coated by the plasma proteins that reach them. Only to exceptional surfaces to which plasma proteins adhere very poorly could platelet adherence be either particularly weak or particularly strong. The endothelial lining might be characteristic of the former, the collagen fiber surface of the latter case.

Activation may involve a mechanical interaction with the substrate. The resistance to deformations induced by flow or by spontaneous or induced cell-shape changes may play the important role in activation.

A BIOLOGIST'S VIEW

Leo Vroman

Interface Laboratory
Veterans Administration Hospital
Brooklyn, New York 11209

We had arranged the time for the speakers at the conference on which this volume is based more or less in sequence of their concern with entities of increasing size, from molecules to thrombi. Our intention was to suggest that blood, meeting a new surface, will react first with its smallest elements and then with larger and larger ones. The immediate response of blood to our introduction of a man-made material would be perhaps some reorientation of the blood's water at the material's surface and the rapid migration of some plasma ions, to be followed by the deposition of certain plasma proteins. The selection of specific proteins out of thousands for adsorption, orientation, and conformational changes at the surface, being dictated by properties of the lifeless matter we introduced, would all be events within the realm of physicists. However, the effect of these events on the activity of the adsorbed proteins is, of course, a biochemical subject. So is the subsequent, often enzymatic interaction of the bulk plasma with the film it has deposited.

At some time during these later events, formed elements of the blood will arrive. They will interpret the resulting surface as they find it, in their own "language." This language is determined by their membrane structure; it will dictate whether or not the platelet or white cell will adhere, and, to a degree, what it will do next. For example, the adhering platelet will or will not spread or cause other platelets to adhere to itself, and the adhering granulocyte will or will not spread or crawl. These decisions have a more biological flavor, and their consequences may grow to become medical problems.

It is my impression that there are at least three distinct surface/protein interactions, each with its own visible consequence: adsorption of factor XII in a certain position may lead to clotting, adsorption of fibrinogen in a certain position may lead to platelet adhesion, and adsorption of specific globulins in a certain position may lead to granulocyte adhesion. The movements of these formed elements, being large enough for live display microscopically, somehow seem slower than the molecular reactions that steer them, because our biological observations are made at a distance that allows simple conclusions, from a far vantage point where only the slowly shifting statistical means of rapid molecular events can be seen, tempting us to slow our observations and conclusions as well.

This, I feel, is a severe error. I shall call it our *first error;* it seems typical for a kind of naïve biology and resembles an error of early physics. It makes us believe that less knowledge is needed to understand larger systems (even though most living things increase in complexity with size), so that for the understanding of entire human societies almost no knowledge would be needed at all. No, the molecular substrate of life never tires and never slows down by growing simpler; worse than in physics, it is booby-trapped with amplifying systems that quite unexpectedly can promote an unobservably minor event to become the master of a giant one. The live blood, by amplifying unnoticed heterogeneities on a seemingly uniform surface, may thus cover this surface with an incomprehensibly heterogeneous garden of fibrin strands, platelet groups, and granulocytes. How much more incomprehensible must be the interface between two living things, such as endothelium and blood!

Red blood cells, as Dr. Silberberg has pointed out, present a very large total surface area to the rest of the blood without being thrombogenic. Compared to the endothelial surface, the red cell membrane seems simple. If we could only understand it, could we then incorporate its nonthrombogenic properties in biomaterials? Hidden in this line of thinking is the *second error* against biology: the hope of isolating one part of life to show us its normal properties without interference by the rest of life. Let us follow the early life of a red cell. It forms in the bone marrow, surrounded by many dissolved proteins, and then somehow slips through a small pore somewhere that perhaps massages it into the blood stream. There, the cell slowly loses its residual reticulum. It does not spend a single moment without being surrounded by proteins, and its birth is very unlike the introduction of any form of man-made material into the bloodstream.

As we showed during this conference, the study of washed cells and platelets may be very interesting, but no cell has ever been "clean" before. Isolated behavior is abnormal behavior; neither blood separated from the body nor a blood cell separated from the blood behaves as if living *in vivo*. This should not surprise a biologist used to observing the effect of his presence on what he tries to observe; but the blood is such a leaky tissue that on the one hand it lets us take samples with deceptive meekness, while on the other hand it has developed such an elaborate system to defend itself against such leaks that we shall never catch it unprepared.

Several paradoxical findings indicate blood *in vivo* is unlike blood *in vitro*. For example, negatively charged surfaces activate factor XII, but negatively charged cells and blood vessel walls do not. Fibrinogen seems present on blood cell surfaces, but only *in vitro* does it seem to form a film that causes platelet adhesion. A third example: platelets in a freshly drawn sample of blood were reported to be retained more by a glass bead column than were platelets in a sample that had been "disturbed" shortly before testing. But a freshly drawn sample of blood must have been subjected to at least as much disturbing flow *in vivo* before it was drawn. Perhaps even identical flow patterns have different effects inside and outside us.

As a biologist, I find myself standing between clear physical principles and clear medical evidence, without a clear connection between the two in the involved world in which I live. I have said that the one property that renders the endothelial lining nonthrombogenic is its complexity; it cannot be imitated. Materials and devices compatible with blood must be searched for on the basis of some principle or other, if only to limit the search. The best a biologist can do, I think, is interpret the blood's opinion of these principles.

A CLINICIAN'S VIEW

Edwin W. Salzman

Department of Surgery
Harvard Medical School
Beth Israel Hospital
Boston, Massachusetts 02215

For the clinician the proceedings of the past several days have been a stimulating and provocative intellectual exercise, the ultimate practical value of which is potentially great but not yet calculable. One must applaud the elegant work that has been presented and the attempts to grapple with important problems at a basic level. Unfortunately, these are difficult questions, and the clinician cannot wait for complete understanding of fundamental processes. The demands of patient care and the need to treat disease in real-life situations force the practitioner to compromise and to use whatever effective means are available to him, however imperfect or poorly understood. Physicians treated dropsy with foxglove long before they could measure blood levels of digitalis by radioimmunoassay. Similarly they were quick to attack renal failure by passing blood through a sausage casing in a washpan even though the apparatus available for this enterprise was crude, and the artificial circulation was far from inert toward the blood.

Thanks to a friendly evolution, the human organism has great capacity to tolerate physiologic insults. This resilience deserves credit for the success of many of our current practices in which blood comes in contact with artificial surfaces. Despite the unavailability of truly bland surfaces, there have been dramatic achievements in cardiac surgery, in implanted prosthetic devices, and in hemodialysis, and they are cause for satisfaction and pride. They are, however, only stop-gap measures, and further advances will require improved basic understanding. It is in this area that we hope this conference will have its greatest impact.

Such elegant contributions as those of Dr. Ratnoff, Dr. Kaplan, and Dr. Hemker, with their emphasis on positive feedback in the earliest activation steps in plasma clotting, have enormous implications for consideration of disease processes, where such insights force us to regard blood coagulation as an example of the response of blood to injury rather than simply as a way of plugging holes. Further, they offer new prospects for therapeutic intervention by identifying additional potential control points for modulation by drugs and perhaps by surfaces.

The same can be said for studies of the effects of surface contact on platelet function. The demonstration that platelet activation by surfaces has many features in common with the much more extensively studied effects of soluble agents on platelets allows a rational approach to the use of pharmacologic agents to modify blood-surface interactions and permits one to bring to bear on examination of surface-induced effects on platelets the enormous body of knowledge that now exists concerning basic biochemistry and physiology of the platelet.

The discussions of white cell activities were exciting and of great potential importance. That leukocytes participate in the reactions of blood with surfaces is not a new observation. It was suggested years ago that the appearance of white cells on a surface after an initial period of intense platelet activity and before a later phase of relative blandness might have more than casual significance. Participation of leukocytes in a passivation process *in vivo* after implantation of prosthetic devices must be important. One may hope that renewed interest in leukocyte-surface interaction may lead to new understanding.

There is much activity directed toward the response of the vessel wall to injury, an area of obvious importance for understanding atherosclerosis and processes of vascular repair. Where this new knowledge will have implications for artificial devices is not clear at the moment, but, as a minimum, improved management of disease processes for which prosthetics are employed may be expected.

If one might speak critically, it does seem that materials science has received somewhat light treatment here, perhaps because of the difficulties of advancing in this area where methodology is so important and so limiting. Available techniques for exploration of surface chemistry lack resolution to deal with events occurring at the molecular level. Perhaps complete understanding of this problem is impossible with current techniques. We do begin to see a glimmer of insight into the rules that govern interactions of blood with surfaces and the influence of fluid mechanics on these phenomena. Further explorations here are to be encouraged.

In summary, I might say that clinicians will look to serious workers in this field to help us proceed on two levels. We will continue to use artificial devices clinically where the need exists and where the state of knowledge, however imperfect, suggests that practices available are effective and tolerable, with side effects that are minor or at least secondary compared with the gravity of the patient's illness. On the other hand, we will look for improvements in design of these devices on the basis of rational theory, encouraging fundamental research into the basic processes with exploration even into the details of molecular events when methodology is sufficient to examine these aspects.

On behalf of the participants, I thank Dr. Leonard and Dr. Vroman for what have been a most fascinating and provocative three days.